E. H. Estey · S. H. Faderl · H. M. Kantarjian

Hematologic Malignancies: Acute Leukemias

Wolfgang Meyer 03/08

E.H. Estey · S.H. Faderl · H.M. Kantarjian

Hematologic Malignancies: Acute Leukemias

With 44 Figures and 51 Tables

Springer

E. H. Estey
Department of Leukemia
The University of Texas
MD Anderson Cancer Center
Houston, Texas, USA

H. M. Kantarjian
Department of Leukemia
The University of Texas
MD Anderson Cancer Center
Houston, Texas, USA

S. H. Faderl
Department of Leukemia
The University of Texas
MD Anderson Cancer Center
Houston, Texas, USA

ISBN 978-3-540-72302-8 Springer Berlin Heidelberg New York

Library of Congress Control Number: 2007932731

Springer is a part of Springer Science+Business Media

springer.com

Editor: Dr. Ute Heilmann, Heidelberg, Germany
Desk editor: Meike Stoeck, Heidelberg, Germany
Production: LE-TEX Jelonek, Schmidt & Vöckler GbR, Leipzig, Germany
Typesetting: K+V Fotosatz GmbH, Beerfelden, Germany
Cover design: Erich Kirchner, Heidelberg, Germany

21/3180/YL – 5 4 3 2 1 0 – Printed on acid-free paper

Table of Contents

Contributors

S. Abutalib
Section of Hematology-Oncology
University of Illinois
Chicago, IL, USA

A.S. Adelman
Department of Biostatistics, Bioinformatics
and Epidemiology
Medical University of South Carolina
Charleston, SC, USA

M. Albitar
Quest Diagnostics Nichols Institute
San Juan Capistrano, CA, USA

R.H. Alvarez
Department of Cancer Medicine, Unit 10
University of Texas
M.D. Anderson Cancer Center
Houston, TX, USA

J. Anastasi
Section of Hematology/Oncology
Department of Medicine
and Department of Pathology
Cancer Research Center
University of Chicago
Chicago, IL, USA

R. Arnold
Johann Wolfgang Goethe-University
Medical Department II
Frankfurt, Germany

A. Böhme
Johann Wolfgang Goethe-University
Medical Department II
Frankfurt, Germany

P. Casassus
Service d'hématologie clinique
Hôpital Avicennes
Université Paris XIII
Bobigny, France

R. Champlin
Department of Blood
and Marrow Transplantation
University of Texas
M.D. Anderson Cancer Center
Houston, TX, USA

J.E. Cortes
Department of Leukemia
The University of Texas
M.D. Anderson Cancer Center
Houston, TX, USA

B. Deschler
Medical Center
Department of Hematology and Oncology
University of Freiburg
Freiburg, Germany

E.H. Estey
Department of Leukemia
University of Texas
M.D. Anderson Cancer Center
Houston, TX, USA

S. H. Faderl
Department of Leukemia
The University of Texas
M.D. Anderson Cancer Center
Houston, TX, USA

P. Fenaux
Service d'hématologie clinique
Hôpital Avicennes
Université Paris XIII
Bobigny, France

D. Fiere
Groupe d'Etude et de Traitement de la Leucémie
Aiguë Lymphoblastique de l'Adulte
(GET-LALA Group)
Hematology Department
Edouard Herriot Hospital
Lyon, France

R. Fietkau
Johann Wolfgang Goethe-University
Medical Department II
Frankfurt, Germany

O. Frankfurt
Northwestern University Feinberg School
of Medicine
Robert H. Lurie Comprehensive Cancer Center
Chicago, IL, USA

M. Freund
Johann Wolfgang Goethe-University
Medical Department II
Frankfurt, Germany

A. Ganser
Johann Wolfgang Goethe-University
Medical Department II
Frankfurt, Germany

S. Giralt
Section of Blood and Marrow Transplantation
The University of Texas
M.D. Anderson Cancer Center
Houston, TX, USA

N. Gökbuget
Johann Wolfgang Goethe-University
Medical Department II
Frankfurt, Germany

F. D. Groves
Department of Epidemiology
and Population Health
School of Public Health and Information Sciences
University of Louisville
Louisville, KY, USA

D. Head
Department of Pathology
Vanderbilt University School of Medicine
Nashville, TN, USA

D. Hoelzer
Johann Wolfgang Goethe-University
Medical Department II
Frankfurt, Germany

H. M. Kantarjian
Department of Leukemia
The University of Texas
M.D. Anderson Cancer Center
Houston, TX, USA

P. Kebriaei
Section of Blood and Marrow Transplantation
The University of Texas
M.D. Anderson Cancer Center
Houston, TX, USA

M. Kneba
Johann Wolfgang Goethe-University
Medical Department II
Frankfurt, Germany

M. Kryzstof
Division of Hematology and Oncology
Arthur G. James Cancer Hospital
Ohio State University
Columbus, OH, USA

N. Lamanna
Memorial Sloan-Kettering Cancer Center
New York, NY, USA

R. A. Larson
Section of Hematology/Oncology
Department of Medicine
and Department of Pathology
Cancer Research Center
University of Chicago
Chicago, IL, USA

T. Lipp
Johann Wolfgang Goethe-University
Medical Department II
Frankfurt, Germany

M. Lübbert
Medical Center
Department of Hematology and Oncology
University of Freiburg
Freiburg, Germany

W. D. Ludwig
Johann Wolfgang Goethe-University
Medical Department II
Frankfurt, Germany

G. Maschmeyer
Johann Wolfgang Goethe-University
Medical Department II
Frankfurt, Germany

D. Messerer
Johann Wolfgang Goethe-University
Medical Department II
Frankfurt, Germany

J. P. Radich
Clinical Research Division
Fred Hutchinson Cancer Research Center
Seattle, WA, USA

V. Ribrag
Service d'hématologie
Institut Gustave Roussy
Villejuif, France

H. Rieder
Johann Wolfgang Goethe-University
Medical Department II
Frankfurt, Germany

O. Sala-Torra
Clinical Research Division
Fred Hutchinson Cancer Research Center
Seattle, WA, USA

B. L. Sanford
Section of Hematology/Oncology
Department of Medicine
and Department of Pathology
Cancer Research Center
University of Chicago
Chicago, IL, USA

W. Stock
Department of Medicine and University
of Chicago Cancer Research Center
Chicago, IL, USA

M. S. Tallman
Division of Hematology-Oncology
Department of Medicine
Northwestern University,
Feinberg School of Medicine
Chicago, IL, USA

E. Thiel
Johann Wolfgang Goethe-University
Medical Department II
Frankfurt, Germany

D. A. Thomas
Department of Leukemia
The University of Texas
M.D. Anderson Cancer Center
Houston, TX, USA

X. Thomas
Groupe d'Etude et de Traitement de la Leucémie
Aiguë Lymphoblastique de l'Adulte
(GET-LALA Group)
Hematology Department
Edouard Herriot Hospital
Lyon, France

M. von Hassell
Memorial Sloan-Kettering Cancer Center
New York, NY, USA

M. A. Thompson
Department of Pathology
Vanderbilt University School of Medicine
Nashville, TN, USA

D. Wartenberg
Department of Environmental
and Occupational Medicine
Robert Wood Johnson Medical School
Piscataway, NJ, USA

M. Weiss
Memorial Sloan-Kettering Cancer Center
New York, NY, USA

M. Wetzler
Roswell Park Cancer Institute
Elm and Carlton Streets
Buffalo, NY, USA

D. Yu
Section of Hematology/Oncology
Department of Medicine
and Department of Pathology
Cancer Research Center
University of Chicago
Chicago, IL, USA

Part I – Acute Myeloid Leukemia

Therapy of AML

Elihu Estey

Contents

1.1 Introduction

As with any disease, there are three general options for treatment of AML: supportive care only, standard therapy, and investigational therapy. Although, as discussed below, there are instances where the first option is preferable, the natural history of AML typically mitigates against it [1]. Since by definition there is much more information available about standard than about investigational therapy, most patients prefer the former, provided outcome with it is satisfactory. Hence, this review will begin by describing standard therapy, with emphasis on the factors that predict success following its use. Subsequent discussion will focus on investigational options of potential use for patients in whom results with standard therapy are poor.

The criteria for a diagnosis of AML have changed with publication of a report sponsored by the WHO [2]. Previous criteria were those of the FAB group and required a minimum of ≥30% blasts [3]. The WHO has lowered this to ≥20% blasts, in the process eliminating the myelodysplastic syndrome refractory anemia with excess blasts in transformation (RAEB-t). Although data mentioned below suggest that blast counts between 10–100% are not themselves independent predictors of outcome, we will adhere to the WHO criterion in the material that follows.

1.2 Standard Therapy

1.2.1 "3+7"

Standard therapy consists of "induction" and "postremission" phases. The intent of the former is to produce, and of the latter to prolong, a complete remission (CR) defined as a marrow with <5% blasts and peripheral blood with >1000 neutrophils and >100 000 platelets. The importance of CR relates to its ability to prolong survival. Thus, 40 years ago, Freireich et al. [1] documented that patients who achieved CR lived longer than those who did not. The difference in survival time was entirely due to the time spent in CR, suggesting that this difference resulted from achievement of CR rather than from a superior natural history. The risk of relapse from CR is constant for the first 2 years, but once patients have been in CR for 3 years it declines precipitously (to <10%), allowing such patients to be considered potentially cured [4].

For 30 years most patients with AML who have been treated have received remission induction therapy with what is commonly called "3+7." The "3" refers to the 3 days on which patients receive an agent (most commonly an anthracycline such as daunorubicin or idarubicin) that affects topoisomerase II and the "7" to the 7 days of cytosine arabinoside (ara-C) that accompany and follow the anthracycline. If blasts remain in a marrow aspirated 14 days after beginning therapy (day 14), a second course is often administered, with the number of days of anthracycline reduced to 2 and of ara-C to 5. If the day-14 marrow contains very few blasts, the marrow is reaspirated weekly until response (CR or reappearance of blasts) becomes clear.

Upon documentation of CR, patients frequently receive additional courses of anthracycline + ara-C, with a reduction in the doses or in the number of doses. While some such therapy is almost certainly necessary today, the proper amount likely depends on the intensity of the first several courses. For example, a German AML Cooperative Group (AMLCG) trial randomly assigning patients who had received 1 post-CR course to no further therapy or 3 years of maintenance found that the latter prolonged relapse-free survival time (RFS) from 7% to 30% [5]. However, a subsequent randomized AMLCG trial found much less improvement in RFS (28% vs. 35% at 3 years) and no difference in survival when patients in the no-further-therapy group received a more intense induction regimen and one intense post-remission course [6]. Regarding the specific number of postremission courses to administer following a first course of 3+7, the British NCRI (formerly MRC) group found no difference between 4 and 7 courses [7].

1.2.2 Outcome Following 3+7

CR, survival, event-free survival, and relapse-free survival rates are very variable after administration of 3+7; substantial numbers of patients die within a few weeks of beginning therapy and substantial numbers are potentially cured. Thus, speaking of an average outcome is not particularly informative. As with all anti-AML therapy, two general types of variables are associated with outcome: those that predict treatment-related death before response to induction therapy can be evaluated ("TRD") and those that predict true resistance to therapy. The criterion for "early death" is somewhat arbitrary. Very few patients achieve CR before day 21. Thus, deaths before day 21 are true early deaths resulting from supportive care failure. However, half the patients who will achieve CR have done so by day 35. Accordingly, failure in patients who die between days 21 and 35 and who have not achieved CR is due to both failure of supportive care and resistance. Beyond day 35, resistance to therapy becomes increasingly responsible for failure to enter CR. In CR, treatment-related mortality is rare (5–10%) in contrast to relapse from CR (50–100%).

1.2.3 Predictors of TRD

The principal predictor of TRD is pretreatment performance status. Table 1.1 illustrates that the proportion of patients who are bed-ridden most (performance sta-

Table 1.1. Effect of performance status and age on treatment-related death (TRD) rates

Age	Performance status (Zubrod)	Patients	Dead by day 21	Dead by day 35
<50	<3	490	3%	5%
<50	>2	37	32%	46%
50–59	<3	361	4%	7%
50–59	>2	28	25%	38%
60–69	<3	372	7%	11%
60–69	>2	45	43%	50%
70–79	<3	328	8%	17%
70–79	>2	46	52%	68%
80	<2	60	16%	26%
80	>2	10	40%	70%

tus 3), or all (performance status 4) of the time increases with increasing age. However, performance status is more important than age. Thus, while the proportion of patients dead 5 weeks after beginning treatment rises from 5% to 26% as age increases from <50 to ≥80, patients with performance status 3–4 but who are below age 50 have higher TRD rates than more ambulatory patients age ≥80.

Renal and hepatic function may also be more useful in predicting TRD than age. For example, in patients with performance status <2 and calling a bilirubin or creatinine >1.9 abnormal, TRD rates within 35 days of beginning treatment were 5% (43/808), 21% (7/34), 13% (91/688), and 36% (21/58) among, respectively, patients age <60 with normal pretreatment bilirubin and creatinine, patients age <60 with abnormal bilirubin or creatinine, patients age >59 with normal bilirubin and creatinine, and patients age >59 with abnormal bilirubin or creatinine. The ability of various "comorbidity" scales to predict TRD independent of performance status, age, and organ function is also being evaluated [8, 9].

1.2.4 Cytogenetics as the Principal Predictor of Resistance in AML

For many years cytogenetic findings in AML blasts have been the principal predictor of relapse from CR, or failure to achieve CR despite living long enough (e.g., >35 days) to plausibly have done so [10–12]. Three groups can be distinguished. A *better-prognosis* group consists of patients with a pericentric inversion of chromosome 16 [inv 16] or a translocation (t) between chromosomes 8 and 21 (t 8;21); less often there is a t(16;16). Each of these abnormalities disrupts the function of a transcription factor ("core binding factor," CBF) regulating the expression of genes important in hematopoietic differentiation [13]. At most 10% of unselected patients have CBF AML; these patients are typically age <60. A *worse-prognosis* group includes patients with monosomies, or deletions of the long arms, of chromosomes 5 and/or 7 typically accompanied by several additional chromosome abnormalities. Patients with such "–5/–7 AML" constitute 30–40% of all patients, are usually older (>50–60), and disproportionately have "secondary AML," i.e., a history of abnormal blood counts for ≥1 month before the diagnosis of AML ("antecedent hematologic disorder", AHD) or have received alkylating agents for other conditions, e.g., breast or ovarian cancer or lymphoma. Some consider the rare patients with inv (3)/t (3;3), t(6;9), t(6;11), t(11;19) or >3 abnormalities without –5/–7 to belong to the worse prognosis group. The remaining 50–60% of patients primarily consist of the 35–40% of all patients with a normal karyotype; these patients comprise an *"intermediate" prognosis group*, whose prognosis bears more resemblance to the worse- than the better-prognosis group.

1.2.5 Effect of Higher Doses of Ara-C

The significance of cytogenetics applies not only to patients given 3+7 but also to patients given higher doses of ara-C, e.g., 0.4–3 g/m^2/dose; the 0.4–1.5 g/m^2 dose is often called "intermediate-dose ara-C" (IDAC); doses in the 2–3 g/m2 range are known as "high-dose ara-C ("HDAC)"); in particular, the benefit obtained with IDAC/HDAC is proportional to sensitivity to the "standard" doses used in 3+7 (100–200 mg/m^2 daily ×7). In a seminal study randomizing patients in CR among different doses of ara-C [14], Cancer and Leukemia Group B (CALGB) showed that HDAC's biggest impact was in

CBF AML where it produced average cure rates in excess of 50%. In the normal karyotype group, IDAC and HDAC were equivalent, with each superior to standard doses, i.e., those in 3+7. In the worse-prognosis group any differences among HDAC, IDAC, and standard doses were small relative to the poor outcome observed with all three doses. NCRI data suggest that similar results can be obtained in CBF AML with IDAC as with HDAC [10], leading to an NCRI trial randomizing between these 2 doses.

1.2.6 Beyond Cytogenetics

Although cytogenetic findings remain the most important prognostic factor in AML, there is considerable variability in outcome particularly within the intermediate and favorable groups. The presence of (a) secondary AML, (b) "white blood cell index," (c) "secondary" chromosome abnormalities superimposed on the primary abnormalities noted above, and (d) molecular abnormalities such as gene mutations and deregulated gene expression are useful in unravelling this heterogeneity. The poorer outcome in secondary rather than in de novo AML is well known and appears independent of the association between secondary AML and worse-prognosis cytogenetics [15]. Nguyen et al. for the French AML Intergroup found that relapse-free survival in patients with t (8;21) given IDAC (or an allogeneic transplant) varied as a function of a "white blood cell index" defined as [WBC×% marrow blasts]/100 [16]. Long-term RFS was >75% with an index <2.5, 60% with an index 2.5–20, and 30% with an index >20. In general, the presence of secondary chromosome abnormalities has little affect on prognosis. However, the German AML Intergroup and Cancer and Leukemia Group B (CALGB) have shown that trisomy 22 improves relapse-free survival in inv [16] AML [17, 18], while the German group has also shown that a missing Y chromosome is associated with shorter survival t(8;21) [17]. Of more general interest, mutations in receptor tyrosine kinases (RTK), such as *KIT*, and in RAS genes have been found in 25% of cases of inv 16 AML and in 10% of cases of t(8;21) AML; *KIT* mutations appear associated with an inferior prognosis [19–22].

Given its frequency, the normal karyotype group is the one in which prognostic heterogeneity is most problematic. Such patients often have molecular abnormalities involving *FLT3*, *NPM1*, *CEBPA*, *MLL*, *RAS*, *BAALC*, or *EVI,1*. Internal tandem duplications (ITD) within the juxtamembrane domain of the RTK *FLT3* occur in 28–34% of patients with normal karyotype AML and are consistently associated with a significantly inferior outcome [23–27]. An additional 10–15% of these patients have mutations within the activation loop of the second tyrosine kinase domain (TKD) [25, 26, 28, 29]. A recent meta-analysis suggests that *FLT3* TKD mutations also negatively affect RFS, although the British NCRI group has recently reported a favorable effect [30, 31]. The most common somatic gene alterations in AML are mutations in the nucleophosmin (*NPM1*) gene, resulting in cytoplasmic rather than nuclear localization of the *NPM1* protein. *NPM1* mutations have been reported in 48–64% of normal karyotype AML [32–36]. Recent studies have found that overall survival (OS) and relapse-free survival (RFS) are significantly better in *NPM1+/FLT3* ITD– patients contrasted with *NPM1*– and *NPM1+/FLT3* ITD + patients [32–36]. *NRAS/KRAS* mutations occur in approximately 18% of normal karyotype AML [37]. Although no consistent prognostic effect has yet been shown, there may be such an effect after accounting for mutations in other genes, such as dominant negative mutations in the transcription factor *CEBPA* and partial tandem duplications (PTD) in the *MLL1* gene, which occur in 15–18% and 8–11% of normal karyotype cases, respectively. *CEBPA* mutations are associated with superior OS and RFS [38–40], while *MLL1* mutations predict for inferior RFS without significant effect on OS [41–44]. A significant negative prognostic effect on these two outcomes has also been reported in cases with aberrant overexpression of *BAALC*, a gene that is physiologically expressed in brain tissue and in hematopoietic progenitor cells [45, 46].

Genome-wide gene expression profiling based on DNA microarrays has provided additional prognostic information [47–49]. In particular, hierarchical clustering has identified two normal karyotype-predominant classes that differed in OS, and a gene expression predictor emerged as the strongest prognostic factor in multivariate analysis. These findings have been validated prospectively in an independent data set [50].

Table 1.2, based on outcome in younger adults given anthracycline + IDAC/HDAC, provides a prognostic system combining genetic and cytogenetic information. The value of cytogenetics in predicting RFS can also be enhanced by incorporating information regarding response to induction therapy [51].

Table 1.2. Approximate 3-year event-free survival probabilities based on cytogenetic and molecular findings in younger adults treated with anthracycline + IDAC/HDAC

Group	
EFS >75%	t(8;21) with WBC index <2.5 and without kit mutation inv(16), +22 and without kit mutation
EFS 50–75%	Other inv(16) without Kit mutation t(8;21) with WBC index 2.5–20 and without kit mutation Normal karyotype and CEBPA+ Normal karyotype and NPM1+/FLT3 ITD– del(9q)
EFS 25–50%	Inv 16 with kit mutation t(8;21) wit WBC index >20 or with kit mutation t(9;11) Normal karyotype and NPM1–/FLT3 ITD– Normal karyotype and NPM1+ or –/FLT3 ITD+ Normal karyotype and MLL1 PTD+
EFS <20%	inv(3)/t(3;3) t(6;9) t(6;11), t(11;19) abn(12p) +8 +11 +13 +21 –5/–7 not as sole abnormality Complex karyotype

1.2.7 Effect of Allogeneic Stem Cell Transplant (Allo SCT)

Although first used in patients with chemotherapy-resistant AML, the most frequent use of allo SCT has been in patients in first CR. Controversy over whether such patients should receive an allo SCT rather than continue the therapy that produced CR has been unabated for 25 years. A disinterested observer might thus suspect that any differences between chemotherapy and allo SCT, as commonly practiced, must be relatively small.

Examination of the literature suggests that such is the case. Formal comparisons between allo SCT and chemotherapy in first CR typically find that the proportion of patients who do not receive allo SCT, although they have been assigned to the procedure because suitable donors exist, is higher than the proportion of patients without donors who do not receive chemotherapy [52, 53]. It is suspected that patients assigned to a treatment but who do not receive it have worse prognoses than patients who receive the treatment. To avoid such "selection bias," comparisons involve patients with a donor, regardless whether the patients receive allo SCT, and patients without a donor. Such "biologically randomized" comparisons, after eliminating from analysis patients in the no-donor group who have an event in CR before the average patient with a donor is transplanted, typically find that the donor group has longer RFS (despite higher TRD rates) but similar OS [52–55]. Thus, while the rate of TRD + relapse is lower with allo SCT, patients in the no-donor group live longer once relapse has occurred.

In light of the prognostic heterogeneity of AML, it is important to assess whether particular groups do better with allo SCT, in particular patients with "poor prognosis" cytogenetic, or molecular, features, or younger patients (given the effect of age on TRD, which averages 20–25% after allo SCT), Slovak et al. [12] reported that relative risks of death in patients assigned chemotherapy rather than allo SCT were as follows: 2.04 if favorable cytogenetics, 0.70 if intermediate cytogenetics, and 1.82 if unfavorable cytogenetics. However, of relevance in the favorable and intermediate groups, patients assigned chemotherapy received only 1 course of IDAC/HDAC, and of relevance given the small sample sizes (each of the 95% confidence intervals included 1.00) the prognostic heterogeneity of each of the cytogenetic groups may have affected the conclusions. The paper of Burnett et al. [54] seems to address these criticisms given the authors' use of a more intense chemotherapy regimen in their no donor group, and their use of a prognostic index that incorporated information about response to induction into their cytogenetic classification [51]. With sample sizes approximately three-fold greater than those of Slovak et al., they found that the only donor group that had superior OS was the intermediate prognosis group ($p = 0.02$, 56% vs. 45% at 7 years). They noted that "in the absence of an overall survival benefit, this could be a chance subgroup effect, and it would not be valid to conclude that there was definite evidence of benefit." A donor–no donor comparison by Jourdan et al. [55] also found that only the intermediate prognosis donor group had superior OS ($p=0.02$, 55% vs. 70% at 7 years), although the same comment about subgroup effect can be made, in addition to which only 79% in the no-donor group received ≥1 course of IDAC/HDAC, and the authors' prognostic index incorporated WBC count and FAB category, neither commonly recognized as particularly "prognostic," in addition to cytogenetics and response to the first course of treatment. Two groups have used a donor–no donor comparison to examine the effect of allo SCT in patients with poor prognosis molecular abnormalities. The NCRI found equivalent OS and RFS in patients with a FLT3 ITD [56] (68 donor, 114 no-donor patients), while examining patients who were *NPM1*– or *NPM1+/FLT3* ITD + the German-Austrian AML group reported longer RFS in the donor group ($p=0.001$, e.g., 60% vs. 40% at 2 years) [33]; OS was not reported.

All the patients in the Jourdan et al. [55] paper were age <45, while those in the papers of Slovak et al. [12] and Burnett et al. [54] were age <56. Only the latter paper examined the effect of age, finding no difference in OS among patients aged 0–14, 15–34, or 35–56 according to whether they were in the donor or no-donor group. This finding, which contradicts prior belief that patients less than 20–30 years old should receive an allo SCT in first CR, resulted from improvements in chemotherapy (e.g., use of IDAC/HDAC). It is not implausible that similar improvements may eventually affect SCT. For example, TRD rates may be reduced by use of peripheral blood as the stem cell source or by using reduced-dose conditioning regimens (discussed in the section on investigational treatments), thus altering OS in favor of allo SCT. However, there are currently no data indicating that allo SCT prolongs OS in any patient in first CR; furthermore, allo SCT typically has more long-term complications than chemotherapy. If conventional allo SCT is performed, there seems to be no advantage to administer HDAC or other postremission therapy prior to transplantation.

While the donor–no donor comparison approach has obvious value, it tends to mask the value of allo SCT in patients who are fit enough to undergo the procedure. Thus, a transplant–no transplant comparison might also be of interest. Lending credence to performing this type analysis is the NCRI's report that patients with a donor who were not transplanted had similar outcomes as patients without a donor [54]. Of course, if the proportion of patients with a donor who receive allo SCT is sufficiently low, the transplant–no transplant comparison becomes primarily of academic interest. In this regard, it has been shown that even in relatively young patients the impact of allo SCT on the management of AML is quite small [57, 58].

1.2.8 Effect of Autologous Stem Cell Transplant (Auto SCT)

In several of the studies discussed above, patients in the no-donor group were randomized between chemotherapy and auto SCT in first CR. Comparisons of the latter two strategies may be confounded if, as in the NCRI trial, both groups get the same amount of chemotherapy, with the chemotherapy group then stopping treatment, but the auto SCT group then proceeding to auto SCT [59]. Typically studies report longer RFS with auto SCT, but have not found longer OS, either on average or in any subgroup [52, 53]. While there is little doubt that TRD rates with auto SCT will decline thus possibly tilting the OS balance in its favor vis a vis chemotherapy, it is also plausible that this balance might be shifted to favor chemotherapy if new non-SCT, such as those discussed below, reduce the risk of relapse.

1.2.9 Effect of Colony Stimulating Factors (CSFs)

As with auto SCT, the space devoted to a discussion of CSFs in a current review of treatment of AML is much less than would have been the case several years ago, reflecting a decreased interest in such therapy. CSFs and specifically G- and GM-CSF have neither decreased TRD (or serious morbidity) when administered during/after anthracycline + ara-C [60, 61] nor decreased resistance (e.g., by "priming" blasts to the effects of these drugs) when given before/during such therapy [62–64]. An exception was a trial [65] randomizing 640 patients aged 18–60 to receive or not receive G-CSF in conjunction with 2 courses of standard dose ara-C, the first with idarubicin and the second with amsacrine, whose mechanism of action is presumed similar to that of idarubicin. Idarubicin was given on days 6–8, rather than days 1–3 as in the usual 3+7 regimen, and amsacrine on days 4–6, rather than 1–3. The authors hypothesized that delayed administration would prevent interference of the "cell-cycle-dependent synergy" between G-CSF and ara-C. G-CSF did not affect outcome in unfavorable prognosis patients (defined to include those with secondary AML), but improved RFS in intermediate-prognosis patients (as defined by cytogenetics and de novo AML) at 4 years from 33 +/3% to 45 +/ 3%. There currently appear to be few large trials attempting to confirm this result; until then there is no reason to routinely use G- or GM-CSF. Rather, a 3- to 4-day trial of these CSFs might be tried in patients who have developed serious infections while still neutropenic after chemotherapy.

1.2.10 Candidates for "Standard" Therapy

As noted in the introductory paragraph, the fundamental principle underlying treatment of AML is to use the prognostic information illustrated in Tables 1.1, 1.2 to decide which patients are candidates for standard therapy. "Standard therapy" is defined here as therapy whose results are well known. It thus primarily consists of 3+7, of IDAC/HDAC +/– anthracycline, and of allo or auto SCT, as commonly administered, e.g., using cyclophosphamide and busulfan as the preparative regimen. In the following discussion we will focus on cytogenetics assuming that the molecular tests cited in Table 1.2 are routinely unavailable, but will include discussion as to how the latter might affect management. The general algorithm we will use is presented in Table 1.3. In principle, the best way to identify patients at low risk of TRD would almost certainly be via a predictive "model" that incorporates performance status, age, organ function, and various comorbidities [66]. Regrettably however, age is often used alone as a surrogate for risk of TRD. Currently, the significance of this practice is reduced given that investigational drugs are unavailable for patients with poor performance status, abnormal organ function, or significant comorbidities. At any rate we will use ≥60–65 as the age associated with an increased risk of TRD. It should be recognized however that each additional year of age beyond age 18 is associated with a poorer prognosis, i.e., any age cut-off is arbitrary [67].

Table 1.3. General approach to management of AML

Probability of TRD	Probability of resistant AML	Therapy
Low	Low	Standard, including IDAC or HDAC
Low	High	Investigational (high intensity)
High	Low	Standard without IDAC/HDAC
High	High	Investigational (low intensity)

1.2.10.1 Younger Patients (Age <60) with CBF AML

These patients should receive IDAC or HDAC. This recommendation is supported by the CALGB trial described in the section on IDAC/HDAC. There are conflicting data regarding whether, once HDAC is given (with an anthracycline) during induction, further HDAC is of value during postremission therapy. A SWOG trial suggested "yes" [68], an Australasian Leukemia and Lymphoma Group trial suggested "no" [69]. Patients with CBF AML were a minority in both studies' patients; the Australasian, but not the SWOG, study administered etoposide in addition to idarubicin and ara-C. While it is thus difficult to fault a practice administering IDAC/HDAC only as part of postremission therapy, the author believes that the potential benefit from giving IDAC/HDAC during both induction and postremission phases is sufficiently high to justify this practice in patients whose risk of TRD is extremely low, e.g., performance status 1, age <50. Retrospective surveys by CALGB suggest that 3–4 consecutive postremission cycles of HDAC (cumulative dose: 54–72 g/m^2) are superior to one cycle (18 g/m^2) [70, 71]. However, since the patients given only 1 cycle did not receive any other ara-C in remission, the CALGB results speak primarily to the effectiveness of ara-C rather than to value of 3 or 4 postremission cycles of HDAC. Indeed, results of the German AML Intergroup survey [17] suggest that two cycles of HDAC – in combination with an anthracycline or mitoxantrone – are equally effective as 3 or 4, and that there is no prognostic impact of HDAC on RFS in a dose range between 20.8 g/m^2 and 56.8 g/m^2. Furthermore, use of only 1 cycle of HDAC consolidation in the British AML10 study [10] produced results in patients with CBF AML similar to those seen with 3 or 4 postremission courses in the CALGB studies.

Nonetheless, for reasons similar to those explaining his preference for IDAC/HDAC during both induction and postremission therapy, the author would favor administration of 3 or 4 postremission cycles. Neither allo SCT nor auto SCT should be used in the average CBF patient in first CR.

CBF patients with KIT mutations and t(8;21) patients with WBC index >20 have much less favorable outcomes than other patients with similar cytogenetics [19–22] (Table 1.2). Such "poor-prognosis" CBF patients might be candidates for investigational therapy provided large elements of the standard therapy described above are retained in deference to the 25–50% success rate even in such poor-prognosis patients. For example, a tyrosine kinase inhibitor might be added in patients with KIT mutations.

Other candidates for standard therapy are those age <60 (low risk of TRD) with a normal karyotype who have either a CEBPA mutation or have an NPM mutation and have wild-type FLT3 (50–75% success rate, Table 1.2). Given the low-risk of TRD, the author favors use of IDAC/HDAC with anthracycline during both induction and postremission phases.

1.2.11 Candidates for Investigational Therapy

1.2.11.1 Elderly Patients (Age ≥60–65)

Table 1.4 presents results of trials investigating standard therapy in elderly patients. The depicted average median survival times of 10 months make it difficult to recommend standard therapy to many such patients. This is particularly so given the 15–20% risk of TRD occurring during the approximately 1–2 month remission induction period (Table 1.4), noting that some of the trials shown in Table 1.4 limited eligibility to patients with better performance status, normal organ function, and no major infection. Reducing the doses/duration of anthracycline and/or cytarabine has decreased both early mortality and the anti-AML efficacy of treatment, resulting in no improvement in survival [76]. Addition of G-CSF or GM-CSF to an anthracycline + ara-C, substitution of mitoxantrone for an anthracycline, or use of single agent gemtuzumab ozogamycin [77] have also failed to lengthen survival (Table 1.4).

It is useful to attempt to identify groups of older patients for whom standard therapy might be reasonable. Two such groups are patients CBF AML and patients with a normal karyotype, who are age 60–69, have de novo AML, a Zubrod performance status 0–2, normal

Table 1.4. Outcomes in older patients given anthracycline + Ara-C

Study [reference]	Patients	Median survival	Probability survival at 2 years	CR rate	Induction death rate	Comment
ECOG [72]	234, age ≥56	7–8 months	≈ 20%	41%	19%	Results same with daunorubicin, idarubicin, or mitoxantrone and +/– GM-CSF priming
NCRI (formerly MRC), (AML 11) [7]	1314, age ≥56	≈ 12 months	≈ 25%	62%	16%	Results same with 1 or 4 courses post-CR and +/– G-CSF starting 8 days after end induction
SWOG [73]	161, age ≥56	9 months	19%	43%	15%	Survival worse with mitoxantrone + etoposide
HOVON [74]	211, age ≥60	≈ 10 months	≈ 25%	48%	15%	Results same +/– PSC-833
M.D. Anderson [75]	31, age ≥65	≥12 months	≈ 20%	48%	Not given	Ara-C at 1.5 g/m^2 daily ×3; survival worse with single agent gemtuzumab

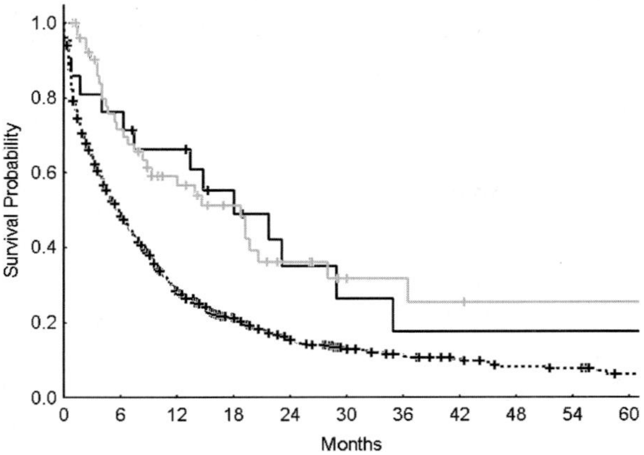

Fig. 1.1. Survival probabilities in three groups of elderly patients. *Black line* denotes patients with inv(16) or t(8;21) (n = 22), *gray line* denotes patients with a normal karyotype and de novo AML who were age 60–69 with a good performance status, normal pretreatment organ function, and no pretreatment infection (n = 54), while *dashed line* denotes other patients (n = 627). The differences between the first two groups, on the one hand, and the third group, on the other ($p < 0.001$), suggest that while standard therapy might be appropriate for the first two groups, it is not for the third group.

values for bilirubin and creatinine, and no pretreatment infection. Both groups had a median survival of 18 months following various cytarabine-containing regimens, as given at M.D. Anderson Hospital (MDA), with only a 5–10% TRD rate (Fig. 1.1). However, the probabilities of being in CR 3 years after initial diagnosis, corresponding to the time when patients can be considered "potentially cured" ranged between 9% and 16%. Given these data, some patients might prefer standard, and other patients investigational, therapy.

The "favorable" elderly patients described above constituted only 8% of the 968 patients age 60 and above given induction therapy at MDA over the past decade. The others had a median survival, when given cytarabine- or anthracycline-containing therapy, of 6 months (Fig. 1.1), with a 6% probability of being in CR at 3 years, and a 25% TRD rate. Thus, I recommend new therapies for the great majority of older patients with untreated AML. The National Comprehensive Cancer Network, a consortium of prominent American cancer centers explicitly cites "clinical trial" as the preferred option in patients with untreated AML age 60 and above [78]. There is of course no assurance that results with investigational therapy will not be worse than those with 3+7. For example, a CALGB study in older patients was stopped before accrual was completed because patients randomized to the investigational arm (daunorubicin + cytarabine + etoposide + PSC-833) had a higher death rate than patients randomized to the same 3 drugs without PSC-833 [79]. While investigational therapy may thus prove worse than standard, it seems fair to ask: "how much worse than 3+7 can an investigational therapy be." The weight given to the recommendation for investigational therapy should increase as the number of unfavorable prognostic factors (age > 69, adverse cytogenetics, secondary AML, poor performance status, infection, abnormal organ function) increases (see also Table 1.2).

Any discussion of choice of therapy must refer to Sekeres et al.'s observations [80] that 74% of older patients estimated that their chances of cure with 3+7 were at least 50%; in contrast, 85% of their physicians estimated this chance to be < 10%. While the most plausible cause of this discrepancy is patients' natural tendency to believe what they want to believe, there may also be gaps in communication between physicians and patients.

1.2.11.2 Younger Patients (Age < 60) with Chromosome Abnormalities Other Than inv (16) or t(8;21)

Given their median age of 45, these patients would have a very considerable life expectancy if they did not have AML. Hence potential cure is of more significance for them than for older patients (age > 60), whose median age is 70. Figure 1.2 (top) indicates that the probability of being in CR 3 years after starting initial IDAC/HDAC-containing treatment (corresponding to our criterion for potential cure) in the most favorable subset of younger patients with –5/–7 (i.e., patients with de novo AML and a performance status < 3) is 10%. Their median event-free survival is 39 weeks (Fig. 1.2, bottom). Hence the author believes that investigational treatment should be the preferred option in younger patients with –5/–7, recalling that the weight of evidence suggests that these patients are not materially benefited by allo or auto SCT, as typically performed. Exceptions might be made for the rare patients who have –5/–7 as a single abnormality [81].

Younger patients with performance status < 3, de novo AML and other cytogenetic abnormalities (excluding inv 16 and t(8;21) have 3-year EFS that while statistically different than those in comparable -5/-7 patients

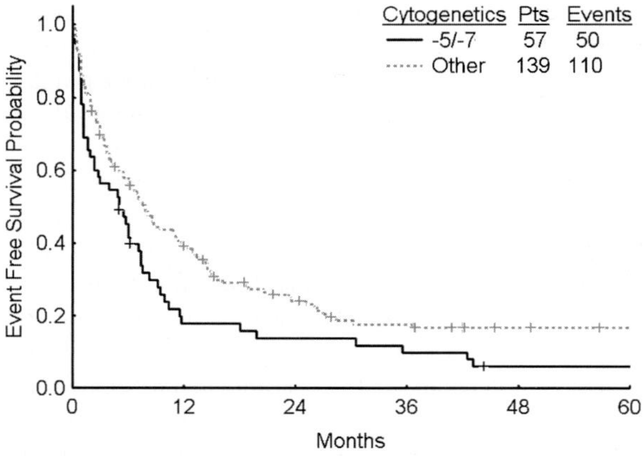

Fig. 1.2. Event-free survival probabilities following IDAC- or HDAC-containing regimens in patients age <60 with performance status <2 and with de novo AML (M.D. Anderson data 1991–2005). Despite these "favorable" features, outcome (particularly EFS at 3 years) in patients with "–5/–7" is such that investigational therapies are the preferred option. Although outcome is somewhat better in patients with other cytogenetic abnormalities (inv 16 and t(8;21) excluded) (p=0.02 for both EFS and OS), there is sufficient qualitative similarity between the two groups that the investigational therapy is also the preferred option in the other cytogenetic abnormality group.

are not materially different (e.g., 17% EFS at 3 years; Fig. 1.2 top). Hence, despite their median event-free survival of 74 weeks (Fig. 1.2), I believe that the preferred option in these patients is also investigational therapy. Obviously some would disagree with what is essentially a subjective view and believe that these patients are candidates for standard as well as investigational treatment. It is noteworthy however that phase 2 studies of new drugs are routinely performed in untreated patients with pancreas, or metastatic lung cancer, diseases in which median event-free survival is not materially different than the 74-week figure noted here.

1.2.12 Candidates for Either Standard or Investigational Therapy

1.2.12.1 Younger Patients with a Normal Karyotype

M.D. Anderson data (326 patients treated since 1990 with IDAC/HDAC-containing therapy) indicate that these patients have a 3-year event-free survival probability of 26%. It is not implausible that some patients when given this information would choose standard therapy, assuming correctly that investigational therapy could be worse. Certainly given the reasonable success rate observed with standard therapy, investigational therapy in these patients should be based on standard therapy, a constraint that is less applicable for the patients described above in whom investigational therapy is the preferred option, particularly elderly patients and those young patients with –5/–7. In light of the relatively low risk of TRD, and the CALGB data suggesting the superiority of IDAC to standard doses of ara-C [14], IDAC should be included in either induction or postremission phases or both.

Young patients with a normal karyotype are a group for whom the molecular information outlined in Table 1.2 will be particularly important. For example, the presence of a FLT3 ITD would weigh the choice toward investigational therapy, while an NPM or CEBA mutation would favor the standard therapy option.

1.2.13 When Should Therapy Start?

At least several days are needed for results of cytogenetic and molecular studies to become available. However, patients with high (>100 000) or rapidly rising WBC counts or a somewhat lower count (>10 000–20 000) and symptoms of lung or brain involvement require immediate institution of definitive therapy, which should not be delayed by leukapheresis or use of hydroxyurea. However, in other patients delaying therapy to await cytogenetic and molecular results may be feasible. Knowledge of such results prior to beginning induction therapy is less important in younger patients since the risk of TRD is low, and investigational therapy could be given when results of induction therapy, and of cytogenetic/molecular tests, are known. However, initiation of investigational therapy only in CR is not optimal since it is known that the type of therapy used for induction has a powerful influence on outcome in CR (see, for example, [82, 83]). Older patients have higher rates of TRD, and hence the desirability of delaying a therapy that is unlikely to be successful (e.g., if the patient has –5/–7) is even greater. Older patients usually do not present with features demanding immediate therapy, making it possible to delay therapy for cytogenetic results. Among 197 patients presenting to MDA with WBC <50 000, multivariate analysis indicated that age and unfavorable cytogenetics were independent predictors of CR, but that days from MDA diagnosis to start of treatment (delay) was not [84]. A delay of >9 days occurred in only 25% of patients. However, since 2000, survival is equivalent in the 49 patients age ≥60 beginning treatment >1 month from MDA diagnosis and in the 560 similarly aged patients beginning treatment sooner. Although selection bias may influence these findings, which are in contrast to those reported by the ECOG [72], they suggest that the risk of waiting to obtain results that might influence choice of therapy is less than the risk of giving therapy that is unlikely to be successful and may, as with 3+7 in older patients, be associated with significant rates of TRD. Furthermore, both the ECOG and MDA studies undoubtedly underestimate the interval from diagnosis to treatment since neither account for the interval from diagnosis by referring physicians to confirmation of diagnosis at the tertiary center.

1.2.14 Patients for Whom Investigational Therapy is Unavailable

It is important to recognize that, for logistical or financial reasons, investigational therapies are unavailable for many patients. The major group for whom ability to access new drugs is problematic are patients at high risk of TRD, e.g., older patients and patients with performance status 3–4. The options for these patients are 3+7, low-dose ara-C (LDAC, e.g., 20 mg bid×10–14 days by subcutaneous injection every 4–6 weeks), or "supportive care." An EORTC study randomly assigned patients age >65 to immediate 3+7 or to observation/supportive care, with use of chemotherapy (hydroxyurea or LDAC) if blood counts worsened or symptoms developed [85]. Median survival was 21 weeks in the 3+7 arm and 10 weeks in the observation arm, and the number of days spent in hospital was essentially identical. However, 80% of the 60 patients enrolled had a performance status <3, and all patients had relatively normal organ function. Furthermore, 50% of the patients randomized to observation had to begin therapy within 1 month, suggesting that they were on the verge of progression when randomized. Thus, data from this trial can be used to support immediate 3+7 only in patients who are relatively fit and likely to progress. In its AML14 trial in patients age >60 not considered fit for 3+7 by community physicians, the NCRI terminated randomization between LDAC and hydroxyurea because of longer survival (medians of 6 vs. 4 months) with LDAC [86]; number of days in hospital were similar. However similar to the EORTC trial, only 12% of the patients had a performance status of 3–4, with another 18% having a performance status of 2; furthermore, it is unclear, although likely, that hydroxyurea and supportive care are exchangeable. Finally, Tilly et al. found equivalent survival in older patients randomized between LDAC and 3+7, but with less time spent in hospital in the LDAC group; patients with abnormal organ function or poor performance status were excluded [87].

Although the differences in survival between LDAC, 3+7, and supportive care are thus relatively modest, it appears reasonable to administer LDAC to older patients who are unable to receive investigational therapy but have a performance status of Zubrod 0–2, and relatively preserved organ function. Because higher doses of ara-C produce better outcomes in patients with a normal karyotype, use of 3+7 rather than LDAC should be strongly considered in such patients. In contrast, in patients with poor performance status or age ≥80, supportive care should be the first option given the TRD rates listed in Table 1.1 and the absence of data suggesting benefit from LDAC or 3+7. Similarly, a low and stable WBC would add support to a choice of supportive care, since experience suggests that at least some such older patients can survive for 1–2 years without undue morbidity.

1.2.15 Investigational Therapies

1.2.15.1 Not Involving SCT

Table 1.5 [88–100] lists various investigational agents in clinical trial. I will divide these into "noncytotoxic" (NCT) and "cytotoxic" (CT). Examples of the former are tipifarnib, flt3 inhibitors such as PKC412 and CEP701, hypomethylating agents such as decitabine, and agents such as oblimersen that act to accelerate the apoptosis of AML blasts. Examples of CT agents are clofarabine and cloretazine. Although NCT, but not CT, agents are often viewed as "targeted," it should be kept in mind that CRs following use of standard CT agents result from the greater sensitivity of AML blasts than normal cells, i.e., targeting. Clinically the principal differences between NCT and CT agents are the lower presumably TRD rates with NCT, consequent to lack of effect on organs such as the lung or gut. Table 1.5 illustrates that CR rates seem highest when NCT drugs

Table 1.5. Examples of new drugs being tested in AML

Drug class	Example	Patients	CR rate	Response <CR rate	Effect on survival	Ref.
Farnesyl-transferase inhibitor	Tipifarnib	170 untreated, median age 73	18%	16%	Median 5.6 months	[88]
FLT3 inhibitor	PKC412	20 relapsed/refractory	5%	35–70%	Not stated	[89]
	CEP701	14 relapsed	0%	36%	Not stated	[90]
		24 untreated age >65 & not considered fit for more standard therapy	0%	32%	Not stated	[91]
Proteosome inhibitor	Bortezomid (+ idarubicin & cytarabine)	12 untreated (age >60) and relapsed	33%	42%	Not stated	[92]
Hypomethylating agent	Decitabine	36 with MDS	28%	59%	Mortality rate at 8 weeks 7% vs 26% with AML-type therapy	[93]
	Decitabine + all-trans retinoic acid (ATRA)	29 age >60 and not eligible for standard induction for untreated AML	14%	17%	Median 7.5 months	[94]
Nucleoside analog	Clofarabine	28 untreated age >70, or >60 & not considered fit for more standard therapy	59%	11%	19% induction mortality rate	[95]
Alkylating agent	Cloretazine	28 relapsed/refractory	4%	Not given	Median survival 9 weeks	[96]
Enhancer of apoptosis	Bcl-2 antisense (oblimeresen sodium) (+daunorubicin & cytarabine)	29 untreated age >60	48%	10%	Not stated	[97]
P glycoprotein inhibitor	Zosuquidar (+daunorubicin & cytarabine)	16 untreated and relapsed	69%	6%	Median 18 months	[98]

are combined with standard CT agents, or when the new agent (e.g., clofarabine) bears some resemblance to traditional CT. Nonetheless, patients at high risk of TRD might still initially receive NCT given the risk of TRD with CT (Table 1.3). In contrast, patients at lower risk of TRD might begin therapy with a combination of an NCT agent and standard CT or with an investigational CT agent (Table 1.3). This is particularly the case since much of the morbidity and mortality associated with AML results from bone marrow failure, which is most rapidly reversed by producing a CR; indeed, as discussed below, it appears that responses <CR are less effective at prolonging survival than is CR.

Table 1.5 (continued)

Drug class	Example	Patients	CR rate	Response <CR rate	Effect on survival	Ref.
Anti CD33 antibody attached to toxin	Gemtuzumab ozogamycin [GO] (+daunorubicin & cytarabine or + fludarabine & cytarabine & idarubicin)	64 untreated age <60	84%	–	80% alive with median follow-up (f/u) of 8 months	[99]
	GO (+ daunorubicin + cytarabine)	53 untreated age <60	83%	–	68% alive with median f/u 9 months	[100]
	GO (+cytarabine) Gemtuzumab ozogamycin	21 age >60	43%	–	48% alive with median f/u 7 months	

Not all investigational therapies need involve new drugs. For example, for many years it was thought that no more than 60 mg/m^2 of daunorubicin could be given daily×3 when combined with standard dose ara-C. However, perhaps reflecting improvements in supportive care, data from CALGB indicate that the MTD is ≥90 mg/m^2 daily×3 when given with standard dose ara-C + etoposide. This result has prompted an ECOG trial randomizing patients among the 60 and 90 mg/m^2 daily×3 schedules [101]. By analogy to ara-C this approach might be most useful in young patients with normal karyotype or CBF AML.

There is little doubt of the existence of myeloid leukemia-specific antigens. These antigens underlie the graft-versus-leukemia (GVL) effect. The most obvious proof of the existence of GVL is the reinduction of remission by donor lymphocyte infusions after failure of SCT [102]. An example of a leukemia-associated antigen is PR1, an epitope of proteinase 3 (PRTN3), a serine protease expressed in the azurophilic granules of myeloid leukemia cells (CML and AML) at two- to five-fold the amount found in normal myeloid cells. Molldrem et al. suggested that failure of myeloid leukemia patients to spontaneously develop an immune response PR1 resulted from overexpression of PRTN3 leading to apoptosis of PR1-specific high-avidity cytotoxic T-lymphocytes (CTL) [103]. Vaccination with PR1 has been studied under the hypothesis that it might increase PR1 immunity if done when the number of AML blasts had been reduced, e.g., following chemotherapy. Clinical responses have followed PR1 vaccination of patients with AML [104] and have occurred only in patients in whom there was at least a two-fold increase in the number of PR1-specific CTL; in contrast there was no relation between response and the number of CTL directed against the "control" antigen PP65. Immune response was indeed more common in patients who had minimal residual, rather than overt, disease when beginning vaccination. A trial in which patients in CR will be randomized to receive or not receive PR1 vaccine was initiated in late 2006. Wilms tumor antigen-1 (WT-1) is also an AML-specific antigen; a vaccine against WT-1 has produced responses in early phase trials [105, 106].

1.2.15.2 RIC SCT

As noted above, TRD is a major reason that survival after allo SCT is not superior to that seen with CT. The use of reduced intensity conditioning (RIC) is intended to address this problem. Although it was believed that much of the efficacy of allo SCT stemmed from the high doses of chemotherapy/radiation made possible by the transplant, current thinking assigns more of a role to GVL. If GVL, not high dose chemotherapy, is the principal mediator of the effectiveness of allo SCT, it becomes feasible to employ RIC SCT ("minitransplant"), thus reducing TRD. Tibes et al. described a systematic attempt to perform minitransplants in first CR in all MDA patients age ≥50 with an abnormal karyotype and a sibling or matched, unrelated donor [107]. Matching for known prognostic factors suggested that the 14 who were transplanted had better outcomes than the 83 who were not, but these 14 represented only 5% of all treated patients age >50 with abnormal karyotypes. These results question the general applicability of minitransplant and suggest that it might be done before patients enter first CR so as to increase the number of patients who might be candidates given the low CR rates in older patients (and high-risk younger patients). For example, older patients might initially receive an NCT agent. While waiting to see this agent's effect, a donor search might be completed, as might various logistical arrangements. Minitransplant would be performed once the response to the NCT agent is known.

1.2.15.3 SCT

An important development has been the introduction of new radioimmuno-conjugates as part of the pretransplant preparative regimen [108]. For example, Pagel et al. have shown that addition of ^{131}I-anti CD45 antibody to a busulfan/cyclophosphamide (Bu/Cy) conditioning regimen may improve outcome of allo SCT in first CR relative to that seen with Bu/Cy [107].

1.2.16 New Response Criteria

For many years response to induction therapy for AML was classified as CR or no CR. As seen in Table 1.5, responses less than CR have recently been recognized [109]. An example is CRp, i.e., CR with incomplete platelet recovery. Attaining CRp suggests that a treatment is more "active" than if, despite survival time sufficiently long to observe CR or CRp, neither response occurred ("resistant"). However, it is also important to assess whether CRp conveys clinical benefit, i.e., lengthens survival relative to resistant. This appears to be the case [110]; however, little information is available regarding responses such as "hematologic improvement" or "marrow CR."

1.2.17 Therapy for Relapsed or Refractory AML

Most patients with AML will require "salvage therapy" because of failure to enter CR after initial treatment ("primary refractory") or, more typically, relapse after a brief CR. As with therapy for untreated disease, the type of salvage therapy administered should depend on expected outcome with standard salvage regimens such as high-dose ara-C or fludarabine + ara-C. The factors most predictive of response are the duration of the previous remission (zero in primary refractory patients) and the number of previous salvage attempts [111, 112]. If the first CR lasted less than 6 months to 1 year, standard regimens produce CR rates averaging 10–20% when used as first salvage and <5% in > first salvage. In contrast, first salvage CR rates in patients with first CRs >1-year average 40–50%. Accordingly, the first treatment option in patients with short first CRs or who are receiving > first salvage is investigational therapy. If such therapy is not available, an argument can be made for a supportive care only approach. A stronger case for standard regimens can be made in patients with longer first CRs. Allo SCT can also be used for salvage or in second CR. Its potential value is suggested by Wong et al.'s observation [113] that survival in 135 patients who were either primary refractory or beyond first salvage was similar to that reported by Breems et al. [114] in 507 first salvage, nonprimary refractory patients, who presumably had a better prognosis than Wong et al.'s patients, but only 20% of whom received an allo SCT. Outcome of allo SCT is clearly better in second CR than in first relapse, often prompting a desire to postpone the procedure until second CR. Nonetheless, allo SCT in first relapse may still be superior to chemotherapy in first relapse (the real comparison of interest), even in the presence of circulating blasts, which is associated with a much greater reduction in the effectiveness of allo SCT than in the effectiveness of chemotherapy [113]. Of course, as with allo SCT in first CR, various selection biases likely affect these conclusions.

1.2.18 Treatment of Minimal Residual Disease (MRD)

Most patients ostensibly in remission have residual AML that eventually becomes apparent, leading to diagnosis of "relapse." Detection of MRD would in principle permit treatment to be changed before relapse and to be discontinued in patients with levels of MRD sufficiently low that relapse is very unlikely. Since relapse can only be diagnosed when >5% blasts are present in the marrow, the sensitivity of morphologic examination of the marrow for detection of relapse is only 1 in 20. In contrast, if 30 metaphases are examined, cytogenetic examination has a sensitivity of 1 in 30, while fluorescent in situ hybridization typically has a sensitivity of 1 in 500. Polymerase chain reaction (PCR) techniques allow detection of transcripts of such fusion genes as *RUNX1-CBFA2T1, CBFB-MYH11*, or *PML-RARα* (characteristic of acute promyelocytic leukemia) at a frequency of ≤10(−4). Assays for NPM1 have been proposed as another means of MRD detection [114].

Although the molecular abnormalities described above are not detectable even at diagnosis in many patients, all patients may have blasts characterized by aberrant surface marker expression; for example, the same blast may display markers characteristic of both an early and a later stage of differentiation. These patterns are quite specific for AML, as opposed to normal blasts. Once detected at diagnosis, such leukemia-associated immunophenotypes (LAIPs) can thus be used to serially assess MRD. Flow cytometric methods allow detection of 1 cell expressing an LAIP among 1 000–10 000 normal marrow cells [115].

The detection of MRD does not necessarily mean relapse is inevitable. Hence, although more sensitive methods of MRD detection will lead to more sensitivity for diagnosis of subsequent relapse, specificity must also be assured before using a method of MRD detection to guide clinical decisions. Currently, flow cytometry to detect LAIP appears to be both reasonably sensitive and specific [116, 117]. Thus, Kern et al. reported that the change in the number of LAIP+ cells between diagnosis and the end of either induction or consolidation therapy predicted subsequent RFS independent of cytogenetics and in both patients with intermediate or unfavorable cytogenetics [116].

1.2.19 Clinical Issues

Several practices which may have little effect on mortality, but considerable effect on patients' lives, should be mentioned:

1. Hospitalization. Given the more serious nature of hospital-acquired than community-acquired infection, routine hospitalization during induction or postremission therapy should be discouraged. In addition to the possibility of infection being passed from one hospitalized patient to another by medical personnel who fail to wash their hands, it has been pointed out that hospital water distribution systems may serve as reservoirs of aspergillus and other molds that are aerosolized and subsequently inhaled. The possibility of hospitalization in the typical "reverse isolation" room has little effect on this recommendation.
2. Masks and avoidance of crowds. The advice to avoid crowds flies in the face of observations that bacteria and fungi, rather than viruses, are the typical causes of infection. The bacteria are invariably residents of the patients' own skin (e.g., staph), mouth (pseudomonas maltophilia), or intestines (gram-negative bacilli). The fungi are similarly found on the skin (candida) or are airborne (aspergillus). However, it is unlikely that masks will restrict entry of aspergillus into the nose.
3. Fresh fruits and vegetables. Because there is no evidence that avoidance of these foods lessens the risk of infection, we are conducting a randomized trial in which patients are either encouraged to eat fresh fruits and vegetables or advised not to eat them. Similarly, there are no data suggesting that exposure to flowers or plants is detrimental.
4. Antidepressants. It is the author's opinion that symptoms such as persistent nausea or lack of appetite after completion of chemotherapy are often symptoms of depression. Another perhaps underappreciated cause is antibiotics. Megesterol acetate ("megace") may also be useful to promote appetite.

1.2.20 New Approaches to Clinical Trials in AML [118]

Randomized trials in patients with AML typically enroll 100–200 patients per treatment arm. Such numbers are needed to have 80% power (type 2 error 20%) to detect frequently small absolute differences with a false positive rate (type 1 error) <5%. These rates are sensible when studying a new drug in a disease where standard treatment is reasonably good, and thus where the principal concern is to prevent use of a falsely promising drug that might usurp standard therapy. In contrast, AML is a disease for which there is often no satisfactory treatment. Thus, there may be more reason to protect against a false negative than a false positive result. At the least, it might be reasonable to specify type 1 and type 2 errors of 20% each. Such a change together with an interest in detecting only larger, more clinically meaningful, differences would enable fewer patients to be entered per treatment arm, thus allowing more treatments to be studied [119]. While such trials would be nominally "underpowered," this ignores the false negative rate inherent in the selection of which, of many, investigational regimens to study. For example, if there are three potential regimens that could be investigated and if preclinical rationale is an imperfect predictor of clinical results, limiting investigation to one regimen potentially entails a false negative rate of 67%. In particular, the most egregious false negative results when a treatment is not studied at all [119]. This is problematic since, although by no means exhaustive, Table 1.5 lists nine different classes of drugs undergoing investigation. Use of each class rests on a presumably sound preclinical rationale, and each class may contain many drugs. Furthermore, there may eventually be combinations of drugs across classes.

Patients with poor performance status or other factors likely to increase TRD are often ineligible for clinical trials, although the development of new NCT agents might particularly benefit such patients. Even when eligible, patients may be excluded because it is believed they will do poorly. Although the extent of this subtler form of selection bias is unknown, papers reporting results of clinical trials only infrequently note that consecutive patients were entered and treated. Obviously the greater the extent of such bias the less likely it becomes that results will be reproducible in a more representative group of patients.

References

1. Freireich EJ, Gehan EA, Sulma D, et al. (1961) The effect of chemotherapy on acute leukemia in the human. J Chron Dis 14: 593–608
2. Jaffe ES, Harris NL, Stein H, Vardiman JW (eds) (2001) World Health Organization Classification of Tumours. Pathology and Genetics of Tumours of Haematopoietic and Lymphoid Tissues. IARC Press, Lyon
3. Bennett JM, Catovsky D, Daniel MT, Flandrin G, Galton DA, Gralnick HR (1985) Proposed revised criteria for the classification of acute myeloid leukemia. A report of the French-American-British Cooperative Group. Ann Intern Med 103:620–625
4. de Lima M, Strom S, Keating M, et al. (1997) Implications of potential cure in acute myelogenous leukemia: Development of subsequent cancer and return to work. Blood 90:4719–4724
5. Buchner T, Urbanitz D, Hiddemann W, et al. (1985) Intensified induction and consolidation with or without maintenance chemotherapy for acute myeloid leukemia (AML): Two multicenter studies of the German AML Cooperative Group. J Clin Oncol 3:1583–1589
6. Buchner T, Hiddemann W, Berdel B (2001) Requestioning the role of prolonged maintenance chemotherapy in AML: A randomized trial by the German AML Cooperative Group. Blood 98:462a
7. Goldstone AH, Burnett AK, Wheatley K, Smith AG, Hutchinson RM, Clark RE (2001) Attempts to improve treatment outcomes in AML in older patients: The results of the United Kingdom Medical Research Council AML11 trial. Blood 98:1302–1311
8. Charlson ME, Pompei P, Ales KL, et al. (1987) A new method of classifying prognostic comorbidity in longitudinal studies: Development and validation. J Chr Dis 40:373–383
9. Sorror MI, Maris MB, Storer B, et al. (2004) Comparing morbidity and mortality of HLA-matched unrelated donor hematopoietic cell transplantation after nonmyeloablative and myeloablative conditioning: Influence of pretransplantation comorbidities. Blood 104:961–968
10. Grimwade D, Walker H, Oliver F, et al. (1998) The importance of diagnostic cytogenetics on outcome in AML: Analysis of 1,612 patients entered into the MRC AML 10 trial. The Medical Research Council Adult and Children's Leukemia Working Parties. Blood 92:2322–2333
11. Grimwade D, Walker H, Harrison G, et al. (2001) The predictive value of hierarchical cytogenetic classification in older adults with acute myeloid leukemia: Analysis of 1065 patients entered into the United Kingdom Medical Research Council AML 11 trial. Blood 98:1312–1320
12. Slovak ML, Kopecky KJ, Cassileth PA, et al. (2000) Karyotypic analysis predicts outcome of preremission and postremission therapy in adult acute myeloid leukemia: A Southwest Oncology Group/Eastern Cooperative Oncology Group Study. Blood 96:4075–4083
13. Downing JR (2003) The core-binding factor leukemias: Lessons learned from murine models. Curr Opin Genet Dev 13:48–54
14. Bloomfield CD, Lawrence D, Byrd JC, et al. (1998) Frequency of prolonged remission duration after high-dose cytarabine intensification in acute myeloid leukemia varies by cytogenetic subtype. Cancer Res 58:4173–4179
15. Goldstone AH, Burnett AK, Avivi I, et al. (2002) Secondary AML has a worse outcome than de novo AML even taking into account cytogenetics and age. AML 10,11,12 MRC trials. Blood 100:88a (abstr)
16. Nguyen S, Leblanc T, Fenaux P, et al. (2002) A white blood cell index as the main prognostic factor in t(8;21) acute myeloid leukemia (AML): A survey of 161 cases from the French AML Intergroup. Blood 99:3517–3523
17. Schlenk RF, Benner A, Krauter J, et al. (2004) Individual patient data-based meta-analysis of patients aged 16–60 years with core binding factor acute myeloid leukemia: A survey of the German Acute Myeloid Leukemia Intergroup. J Clin Oncol 15:3741–3750
18. Marcucci G, Mrózek K, Ruppero AS, et al. (2005) Prognostic factors and outcome of core binding factor acute myeloid leukemia patients with t(8;21) differ from those of patients with inv(16): A Cancer and Leukemia Group B Study. J Clin Oncol 23:5705–5717

19. Care RS, Valk PJ, Goodeve AC, et al. (2003) Incidence and prognosis of c-KIT and FLT3 mutations in core binding factor (CBF) acute myeloid leukaemias. Br J Haematol 121:775–777
20. Carioli R, Beghini A, Grillo G, et al. (2006) Prognostic impact of c-KIT mutations in core binding factor leukemias: An Italian retrospective study. Blood 107:3463–3468
21. Schnittger S, Kohl TM, Haferlach T, et al. (2006) KIT-D816 mutations in AML1-ETO positive AML are associated with impaired event-free and overall survival. Blood 107:1791–1799
22. Paschka P, Marcucci G, Ruppert A, et al. (2006) Mutations of KIT tyrosine kinase (TK) gene predict relapse in adult patients (pts) with core binding factor acute myeloid leukemia (CBF AML): A cancer and leukemia group B (CALGB) study. Proc Am Soc Clin Oncol 24:1 (abstr)
23. Yokota S, Kiyoi H, Nakao M, et al. (1997) Internal tandem duplication of the FLT3 gene is preferentially seen in acute myeloid leukemia and myelodysplastic syndrome among various hematological malignancies: A study on a large series of patients and cell lines. Leukemia 10:1605–1609
24. Kottaridis PD, Gale RE, Frew ME, et al. (2001) The presence of a FLT3 internal tandem duplication in patients with acute myeloid leukemia (AML) adds important prognostic information to cytogenetic risk group and response to the first cycle of chemotherapy: Analysis of 854 patients from the United Kingdom Medical Research Council AML 10 and 12 trials. Blood 98:1752–1759
25. Fröhling S, Schlenk RF, Breitruck J, et al. (2002) Prognostic significance of activating FLT3 mutations in younger adults (16 to 60 years) with acute myeloid leukemia and normal cytogenetics: A study of the AML Study Group Ulm. Blood 100:4372–4380
26. Thiede C, Steudel C, Mohr B, et al. (2002) Analysis of FLT3-activating mutations in 979 patients with acute myelogenous leukemia: Association with FAB subtypes and identification of subgroups with poor prognosis. Blood 99:4326–4335
27. Whitman SP, Archer KJ, Feng L, et al. (2001) Absence of the wild-type allele predicts poor prognosis in adult de novo acute myeloid leukemia with normal cytogenetics and the internal tandem duplication of FLT3: A cancer and leukemia group B study. Cancer Res 61:7233–7239
28. Yamamoto Y, Kiyoi H, Nakano Y, et al. (2001) Activating mutation of D835 within the activation loop of FLT3 in human hematologic malignancies. Blood 97:2434–2439
29. Fröhling S, Scholl C, Gilliland DG, Levine RL (2005) Genetics of myeloid malignancies – Pathogenetic and clinical implications. J Clin Oncol 23:6285–6295
30. Yanada M, Matsuo K, Suzuki T, Kiyoi H, Naoe T (2005) Prognostic significance of FLT3 internal tandem duplication and tyrosine kinase domain mutations for acute myeloid leukemia: A meta-analysis. Leukemia 19:1345–1349
31. Mead A, Linch D, Hills R, et al. (2005) Favorable prognosis associated with FLT3 tyrosine kinase domain mutations in AML in contrast to the adverse outcome associated with internal tandem duplications. Blood 106:334 (abstr)
32. Falini B, Mecucci C, Tiacci E, et al. (2005) Gimema Acute Leukemia Working Party. Cytoplasmic nucleophosmin in acute myelogenous leukemia with a normal karyotype. N Engl J Med 352:254–266
33. Döhner K, Schlenk RF, Habdank M, et al. (2005) Mutant nucleophosmin (NPM1) predicts favorable prognosis in younger adults with acute myeloid leukemia and normal cytogenetics – Interaction with other gene mutations. Blood 106:3740–3746
34. Verhaak RGW, Goudswaard CS, van Putten W, et al. (2005) Mutations in nucleophosmin NPM1 in acute myeloid leukemia (AML): Association with other genetic abnormalities and previously established gene expression signatures and their favorable prognostic significance. Blood 106:3747–3754
35. Schnittger S, Schoch C, Kern W, et al. (2005) Nucleophosmin gene mutations are predictors of favorable prognosis in acute myelogenous leukemia with a normal karyotype. Blood 106: 3733–3739
36. Suzuki T, Kiyoi H, Ozeki K, et al. (2005) Clinical characteristics and prognostic implications of NPM1 mutations in acute myeloid leukemia. Blood 106:2854–2861
37. Bowen DT, Frew ME, Hills R, et al. (2005) RAS mutation in acute myeloid leukemia is associated with distinct cytogenetic subgroups but does not influence outcome in patients < 60 yrs. Blood 106:2113–2119
38. Preudhomme C, Sagot C, Boissel N, et al. (2002) Favorable prognostic significance of CEBPA mutations in patients with de novo acute myeloid leukemia: A study from the Acute Leukemia French Association (ALFA). Blood 100:2717–2723
39. Barjesteh van Waalwijk van Doorn-Khosrovani S, Erpelinck C, Meijer J, et al. (2003) Biallelic mutations in the CEBPA gene and low CEBPA expression levels as prognostic markers in intermediate-risk AML. Hematol J 4:31–40
40. Fröhling S, Schlenk RF, Stolze I, et al. (2004) CEBPA mutations in younger adults with acute myeloid leukemia and normal cytogenetics: Prognostic relevance and analysis of cooperating mutations. J Clin Oncol 22:624–633
41. Caligiuri MA, Schichman SA, Strout MP, et al. (1994) Molecular rearrangement of the ALL-1 gene in acute myeloid leukemia without cytogenetic evidence of 11q23 chromosomal translocations. Cancer Res 54:370–373
42. Caligiuri MA, Strout MP, Lawrence D, et al. (1998) Rearrangement of ALL1 (MLL) in acute myeloid leukemia with normal cytogenetics. Cancer Res 58:55–59
43. Döhner K, Tobis K, Ulrich R, et al. (2002) Prognostic significance of partial tandem duplications of the MLL gene in adult patients 16 to 60 years old with acute myeloid leukemia and normal cytogenetics: A study of the Acute Myeloid Leukemia Study Group Ulm. J Clin Oncol 20:3254–3261
44. Steudel C, Wermke, Schaich M, et al. (2003) Comparative analysis of MLL partial tandem duplication and FLT3 internal tandem duplication mutations in 956 adult patients with acute myeloid leukemia. Genes Chromosomes Cancer 37:237–251
45. Baldus CD, Tanner SM, Ruppert AS, et al. (2003) BAALC expression predicts clinical outcome of de novo acute myeloid leukemia patients with normal cytogenetics: A Cancer and Leukemia Group B Study. Blood 102:1613–1618
46. Bienz M, Ludwig M, Mueller BU, et al. (2005) Risk assessment in patients with acute myeloid leukemia and a normal karyotype. Clin Cancer Res 11:1416–1424
47. Bullinger L, Valk PJM (2005) Gene expression profiling in acute myeloid leukemia. J Clin Oncol 23:6296–6305
48. Bullinger L, Döhner K, Bair E, et al. (2004) Use of gene expression profiling to identify prognostic subclasses in adult acute myeloid leukemia. N Engl J Med 350:1605–1616

49. Valk PJ, Verhaak RG, Beijen MA, et al. (2004) Prognostically useful gene-expression profiles in acute myeloid leukemia. N Engl J Med 350:1617–1628
50. Marcucci G, Radmacher MD, Ruppet AS, et al. (2005) Independent validation of prognostic relevance of a previously reported gene-expression signature in acute myeloid leukemia with normal cytogenetics: A Cancer and Leukemia Group B Study. Blood 106:755 (abstr)
51. Wheatley K, Burnett AK, Goldstone AH, et al. (1999) A simple, robust, validated and highly predictive index for the determination of risk-directed therapy in acute myeloid leukaemia derived from the MRC AML 10 trial. United Kingdom Medical Research Council's Adult and Childhood Leukaemia Working Parties. Br J Haematol 107:69–79
52. Cassileth PA, Harrington DP, Appelbaum FR, et al. (1998) Chemotherapy compared with autologous or allogeneic bone marrow transplantation in the management of acute myeloid leukemia in first remission. N Engl J Med 339:1649–1656
53. Zittoun RA, Mandelli F, Willemze R, et al. (1995) Autologous or allogeneic bone marrow transplantation compared with intensive chemocherapy in AML. N Engl J Med 332:217–223
54. Burnett AK, Wheatley K, Goldstone AH, et al. (2002) The value of allogeneic bone marrow transplant in patients with acute myeloid leukaemia at differing risk of relapse: Results of the UK MRC AML 10 trial. Br J Haematol 118:385–400
55. Jourdan E, Boiron J, Dastugue N, et al. (2005) Early allogeneic stem-cell transplantation for young adults with acute myeloblastic leukemia in first complete remission: An intent-to-treat long-term analysis of the BGMT experience. J Clin Oncol 23: 7676–7684
56. Gale R, Hills R, Kottaridis PD, et al. (2005) No evidence that FLT3 status should be considered as an indicator for transplantation in acute myeloid leukemia (AML): An analysis of 1135 patients excluding promyelocytic leukemia from the UK MRC AML10 and 12 trials. Blood 106:3658–3665
57. Berman E, Little C, Gee T, et al. (1992) Reasons that patients with AML do not undergo allogeneic bone marrow transplantation. N Engl J Med 326:156–160
58. Proctor SJ, Taylor PRA, Stark A, et al. (1995) Evaluation of the impact of allogeneic transplant in first remission on an unselected population of patients with AML aged 15–55 years. Leukemia 9:1246–1251
59. Burnett AK, Goldstone AH, Stevens RM, et al. (1998) Randomized comparison of addition of autologous bone-marrow transplantation to intensive chemotherapy for acute myeloid leukaemia in first remission: Results of MRC AML 10 trial. UK Medical Research Council Adult and Children's Leukaemia Working Parties. Lancet 351:700–708
60. Stone RM, Berg DT, George SL, et al. (1995) Granulocyte-macrophage colony-stimulating factor after initial chemotherapy for elderly patients with primary AML. N Engl J Med 332:1671–1677
61. Godwin JE, Kopecky KJ, Head DR, et al. (1998) A double blind placebo controlled trial of G-CSF in elderly patients with previously untreated AML: A Southwest Oncology Group Study 9031. Blood 91:3607–3615
62. Zittoun R, Suciu S, Mandelli F, et al. (1996) Granulocyte-macrophage colony-stimulating factor associated with induction treatment of AML: A randomized trial by the European Organization for Research and Treatment of Cancer Leukemia Cooperative Group. J Clin Oncol 14:2150–2159
63. Lowenberg B, Boogaerts MA, Daenen SMGJ, et al. (1997) The value of different modalities of GM-CSF applied during or after induction therapy of AML. J Clin Oncol 15:3496–3506
64. Lowenberg B, Suciu S, Archimbaud E, et al. (1997) Use of recombinant GM-CSF during and after remission induction chemotherapy in patients aged 61 years and older with acute myeloid leukemia: Final report of AML-21, a phase III randomised study of the EORTC-LCG and HOVON groups. Blood 90:2952–2961
65. Lowenberg B, van Putten W, Theobald M, et al. (2003) Effect of priming with granulocyte colony-stimulating factor on the outcome of chemotherapy for acute myeloid leukemia. N Engl J Med 349:743–752
66. Estey E, Smith T, Keating M, et al. (1989) Prediction of survival during induction therapy in patients with newly diagnosed AML. Leukemia 3:257–263
67. Thall P, Estey E (2001) Graphical methods for evaluating covariate effects in the Cox model. In: Crowley J (ed) Handbook of statistics in clinical oncology. Marcel Dekker, New York, pp 411–433
68. Weick J, Kopecky K, Appelbaum F, et al. (1996) A randomised investigation of high-dose versus standard-dose cytosine arabinoside with daunorubicin in patients with previously untreated acute myeloid leukemia: A Southwest Oncology Group Study. Blood 88:2841–2851
69. Bradstock KF, Matthews JP, Lowenthal RM, et al. (2005) A randomised trial of high- versus conventional-dose cytarabine in consolidation chemotherapy for adult de novo acute myeloid leukemia in first remission after induction therapy containing high-dose cytarabine. Blood 105:481–488
70. Byrd JC, Dodge RK, Carroll A, et al. (1999) Patients with t(8;21)(q22; q22) and acute myeloid leukemia have superior failure-free and overall survival when repetitive cycles of high-dose cytarabine are administered. J Clin Oncol 17:3767–3775
71. Byrd JC, Ruppert AS, Mrózek K, et al. (2004) Repetitive cycles of high-dose cytarabine benefit patients with acute myeloid leukemia and inv(16)(p13q22) or t(16;16)(p13; q22): Results from CALGB 8461. J Clin Oncol 22:1087–1094
72. Rowe JM, Neuberg D, Friedenberg W, et al. (2004) A phase 3 study and of priming with GM-CSF in older adults with AML: A trial by the Eastern Cooperative Oncology Group. Blood 103:479–485
73. Anderson JE, Kopecky KJ, Willman CL, et al. (2002) Outcome after induction chemotherapy for older patients with AML is not improved with mitoxantrone and etoposide compared to daunorubicin and cytarabine: A Southwest Oncology Group Study. Blood 100:3869–3876
74. Van der Holt B, Lowenberg B, Burnett AK, et al. (2005) The value of the MDR1 reversal agent PSC-833 in addition to daunorubicin and cytarabine in the treatment of elderly patients with previously untreated AML in relation to MDR1 status at diagnosis. Blood 105:2646–2654
75. Estey EH, Thall PF, Giles FG, et al. (2002) Gemtuzumab ozogamycin with or without interleukin 11 in patients 65 years of age or older with untreated AML or high-risk MDS: Comparison with idarubicin plus high-dose continuous infusion cytosine arabinoside. Blood 99:4343–4349
76. Kahn SB, Begg CB, Mazza JJ, Bennett JM, Bonner H, Glick JH (1984) Full dose vs. attenuated daunorubicin, cytosine arabinoside and

6-thioguanine in the treatment of acute non-lymphocytic leukemia in the elderly. J Clin Oncol 2:865–870
77. Amadori S, Suciu S, Stasi R, et al. (2005) Gemtuzumab ozogamycin as single-agent treatment for frail patients age 61 years of age and older with acute myeloid leukemia: Final results of AML-15B, a phase 2 study of the European Organization for Research and Treatment of Cancer and Gruppo Italiano Malattie Ematologiche dell' Adulto Leukemia Groups. Leukemia 19: 1768–1773
78. National Comprehensive Cancer Network (NCCN) (2003) AML Panel. AML clinical practice guidelines. Journal of the NCCN, vol 1, 4:520–539
79. Baer MR, George SL, Dodge RK, et al. (2002) Phase 3 study of the multidrug resistance modulator PSC-833 in previously untreated patients 60 years of age and older with acute myeloid leukemia: Cancer and Leukemia Group B Study 9720. Blood 100:1224–1232
80. Sekeres MA, Stone RM, Zahrieh D, et al. (2004) Decision-making and quality of life in older adults with AML or advanced MDS. Leukemia 18:809–816
81. Estey E, Pierce S, Keating M (2000) Identification of a group of AML/MDS patients with a relatively favorable prognosis who have chromosome 5 and/or 7 abnormalities. Haematologica 85:246–249
82. Bishop JF, Lowenthal RM, Joshua D, et al., for the Australian Leukemia Study Group (1990) Etoposide in acute nonlymphocytic leukemia. Blood 75:27–32
83. Bishop J, Matthews J, Young G, et al. (1996) A randomised trial of high-dose cytarabine in induction in acute myeloid leukemia. Blood 87:1710–1717
84. Estey E, Wang X-M, Thall P, et al. (2004) Plausibility of delaying induction therapy in untreated AML. Blood 104:879a (abstr)
85. Lowenberg B, Zittoun R, Kerkhofs H, et al. (1989) On the value of intensive remission induction therapy in elderly patients of 65 + years with AML: A randomized phase III study of the European Organization for Research and Treatment of Cancer Group. J Clin Oncol 7:1268–1274
86. Burnett AK, Milligan D, Prentice AG, et al. (2004) Low dose ara-C versus hydroxyurea with or without retinoid in older patients not considered fit for intensive chemotherapy: The UK NCRI AML14 trial. Blood 104:872a (abstr)
87. Tilly H, Castaigne S, Bordessoule D, et al. (1990) Low dose cytarabine vs. intensive chemotherapy in the treatment of acute nonlymphocytic leukemia in the elderly. J Clin Oncol 8:272–279
88. Lancet J, Gotlib J, Gojo I, et al. (2004) Tipifarnib (ZARNESTRA^{TM}) in previously untreated poor-risk AML of the elderly: Updated results of a multicenter phase 2 trial. Blood 104:874a (abstr)
89. Stone R, DeAngelo D, Klimek V, et al. (2005) Patients with acute myeloid leukemia and an activating mutation in FLT3 respond to a small-molecule FLT3 tyrosine kinase inhibitor, PKC412. Blood 105:54–60
90. Smith D, Levis M, Beran M, et al. (2004) Single-agent CEP-701, a novel FLT3 inhibitor, shows biologic and clinical activity in patients with relapsed or refractory acute myeloid leukemia. Blood 103:3669–3676
91. Knapper S, Burnett A, Kell J, et al. (2004) A phase II trial of the FLT3 inhibitor CEP701 as first line treatment for older patients with acute myeloid leukemia not considered fit for intensive chemotherapy. Blood 104:864a (abstr)
92. Attar E, DeAngelo D, Ballen K, et al. (2004) Phase I dose escalating trial of bortezomib (in combination with idarubicin and cytarabine in patients with acute myeloid leukemia. Blood 104: 1799a (abstr)
93. Kantarjian H, Ravandi F, O'Brien S, et al. (2004) Decitabine low-dose schedule (100 mg/m^2/course) in myelodysplastic syndrome. Comparison of 3 different dose schedules. Blood 104: 1437a (abstr)
94. Lubbert M, Ruter B, Schmid M, et al. (2005) Continued low-dose decitabine is an active first-line treatment of older AML patients: First results of a multicenter phase II study. Blood 106:527a (abstr)
95. Burnett A, Russell N, Kell J, Milligan D, Culligan D (2004) A phase 2 evaluation of single agent clofarabine as first line treatment for older patients with AML who are not considered fit for intensive chemotherapy. Blood 104:869a (abstr)
96. Giles F, Thomas D, Garcia-Manero G, et al. (2004) A phase I and pharmacokinetic study of VNP40101M, a novel sulfonylhydrazine alkylating agent, in patients with refractory leukemia. Clin Cancer Res 10:2908–2917
97. Marcucci G, Stock W, Dai G, et al. (2005) Phase I study of oblimersen sodium, an antisense to Bcl-2, in untreated older patients with acute myeloid leukemia: Pharmacokinetics, pharmacodynamics, and clinical activity. J Clin Oncol 23:3404–3411
98. Gerrard G, Payne E, Baker RJ, et al. (2004) Clinical effects and P-glycoprotein inhibition in patients with acute myeloid leukemia treated with zosuquidar trihydrochloride, daunorubicin and cytarabine. Haematologica 89:782–790
99. Kell W, Burnett A, Chopra R, et al. (2003) A feasibility study of simultaneous administration of gemtuzumab ozogamicin with intensive chemotherapy in induction and consolidation in younger patients with acute myeloid leukemia. Blood 102: 4277–4283
100. De Angelo D, Stone RM, Durant S, et al. (2003) Gemtuzumab ozogamicin (Mylotarg) in combination with induction chemotherapy for the treatment of patients with de novo acute myeloid leukemia: Two age-specific phase 2 trials. Blood 102:100a (abstr)
101. Kolitz J, George S, Dodge R, et al. (2004) Dose escalation studies of cytarabine, daunorubicin, and etoposide with and without multidrug resistance modulation with PSC-833 in untreated adults with acute myeloid leukemia younger than 60 years: Final induction results of cancer and leukemia group B study 9621. J Clin Oncol 22:4290–4301
102. Kolb HJ, Schattenberg A, Goldman JM, et al. (1995) Graft-versus-leukemia effect of donor lymphocyte transfusions in marrow grafted patients. European Group for Blood and Marrow Transplantation Working Party Chronic Leukemia Blood 86:2041–2050
103. Molldrem JJ (2006) Vaccination for leukemia. Biol Blood Marrow Transplant 12:13–18
104. Qazilbash M, Wieder E, Rios R, et al. (2004) Vaccination with the PR1 leukemia-associated antigen can induce complete remission in patients with myeloid leukemia. Blood 104:259 (abstr)
105. Azuma T, Makita M, Ninomiya K, et al. (2002) Identification of a novel WT-1-derived peptide which induces human leukocyte antigen-A24-restricted anti-leukaemia cytotoxic T lymphocytes. Brit J Haematol 116:601–603

106. Keilholz U, Scheibenbogen C, Letsch A, et al. (2005) WT1-peptide vaccination shows high immunogenicity and clinical activity in patients with acute myeloid leukemia. Blood 106:122a (abstr)
107. Tibes R, de Lima M, Estey E, Shahjahan R, Champlin R (2005) Non-myeloablative HSCT in elderly AML/MDS patients in first CR. Proc Am Soc Clin Oncol ASCO abstract # 6655
108. Pagel J, Appelbaum F, Eary J (2006) 1311-anti-CD45 antibody plus busulfan and cyclophosphamide before allogeneic hematopoietic cell transplantation for treatment of acute myeloid leukemia in first remission. Blood 107:2184–2191
109. Sievers EL, Larson RA, Stadtmauer EA, et al. (2001) Efficacy and safety of gemtuzumab ozogamicin in patients with CD33-positive AML in first relapse. J Clin Oncol 19:3244–3254
110. Estey E, Garcia-Manero G, Giles F, Cortes J, O'Brien S, Kantarajian H (2005) Clinical relevance of CRp in untreated AML. Blood 106 (abstr)
111. Estey E (2000) Treatment of relapsed and refractory acute myeloid leukemia. Leukemia 14:476–479
112. Breems D, Van Putten W, Huijgens P, et al. (2005) Prognostic index for adult patients with acute myeloid leukemia in first relapse. J Clin Oncol 23:1969–1978
113. Wong R, Shajahan M, Wang X, et al. (2005) Prognostic factors for outcomes of patients with refractory or relapsed acute myelogenous leukemia or myelodysplastic syndromes undergoing allogeneic progenitor cell transplantation. Biol Blood Marrow Transplant 11:108–114
114. Gorello P, Cazzaniga G, Alberti F, et al. (2006) Quantitative assessment of minimal residual disease in acute myeloid leukemia carrying nucleophosmin (NPM1) gene mutations. Leukemia Mar 16 [Epub ahead of print]
115. Vidriales M, San Miguel J, Orfao A, et al. (2003) Minimal residual disease monitoring by flow cytometry. Best Pract Res Clin Haematol 16(4):599–612
116. Kern W, Voskova D, Schoch C, et al. (2004) Determination of relapse risk based on assessment of minimal residual disease during complete remission by multiparameter flow cytometry in unselected patients with acute myeloid leukemia. Blood 104:3078–3085
117. San Miguel J, Vidriales M, Lopez-Berges C, et al. (2001) Early immunophenotypical evaluation of minimal residual disease in acute myeloid leukemia identifies different patient risk groups and may contribute to postinduction treatment stratification. Blood 98:1746–1751
118. Estey E (2004) Clinical trials in AML of the elderly: Should we change our methodology? Leukemia 18:1772–1774
119. Estey E, Thall P (2003) New designs for phase 2 clinical trials. Blood 102:442–448

Diagnosis and Classification of the Acute Myeloid Leukemias (with Discussion of the Role of the Myelodysplastic Syndromes in AML Pathogenesis)

David Head, Mary Ann Thompson

Contents

2.1 Introduction

The Acute Myeloid Leukemias (AML) are a diverse set of phenotypically similar diseases whose classification has been the source of some controversy in recent years. In this chapter we discuss the best current clinically and biologically relevant classification of these diseases, including appropriate laboratory studies for accurate diagnosis and subclassification. Understanding the basis for current classification of AML requires additional knowledge of the Myelodysplastic Syndromes (MDS) and their relationship to a subset of AML, which will also be discussed. Finally, some attention will be devoted to monitoring AML during treatment.

2.2 Classification of AML

For much of the twentieth century classification of AML was based on how leukemic blasts, the predominant cell in the disease process, recapitulate normal hematopoi-

Table 2.1. Morphologic (modified FAB) description of acute myeloid leukemia [1]

M0	AML with no Romanowsky or cytochemical evidence of differentiation
M1	Myeloblastic leukemia with little maturation
M2	Myeloblastic leukemia with maturation
M3	Acute promyelocytic leukemia (APL)
M3h	APL, hypergranular variant
M3v	APL, microgranular variant
M4	Acute myelomonocytic leukemia (AMML)
M4eo	AMML with dysplastic marrow eosinophils
M5	Acute monoblastic leukemia (AMoL)
M5a	AMoL, poorly differentiated
M5b	AMoL, differentiated
M6	"Erythroleukemia"*
M6a	AML with erythroid dysplasia
M6b	Erythroleukemia
M7	Acute megakaryoblastic leukemia (AMkL)

* most M6 is M6a, not erythroleukemia but AML with erythroid dysplasia. M6b, true erythroleukemia, is rare.

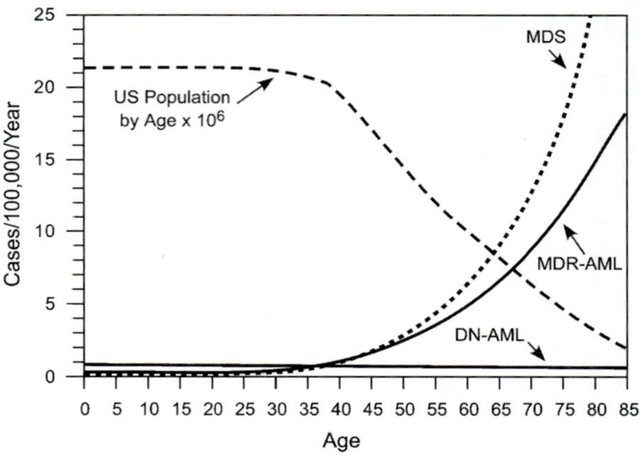

Fig. 2.1. Age incidence of MDS for population at risk (estimated from [2, 143–151]). Note that these curves are approximations. Population-based demographic incidence data are insufficient to describe exactly the relationship of the MDS and MDR-AML curves. The exact slope of the DN-AML curve is uncertain; some data suggest a slight up-slope with progressive age [149].

esis. Are blasts in a given case myeloblasts, monoblasts, megakaryoblasts, etc., and are they un-, minimally, or moderately differentiated. This approach was formalized by the FAB working group in a series of papers beginning in 1976, allowing analysis of its relevance [1] (Table 2.1). As specified in the table, M0 designates AML with minimal morphologic or cytochemical differentiation, M1–2 AML with minimal or moderate granulocytic differentiation, M3 acute promyelocytic leukemia (APL), M4 AML with mixed myelomonocytic differentiation, M5a and M5b monoblastic leukemia with minimal or moderate differentiation, M6a myeloid leukemia with dysplastic background erythropoiesis, M6b acute erythroblastic leukemia, and M7 acute megakaryoblastic leukemia. Unfortunately, subsequent analyses showed a general lack of clinical and biological relevance to this long-standing approach, e.g., failure to predict outcome, partial and imprecise correlation with cytogenetics, failure to predict expression of the membrane pump MDR1, and failure to predict clonality of presentation and remission hematopoiesis. The approach remains a useful shorthand descriptor of myeloblast morphology, but should not be used alone as a classification of AML. Instead, what has become apparent is that the phenotype of AML is divisible into two approximately equal broad pathogenetic groups of disease, which the authors designate DN (de novo)-AML and MDR (myelodysplasia-related)-AML [2]. The median age of AML is in the mid-60s in the US and western Europe, with an exponential age incidence curve with advancing age, most noticeable after age 50 (Fig. 2.1). The age incidence of MDR-AML substantially mimics this exponential curve, while the age incidence of DN-AML is approximately flat for population at risk throughout life (Fig. 2.1). Distinction of DN- versus MDR-AML is very important, as the latter group has MDS-like background hematopoiesis, with poor marrow reserve and the probability of reversion to clonal hematopoiesis (i.e., MDS) during "remission." MDR-AML also has a high frequency of resistance to chemotherapy at presentation. The WHO (World Health Organization) Classification of AML (2001) appropriately adopted this distinction in its first two categories of AML [3] (discussed below). (It should be noted that in its fourth category the WHO Classification confusingly retained a modified FAB AML classification that redundantly overlaps almost completely the first two categories; comments above about the FAB classification apply equally to this fourth category of the WHO classification.)

2.2.1 De Novo AML

DN-AML is the more common AML of children and young to middle age adults, with a median age in the 30s corresponding approximately to the median age of the population [2]. DN-AML occurs with approximately flat incidence throughout life (Fig. 2.1). This flat incidence curve suggests a single rate limiting pathogenetic step in development of disease. To the extent that the molecular pathogenesis of DN-AML has been clarified, cases are characterized by one of a series of recurring genetic abnormalities that block differentiation of hematopoietic precursors [4–7] (Table 2.2). However, as suggested by Gilliland, a block of differentiation alone is insufficient to create the phenotype of AML, and a drive to proliferate, probably coupled with inhibition of apoptosis, is also requisite for the acute leukemia phenotype of DN-AML [8, 9]. Such additional genetic damage has been identified in a large percentage of DN-AML cases. The most common abnormality of this type is mutation of FLT3, a membrane receptor tyrosine kinase that normally in the presence of its ligand drives proliferation and inhibits apoptosis of hematopoietic progenitors [10]. FLT3 mutations in AML constitutively activate its kinase activity in affected hematopoietic precursors. Apparently these effects, coupled with a block of differentiation, combine to generate the AML phenotype. Other mutations have been described that drive proliferation in DN-AML, e.g., activating RAS, cKit, and CSF-1 receptor mutations [11–14]. Both the proliferative drive mutations and the block of differentiation mutations are mutually exclusive of other mutations in each group, suggesting the members of each group contribute the same biologic component to transformation. It should be noted that the two sets of genetic damage appear to occur substantially independently of one another (e.g., FLT3 mutations have been described with each common recurring translocation in DN-AML) [10]. It has been suggested that multiple additional biologic events are necessary to transform normal cells into solid tumor malignancies, but it is unclear if this information is applicable to acute leukemia, and if so whether additional events need be genetic versus epigenetic or physiologic [15, 16]. Virtually all recurring genetic abnormalities identified to date in DN-AML either block differentiation or drive proliferation and inhibit apoptosis.

Table 2.2. Common genetic abnormalities in AML, by risk group[@] [141, 142]

Favorable	Intermediate	Adverse
	Normal karyotype	–5, 5q–*
	+8*,	–7*,
	+6	7q–*
t(8;21)	+21*	
t(15;17)	+22*	Abnormal 3q*
inv(16), t(16;16), 16q–	–Y	Abnormal 9q*
NPM mutation (FLT3–)	12p–	11q23 abnormality**
	NPM mutation (FLT3+)	t(9;22)
	C/EBPα mutation	20q–*
	Other non-complex structural or numerical abnormalities	21q–
		17p abnormality
		t(6;9)
		t(3;21)*
		Complex karyotype* (≥3 unrelated mutations)

* genetic change associated with MDR-AML

** 11q23 deletion is seen in MDR-AML. Most other 11q23 abnormalities are translocations, and occur in DN-AML rather than MDR-AML.

@ It must be noted that most of these designations are for single abnormalities, yet at least 2 genetic mutations appear necessary for transformation, and as shown by the interaction of NPM and FLT3, both affect prognosis. It should also be noted that risk group is dependent on treatment; e.g., APL's risk group may change if ATRA or aggressive anthracycline are not used for treatment.

In the WHO classification of AML (Table 2.3), DN-AML falls under AML with Recurrent Cytogenetic Abnormalities [3] with subclassification based on the common recurring cytogenetic translocations of DN-AML. A limitation of this approach can be seen from the previous paragraph. The classification includes only one of the two known genetic elements required for the leukemic phenotype, yet both elements have biologic, prog-

Table 2.3. WHO classification of AML [3]

AML with recurrent cytogenetic abnormalities
AML with t(8;21)(q22;q22), (*AML1/ETO*)
AML with inv(16)(p13;q22) or t(16;16)(p13;q22), (*CBFβ/MYH11*)
AML with t(15;17)(q22;q12), (*PML/RARα*) (APL)
AML with 11q23 (*MLL*) abnormalities
AML with multilineage dysplasia
With prior myelodysplastic syndrome
Without prior myelodysplastic syndrome
AML and MDS, therapy related
Alkylating agent type
Topoisomerase II inhibitor type
AML, NOS (modified FAB classification)
AML, minimally differentiated
AML without maturation
AML with maturation
Acute promyelocytic leukemia
Acute myelomonocytic leukemia
Acute monoblastic and monocytic leukemia
Acute erythroid leukemia
AML with erythroid dysplasia
True erythroid leukemia
Acute megakaryoblastic leukemia
Acute basophilic leukemia
Acute panmyelosis with myelofibrosis
Myeloid sarcoma

nostic, and potential therapeutic significance. It is not clear how to resolve this limitation in a functional classification of DN-AML. Inclusion of both sets of data, and other as-yet-undefined relevant genetic, epigenetic, or physiologic data, in a classification will become hopelessly complex, yet these details may prove important for understanding the biology of and for treating DN-AML. One solution would be to use the generic term DN-AML for diagnosis of this entire set of diseases, with a template for inclusion of specific events blocking differentiation, driving proliferation, and other data as necessary and available for clinical decisions, biologic studies, and monitoring of disease.

DN-AML has polyclonal background hematopoiesis at presentation, and remissions that restore normal polyclonal hematopoiesis with production of normal peripheral blood counts (reviewed in [2]). Both at presentation and in remission, background hematopoiesis lacks the dysplastic morphology characteristic of MDS. In some instances one of the genetic events required for transformation may remain present in some precursor cells in remission, e.g., persistent positivity for the fusion message *AML1/ETO* during prolonged remission in some patients with AML with t(8;21). The clinical significance of this finding is not completely certain, but such patients may remain in stable remission indefinitely; it should be noted that the fusion protein product in this setting usually appears to block differentiation of affected cells, rather than driving proliferation, supporting the concept that a block of differentiation alone is insufficient for leukemogenesis. As a group DN-AML tends to be responsive to cytotoxic chemotherapy, and that failing, most patients are potential candidates for allogeneic stem cell transplantation due to young median age.

Therapy-related AML mimicking DN-AML occurs in at least two clinical settings. The more common setting is following epipodophyllotoxin chemotherapy, with 11q23/*MLL* translocations or less frequently 21q22/*AML1* translocations [17]. Less commonly, all of the common recurring balanced translocations of DN-AML occur with increased frequency following complex multiagent chemotherapy [18]. These two settings appear to be iatrogenic models of DN-AML pathogenesis.

2.2.2 Myelodysplasia-Related AML

MDR-AML is the common AML of the elderly, comprising the majority of AML cases beyond age 60, with a median age in the 70s [2]. While it does occur in children and young adults, its incidence for population at risk comprises an exponential curve with progressive age, accounting for this feature of the incidence curve of AML as a whole (Fig. 2.1). The exponential curve suggests several random events are required for generation of this set of AML. MDR-AML is characterized by a series of cytogenetic changes shared with MDS (Table 2.2). Despite extensive efforts, the genes affected and the biologic impact of the cytogenetic changes common to MDR-AML and MDS (e.g., –7, 5q–, +8, 20q–, +21) remain unclear. These cytogenetic changes appear to relate to progression of MDS, rather than its initiation, as they are absent in 60% of MDS at presentation, and all of the common cytogenetic changes may appear as clonally selected changes after initial presentation of MDS. Presence of cytogenetic changes characteristic of DN-AML (Table 2.2) precludes diagnosis of MDR-AML. In parallel with DN-AML, the limited data available appear to support the requirement for both a block of differentiation and a drive to proliferate (coupled with inhibition of apoptosis) in the pathogenesis of MDR-AML. Activating RAS [13, 14], FLT3 [10], and C-FMS [11] mutations, all of which drive proliferation through the RAS pathway, are found in some cases of MDR-AML. As in DN-AML, these mutations are mutually exclusive of one another, suggesting they each contribute the same function to transformation. Dysregulated expression of *EVI-1*, which blocks the differentiating effect on hematopoietic precursors of GATA-1, also precedes transformation of MDS to AML in some cases [19], and inactivating mutations of GATA-1 have been described in MDR-AML occurring in Down syndrome children [20]. Thus, available evidence suggests two things. First, acquisition of the MDR-AML phenotype requires a parallel set of genetic damage to that required for the DN-AML phenotype, both resulting in the generic phenotype of AML. Second, in MDR-AML acquisition of this genetic damage appears to derive from the mutator phenotype of MDS, while in DN-AML the flat incidence curve suggests random genetic damage as the cause.

In the WHO classification, MDR-AML is categorized as AML with Multilineage Dysplasia [3]. Acceptance of this basic distinction of MDR-AML and DN-AML (WHO AML with Recurrent Cytogenetic Abnormalities) is an important improvement in AML classification [2]. However, several limitations of the WHO classification deserve discussion. One is semantic. Like AML with Recurrent Cytogenetic Abnormalities (WHO), MDR-AML (AML with Multilineage Dysplasia [WHO]) may have "recurrent cytogenetic abnormalities" (e.g., −7, 5q−, +8, 20q−, +21), rendering the terminology ambiguous (Table 2.2). More importantly, more features than just multilineage background dysplasia should be used to recognize MDR-AML, including the typical cytogenetic changes of MDS and MDR-AML (Table 2.2), history (preceding MDS), and exposure to environmental toxins suspected of causing MDS and MDR-AML. It may be difficult to assess background hematopoiesis for multilineage dysplasia in AML, if the marrow blast percentage is high, further limiting reliance on this sole parameter, and hematopoietic dysplasia is neither always present nor completely specific for MDS and MDR-AML (e.g., relative folate deficiency can cause virtually identical morphologic abnormalities). Finally, lacking more definitive data, patient age is an important parameter; beyond age 60 the presumption should be that a patient has MDR-AML until proven otherwise. Similarly, lacking more definitive data, below age 50 the presumption for treatment purposes should be that a patient has DN-AML, until proven otherwise.

There is no subclassification of MDR-AML in the WHO classification. Clinical subclassification for therapeutic decisions is based in part on cytogenetics (e.g., −8 may convey average risk, −7 or 5Q− high risk) (Table 2.2), but given limited current treatment options and poor outcome in most patients (who are elderly), the significance of this subclassification is limited. As we learn more about the transforming events in MDR-AML we will encounter a similar classification dilemma to DN-AML, i.e., as discussed previously at least two events are necessary for transformation to AML. In parallel with DN-AML, a possible subclassification solution may be to use a generic diagnosis of MDR-AML with a template for inclusion of other data as available and relevant for clinical treatment, biologic analysis, and disease monitoring.

In MDR-AML as a group leukemic blasts tend to be inherently resistant to chemotherapy (e.g., expression of P-glycoprotein at presentation) [21, 22], while background hematopoiesis simultaneously is hypersensitive to chemotherapy, often resulting in prolonged severe cytopenias during induction therapy. The outcome of MDR-AML has improved little in the last 25 years with cytotoxic chemotherapy, and the only significant curative treatment is allogeneic stem cell transplantation. Unfortunately, this treatment is not available for most patients due to an average age in the 70s. MDR-AML has clonal background hematopoiesis at presentation [23], and often has clonal remissions, often with multilineage dysplasia in hematopoietic precursors, with or without the cytogenetic abnormalities present in the leukemia. Thus remissions in MDR-AML appear to represent reversion of the patient to MDS, rather than to normal hematopoiesis, and they are often characterized by persistent cytopenias between chemotherapy dosing, and prolonged severe cytopenias with chemotherapy.

Therapy-related AML mimicking MDR-AML occurs following chemotherapy with agents that cause cross-link DNA damage (alkylating agents, platinum derivatives, and the nitrosoureas) (reviewed in [24]). These settings appear to be iatrogenic models of MDR-AML pathogenesis.

2.3 The Myelodysplastic Syndromes

MDS is an enigmatic and still poorly understood set of diseases that is pathogenetically related to MDR-AML [2]. Separation of MDS from AML is currently based empirically on the marrow blast percentage, rather than an understanding of biological differences in the two sets of disease [25, 26]. Intermediate and high-grade subsets of MDS (see below) are usually fatal with or without transformation to MDR-AML. Understanding the biology and pathogenesis of MDS is critical to improving the differential diagnosis of MDR-AML versus both MDS and DN-AML. Improved understanding might also contribute to improved treatment of MDR-AML and MDS, and possibly to future prevention of progression of MDS to MDR-AML.

The FAB working group standardized classification of MDS into five defined subsets (Table 2.4) [25]. This approach has been improved in the WHO MDS classification, with inclusion of several new subtypes of MDS, and removal of one subtype (chronic myelomonocytic leukemia, CMML) to a new category of Myelodysplastic/Myeloproliferative (MD/MP) diseases (Table 2.5) [26, 27]. For discussion of AML pathogenesis the WHO classification can be reduced to Low Grade (LG) (Refractory Anemia, Refractory Anemia with Ringed Sideroblasts, MDS associated with isolated del(5q) chromosome abnormality [5q− Syndrome]), Intermediate Grade (IG) (Refractory Cytopenia with Multilineage Dysplasia [RCMD]), and high grade (HG) disease (Refractory Anemia with Excess Blasts [RAEB]). MDS, unclassifiable is inserted to capture cases of unilineage granulocytic or megakaryocytic disease, which tend to act as IG/HG disease, rather than like LG disease.

A variety of data (including progressive cytogenetic damage, acquired structural and functional abnormalities in hematopoietic cells, and the high rate of transformation to AML) suggest that IG/HG Grade MDS is a mutator phenotype with inherent genetic instability. As discussed, MDR-AML appears to require both a block of differentiation and a drive to proliferate, but it is doubtful either of these events is the biologic basis of MDS. A solitary drive to proliferate (with associated

Table 2.4. FAB classification of MDS [25]

Refractory anemia
Refractory anemia with ringed sideroblasts
Refractory anemia with excess blasts
Refractory anemia with excess blasts in transformation
Chronic myelomonocytic leukemia

Table 2.5. WHO classification of MDS [26]

Refractory anemia (RA)
Refractory anemia with ringed sideroblasts (RARS)
Refractory cytopenia with multilineage dysplasia (RCMD)
Refractory cytopenia with multilineage dysplasia with ringed sideroblasts
Refractory anemia with excess blasts (RAEB), types −1 and −2
MDS associated with isolated del(5q) chromosome abnormality (5q− syndrome)
MDS, unclassifiable

inhibition of apoptosis) is the apparent cause of chronic myelogenous leukemia (reviewed in [28]) and the other chronic myeloproliferative diseases [29]; these differ from MDS in being proliferative, lacking MDS-type morphologic dysplasia, and lacking MDS-type cytogenetic abnormalities. A solitary block of differentiation in hematopoietic progenitors has no clinical phenotype, except a possible propensity to be transformed by acquisition of a second genetic event that drives proliferation [30]. Both clinical and transgenic examples of each of these possibilities lack the phenotype of MDS, although acquisition of both appears required for MDS to transform to MDR-AML. A plausible hypothesis is that subsets of HG MDS type disease represent acquisition of one of these events superimposed on the underlying phenotype of IG MDS. While IG MDS (RCMD) has relatively short survival (median 2 1/2 years) and frequent progression to AML (11%), it has a normal blast percentage in blood and marrow. HG MDS (RAEB) is characterized by increased marrow blasts, with shortened survival and increased propensity to progress to AML. Thus, RAEB may plausibly but hypothetically represent a block of differentiation superimposed on the biology of IG MDS. The MD/MP diseases (WHO)

(CMML, Juvenile Myelomonocytic Leukemia, and Atypical Chronic Myeloid Leukemia) have mixed features of MDS (dysplasia, shared cytogenetic abnormalities) and the chronic myeloproliferative diseases (proliferation) [27]. A drive to proliferate through mutations leading to increased active RAS has been demonstrated in many MD/MP cases (inactivating ATM mutations [31], activating RAS mutations [32], PTPN11 mutations [33, 34]), yet the cases also share morphology and cytogenetic abnormalities with MDS. In a possibly informative clinical scenario, septic patients with MDS may develop a reversible leukemoid reaction, often with monocytosis and mimicking CMML (apparently due to a physiologic proliferative drive superimposed on MDS). Thus, available data indicate that while both a drive to proliferate and a block of differentiation may contribute to MDS progression, and both are necessary for progression to MDR-AML, neither represents the underlying pathogenesis of MDS. The most tenable hypothesis is that the underlying pathogenic abnormality of IG/HG MDS is its mutator phenotype, which causes random genetic damage, including in some cases a drive to proliferate, block of differentiation, and resultant progression to MDR-AML.

While IG/HG Grade MDS is a mutator phenotype, at least some LG MDS is not. Both 5q− Syndrome and Refractory Anemia with Ringed Sideroblasts, if defined stringently using WHO criteria, have very low rates of progression to AML with survival approaching age-matched peers [35, 36]. While 5q− is one of the most common cytogenetic abnormalities in MDS, in most cases secondary to an underlying mutator phenotype, the specific 5q− Syndrome may represent emergence of a 5q− clone with an associated clonal survival advantage, but a stable biologic state with no underlying mutator phenotype. RARS, defined as unilineage erythroid abnormalities, may have a similar pathogenesis.

Progression of IG/HG MDS to MDR-AML does not represent a continuum, but rather stepwise acquisition of specific genetic events required for transformation, and should equate with a rapid rate of accumulation of primitive precursors (blasts) in the marrow, differing qualitatively from MDS (Fig. 2.2). Thus, separation of MDS and MDR-AML should be based on evidence of transformation, a change in the rate of accumulation of blasts, not just on the marrow blast percentage rising above a threshold (whether 20% or 30%). While it is safe to assume that a high marrow blast percentage (>40–50%) represents transformation to MDR-AML, lower levels require clinical interpretation as to whether the patient's disease has shifted from primary marrow failure to proliferating blasts. If initial data are inconclusive, a repeat marrow after an interval may clarify whether the basic disease process has changed from one of marrow failure (MDS) to a proliferative state (AML) (Fig. 2.2). As our knowledge of these diseases increases, separation of MDS and MDR-AML may eventually include demonstration of specific genetic events leading to transformation, but this is not currently feasible. Finally, this perspective should not be interpreted to mean that MDS with a high blast percentage is a favorable disease; it is lethal with short median survival, but lacking transformation there is little hope for a favorable response to cytotoxic chemotherapy [35, 36].

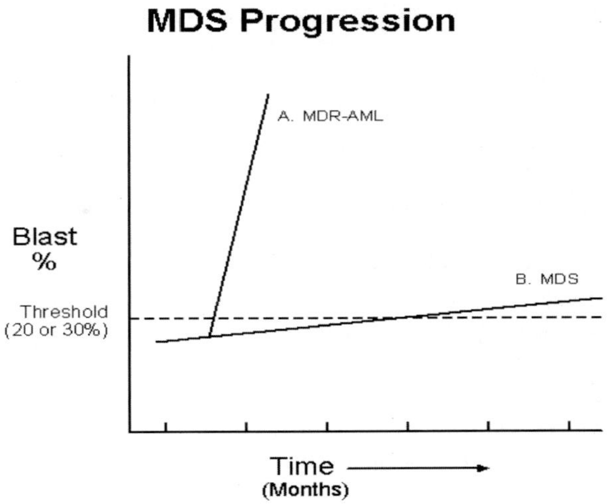

Fig. 2.2. Blast progression over time in MDS. If the blast percentage in marrow rises rapidly (**A**), the case has transformed to AML. In contrast, if the blast percentage rises slowly over months to exceed an artificial threshold (whether 20% or 30%), the case should be considered to be persistent MDS. A single observation of a high blast percentage in this setting may be interpreted as transformation to MDR-AML [152, 153].

2.4 Laboratory Studies for Diagnosis and Monitoring of AML

Accurate diagnosis and classification in AML and MDS are essential for treatment decisions, assessment of prognosis, and correlative biology studies. Initial assessment requires a careful history (work and exposure history, medical and medication history, family history), physical exam, CBC with peripheral smear review, and bone marrow examination to include in addition to routine morphologic assessment flow cytometry, cytogenetics, and selected molecular genetic analyses. It is critical that the bone marrow sample obtained at diagnosis be sufficient for all diagnostic studies, as there is usually only one chance to get complete laboratory studies before commencement of treatment that compromises subsequent analyses. The bone marrow specimen is crucial for confirming acute leukemia, differentiating between AML and acute lymphoblastic leukemia (ALL), and subclassifying both. Therefore, initial samples must be sufficient to support the full panoply of studies required for accurate diagnosis. Fortunately, preliminary studies are largely identical for AML and ALL.

2.4.1 Bone Marrow Sampling

Poor bone marrow sampling presents sufficient recurring problems in diagnosis that a brief review of bone marrow technique is in order. Before performing marrow sampling, neophytes should review on a skeleton the generally neglected anatomy of the posterior iliac crest. It is important to be aware of the extensive innervation of periosteum. With proper technique, appropriate reassurance of the patient with attention to his anxiety, and generous local anesthesia including liberal numbing of periosteum on the posterior iliac crest, the bone marrow procedure is usually well tolerated by adolescents and adults without general anesthesia. If performed poorly and with insufficient local anesthesia, it may approach torture worthy of Torquemada [37]. After appropriate anesthesia, the aspirate needle should be firmly seated on the posterior iliac crest and advanced into the marrow space, the trochar removed, and a volume of marrow quickly aspirated that is sufficient for all diagnostic studies. The one part of the procedure that cannot be anesthetized is the aspiration itself, which produces a dull ache for several seconds. With sufficient circulating blasts, diagnosis of acute leukemia can be made with a peripheral blood sample, but blast populations may vary in blood versus marrow, and when clinical circumstances permit we recommend analysis of a marrow sample for diagnosis.

Aspirate smears should be made expeditiously, using at least two forms of smears because of limitations with all types of smears. A push (actually pull) prep (same technique as a peripheral smear) is easy to perform and generally provides excellent smears, especially in children and young to middle age adults. Cellular morphology is excellent with minimal distortion, but in older patients, packed or empty marrows, or fibrosis, the minimal turbulence with this method may be insufficient to disrupt particles, resulting in few spread cells for review. Coverslip smears also generally provide good cellular morphology, but require manual staining, cannot be individually labeled (introducing the possibility of identification errors), and if improperly performed (too little blood, too much capillary spreading before smearing) may result in extensive disruption of cells. Squash preparations are generally problematic. If done well by experienced individuals they can provide excellent smears, but far too often they result in extensive and nonrandom destruction of cells, compromising interpretation in difficult cases. Staining of smears may be manual, but automated stainers are effective for smears on slides, and more reproducible than manual stains. Wright-Giemsa staining is preferable to the simple historical Wright stain, because of better discrimination of granules and immature cytoplasm; despite labels some standard hematology stain packs now have staining characteristics of the Wright-Giemsa (rather than the Wright) stain. Additional aspirate material may be allowed to clot (clot section) or anticoagulated and filtered with processing of the filtered particles as a tissue section. (The filtrate is then typically used for flow cytometry and other analyses.)

If a core biopsy is obtained, a separate biopsy needle should be used and redirected to avoid aspiration artifact in the specimen. The biopsy needle should be directed slightly anterolaterally toward the anterior iliac crest, down the long axis of bone, allowing a long expanse of bone for sampling. The trochar should not be removed until the needle is seated on the posterior iliac crest. The biopsy should be of sufficient size for adequate evaluation. In a normal adult, a biopsy of approximately 2 cm length should be obtained. Note that immediate subcortical marrow is often not representative of deeper marrow, especially for cellularity. Touch preparations, prepared by gently touching (not smearing) the biopsy on a glass slide, should be made from the biopsy as a fallback for poor aspirate smears, using care to avoid damaging the biopsy. Touch preps are processed similarly to aspirate smears. Additionally, the biopsy needle should be rinsed with RPMI and the rinse saved, as a fallback for flow cytometry and other studies if aspirate material is insufficient.

The particle preparation (clot or filtered particles) and biopsy are fixed, the biopsy decalcified, and both processed as surgical biopsy samples with H&E staining of sections. B5 fixation gives optimal results, but it is an environmental hazard and is being displaced by safer fixatives. The sections are reviewed for cellularity, distribution of immature and mature cells, and focal lesions such as granulomata or tumor. Immunohistochemical staining of sections may help resolve cases with poor aspirate smears, poor flow cytometry, or otherwise ambiguous results, using panels of antibodies similar to those used for flow cytometry. Finally, while morphologic analysis is of primary importance in diagnosis and management of AML, it is extremely important that an ample additional sample be available for flow cytometric, cytogenetic, and selected molecular genetic analyses in every new case of acute leukemia.

2.4.2 Morphologic Review

Microscopic analysis of air-dried Wright-Giemsa stained peripheral blood and marrow aspirate smears remains fundamental to diagnosis of acute leukemia, and provides some information for separation of AML and ALL (e.g., Auer rods, typical APL hypergranular promyelocytes), but other studies (flow cytometry, previously cytochemistry) are usually required for reliable separation of AML and ALL. Presence of multilineage dysplasia in background cells suggests diagnosis of MDR-AML, although we recommend corroboration with history, cytogenetics, and patient age. It is important for the morphologist to realize the range of blasts that may be seen in marrow and peripheral blood in AML, to include myeloblasts in varying stages of differentiation, hypergranular and hypogranular promyelocytes, monoblasts, erythroblasts, and megakaryoblasts, as described in FAB and WHO publications, other atlases, and illustrated in accompanying figures [1, 3] (Figs. 2.3–2.7).

2.4.3 Leukemia Cytochemistry

Cytochemical analysis, critical historically for separation of AML and ALL and for FAB subclassification of AML, has been largely supplanted by flow cytometric characterization of blasts. Selected cytochemistry studies remain useful for resolving difficult cases where lineage remains ambiguous with flow cytometric work up.

2.4.3.1 Myeloperoxidase and Sudan Black

Sudan black (SB) or myeloperoxidase (MPO) stains may be used to confirm myeloid differentiation. SB stains a lipid in myeloid granules, whereas MPO stains that enzyme in myeloid primary granules. Both stains mark myeloblasts, some monoblasts, and eosinophils. Although MPO is the better marker for granulocytic lineage, the enzyme deteriorates rapidly on slides, especially with light exposure, whereas SB staining may be

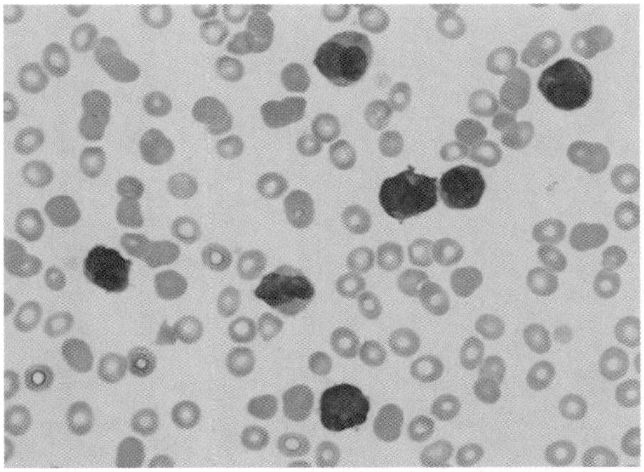

Fig. 2.3. Acute promyelocytic leukemia, microgranular variant (FAB M3v). Peripheral blood smear, Wright's stain.

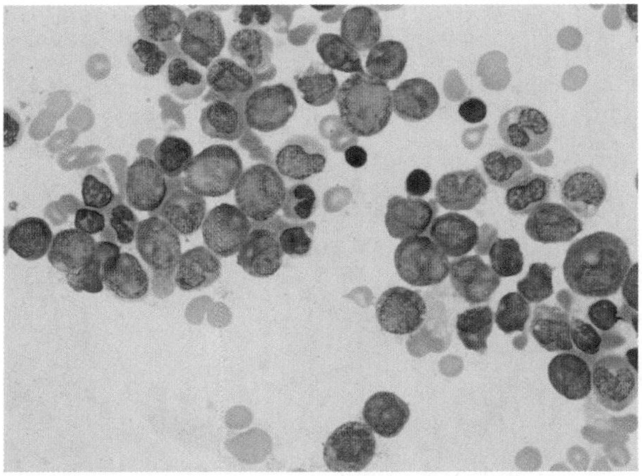

Fig. 2.4. AML with t(8;21), bone marrow aspirate smear (FAB M2). Wright's stain, showing blasts and myelocytes with orange Hoff.

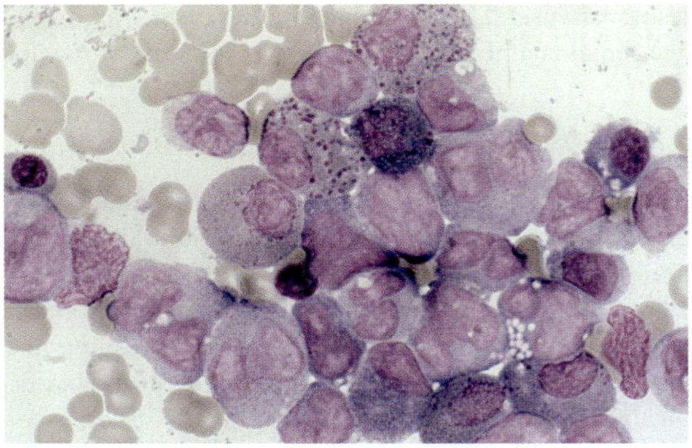

Fig. 2.5. AML with inv(16) (FAB M4Eo). Note the abnormal eosinophilic precursors with orange and basophilic granules. Bone marrow aspirate smear, Wright's stain.

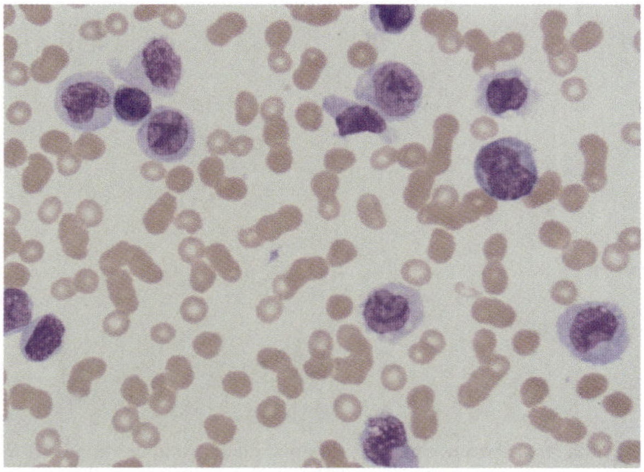

Fig. 2.6. Acute monoblastic leukemia (FAB M5). Peripheral blood smear, Wright's stain.

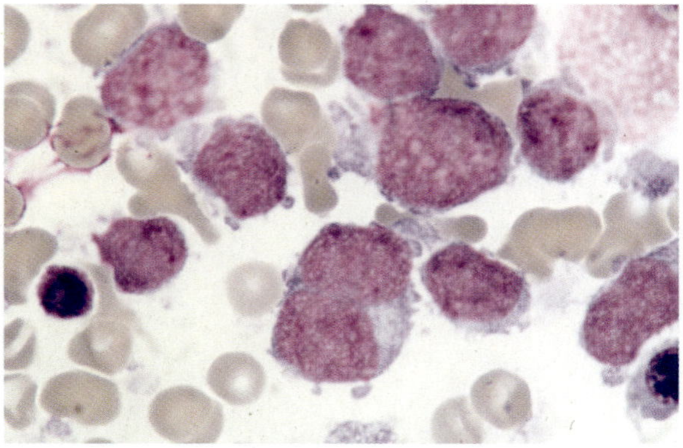

Fig. 2.7. Acute megakaryoblastic leukemia (FAB M7). Bone marrow aspirate smear, Wright's stain. Note cytoplasmic blebbing and the binucleate blast.

performed successfully on smears after several weeks or more. With cytochemistry AML was defined as having greater than 3% SB or MPO positive blasts (FAB), but in practice this requires discretion in application. The intent is that lymphoblasts are negative with these stains, but normal myeloblasts (up to 3%) are present in background hematopoiesis in ALL; in fact this number may be higher in occasional cases of ALL. Auer rods are easier to detect with these stains than with Wright-Giemsa staining. SB may also faintly stain granular ALL, with much less intensity (elephant gray) than myeloblasts or internal control maturing neutrophils (black).

2.4.3.2 Esterase Stains

Naphthol-ASD chloroacetate esterase (a.k.a. specific esterase [SE] or Leder stain) stains a myeloid secondary granule enzyme and also stains mast cells. It is less sensitive than myeloperoxidase but will strongly stain promyelocytes in both the hypergranular and microgranular variants of acute promyelocytic leukemia. Despite its name, "specific" esterase is not completely specific, and stains monoblasts in some cases. Monoblasts and monocytes stain with α-naphthyl butyrate (ANB) esterase and α-naphthyl acetate (ANA) esterase stains (a.k.a. nonspecific esterase, NSE), enzymes found in monocytes/macrophages. NSEs in monocytes are inhibitable by sodium fluoride. Megakaryoblasts also stain with ANA (but not ANB), and this ANA staining is resistant to sodium fluoride inhibition. Some have suggested use of the esterase stains to distinguish monoblastic (NSE positive) from myelomonocytic (SE and NSE positive) leukemia; but this approach is not widely accepted because of the lack of specificity of the "specific" esterase stain. Lymphoblasts, in particular granular lymphoblasts, may also exhibit granular positivity with the esterase stains.

2.4.3.3 Periodic Acid Schiff Stain

The periodic-acid Schiff (PAS) stain marks lymphoblasts in some cases of ALL, staining cytoplasmic glycogen with fine to marked or "block" positivity. However, PAS staining is not specific for ALL. Acute erythroblastic leukemia, erythroblasts in MDS, monoblasts, basophils, and some metastatic tumors (rhabdomyosarcoma, Ewing's sarcoma) may exhibit similar PAS staining.

These stains may be helpful in assigning lineage in ambiguous cases of acute leukemia. However, aside from dysplastic PAS positivity in erythroblasts, they are not helpful in separation of MDR- versus DN-AML.

2.4.4 Flow Cytometry

Immunophenotyping blasts by flow cytometry has become standard for diagnosis of the acute leukemias, in particular for separation of AML and ALL, as well as for recognition of myeloblastic, monoblastic or megakaryoblastic differentiation in leukemic blasts. Variations in details of flow cytometry are beyond the scope of this chapter, but some comments with respect to its application to AML are appropriate. A standard flow cytometric approach for acute leukemia is to use a combination of CD45, side scatter, and forward scatter to recognize an abnormal population consistent with blasts, with blasts usually having reduced CD45 and low side scatter [38]. This population is then characterized with a series of antibodies directed against surface antigens present on immature hematopoietic cells to separate B or T lymphoblasts from blasts with myeloid differentiation, and to delineate lineage commitment of the myeloid blasts. It should be noted again that lineage commitment is not a satisfactory approach for subclassification of AML, but it is useful for confirming diagnosis of AML versus ALL. Commonly used surface antigens for this purpose are: for myeloid differentiation CD13, CD33, CD117, CD16, CD64, CD14, CD11b, CD4(2–), and CD61; for B-lymphoid differentiation CD19, CD79a, CD22, CD20, CD10, and TdT; and for T-lymphoid differentiation CD2, CD7, CD4, CD8, CD1[a], and TdT. None of these antigens singly are lineage-specific, but rather lineage-associated, but unambiguous sets of lineage-associated antigen positivity reliably indicate lineage commitment of blasts. Myeloid blasts can be further characterized as having myeloblastic, monoblastic (CD4+, CD14+, CD64+), or megakaryoblastic (CD61+) differentiation. There are two general approaches to resolve ambiguous cases. One approach, proposed by the European Group for Immunologic Classification of Leukaemia (EGIL), is a scoring system that applies variable weight to surface antigens, plus several cytoplasmic antigens (cytoplasmic [c]CD79a, cCD22, cCD3, and cMPO) [39] (see Table 2.6). This approach requires a score of greater than 2 for confirmation of lineage differentiation. The second approach treats only a limited panel of cytoplasmic markers as definitive for lineage differentiation of blasts: cCD79a or cCD22 for B differentiation, cCD3 for T differentiation, cMPO for myeloid differentiation, and cCD61 for megakaryoblastic differentiation.

Table 2.6. EGIL criteria for immunologic classification of acute leukemia [39]

Score	Myeloid	B-lymphoid	T-lymphoid
2	MPO	CytCD79a*	CytCD3
		CytIgM	anti-TCR$\alpha\beta$
		CytCD22	anti-TCR$\gamma\delta$
	CD117	CD19	CD2
1	CD13	CD20	CD5
	CD33	CD10	CD8
	CD65	CD19	CD10
	CD14	TdT	TdT
0.5	CD15	CD24	CD7
	CD64		CD1a

* also seen in some T-ALL

A score of 2.5 or greater is interpreted as lineage commitment in this system.

Frequent cases of acute leukemia demonstrate "aberrant" expression of antigens typically associated with another lineage of differentiation (e.g., CD19 or CD2 expression by blasts in otherwise typical AML). This expression has little bearing on prognosis of a given case, and does not indicate bilineage differentiation in most such cases of acute leukemia. Such expression may provide a useful marker of leukemic blasts for monitoring treatment of such cases with flow cytometry for low-level residual disease. A small percentage of cases of acute leukemia do demonstrate dual lineage differentiation of blasts, either B-myeloid or T-myeloid. Many such cases demonstrate dual morphology with small lymphoblasts and larger myeloblasts (often more apparent in thicker areas of smears), often with granular differentiation or Auer rods in myeloblasts. In addition, cytochemical stains may demonstrate dual populations, with Sudan black or myeloperoxidase cytochemical positivity in the larger blasts. Confirmation of such dual differentiation requires flow cytometric demonstration of expression of multiple myeloid and either B- or T-lymphoid lineage-associated antigens or lineage-specific cytoplasmic markers. As discussed in the preceding paragraph, there are two general approaches for confirmation of bilineage commitment of blasts, either use of the EGIL scoring system or demonstration of confirmatory cytoplasmic antigen positivity. In this situation cytochemical myeloperoxidase or Sudan black positivity in leukemic blasts can supplement flow cytometric demonstration of myeloid differentiation. Finally, some have recommended the terminology of bilineal acute leukemia for cases with two distinct populations of blasts, versus biphenotypic for cases with expression of markers of two distinct lineages of differentiation on the same blasts. In both settings both populations of blasts usually have a uniform set of genetic abnormalities. Only very rarely are two completely unique sets of genetic abnormalities present in distinct blast populations in acute leukemia, suggesting simultaneous occurrence of two unrelated diseases.

There are several pitfalls and caveats in evaluation of leukemic blasts with flow cytometry. With standard flow cytometric CD45/side scatter gating for a blast population, the position of leukemic promyelocytes tends to merge with the normal granulocyte population, compromising recognition and separation of the two populations in APL. Monoblasts and promonocytes tend to merge with normal monocytes with the same gating, and this separation is further complicated by the presence of few distinguishing cytometric markers between the two populations. Therefore, morphologic correlation is essential when evaluating monoblastic leukemia. Hypogranular granulocytes in MDS and MDR-AML tend to merge with the blast gate, because of decreased side scatter, causing overestimation of the blast percentage in such cases. Elimination of erythroid precursors in processing the sample before flow analysis may falsely elevate the blast percentage by reducing the denominator in the sample. Despite these limitations, flow cytometry has become an indispensable tool for rapid and efficient diagnosis of acute leukemia.

Flow cytometric analysis can be adapted to monitoring minimal residual disease during treatment of AML, with sensitivity of approximately 1 cell in 10^{3-4}, if an informative phenotype differing from normal populations is identified (discussed below). In this capacity this technology may be superior to other approaches because of its speed and cost, but may require greater than the current standard 4-color flow cytometry to be informative and practical in most cases.

A number of reports indicate that demonstration by flow cytometry of aberrant expression, or aberrant timing of expression, of antigens in myeloid progenitors may be a useful adjunct for diagnosis of MDS [40–42]. Such testing is not yet widely used for this purpose in clinical practice, in part because it requires more extensive antigen panels and/or greater than the usual current 4-color flow cytometry for implementation. However, with technical improvements in cytometric equipment such testing could become a valuable adjunct for confirmation of diagnosis of MDS, and similar testing of background hematopoiesis could potentially be used in differential diagnosis of MDR- and DN-AML.

2.4.5 Cytogenetics and Molecular Genetics

Karyotype analysis remains indispensable as a diagnostic tool for acute leukemia, due to its ability to screen the entire complement of chromosomes for large scale abnormalities. In the majority of childhood acute leukemia and 54–78% of adult AML, cytogenetic abnormalities are detected on karyotype analysis of blood or marrow [43]. Cytogenetic studies at diagnosis help separate DN- and MDR-AML, and are currently one of the most valuable prognostic indicators for AML, separating patients into favorable, intermediate, or unfavorable clinical risk groups (Table 2.2). The translocations of AML with Recurrent Cytogenetic Abnormalities (WHO) (Table 2.3) each have prognostic significance: t(8;21), inv(16), and t(15;17) confer favorable risk, 11q23 abnormalities intermediate risk. Of the karyotypic changes associated with MDS or MDR-AML, −5 and −7 are in the adverse risk group, while +8 and +21 are intermediate risk. A second reason that cytogenetic studies should be done on all new AML cases is that treatment options may vary depending on cytogenetic results, particularly with t(15;17) (APL) and t(9;22) (which may indicate myeloid blast crisis of CML).

Molecular diagnostic tools such as fluorescent in situ hybridization (FISH), Southern blotting, and RT-PCR, while more specific and/or sensitive than classic cytogenetics, require focus on specific genes for testing, rather than providing a screening tool for multiple abnormalities. However, there is a role for these directed tests to increase detection sensitivity for the common translocations, additions, and deletions of AML, to confirm translocation breakpoints detected by karyotyping, and to detect cytogenetically silent genetic abnormalities [e.g., t(12;21) of ALL, FLT3 internal tandem repeats, *C/EBPα* mutations]. In addition to karyotyping, most academic centers use FISH or RT-PCR to test for *PML/RARα*, *CBFβ/MYH11*, *AML1/ETO*, and *MLL* disruption, and often use FISH to search for −7, 5q−, and +8. Although these examples are usually detected by classic karyotype analysis, poor viability and inability to obtain metaphase spreads may compromise karyotype analysis, and cryptic insertional translocations occur that cannot be detected by karyotype analysis. An additional advantage of FISH is that it can be performed on paraffin sections of nondecalcified tissue, such as bone marrow particle sections. Thus, in AML cases with a negative karyotype FISH or RT-PCR is recommended for some common abnormalities. For the more common translocations, the following are estimates of the percentage of cases missed if only karyotype analysis is performed: *AML1/ETO*, 6% [44]; *CBFβ/MYH11*, 4% [45]; *PML/RARα*, 15% [46]. These cases include those where karyotype analysis was unsuccessful, as well as cases with cryptic translocations. With the additional methods of testing the overall incidence of the major recurring translocations in AML in the US and western Europe, from age 2 to middle age, are: *MLL* (11q23): 3–7%, *AML1/ETO*: 14%, *PML/RARα*: 10–15%, *CBFβ/MYH11*: 10% [47]. (It should be noted that there is heterogeneous distribution of some of these translocations; e.g. a high incidence of t(15;17) has been described in both northern Italy and in Latinos in the Los Angeles area in the US.) FISH and PCR each have distinct advantages for detection of recurring translocations, and the optimal test depends on the molecular biology of the particular translocation. If there are multiple possible break-points for a translocation, FISH is preferable, as large (approximately 100 kbp) FISH probes can span multiple breakpoints, whereas for PCR several reactions with multiple primer pairs would be required. If there are multiple possible fusion partners, as with *MLL* abnormalities, a FISH break-apart probe can detect disruption of the locus by any translocation. On the other hand, PCR is more sensitive than FISH, with the ability to detect 1 in 10^{4-5} cells, while the maximal reliable sensitivity of FISH appears in the range of 2 to 5 in 10^3 with double break-apart/fusion probes [48]. PCR sensitivity is especially suited over FISH for detection of minimal residual disease, if presence of a target is confirmed at diagnosis.

2.4.6 Specific Recurring Genetic Abnormalities of AML

A variety of specific genetic abnormalities have been described in patients with AML, some of which appear to block differentiation, while others drive proliferation and inhibit apoptosis. Abnormalities of each functional group appear to be mutually exclusive of other abnormalities of the same group, but as discussed previously, abnormalities of both groups appear necessary to create the acute leukemia phenotype. As stated previously, despite extensive efforts specific genetic abnormalities caused by the major chromosomal abnormalities typical of MDS and MDR-AML (i.e., −7, 5q−, +8, 20q−, +21, etc.) that contribute to disease pathogenesis remain unknown.

2.4.6.1 Retinoic Acid Receptor Translocations

The successful treatment of acute promyelocytic leukemia with retinoic acid (RA) is a stunning example of the potential power of molecular medicine. As the association between t(15;17) (q22;q21) and APL was known, the report [49] that oral all trans-retinoic acid (ATRA) induced complete remission in APL led quickly to demonstration that t(15;17) involves the retinoic acid receptor *α* gene (*RARα*) at chromosome 17q21 [50–52]. Recognition of APL morphology remains important to alert clinicians to the potential of a concomitant hemorrhagic diathesis, to direct appropriate diagnostic studies, and to raise the possibility of directed treatment possibilities [3, 53–55]. The hypergranular variant of APL (M3h) has distinctive hypergranular blasts with a reddish color shift of granules, bilobed grooved nuclei, frequent Auer rods, and faggot cells with multiple Auer rods. The microgranular variant (M3v) (Fig. 2.3) has similar bilobed nuclei, but few obvious granules with Romanowsky staining. Flow cytometric findings demonstrate standard myeloid markers, but blasts are usually negative for CD34 and HLA-DR, and often aberrantly positive for CD2.

Of four 17q21 translocations involving *RARα*, the most common is t(15;17), in which the 5′ portion of the major fusion protein is encoded by the *PML* (Pro-Myelocytic Leukemia) gene at 15q22, and the 3′ portion is encoded by the *RARα* gene at 17q21. The breakpoint in *RARα* is invariant in intron 2, incorporating in the fusion protein the C-terminal portion of *RARα* including its DNA-binding, ligand-binding, dimerization, and repression domains. There are three breakpoint regions in *PML*. The most common, bcr-1 in intron 6, includes the first 6 exons of *PML*, and is designated *PML(L)/RARα* [56]. The second, bcr-3 in intron 3, generates a shorter transcript, *PML(S)/RARα*. The third, bcr-2, occurs within exon 6. RT-PCR using a single 3′ RAR*a* primer and 2 PML primers to encompass the breakpoint sequences in introns 3 and 6 detects all 3 transcripts. FISH will also detect all *PML/RARa* fusion gene variants.

RAR*a* is half (with RXR) of a heterodimer ligand-dependent nuclear membrane receptor which mediates the cellular effects of RA. The heterodimer binds to RA response elements (RAREs) in the promoters of many genes important in myeloid differentiation. In the absence of RA, wild-type RAR*a*/RXR on RAREs binds to the corepressor proteins SMRT, N-CoR, mSin3, and histone deacetylases. Deacetylation of histone at the promoter, mediated by this complex, results in transcriptional repression. Physiologic concentration retinoic acid (10^{-8} M) causes a conformational change of the receptor, release of corepressors, and recruitment of a coactivator complex (SRC-1) which associates with histone acetyltransferases [57]. This new complex mediates acetylation of histones at the promoter, relaxes chromatin conformation, and allows transcription to proceed (reviewed in [58]).

PML/RAR*a* also heterodimerizes with RXR and binds to RAREs, competing with RAR*a*/RXR in a dominant negative manner. In the absence of ligand, PML/RAR*a* (via its 3′ RAR*a* portion) binds corepressor proteins similarly to RAR*a*, but requires pharmacologic concentration ATRA (10^{-6} M) to release them and bind to the coactivator complex, the mechanistic basis for the induction of differentiation of leukemic cells in APL with pharmacologic dosage of ATRA [7, 57].

Studies of variant RAR*a* translocation t(11;17)(q23;q21) cases of AML [6, 7] have furthered understanding of the mechanism of response of APL to ATRA. Patients with t(11;17) AML are resistant to treatment with pharmacologic dosage ATRA. The fusion partner gene on chromosome 11q23 encodes PLZF, a transcriptional repressor that contributes a second corepressor binding site to the fusion protein. Although pharmacologic dosage ATRA induces release of corepressors from the RAR*a* portion of the fusion protein, those binding to PLZF are unaffected [57–59]. Addition of Trichostatin A, which inhibits the deacetylase activity of PLZF-associated corepressors [7, 60], allows induction of differentiation to proceed.

Finally, two additional RAR*a* translocations, both of which are ATRA responsive, are associated with APL. With t(5;17)(q35;q21), nucleophosmin (*NPM*) is fused with *RARa*, contributing an oligomerization domain [61]. With t(11;17)(q13;q21) the *NUMA* gene is fused to *RARa*. The NUMA protein is involved in the mitotic process and also contributes a coiled-coil dimerization domain [62]. Thus, all translocation partners of *RARa* encode proteins with multimerization domains, and all these translocations appear to contribute a block of differentiation to leukemia pathogenesis.

2.4.6.2 Core Binding Factor Mutations

The core binding factor translocations include t(8;21)(q22;q22) which produces the AML1/ETO fusion protein [63] and inv(16), which produces the CBF*β*/MYH11 fusion protein [64]. The murine counterpart of *AML1* (*RUNX1, CBFa1*) was first described as part of the heterodimer core binding factor (CBF) which binds to a core enhancer sequence of the Molony leukemias virus LTR. Inversion (16)(p13;q22) and t(16;16)(p13;q22) disrupt the other component of CBF, non-DNA binding CBF*β*. The core enhancer sequence is found in the promoter region of a number of human genes, including B-cell tyrosine kinase [65], T cell receptors *a* and *β* [66], the cytokines IL3 [67] and GM-CSF [68], and the granulocyte proteins MPO and neutrophil elastase [69]. Core binding factor translocations appear to contribute a block of differentiation to leukemia pathogenesis.

Core binding factor is essential for hematopoietic development. Knockout of either *AML1* [70] or *CBFβ* [71] in mice results in fetal death at E11.5–12.5 due to absence of fetal hematopoiesis. Transgenic experiments have demonstrated that AML1 is essential for development of hematopoietic stem cells in the aorta/gonadal/mesodermal region, the source of definitive hematopoiesis [72]. The essential role of AML1 in hematopoietic development appears to be through its function as a transcriptional activator.

AML1 is located on chromosome 21q22.3 and comprised of 12 exons over 260 kb of DNA, with 4 different transcripts by alternative splicing [73]. The runt homology domain (RHD) in the N-terminal portion of the protein, homologous to the *Drosophila runt* protein [74], is a sequence specific DNA binding domain. This domain is mutated in the uncommon autosomal dominant inheritance syndrome of familial platelet disorder with predisposition to AML (FPD-AML) and in AML associated with AML1 point mutations [75, 76]. CBF*β* interacts via this domain and changes the conformation of AML1 to increase its DNA binding affinity [77]. C-terminal to the RHD are potential MAP kinase phosphorylation sites, followed by three activation domains, a nuclear matrix target signal, a dimerization domain, and sequences recognized by corepressor proteins (reviewed in [5]).

The *ETO* gene, cloned from the t(8;21) fusion [63], is the mammalian homologue of the *Drosophila nervy* gene [78]. ETO is expressed in CD34+ progenitor cells but not in more differentiated hematopoietic cells [79]. ETO does not appear to bind DNA specifically. However, it may act as a corepressor protein [80], as it associates with N-CoR and mSin3A, and directly binds to the class I HDACs (HDAC-1, HDAC-2, and HDAC-3) [81].

In t(8;21) the breakpoint in *AML1* is between exons 5 and 6 [82], yielding a fusion protein with the N-terminal 177aa of AML1 [63] including the DNA binding domain, but lacking the C-terminal activation domains, corepressor interaction sites, and nuclear localization signals of wild-type AML1 [5]. The breakpoint in the *ETO* gene occurs in the introns between the first two alternative exons of *ETO*, resulting in the inclusion of almost all of the coding region for ETO in the fusion transcript [63]. The AML1/ETO protein binds to the same DNA sequence as AML1, heterodimerizes with CBFβ [83], and acts as a dominant negative inhibitor of wild-type AML1. AML1/ETO can also function as an active transcriptional repressor through its association with HDACs (via ETO). Targets of AML1/ETO repression are presumed to include genes important for granulocyte differentiation. In addition, AML1/ETO may indirectly repress p53 by repressing $p19^{ARF}$ [84], an antagonist of the p53 inhibitor MDM2 [85]; thus reduced p53 checkpoint control might contribute to t(8;21) leukemogenesis. Since observed breakpoints in *AML1* and *ETO* are clustered, RT-PCR using single *AML1* and *ETO* primers should detect the translocation in all cases. In addition, an *AML1/ETO* dual color, dual fusion probe is available for FISH. Other mutations involving AML1 have been described in AML and MDS. The uncommon t(3;21) involves the *AML1* gene and has been described in the setting of AML and MDS following alkylating agent chemotherapy. In addition, several mutations of *AML1* have been identified in FPD-AML and in random cases of AML, including nonsense mutations and intragenic deletion of one allele of *AML1*. Finally, a minority of AML following epipodophyllotoxin chemotherapy are characterized by *AML1* translocations.

AML with t(8;21) is a favorable prognostic subtype of AML, particularly with regimens containing high-dose cytosine arabinoside. The majority of AML with t(8;21) demonstrates differentiation of blasts (M2 morphology) with cytoplasmic granules and Auer rods [3, 86]. In Romanowsky stained marrow smears maturing neutrophils from these patients may have characteristic salmon pink cytoplasm in the Golgi zone (Fig. 2.4) and pseudo Pelger-Huet nuclei. Flow cytometry often reveals aberrant expression of CD19 or CD56.

Inv(16) and t(16;16) result in fusion of the first 165aa of CBFβ to the C-terminal coiled-coil region of MYH11 [64]. The C-terminal region of MYH11 associates with mSin3a and HDAC8, contributing the transcriptional corepressor activity of the fusion protein. Presumably CBFβ/MYH11, which cannot bind DNA on its own, interacts with AML1 to form a transcriptional repressor complex [4].

Inversion 16 AML often associates with myelomonocytic leukemia with dysplastic eosinophils in marrow with purple as well as orange granules (M4Eo) [3, 87]. These abnormal granules are evident especially in eosinophilic myelocytes (Fig. 2.5). Cytogenetic detection of Inv(16) is subtle and may be missed with traditional standard Giemsa banding karyotype analysis. A common secondary abnormality, trisomy 22, or characteristic dysplastic eosinophils in smears, should prompt RT-PCR for *CBFβ*/MYH11. Most *CBFβ* breakpoints occur in intron 5; breakpoints in 7 different exons have been reported in *MYH11*, but type A accounts for 90% of cases. Primers appropriate for these most common breakpoints are used for RT-PCR.

2.4.6.3 MLL Abnormalities

The mixed lineage leukemia gene (*MLL*) (a.k.a. *HRX* or *ALL1*), a transcriptional activator frequently rearranged in infant leukemia, subtypes of therapy-related leukemia, and mixed lineage leukemia, maps to chromosome 11q23 (reviewed in [88, 89]). The gene consists of 34 exons over 100 kb, encoding a 3969 aa protein [90]. *MLL* has homology with *trithorax*, a Drosophila transcriptional regulator which positively regulates homeobox genes [91], a large family of developmental regulator genes essential for growth and differentiation, named for a shared homeobox sequence motif [92]. Wild-type MLL is responsible for maintenance of homeobox gene expression during development [93].

MLL abnormalities are found in 5–10% overall of patients with ALL and AML, and usually associate with poor prognosis with current treatments [94]. In a study of 550 cases of acute leukemia and MDS with 11q23 rearrangements, 16% involved additions, duplications, and inversions, with an internal tandem duplication being the most common alteration [95]. Of the remaining, translocation with 30 different reciprocal partner loci were identified [96]. The two most common translocations with AML were t(9;11) (*MLL/AF9*), and t(6;11) (*MLL/AF6*). As the name implies, MLL is often found with mixed lineage leukemias in which blasts express both myeloid and lymphoid markers. This association, and the presence of *MLL* abnormalities in both ALL and AML cases, suggest that the genetic error may take place in an uncommitted hematopoietic stem cell. Myelomonocytic or monoblastic morphology (M4 or M5 morphology) are common in AML with MLL abnormalities (Fig. 2.6), but a variety of other morphologies are also seen [95]. Most, but not all, MLL translocations are restricted to DN-AML, but 11q23 deletion is found in MDR-AML, and t(11;16)(q23;p13) that results in a fusion of *MLL* and *CBP* (CREB enhancer binding protein) has been described in cases of therapy-related MDS and AML. MLL abnormalities appear to contribute a block of differentiation to leukemia pathogenesis.

The breakpoints of *MLL* usually occur between exons 5 and 11 [97], fusing the N terminal approximately 1400 amino acids of the MLL protein to a C-terminal partner [89]. Due to the complexity of breakpoints and fusion partners, the best method of detecting *MLL* rearrangements is FISH with an *MLL* break apart probe. RT-PCR multiplex approaches detect only the more common *MLL* translocations, and single primer set RT-PCR is impractical unless the putative partner gene is suggested by a cytogenetic translocation.

MLL rearrangements are associated with several unique types of leukemia. In infant acute leukemia (birth to 1 year) there is a 60–80% incidence of 11q23 rearrangement in both AML and ALL [98]. In therapy-related acute leukemias with epipodophyllotoxin inhibitors of topoisomerase II, usually AML, there is an 80–90% incidence of *MLL* rearrangements, particularly t(9;11)(p21–22;q23) and t(11;19)(q23;p13) (most of the remainder involving *AML1*) [96, 99]. Topoisomerase II unwinds DNA during replication and transcription by producing double-strand nicks in the DNA, after which the ends are rejoined by a ligase activity of topoisomerase II. Topoisomerase II inhibitors such as epipodophyllotoxins inhibit this ligase function so that DNA free ends accumulate, triggering apoptotic events, but also apparently facilitating occurrence of translocations through religation errors. In the *MLL* gene there are 11 sites similar to topoisomerase II consensus binding sites in breakpoint cluster areas. Infant leukemia with *MLL* translocations has a similar distribution of breakpoints to therapy related disease, whereas sporadic cases have more random breakpoints [100]. This observation has triggered speculation that in utero exposure to environmental topoisomerase II inhibitors such as flavenoids may have a role in the etiology of infant leukemia [101], although this remains unsubstantiated.

2.4.6.4 C/EBP*α*

C/CAAT enhancer binding protein *α* (C/EBP*α*) is a transcription factor that regulates granulocytic differentiation [102]. The gene produces two proteins using alternative start sites. The larger and predominant 42 kDa protein consists of two N-terminal transactivating domains, with a C-terminal bZIP domain consisting of a basic (b) region that mediates DNA sequence binding and a leucine zipper (ZIP) domain that mediates dimerization [103]. The shorter 30 kDa protein is transcribed from an alternative internal start site, and retains its bZIP domain but lacks the first transactivation domain; it thus retains the ability to dimerize with the long form, but inhibits transactivation by the dimer. The importance of C/EBP*α* in granulocyte differentiation is supported by the lack of granulocyte differentiation in *CEBPA* knockout mice [104], while its conditional expression triggers granulocyte differentiation in bipotential precursors [105]. C/EBP*α* transactivates the genes for G-CSF and GM-CSF receptors, and several granulocyte-specific proteins. Cytogenetically silent mutations of *CEBPA* have been identified in about 8% of AML cases, and are of two types: C-terminal bZIP domain mutations and N-terminal truncating mutations that lead to enhanced production of the 30 kDa protein [106–108]. The former inhibit dimerization and DNA binding. The latter dimerize with the long form, but inhibit transactivation by the dimer, functioning in a dominant negative manner. *CEBPA* mutations are found predominantly in AML with differentiation (M2), similar to AML1 mutations, interesting in that C/EBP*α* interacts with CBF to mediate AML differentiation. Some cases also have associated eosinophilia (M2Eo). Mutation of *CEBPA* has also been described in one family with a familial AML syndrome [109]. Approximately one third of AML with *CEBPA* mutations also have *FLT3* mutations. Data suggest that AML with *CEBPA* mutation and lacking *FLT3* mutation is favorable risk disease, remaining cases falling in the intermediate risk AML category (Table 2.2).

2.4.6.5 GATA1

GATA1 is a zinc finger transcription factor that regulates erythroid and megakaryocytic differentiation. Familial mis-sense mutations in *GATA1* results in a syndrome of dyserythropoietic anemia and thrombocytopenia, while conditional knockout of *GATA1* in megakaryocyte precursors in mice leads to thrombocytopenia and megakaryoblast proliferation. In acute megakaryoblastic leukemia (AMkL) (Fig. 2.7) that occurs in Down Syndrome (DS) children, mutations of *GATA1* have been described in all tested cases [20, 110, 111]. Similar mutations have also been described in transient myeloproliferative disorder (TMD) in the neonatal period in DS patients [110]. About one third of DS patients with TMD later develop AMkL, and identical *GATA1* mutations have been identified in such patients in both TMD and subsequent AMkL. The described mutations result in transcription of a truncated form of *GATA1* that lacks its N-terminal transactivation domain, presumably contributing to the block of differentiation in the patients' leukemic cells. During the intervening period between TMD and AMkL these patients are hematologically normal. In a separate scenario, some patients with MDS and –7 develop translocations at 3q26 prior to progression to MDR-AML. Some of these translocations lead to dysregulated transcription of *EVI1*, a gene not normally expressed in hematopoietic cells. EVI1 is an antagonist of GATA1, with an identical sequence-specific DNA binding domain. Thus, dysregulated expression of EVI1 is presumed to block GATA1-mediated differentiation, contributing to leukemogenesis in this setting. There are no other specific morphologic or clinical correlates to the 3q26 translocations [112].

2.4.6.6 FLT3

FLT3 is possibly the single most commonly mutated gene in AML (reviewed in [10]). Originally cloned from CD34+ hematopoietic stem cells, it encodes a type III receptor tyrosine kinase in the PDGF receptor family. FLT3 ligand (FL), a type I transmembrane protein expressed on the surface of support and hematopoietic cells in the bone marrow, stimulates growth of immature myeloid cells and stem cells [113]. FL binding induces FLT3 dimerization and activation by cross-phosphorylation on intracytoplasmic tyrosine residues. The activated kinase then phosphorylates intermediates in downstream signal transduction pathways. Two types of activating *FLT3* mutations have been identified. The most common are internal tandem repeat duplications (ITD), in which head-to-tail duplications of various lengths and positions occur in the juxtamembrane (JM) portion of the molecule [114]. These may occur due to DNA replication errors as a result of a potential palindromic intermediate that may form at that site [115]. The juxtamembrane domain is an autoinhibitory domain whose function is blocked by autophosphorylation [10]. The in frame insertions in the JM domain produce mutant proteins which are constitutively activated by autodimerization and phosphorylation in the absence of ligand [115]. The second type of mutations are activation loop point mutations, usually an Asp825-Tyr substitution resulting from a point mutation. Usually the activation loop inhibits access of ATP and substrate to the kinase domain until phosphorylation occurs as a result of ligand binding. The activation loop mutations again produce a constitutively active FLT3 protein [10]. Interestingly, FLT3 activity on downstream signal transduction intermediates is altered by these mutations. Ligand-activated wild-type FLT3 stimulates proliferation via activation of the Ras/Raf/MAP kinase pathway. In contrast, FLT3-ITD only weakly activates MAP kinase, but strongly activates STAT5 [116].

The frequency of FLT3-ITD in adult AML is 24%, 10–15% in pediatric AML (reviewed in [10]). FLT3-ITD is detected very frequently in APL, but has been detected in all DN-AML subtypes, and in MDR-AML. The frequency is very low in MDS and ALL. In contrast, the FLT3 activation loop mutation is found in 7% of AML, 3% of MDS, and 3% of ALL [117]. FLT3-ITD is readily detected by PCR of genomic DNA using primer pairs that span the internal tandem repeat region, the amplified abnormal product being easily detected by agarose gel electrophoresis.

The expression of FLT3 may be the most significant current prognostic factor for poor outcome in patients less than 60 years old. In a study of 91 pediatric AML patients, event-free survival at 8 years was 7% for patients with FLT3-ITD compared to 44% for patients with wild-type FLT3 [118]. In adults with AML from 16 to 60 years with otherwise normal cytogenetics, presence of FLT3-ITD significantly decreased the length of remission and overall survival [119].

As with BCR-ABL for CML, the contribution of a constitutively active FLT3 tyrosine kinase to the pathogenesis of AML introduces the possibility of selective kinase inhibition as a specific treatment strategy. Small molecule FLT3 kinase inhibitors that bind to the ATP recognition domain of the enzyme have been identified, and several have been tested in phase I clinical trials [120], with limited frequency and duration of responses. Their use combined with traditional chemotherapy or combined with other classes of inhibitors is being investigated.

2.4.6.7 Other Tyrosine Kinase and RAS Mutations in AML

Recurring mutations have been described in AML in other members of the PDGF receptor tyrosine kinase family. Mutation of cKIT occurs in about 50% of CBF-mutated (AML1 or CBFβ) AML cases. In addition [12], activating RAS mutations have been described in 19% of AML [13, 14], and activating mutations of cFMS [11] have been described in AML, primarily with M4 or M5 morphology. Interestingly, the PDGF receptor tyrosine kinase family functions to drive proliferation through RAS, and RAS, cKIT, cFMS, and FLT3 mutations appear to be mutually exclusive in AML, suggesting all are contributing the same function in leukemogenesis.

2.4.6.8 Nucleophosmin

Nucleophosmin (NPM) is a molecular chaperone that shuttles between cytoplasm and nucleus, with particular nucleolar concentration of protein [121]. While NPM appears to function to transport preribosomal particles from the nucleolus to cytoplasm, other functions have also been described, including regulation of centrosome duplication, regulation of p53, and functional regulation and stabilization of p19^{ARF} (reviewed in [122]). *NPM* is disrupted by the t(2;5) translocation of anaplastic large cell lymphoma [123], as well as two uncommon translocations in AML, t(5;17)(q25;q21) creating the chimeric fusion gene *NPM/RARα*[61] and t(3;5)(q25;q34) creating the chimeric fusion gene *NPM/MLF1* [124]. The precise role of NPM in leukemogenesis in these translocations remains to be determined. Cytogenetically silent mutations of *NPM* have now been identified in 35% of DN-AML; they appear to be absent in MDR-AML [122, 125, 126]. The mutations were first identified by abnormal subcellular localization of NPM, with relocation from its normal predominant nucleolar location to cytoplasmic localization. Sequence analysis subsequently identified mutations in exon 12 of NPM, with each mutation causing a frame-shift resulting in replacement of C-terminal amino acids with an identical 5 amino acid terminal sequence. The mutations were heterozygous, appearing to function in a dominant manner, presumably through heterodimerization with normal NPM, to cause relocation of both normal and abnormal NPM to cytoplasm. These NPM mutations have been verified in a variety of morphologic AML subtypes (excluding APL, AMkL, and AMML with eosinophilia). Almost half of NPM-mutated cases also have FLT3 mutation (33%); despite this association, NPM mutation appeared to convey favorable response to induction chemotherapy [126]. A possible mechanism by which NPM mutation contributes to leukemogenesis remains undefined. Its frequent association with FLT3 mutation suggests it does not function to drive proliferation of leukemic cells, while in translocations it partners with both ALK1 (another tyrosine kinase, in anaplastic large cell lymphoma) and RARα.

2.4.6.9 Summary of Morphologic-Genetic Correlates in AML

The acquired abnormalities in AML that block differentiation correlate to a variable extent with specific morphologic changes. The best correlations are for *RARα* translocations and *GATA1* mutations. The t(15;17) correlates highly with APL morphology, but the correlation is not absolute, as 5–10% of APL cases, depending in part on the skill and experience of the morphologist, lack t(15;17) or other *RARα* translocations [3, 53–55]. A skilled morphologist can sometimes predict an APL case will lack *PML/RARα*, because of lack of bilobed grooved nuclei, lack of a red color-shift in dysplastic granules with Romanowsky staining, or less intense or larger granulation than in typical APL cases. In addition, 1–2% of cases with *PML/RARα* are AML with minimal to moderate differentiation, and lack APL morphology. There is a spectrum from hypergranular to microgranular morphology in sets of APL cases, with frequent morphologically-intermediate cases that behave clinically like classic hypergranular APL (e.g., low WBC counts, low level of peripheral blood blasts). Microgranular morphologic features tend to be more prevalent in peripheral smears than in marrow (Fig. 2.3). Attempts to correlate hypergranular versus microgranular morphology in APL with specific PML breakpoints have been inconsistent, and an explanation for the variable morphology remains obscure. AML with t(11;17) frequently has more differentiated morphology than APL, resembling myelocytes [54, 55]. *GATA1* mutations are substantially restricted to AMkL (Fig. 2.7) in DS patients [20, 110, 111]. Other morphogenetic correlates are less precise. AML with t(8;21) typically demonstrates granulocytic differentiation, and may have a striking orange Hoff (Fig. 2.4), but exceptions are frequent (about 20% of cases) [3, 86]. AML with inv(16) or t(16;16) typically has myelomonocytic morphology with dysplastic marrow eosinophils that contain distinctive basophilic as well as eosinophilic granules (Fig. 2.5), but exceptions are very frequent (about 40% of cases) [3, 87]. MLL and NPM mutations correlate partially with monoblastic or myelomonocytic differentiation (Fig. 2.6). MLL also correlates partially with minimally differentiated and biphenotypic acute leukemia. It must be re-emphasized that most of these correlations are partial, and while of biological interest in understanding the contributions of specific genes to normal and disrupted hematopoiesis, do not substitute for cytogenetic and molecular characterization of cases.

2.4.6.10 Summary of Identified Genetic Mutations in AML

Most recurring mutations described to date in AML appear to contribute to leukemogenesis by either blocking differentiation (RARα, AML1, CBFβ, MLL, C/EBPα, GATA1) or by driving proliferation (FLT3, RAS, cKIT, cFMS). The mutations in each set appear to be mutually exclusive of other mutations in that set, suggesting that members of each set are providing the same function to leukemogenesis. Some specific mutations appear to convey favorable prognosis (PML/RARα, AML1, CBFβ, possibly C/EBPα and NPM), while others may convey an unfavorable prognosis (FLT3, -7, -5) (Table 2.2). Molecularly targeted therapy is in use (ATRA for APL with PML/RARα, cKIT inhibitors) or in development (FLT3 and RAS inhibitors) for some of these mutations, with others predictably to follow. These observations reinforce previously cited subclassification issues for DN- and MDR-AML, as specific genetic information beyond the recurring translocations of DN-AML will become progressively more necessary for guiding therapy and prognostication in individual cases of AML.

Some genetic events contribute to diagnostic separation of DN- and MDR-AML. The recurring translocations characteristic of DN-AML essentially exclude diagnosis of MDR-AML. Although not routinely tested for, NPM and C/EBPα mutations appear to be restricted to DN-AML. The recurring cytogenetic changes of MDS, if present in AML, presumptively identify MDR-AML cases, with the caveat that the recurring DN-AML translocations, if present, supercede the MDS-type changes in significance for classification. As both DN-AML and MDR-AML appear to require similar sets of events for transformation, it seems unlikely that these events alone will explain the consistent differences in clinical outcome in the two groups. Instead, the differences appear to relate to the apparent random pathogenesis of DN-AML (relatively flat incidence curve) versus the relationship of MDR-AML to MDS. Specific genetic events that define most MDR-AML cases have not been defined, and the genetic and pathogenetic basis of MDS remains obscure.

2.4.7 Microarray Analysis of Acute Leukemia

Microarray analysis, or gene expression profiling, provides a snapshot of transcription levels of a large number of genes in a tissue at any one time, giving a more global view of gene expression than provided by traditional Northern blot or PCR analysis of selected single gene expression. There are two general approaches to microarray analysis, both entailing reverse transcription of RNA prepared from tissue samples to fluorochrome-labeled cDNA. In one approach (Affymetrix), labeled cDNA is hybridized to oligonucleotide arrays containing sequence from 5,000 or more genes. The expression value for each gene is presented both numerically and visually as a color showing expression higher or lower than the mean of all samples. In the second approach a mix of test sample and reference cDNA labeled with different fluorochromes is hybridized to a cDNA chip containing an array of selected cDNAs, with the test sample expression value for each gene displayed both numerically and compared to the reference sample [127].

The aims of microarray studies in AML to date have been several: (1) discovery of groups of genes whose expression allows subclassification of AML, (2) discovery of sets of genes that predict prognosis, and (3) discovery of sets of genes instructive as to the pathogenesis of AML. Potential pitfalls include that critical mRNAs may be expressed only transiently, and may be missed in analysis of a large population of unsynchronized cells, or expressed at low levels below the sensitivity of the test system. In addition, results have proven to be heavily dependent on methodology (chip selection) and methods used for statistical analysis.

In microarray studies which have grouped patients with AML on the basis of gene expression signatures, most clusters correspond to the common recurrent translocations or known mutations [128]. Valk et al. [129] (Affymetrix U133A chip with 13,000 unique genes, unsupervised cluster analysis) analyzed blood or bone marrow from 285 patients with AML and identified 16 groups. Patients with the recurrent translocations t(8;21), t(15;17), and inv(16) formed clearly defined clusters, those with 11q23 translocations were in two clusters, and those with t(15;17) formed two groups correlating with presence or absence of FLT3 mutations. Otherwise, FLT3 mutation correlated with no single gene expression signature. Two clusters of patients had high percentages of cases with C/EBPα mutations. Ross et al. (Affymetrix U133A chip, unsupervised two-dimensional hierarchical clustering analysis) demonstrated in 130 cases of pediatric AML clustering of cases with three of the common recurring translocations (*AML1/ETO*, *PML/RARα*, and *MLL*); however, inv(16) cases did not cluster as well as in the adult study [130].

Bullinger et al. [131] (cDNA microarrays, unsupervised hierarchical clustering) analyzed blood or marrow from 116 adults with AML, grouping cases with similar gene expression signatures. The most tightly grouped set was t(15;17), while t(8;21) and inv(16) fell into several clusters. Cases with a normal karyotype formed two separate clusters, one with a high incidence of FLT3 mutations. Additional statistical analysis allowed identification of a 133-gene clinical outcome predictor, validated on an independent test set, which was a strong independent predictor for survival. Genes associated with poor outcome included several homeobox genes (*HOXB2*, *HOXB5*, *PBX3*, *HOXA4*, and *HOXA10*), which were expressed in cases with diverse cytogenetic abnormalities.

Wilson et al. [132] (Affymetrix HG_U95Av2 oligonucleotide microarrays, VxInsight unsupervised cluster analysis) analyzed 170 AML samples and reported the only study in which recurrent cytogenetic abnormalities are not tightly clustered. Their analysis produced 6 clusters with distinct gene expression signatures, with most recurrent cytogenetic abnormalities falling in one cluster. The cluster with the best outcome had a high prevalence of NPM mutations, previously associated with a good prognosis. The cluster of patients with the poorest outcome demonstrated high expression of genes involved in immune regulation (IRF4, IL10R, and MALT).

Bourquin et al. [133] (Affymetrix U133A microchip, agglomerative hierarchical clustering), contrasting acute megakaryocytic leukemia (AMKL) in Down syndrome (DS) versus non-DS children, demonstrated distinct gene expression signatures in the two groups. Some genes overexpressed in DS-AMKL are encoded on the triplicated chromosome 21, for example *AML1*. Most patients with DS-AMKL have a mutation in the transcriptional regulator GATA1; analysis of GATA1-responsive genes in the DS-AMKL samples shows some activation targets of GATA1 (BACH1, LKF1) are overexpressed in DS-AMKL, but some repression targets of GATA1 (KIT, MYC, and GATA2) are also overexpressed in DS-AMKL, indicating possible aberrant transcriptional regulation by the mutated GATA1.

In summary, these microarray studies demonstrate differing effects of recurring genetic abnormalities in shaping gene expression in individual cases of AML. However, to date microarray data do not correlate tightly enough to replace standard genetic methods, have yet to provide significant insights to AML pathogenesis, and have not significantly improved AML classification. They may ultimately contribute discovery of additional prognostic indicators for AML.

2.4.8 Detection of Minimal Residual Disease (MRD)

Assessment of residual disease in AML may be useful for monitoring response to chemotherapy and for early detection of disease relapse. The three major methods of detecting MRD are PCR, flow cytometry, and FISH analysis. Up to 40–50% of AML has a specific translocation that can be monitored by RT-PCR [134]. Use of quantitative RT-PCR (Q-RT-PCR) of RNA fusion transcripts of the major recurrent translocations (*PML/*

RARα, *AML1/ETO*, *CBFβ/MYH11*), is an established technique sensitive to detection of 1 in 10^{4-5} cells [134]. In this setting Q-RT-PCR has minimal background, as these aberrant transcripts are not present in normal cells. Q-RT-PCR may also be used in patients with no fusion transcript, but other mutant phenotypes, e.g., *FLT3* mutation, partial tandem duplication of *MLL* (MLL-PTD), and *NPM* mutations [48, 135, 136]. A disadvantage of *FLT3* mutation as a target is that it is not stable during the course of the disease in about 4% of patients, and levels of transcript per cell may increase during disease progression [136]. The latter disadvantage may be overcome by using a DNA template to quantify presence of the *FLT3* mutations by PCR. In addition, detection of transcripts abnormally overexpressed in AML (e.g., WT1 and PRAME) has been utilized for MRD assessment [48], but these transcripts are not leukemia specific, limiting their utility.

FISH may be used to detect residual cells bearing translocations, with probes commercially available for all the recurrent translocations. However, the sensitivity is limited by a false positivity rate of up to 5%, depending on probe selection, due to the probability of chance apposition of fluorescent signals on overlapping chromosomes. Dual break-apart fusion probes may lower the false positivity rate by a log, but still do not allow sensitivity of 1 cell in 10^3.

Multicolor flow cytometry is the third method of detection of MRD in AML. Although flow assessment of MRD is well established in ALL, it is more difficult in AML to identify a leukemia-associated aberrant immunophenotype (LAIP) [135]. With use of 4-color flow cytometry and a large enough panel of antibodies, LAIP can be detected in 65–75% of adult cases of AML and 85% of pediatric cases of AML with a sensitivity of up to 1 cell in 10^4, depending on the rarity of the particular LAIP among normal myeloid populations [135, 136]. The aberrant phenotype may take the form of crosslineage expression of antigens, lack or overexpression of an antigen, or asynchronous expression of antigens. Although this method is applicable to a larger percentage of patients than PCR, and is more rapid and much cheaper to perform, a drawback is that there is immunophenotypic variation may occur in some AML cases during the course of the disease [136].

Clinical studies have demonstrated the relevance of long-term monitoring of MRD during remission in APL, using Q-RT-PCR of the *PML/RARα* transcript [135–137]. A steady increase in transcript levels by Q-RT-PCR at two consecutive 3-month time points is predictive of an impending hematologic relapse [138]. The median time by which molecular relapse predates hematologic relapse is approximately 3 months, and recent clinical trials have shown that treatment at molecular, rather than hematologic, relapse may improve overall clinical outcome [135, 137]. Trials have also demonstrated that patients with a higher level of PML-RARα after consolidation have an increased relapse rate, a decrease of transcript by greater than 2 logs generally correlating with a positive outcome.

Clinical trials in AML other than APL are ongoing to assess the validity of treatment decisions based upon MRD detection at the end of induction and after consolidation therapy. Critical thresholds may vary with both the genotype of disease in individual cases and with overall treatment strategies. For example, a greater than 2-log decrease in transcript by the end of consolidation therapy appears to predict good outcome in both APL and AML with t(8;21), although the absolute amount of transcript goes to zero quite rapidly in APL, whereas low levels of *AML1/ETO* transcript may persist for a long time after cessation of therapy [48].

Other unresolved issues are the utility of long-term monitoring of AML other than APL for early detection and intervention for relapse, the optimal time interval between testing for such monitoring, and the validity of monitoring blood vs. marrow. Transcript levels are typically up to 1 log lower in blood compared to marrow [136, 139, 140]. We anticipate that MRD assessment of early therapeutic response by Q-RT-PCR or flow cytometry will become standard care in AML. However, in patients other than APL the role of long-term monitoring in remission with preemptive treatment of early relapse remains to be established.

2.5 Summary

An array of testing to include morphology, flow cytometric immunophenotyping, cytogenetics, and increasingly molecular genetics is necessary to diagnose and subclassify AML. Careful attention is required to assure an adequate sample is obtained at diagnosis to accomplish this array of testing. Expanding knowledge of the genetic basis of AML will continue to complicate diagnostic requirements and classification, as increased understanding of biology progresses to therapy directed at specific genetic targets in AML. The most important diagnostic and classification issues are distinction of DN- versus MDR-AML (because of the fundamental biologic differences in the two sets of disease), and recognition of specific genetic subsets of disease amenable to targeted therapy (e.g., APL). Monitoring early response and adjusting treatment will require repeat analysis with a subset of testing, to include morphology and either flow cytometry or high sensitivity molecular testing (i.e., Q-RT-PCR or similar technology). A role for long-term monitoring of MRD remains to be established, except in APL, and microarray analysis of AML has of yet no demonstrated clinical application. Finally, there is a great need for better understanding of the pathogenesis of MDS and MDR-AML, about which we remain substantially ignorant. While we continue to make substantial progress in understanding and treating DN-AML, MDS and MDR-AML remain enigmatic diseases and treatment results for MDR-AML remain dismal in the absence of stem cell transplantation.

References

1. Bennett JM, Catovsky D, Daniel MT, et al. (1976) Proposals for the classification of the acute leukaemias. French-American-British (FAB) co-operative group. Br J Haematol 33(4):451–458
2. Head DR (1996) Revised classification of acute myeloid leukemia. Leukemia 10(11):1826–1831
3. Brunning RD, Matute E, Harris NL, et al. (2001) Acute myeloid leukemias. In: Jaffe EJ HN, Stein H, Vardiman JW (eds) World Health Organization Classification of Tumours: Pathology and genetics of tumours of haematopoietic and lymphoid tissues. IARC Press, Lyon, pp 75–105
4. Durst KL, Lutterbach B, Kummalue T, et al. (2003) The inv(16) fusion protein associates with corepressors via a smooth muscle myosin heavy-chain domain. Mol Cell Biol 23:607–619
5. Licht JD (2001) AML1 and the AML1-ETO fusion protein in the pathogenesis of t(8;21) AML. Oncogene 20:5660–5679
6. Licht JD, Chomienne C, Goy A, et al. (1995) Clinical and molecular characterization of a rare syndrome of acute promyelocytic leukemia associated with translocation (11;17). Blood 85:1083
7. Lin RJ, Nagy L, Inoue S, et al. (1998) Role of the histone deacetylase complex in acute promyelocytic leukemia. Nature 391:811
8. Gilliland DG (1998) Molecular genetics of human leukemia. Leukemia (Suppl) 1:S7–12
9. Gilliland DG (2002) Molecular genetics of human leukemias: new insights into therapy. Semin Hematol 39(4 Suppl 3):6–11
10. Gilliland DG, Griffin JD (2002) The roles of FLT3 in hematopoiesis and leukemia. Blood 100:1532–1542
11. Blume-Jensen P, Hunter T (2001) Oncogenic kinase signalling. Nature 411(6835):355–365
12. Gari M, Goodeve A, Wilson G, et al. (1999) c-kit proto-oncogene exon 8 in-frame deletion plus insertion mutations in acute myeloid leukaemia. Br J Haematol 105(4):894–900
13. Neubauer A, Dodge RK, George SL, et al. (1994) Prognostic importance of mutations in the ras proto-oncogenes in de novo acute myeloid leukemia. Blood 83(6):1603–1611
14. Radich JP, Kopecky KJ, Willman CL, et al. (1990) N-ras mutations in adult de novo acute myelogenous leukemia: prevalence and clinical significance. Blood 76(4):801–807
15. Hahn WC, Weinberg RA (2002) Modelling the molecular circuitry of cancer. Nat Rev Cancer 2(5):331–341
16. Hahn WC, Weinberg RA (2002) Rules for making human tumor cells. N Engl J Med 347(20):1593–1603
17. Pui CH, Ribeiro RC, Hancock ML, et al. (1991) Acute myeloid leukemia in children treated with epipodophyllotoxins for acute lymphoblastic leukemia. N Engl J Med 325(24):1682–1687
18. Sandoval C, Pui CH, Bowman LC, et al. (1993) Secondary acute myeloid leukemia in children previously treated with alkylating agents, intercalating topoisomerase II inhibitors, and irradiation. J Clin Oncol 11(6):1039–1045
19. Morishita K, Suzukawa K, Taki T, et al. (1995) EVI-1 zinc finger protein works as a transcriptional activator via binding to a consensus sequence of GACAAGATAAGATAAN1–28 CTCATCTTC. Oncogene 10(10):1961–1967
20. Wechsler J, Greene M, McDevitt MA, et al. (2002) Acquired mutations in GATA1 in the megakaryoblastic leukemia of Down syndrome. Nat Genet 32(1):148–152
21. Leith CP, Kopecky KJ, Chen IM, et al. (1999) Frequency and clinical significance of the expression of the multidrug resistance proteins MDR1/P-glycoprotein, MRP1, and LRP in acute myeloid leukemia: A Southwest Oncology Group Study. Blood 94(3):1086–1099
22. Leith CP, Kopecky KJ, Godwin J, et al. (1997) Acute myeloid leukemia in the elderly: assessment of multidrug resistance (MDR1) and cytogenetics distinguishes biologic subgroups with remarkably distinct responses to standard chemotherapy. A Southwest Oncology Group study. Blood 89(9):3323–3329
23. Fialkow PJ, Singer JW, Raskind WH, et al. (1987) Clonal development, stem-cell differentiation, and clinical remissions in acute nonlymphocytic leukemia. N Engl J Med 317(8):468–473
24. Levine EG, Bloomfield CD (1992) Leukemias and myelodysplastic syndromes secondary to drug, radiation, and environmental exposure. Semin Oncol 19(1):47–84
25. Bennett JM, Catovsky D, Daniel MT, et al. (1982) Proposals for the classification of the myelodysplastic syndromes. Br J Haematol 51(2):189–199
26. Brunning RD, Bennett JM, Flandrin G, et al. (2001) Myelodysplastic syndromes. In: Jaffe EJ HN, Stein H, Vardiman JW (eds) World Health Organization Classification of Tumours: Pathology and genetics of tumours of haematopoietic and lymphoid tissues. IARC Press, Lyon, pp 61–73
27. Vardiman JW, Pierre R, Bain B, et al. (2001) Myelodysplastic/myeloproliferative diseases. In: Jaffe EJ HN, Stein H, Vardiman JW (eds) World Health Organization Classification of Tumours: Pathology and genetics of tumours of haematopoietic and lymphoid tissues. IARC Press, Lyon, pp 45–59
28. Ren R (2005) Mechanisms of BCR-ABL in the pathogenesis of chronic myelogenous leukaemia. Nat Rev Cancer 5(3):172–183

29. James C, Ugo V, Le Couedic JP, et al. (2005) A unique clonal JAK2 mutation leading to constitutive signalling causes polycythaemia vera. Nature 434(7037):1144–1148
30. Wiemels JL, Xiao Z, Buffler PA, et al. (2002) In utero origin of t(8;21) AML1-ETO translocations in childhood acute myeloid leukemia. Blood 99(10):3801–3805
31. Arico M, Biondi A, Pui C (1997) Juvenile myelomonocytic leukemia. Blood 90(2):479–488
32. Flotho C, Valcamonica S, Mach-Pascual S, et al. (1999) RAS mutations and clonality analysis in children with juvenile myelomonocytic leukemia (JMML). Leukemia 13(1):32–37
33. Loh ML, Vattikuti S, Schubbert S, et al. (2004) Mutations in PTPN11 implicate the SHP-2 phosphatase in leukemogenesis. Blood 103(6):2325–2331
34. Tartaglia M, Niemeyer CM, Fragale A, et al. (2003) Somatic mutations in PTPN11 in juvenile myelomonocytic leukemia, myelodysplastic syndromes and acute myeloid leukemia. Nat Genet 34(2):148–150
35. Cermak J, Michalova K, Brezinova J, et al. (2003) A prognostic impact of separation of refractory cytopenia with multilineage dysplasia and 5q– syndrome from refractory anemia in primary myelodysplastic syndrome. Leuk Res 27(3):221–229
36. Dunkley SM, Manoharan A, Kwan YL (2002) Myelodysplastic syndromes: prognostic significance of multilineage dysplasia in patients with refractory anemia or refractory anemia with ringed sideroblasts. Blood 99(10):3870–3871; author reply 3871
37. Wikipedia. Tomás de Torquemada. www.wikipedia.com
38. Stelzer GT, Shults KE, Loken MR (1993) CD45 gating for routine flow cytometric analysis of human bone marrow specimens. Ann NY Acad Sci 677:265–280
39. Matutes E, Morilla R, Farahat N, et al. (1997) Definition of acute biphenotypic leukemia. Haematologica 82(1):64–66
40. Kussick SJ, Wood BL (2003) Using 4-color flow cytometry to identify abnormal myeloid populations. Arch Pathol Lab Med 127(9):1140–1147
41. Miller TL, Stelzer G (2001) Contributions of flow cytometry to the analysis of the myelodysplastic syndrome. Clin Lab Med 21(4):811–828
42. Stetler-Stevenson M, Arthur DC, Jabbour N, et al. (2001) Diagnostic utility of flow cytometric immunophenotyping in myelodysplastic syndrome. Blood 98(4):979–987
43. Mrozek K, Heinonen K, Bloomfield CD (2001) Clinical importance of cytogenetics in acute myeloid leukaemia. Best Pract Res Clin Haematol 14:19–47
44. Andrieu V, Radford-Weiss I, Troussard X, et al. (1996) Molecular detection of t(8;21)/AML1-ETO in AML M1/M2: Correlation with cytogenetics, morphology and immunophenotype. Br J Haematol 92(4):855–865
45. Langabeer SE, Walker H, Gale RE, et al. (1997) Frequency of CBF beta/MYH11 fusion transcripts in patients entered into the U.K. MRC AML trials. The MRC Adult Leukaemia Working Party. Br J Haematol 96(4):736–739
46. Grimwade D (1999) The pathogenesis of acute promyelocytic leukaemia: Evaluation of the role of molecular diagnosis and monitoring in the management of the disease. Br J Haematol 106(3):591–613
47. Bagg A, Arber DA (2003) USCAP Short Course #49 (syllabus)
48. Raanani P, Ben-Bassat I (2004) Detection of minimal residual disease in acute myelogenous leukemia. Acta Haematologica 112:40–54
49. Huang ME, Ye YC, Chen SR, et al. (1988) Use of all trans retinoic acid in the treatment of acute promyelocytic leukemia. Blood 72:567–572
50. Borrow J, Goddard AD, Sheer D, et al. (1990) Molecular analysis of acute promyelocytic leukemia breakpoint cluster region on chromosome 17. Science 249:1577–1580
51. de Thé H, Chomienne C, Lanotte M, et al. (1990) The t(15;17) translocation of acute promyelocytic leukaemia fuses the retinoic acid receptor a gene to a novel transcribed locus. Nature 347:558–561
52. Longo L, Pandolfi PP, Biondi A, et al. (1990) Rearrangements and aberrant expression of the RARα gene in acute promyelocytic leukemia. J Exp Med 172:1571–1575
53. Cantu-Rajnoldi A, Biondi A, Jankovic M, et al. (1993) Diagnosis and incidence of acute promyelocytic leukemia (FAB M3 and M3 variant) in childhood. Blood 81(8):2209–2210
54. Grimwade D, Biondi A, Mozziconacci MJ, et al. (2000) Characterization of acute promyelocytic leukemia cases lacking the classic t(15;17): Results of the European Working Party. Groupe Francais de Cytogenetique Hematologique, Groupe de Francais d'Hematologie Cellulaire, UK Cancer Cytogenetics Group and BIOMED 1 European Community-Concerted Action "Molecular Cytogenetic Diagnosis in Haematological Malignancies." Blood 96(4):1297–1308
55. Sainty D, Liso V, Cantu-Rajnoldi A, et al. (2000) A new morphologic classification system for acute promyelocytic leukemia distinguishes cases with underlying PLZF/RARA gene rearrangements. Group Francais de Cytogenetique Hematologique, UK Cancer Cytogenetics Group and BIOMED 1 European Community-Concerted Action "Molecular Cytogenetic Diagnosis in Haematological Malignancies." Blood 96(4):1287–1296
56. Geng JP, Tong JH, Dong S, et al. (1993) Localization of the chromosome 15 breakpoints and expression of multiple PML-RAR alpha transcripts in acute promyelocytic leukemia: A study of 28 Chinese patients. Leukemia 7:20–26
57. Guidez F, Ivins S, Zhu J, et al. (1998) Reduced retinoic acid-sensitivities of nuclear receptor co-repressor binding to PML- and PLZF-RARα underlie molecular pathogenesis and treatment of acute promyelocytic leukemia. Blood 91:2634
58. Melnick A, Licht JD (1999) Deconstructing a disease: RARα, its fusion partners, and their roles in the pathogenesis of acute promyelocytic leukemia. Blood 93:3167–3215
59. He LZ, Guidez F, Triboli C, et al. (1998) Distinct interactions of PML-RARa and PLZF-RARα with co-repressors determine differential responses to RA in APL. Nat Genet 18:126
60. Grignani F, De Metteis S, Nervi C, et al. (1998) Fusion proteins of the retinoic acid receptor-α recruit histone deacetylase in promyelocytic leukemia. Nature 391:815
61. Redner RL, Rush EA, Faas S, et al. (1996) The t(5;17) variant of acute promyelocytic leukemia expresses a nucleophosmin-retinoic acid receptor fusion. Blood 87:882
62. Wells RA, Catzavelos C, Kamel-Reid S (1997) Fusion of retinoic acid receptor alpha to NuMA, the mitotic apparatus protein, by a variant translocation in acute promyelocytic leukaemia. Nat Genet 17:109

63. Erickson P, Gao J, Chang KS, et al. (1992) Identification of breakpoints in t(8;21) acute myelogenous leukemia and isolation of a fusion transcript, AML1/ETO, with similarity to Drosophila segmentation gene, runt. Blood 80:1825–1831
64. Liu P, Tarle SA, Hajra A, et al. (1993) Fusion between transcription factor CBFbeta/PEBP2 beta and a myosin heavy chain in acute myeloid leukemia. Science 261:1041–1044
65. Libermann TA, Pan Z, Akbarali Y, et al. (1999) AML1 (CBFalpha2) cooperates with B cell-specific activating protein (BSAP/PAX5) in activation of the B cell-specific BLK gene promoter. J Biol Chem 274(35):24671–24676
66. Bruhn L, Munnerlyn A, Grosschedl R (1997) ALY, a context-dependent coactivator of LEF-1 and AML1 is required for TCRalpha enhancer function. Genes Dev 11:640–653
67. Uchida H, Zhang J, Nimer S (1997) AML1A and AML1B can transactivate the human IL-3 promoter. J Immunol 158:2251–2258
68. Takahashi A, Satake M, Yamaguchi-Iwai Y, et al. (1995) Positive and negative regulation of granulocyte-macrophage colony-stimulating factor promoter activity by AML1-related transcription factor, PEBP2. Blood 86(2):607–616
69. Nuchprayoon I, Meyers S, Scott LM, et al. (1994) PEBP2/CBF, the murine homolog of the human myeloid AML1 and PEBP2 beta/CBF beta proto-oncoproteins, regulates the murine myeloperoxidase and neutrophil elastase genes in immature myeloid cells. Mol Cell Biol 14(8):5558–5568
70. Okuda T, van Deursen J, Hiebert SW, et al. (1996) AML1, the target of multiple chromosomal translocations in human leukemia, is essential for normal fetal liver hematopoiesis. Cell 84: 321–330
71. Wang Q, Stacy T, Miller JD, et al. (1996) The CBFbeta subunit is essential for CBFalpha2 (AML1) function in vivo. Cell 87:697–708
72. North T, Gu TL, Stacy T, et al. (1999) Cbfa2 is required for the formation of intra-aortic hematopoietic clusters. Development 126:2563–2575
73. Miyoshi H, Ohira M, Shimizu K, et al. (1995) Alternative splicing and genomic structure of the AML1 gene involved in acute myeloid leukemia. Nucleic Acids Res 23:2762–2769
74. Levanon D, Negreanu V, Bernstein Y, et al. (1994) AML1, AML2, and AML3, the human members of the runt domain gene-family: cDNA structure, expression, and chromosomal localization. Genomics 23(2):425–432
75. Michaud J, Wu F, Osato M, et al. (2002) In vitro analyses of known and novel RUNX1/AML1 mutations in dominant familial platelet disorder with predisposition to acute myelogenous leukemia: Implications for mechanisms of pathogenesis. Blood 99(4): 1364–1372
76. Osato M, Asou N, Abdalla E, et al. (1999) Biallelic and heterozygous point mutations in the runt domain of the AML1/PEBP2alphaB gene associated with myeloblastic leukemias. Blood 93:1817–1824
77. Tahirov TH, Inoue-Bungo T, Morii H, et al. (2001) Structural analyses of DNA recognition by the AML1/Runx-1 Runt domain and its allosteric control by CBFbeta. Cell 104(5):755–767
78. Feinstein PG, Kornfeld K, Hogness DS, et al. (1995) Identification of homeotic target genes in Drosophila melanogaster including nervy, a proto-oncogene homologue. Genetics 140:573–586
79. Erickson PF, Dessev G, Lasher RS, et al. (1996) ETO and AML1 phosphoproteins are expressed in CD34+ hematopoietic progenitors: implications for t(8;21) leukemogenesis and monitoring residual disease. Blood 88(5):1813–1823
80. Melnick A, Licht JD (2002) Histone deacetylases as therapeutic targets in hematologic malignancies. Curr Opin Hematol 9:322–332
81. Amann JM, Nip J, Strom DK, et al. (2001) ETO, a target of t(8;21) in acute leukemia, makes distinct contacts with multiple histone deacetylases and binds mSin3A through its oligomerization domain. Mol Cell Biol 21:6470–6483
82. de Greef GE, Hagemeijer A, Morgan R, et al. (1995) Identical fusion transcript associated with different breakpoints in the AML1 gene in simple and variant t(8;21) acute myeloid leukemia. Leukemia 9:282–287
83. Meyers S, Downing JR, Hiebert SW (1993) Identification of AML1 and the (8;21) translocation protein (AML1/ETO) as sequence-specific DNA-binding proteins: the runt homology domain is required for DNA binding and protein-protein interactions. Mol Cell Biol 13(10):6336–6345
84. Linggi B, Muller-Tidow C, van de Locht L, et al. (2002) The t(8;21) fusion protein, AML1-ETO, specifically represses the transcription of the p14ARF tumor suppressor in acute myeloid leukemia. Nat Med 8:743–750
85. Zhang X, Ren R (1998) Ber-Abl efficiently induces a myeloproliferative disease and production of excess interleukin-3 and granulocyte-macrophage colony-stimulating factor in mice: A novel model for chronic myelogenous leukemia. Blood 92:3829–3840
86. Downing JR, Head DR, Curcio-Brint AM, et al. (1993) An AML1/ETO fusion transcript is consistently detected by RNA-based polymerase chain reaction in acute myelogenous leukemia containing the (8;21)(q22;q22) translocation. Blood 81(11):2860–2865
87. Shurtleff SA, Meyers S, Hiebert SW, et al. (1995) Heterogeneity in CBF beta/MYH11 fusion messages encoded by the inv(16) (p13q22) and the t(16;16)(p13;q22) in acute myelogenous leukemia. Blood 85(12):3695–3703
88. Dimartino JF, Cleary ML (1999) MLL rearrangements in haematological malignancies: Lessons from clinical and biological studies. Br J Haematol 106:614–626
89. Ernst P, Wang J, Korsmeyer SJ (2002) The role of MLL in hematopoiesis and leukemia. Curr Opin Hematol 9:282–287
90. Ayton PM, Cleary ML (2001) Molecular mechanisms of leukemogenesis mediated by MLL fusion proteins. Oncogene 20:5695–5707
91. Ingham PW (1998) Trithroax and the regulation of homeotic gene expression in Drosophila: a historical perspective. Int J Dev Biol 42:423–429
92. Gehring WJ, Affolter M, Burglin T (1994) Homeodomain proteins. Ann Rev Biochem 63:487–526
93. Yu BD, Hanson RD, Hess JL, et al. (1998) MLL, a mammalian trithroax-group gene, functions as a transcriptional maintenance factor in morphogenesis. Proc Natl Acad Sci 1998:10632–10636
94. Heim S, Mitelman F (1995) Cancer cytogenetics: Chromosomal and molecular aberrations of tumor cells, 2nd edn. Wiley, New York
95. Harrison CJ, Cuneo A, Clark R, et al. (1998) Ten novel 11q23 chromosomal partner sites. European 11q23 workshop participants. Leukemia 12(5):811–822
96. Secker-Walker LM (1998) General report on the European Union Concerted Action Workshop on 11q23, U.K., May 1997. Leukemia 12:776–778

97. Gu Y, Nakamura T, Adler H, et al. (1992) The t(4;11) chromosome translocation of human acute leukemias fuses the ALL-1 gene, related to Drosophila trithroax, to the AF-4 gene. Cell 71:701–708
98. Rubnitz JE, Link MP, Shuster JJ, et al. (1994) Frequency and prognostic significance of HRX rearrangements in infant acute lymphoblastic leukemia; a Pediatric Oncology Group study. Blood 84:570–573
99. Hunger SP, Tkachuck MD, Amylon MP, et al. (1993) HRX involvement in de novo and secondary leukemias with diverse chromosome 11q23 abnormalities. Blood 81:3197–3203
100. Cimino G, Rapanotti MC, Biondi A, et al. (1997) Infant acute leukemias show the same biased distribution of ALL1 gene breaks as topoisomerase II related secondary leukemias. Cancer Res 57:2879–2883
101. Ross JA, Potter JD, Reaman GH, et al. (1996) Maternal exposure to potential inhibitors of DNA topoisomerase II and infant leukemia (United States): A report from the Children's Cancer Group. Cancer Causes Control 7:581–590
102. Tenen DG, Hromas R, Licht J, et al. (1997) Transcription factors, normal myeloid development, and leukemia. Blood 90(2):489–519
103. Vinson CR, Sigler PB, McKnight SL (1989) Scissors-grip model for DNA recognition by a family of leucine zipper proteins. Science 246(4932):911–916
104. Zhang DE, Zhang P, Wang ND, et al. (1997) Absence of granulocyte colony-stimulating factor signaling and neutrophil development in CCAAT enhancer binding protein alpha-deficient mice. Proc Natl Acad Sci USA 94(2):569–574
105. Radomska HS, Huettner CS, Zhang P, et al. (1998) CCAAT/enhancer binding protein alpha is a regulatory switch sufficient for induction of granulocytic development from bipotential myeloid progenitors. Mol Cell Biol 18(7):4301–4314
106. Gombart A, Hofmann WK, Kawano S, et al. (2002) Mutations in the gene encoding the transcription factor CCAAT/enhancer binding protein alpha in myelodysplastic syndromes and acute myeloid leukemias. Blood 99(4):1332–1340
107. Pabst T, Mueller BU, Zhang P, et al. (2001) Dominant-negative mutations of CEBPA, encoding CCAAT/enhancer binding protein-alpha (C/EBPalpha), in acute myeloid leukemia. Nat Genet 27(3):263–270
108. Preudhomme C, Sagot C, Boissel N, et al. (2002) Favorable prognostic significance of CEBPA mutations in patients with de novo acute myeloid leukemia: A study from the Acute Leukemia French Association (ALFA). Blood 100(8):2717–2723
109. Smith ML, Cavenagh JD, Lister TA, et al. (2004) Mutation of CEBPA in familial acute myeloid leukemia. N Engl J Med 351(23):2403–2407
110. Greene ME, Mundschau G, Wechsler J, et al. (2003) Mutations in GATA1 in both transient myeloproliferative disorder and acute megakaryoblastic leukemia of Down syndrome. Blood Cells Mol Dis 31(3):351–356
111. Gurbuxani S, Vyas P, Crispino JD (2004) Recent insights into the mechanisms of myeloid leukemogenesis in Down syndrome. Blood 103(2):399–406
112. Soderholm J, Kobayashi H, Mathieu C, et al. (1997) The leukemia-associated gene MDS1/EVI1 is a new type of GATA-binding transactivator. Leukemia 11(3):352–358
113. Brasel K, Escobar S, Anderberg R, et al. (1995) Expression of the Flt3 receptor and its ligand on hematopoietic cells. Leukemia 9:1212–1218
114. Nakao M, Yokota S, Iwai T, et al. (1996) Internal tandem duplication of the flt3 gene found in acute myeloid leukemia. Leukemia 10:1911–1918
115. Kiyoi H, Towatari M, Yokota S, et al. (1998) Internal tandem duplication of the FLT3 gene is a novel modality of elongation mutation which causes constitutive activation of the product. Leukemia 12:1333–1337
116. Mizuki M, Fenski R, Halfter H, et al. (2000) Flt3 mutations from patients with acute myeloid leukemia induce transformation of 32D cells mediated by the Ras and STAT5 pathways. Blood 96:3907–3914
117. Yamamoto Y, Kiyoi H, Nakano Y, et al. (2001) Activating mutation of D835 within the activation loop of FLT3 in human hematologic malignancies. Blood 97:2434–2439
118. Meshinchi S, Woods WG, Stirewalt DL, et al. (2001) Prevalence and prognostic significance of Flt3 internal tandem duplication in pediatric acute myeloid leukemia. Blood 97:89–94
119. Fröhling S, Schlenk RF, Breitruck J, et al. (2002) Prognostic significance of activating FLT3 mutations in younger adults (16 to 60 years) with acute myeloid leukemia and normal cytogenetics: A study of the AML Study Group Ulm. Blood 100:4372–4380
120. Sawyers CL (2002) Finding the next Gleevec, FLT3-targeted kinase inhibitor therapy for acute myeloid leukemia. Cancer Cell 1:413–415
121. Ruggero D, Pandolfi PP (2003) Does the ribosome translate cancer? Nat Rev Cancer 3(3):179–192
122. Grisendi S, Pandolfi PP (2005) NPM mutations in acute myelogenous leukemia. N Engl J Med 352(3):291–292
123. Morris SW, Kirstein MN, Valentine MB, et al. (1995) Fusion of a kinase gene, ALK, to a nucleolar protein gene, NPM, in non-Hodgkin's lymphoma. Science 267(5196):316–317
124. Yoneda-Kato N, Look AT, Kirstein MN, et al. (1996) The t(3;5)(q25.1;q34) of myelodysplastic syndrome and acute myeloid leukemia produces a novel fusion gene, NPM-MLF1. Oncogene 12(2):265–275
125. Boissel N, Renneville A, Biggio V, et al. (2005) Prevalence, clinical profile, and prognosis of NPM mutations in AML with normal karyotype. Blood 106(10):3618–3620
126. Falini B, Mecucci C, Tiacci E, et al. (2005) Cytoplasmic nucleophosmin in acute myelogenous leukemia with a normal karyotype. N Engl J Med 352(3):254–266
127. Lockhart DJ, Winzeler EA (2000) Genomics, gene expression and DNA arrays. Nature 405(6788):827–836
128. Valk PJ, Delwel R, Lowenberg B (2005) Gene expression profiling in acute myeloid leukemia. Curr Opin Hematol 12:76–81
129. Valk PJ, Verhaak RG, Beijen MA, et al. (2004) Prognostically useful gene-expression profiles in acute myeloid leukemia. N Engl J Med 350:1617–1628
130. Ross ME, Mahfouz R, Onciu M, et al. (2004) Gene expression profiling of pediatric acute myelogenous leukemia. Blood 104:3679–3687
131. Bullinger L, Dohner K, Bair E, et al. (2004) Use of gene-expression profiling to identify prognostic subclasses in adult acute myeloid leukemia. N Engl J Med 350:1605–1616

132. Wilson CS, Davidson GS, Martin SB, et al. (2006) Gene expression profiling of adult acute myeloid leukemia identifies novel biologic clusters for risk classification and outcome prediction. Blood 108:685–696
133. Bourquin JP, Subramanian A, Langebrake C, et al. (2006) Identification of distinct molecular phenotypes in acute megakaryoblastic leukemia by gene expression profiling. Proc Natl Acad Sci USA 103:3339–3344
134. Jaeger U, Kainz B (2003) Monitoring minimal residual disease in AML: The right time for real time. Ann Hematol 82:139–147
135. Goulden N, Virgo P, Grimwade D (2006) Minimal residual disease directed therapy for childhood acute myeloid leukaemia: The time is now. Br J Haematol 134:273–282
136. Kern W, Schoch C, Haferlach T, et al. (2005) Monitoring of minimal residual disease in acute myeloid leukemia. Crit Rev Oncol Hematol 56:283–309
137. Lo-Coco F, Romano A, Mengarelli A, et al. (2002) Molecular monitoring of hematologic malignancies: current and future issues. Semin Hematol 39(Suppl 1):14–17
138. Reiter A, Lengfelder E, Grimwade D (2004) Pathogenesis, diagnosis, and monitoring of residual disease in acute promyelocytic leukaemia. Acta Haematol 112:55–67
139. Cheson BD, Bennett JM, Kopecky KJ, et al. (2003) Revised recommendations of the International Working Group for diagnosis, standardization of response criteria, treatment outcomes, and reporting standards for therapeutic trials in acute myeloid leukemia. J Clin Oncol 21:4642–4649
140. Schnittger S, Schoch C (2005) Quantitative PCR based minimal residual disease detection in core binding factor leukemias: Prognostication and guiding of therapy. Leukemia Res 30:657–658
141. Grimwade D, Walker H, Oliver F, et al. (1998) The importance of diagnostic cytogenetics on outcome in AML: Analysis of 1,612 patients entered into the MRC AML 10 trial. The Medical Research Council Adult and Children's Leukaemia Working Parties. Blood 92(7):2322–2333
142. Slovak ML, Kopecky KJ, Cassileth PA, et al. (2000) Karyotypic analysis predicts outcome of preremission and postremission therapy in adult acute myeloid leukemia: A Southwest Oncology Group/Eastern Cooperative Oncology Group Study. Blood 96(13):4075–4083
143. Aul C, Gattermann N, Schneider W (1992) Age-related incidence and other epidemiological aspects of myelodysplastic syndromes. Br J Haematol 82(2):358–367
144. Cartwright RA, McNally RJQ, Rowland DJ, et al. (1997) The descriptive epidemiology of leukaemia and related conditions in parts of the United Kingdom, 1984–1993. Leukemia Research Fund, London
145. Hasle H, Kerndrup G, Jacobsen BB (1995) Childhood myelodysplastic syndrome in Denmark: Incidence and predisposing conditions. Leukemia 9(9):1569–1572
146. Hasle H, Wadsworth LD, Massing BG, et al. (1999) A population-based study of childhood myelodysplastic syndrome in British Columbia, Canada. Br J Haematol 106(4):1027–1032
147. Passmore SJ, Chessells JM, Kempski H, et al. (2003) Paediatric myelodysplastic syndromes and juvenile myelomonocytic leukaemia in the UK: A population-based study of incidence and survival. Br J Haematol 121(5):758–767
148. Radlund A, Thiede T, Hansen S, et al. (1995) Incidence of myelodysplastic syndromes in a Swedish population. Eur J Haematol 54(3):153–156
149. Schnittger S, Schoch C, Kern W, et al. (2003) Acute myeloid leukemia with recurring chromosome abnormalities as defined by the WHO-classification: Incidence of subgroups, additional genetic abnormalities, FAB subtypes and age distribution in an unselected series of 1,897 patients with acute myeloid leukemia. Haematologica 88(3):351–352
150. Smith MT, Linet MS, Morgan GJ (2002) Causative agents in the etiology of myelodysplastic syndromes and the acute myeloid leukemias. In: Brand JM (ed) The myelodysplastic syndromes, pathobiology and clinical management. Marcel Dekker, New York, pp 29–63
151. Stevens RG (1986) Age and risk of acute leukemia. J Natl Cancer Inst 76(5):845–848
152. Head DR (2000) Reply: Problematic WHO reclassification of myelodysplastic syndrome. J Clin Oncol 18:3451–3452
153. Head DR (2002) Proposed changes in the definitions of acute myeloid leukemia and myelodysplastic syndrome: Are they helpful? Curr Opin Oncol 14(1):19–23

Acute Myeloid Leukemia: Epidemiology and Etiology

Barbara Deschler, Michael Lübbert

Contents

3.1 Epidemiology

3.1.1 Introduction

Although acute leukemias are infrequent diseases, they are highly malignant neoplasms responsible for a large number of cancer-related deaths. Acute myeloid leukemia (AML) is the most common type of leukemia in adults, yet continues to have the lowest survival rate of all leukemias. While results of treatment have improved steadily in younger adults over the past 20 years, there have been limited changes in survival among individuals of age >60 years [1, 2].

3.1.2 Incidence

It is estimated that 44 240 individuals in the USA will be diagnosed with one form of leukemia. Approximately 21 790 will die of their disease [6]. Although the incidence of acute leukemias accounts for less than 3% of all cancers, these diseases constitute the leading cause of death due to cancer in children and persons younger than 39 years of age [3–5].

AML accounts for approximately 25% of all leukemias in adults in the West and constitutes the most frequent form of leukemia [3, 6]. Worldwide, the incidence of AML is highest in the USA, Australia, and Western Europe. The age-adjusted incidence rate of AML in the USA is approximately 3.7 per 100 000 persons (= 2.6 per 100 000 when age-adjusted to the world standard population) [6]. In the USA, 13 410 men and women (7060 men and 6350 women) are estimated to be newly diagnosed with AML in 2007 [6]. Figure 3.1 shows age-standardized incidence rates stratified by various countries [7].

3.1.3 Age

Leukemia is the most common cancer diagnosis in children who are younger than 15 years, with an overall incidence of 4.3/100 000 in the USA [8]. In this age group, however, acute lymphocytic leukemia (ALL) is about five times more common than AML, thus accounting

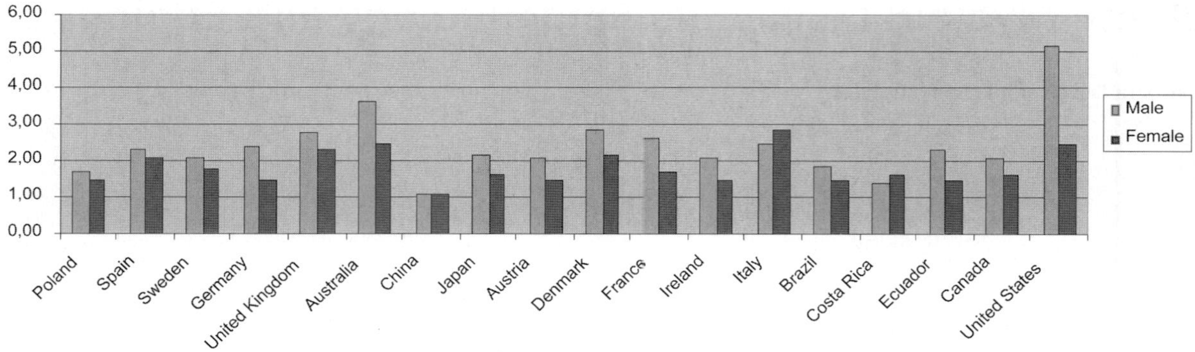

Fig. 3.1. Age-standardized world incidence rates of AML 1997 [92].

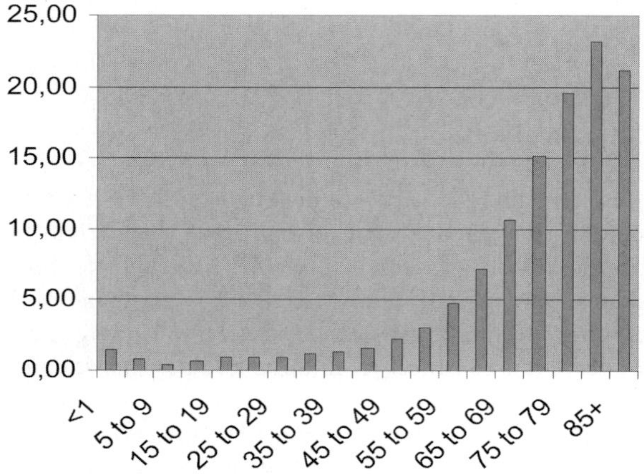

Fig. 3.2. Age-specific incidence of AML: USA 2000–2004 [6].

for about 76% of all childhood leukemia diagnoses. Conversely, AML makes up only 15–20% of cases in those aged 15 years or younger [9]. The peak incidence rate occurs in the first year of life and then decreases steadily up to the age of 4 years. The incidence rate remains relatively constant in childhood and early adulthood [10].

AML is thus a disease of older adults (see Fig. 3.2). The distribution of prevalent cases of all leukemias in the UK shows that 42.8% of patients are above the age of 65 years [11]. Patients newly diagnosed with AML have a median age of 65 years [12]. It is rare before the age of 40; thereafter the incidence increases progressively with age.

From 2000–2004, the US incidence rate in people under the age of 65 was only 1.7 per 100 000, while the incidence rate in people aged 65 or over was 16.8 per 100 000 (Fig. 3.2) [6]. Therefore, of the estimated 13 400 new AML diagnoses in the US, over half will affect patients 60 years of age or older, a population considered "elderly" in leukemia literature.

The high incidence and poor prognosis of AML in the elderly is suspected to be based on the frequent progression of myelodysplastic syndromes (MDS) to AML, an increased incidence of MDS with age appears to explain both. The common AML subtype in the elderly shares characteristics with AML that follows MDS, Fanconi's anemia, alkylating agent chemotherapy (see also Sect. "Etiology" below), and an estimated 10–15% of AML in younger patients. It has been referred to as MDS-related AML and is characterized by common cytogenetic abnormalities shared with MDS, and frequent multilineage dysplastic morphology in the residual hematopoietic precursor cells. A higher frequency of unfavorable biologic and prognostic factors, rather than age per se, is thus the major determinant for the inferior prognosis for elderly patients. By contrast, AML with genotypes typical of younger patients, which may be considered as true de novo AML, has an approximately constant incidence throughout lifetime, also in progressive age groups. Five percent of elderly patients with AML are estimated to belong to the true de novo AML-group, which shows consistency with the incidence in younger patients [13].

Although incidence rates for AML have been near stable over time among the different age groups, there is a slight increase among the oldest group [14].

3.1.4 Gender and Ethnicity

The incidence of AML varies to a certain degree with gender and race. In the SEER data base for children aged 1–4 years there is an incidence rate of 0.9 per 100 000 for boys and 0.8 for girls [6]. In the first few years of life, the incidence of AML in whites is three-fold higher than in blacks; however, blacks have slightly higher rates of AML among children 3 years of age and older [16].

In most countries a slight male predominance of AML in adults has been documented. In 2004, the US age-adjusted incidence rate of AML was 3.6 per 100 000 for both sexes, 4.5 per 100 000 for males, and 3.0 per 100 000 for females [6]. The incidence rate of US males is substantially higher than the incidence rates of males in all other countries (Fig. 3.1).

In the USA between 2000 and 2004, AML was more common in whites (3.7 per 100 000) than in blacks (3.2 per 100 000).

3.1.5 Mortality

Untreated AML is a fatal disease. Although it is possible to support patients for a certain period (median survival: 11–20 weeks) [16, 17], patients not receiving specific treatment ultimately succumb to the leading complications associated with bone marrow failure, such as infection and hemorrhage. Patients typically seek medical attention for symptoms related to infection or bleeding. These patients require immediate therapeutic intervention. Some patients are not candidates for cytotoxic therapy, because of older age and/or poor performance status or other active severe medical comorbidities that complicate their care. In such settings, a supportive strategy may be most appropriate [18]. Firm stratification criteria for decision-making in this setting are not uniformly established and patient- and disease-specific risk assessment has become an additional area of investigation [19].

After long-term increases or mostly level trends that date from the 1930s, death rates for all leukemias were decreasing in the 1990s in the USA and Europe [20, 21]. In 2000–2004, the US age-adjusted mortality rate of AML was 2.7 per 100 000. As is the case with incidence, the mortality associated with AML varies with age, gender, and race. Mortality rates in the USA increase with age. Between 1996 and 2000, the age-adjusted mortality rate showed its peak at 17.6 per 100 000 in people aged 80–84.

The mortality rate for males is higher than that for females, with the US age-adjusted mortality rate at 3.5 per 100 000 for males and 2.2 per 100 000 for females in (2000–2004). AML mortality has for several years been greater in whites than in blacks. The US age-adjusted mortality rate was 2.8 per 100 000 for whites and 2.2 per 100 000 for blacks in the years 2000–2004 [6]. It is estimated that 7800 adults will have died of AML in 2003 in the USA [12, 22].

3.1.6 Survivorship I

A comprehensive report on the total leukemia incidence and survival in the USA covered the period 1973–1990 [23]. Overall survival rates for all leukemia (including chronic leukemia) patients improved only slightly when comparing the periods 1974–1976 and 1983–1989, but were consistently higher in whites compared with blacks, with little gender difference. When analyzing survival rates in more detail, it was found that in comparing the period 1974–1983 with 1984–1993, overall survival rates improved steadily among all races/age groups younger than the age of 45 years. However, for blacks 45 years or older, there was little improvement in overall survival. In particular, for blacks older than 65 years, survival rates for leukemia were decreasing, which was not observed in earlier data [14]. The reasons for these gender and racial differences seen in leukemia (including all subtypes) remain unclear.

The overall US survival rate associated with AML from 1992–1998 was approximately 20% [22].

Figures 3.3–3.5 depict 5-year survival rates stratified by age, gender, and race. The 5-year relative survival rate was highest for those who were younger and female. In AML, however, as opposed to the entire group of leukemias, blacks had a slightly better 5-year relative survival rate than whites (20.8 vs. 18.2%) in several areas of the United States [6].

Survival rates have increased in the last decade among younger groups (from 9% in the 1980s to 35% in the 1990s), but have not changed in the older group. Research now focuses increasingly on improving outcome in the patient group mainly affected by the disease.

In a large Italian population-based study (n = 1005), median survival of patients aged > 60 years with AML either treated with supportive or aggressive therapy was 5 and 7 months, respectively. In patients > 70 years,

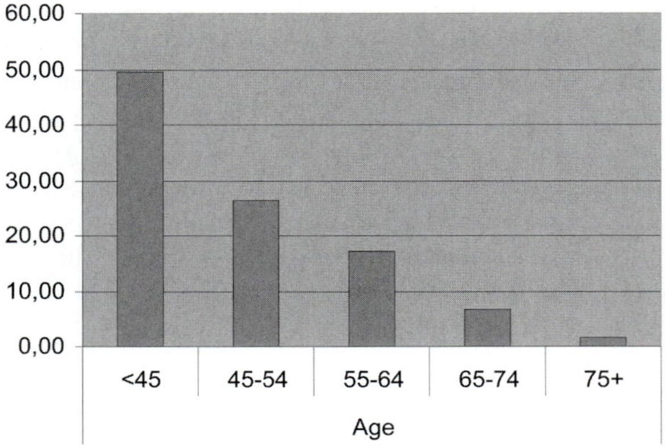

Fig. 3.3. Age associated with 5-year relative survival: USA 1996–2003 [6].

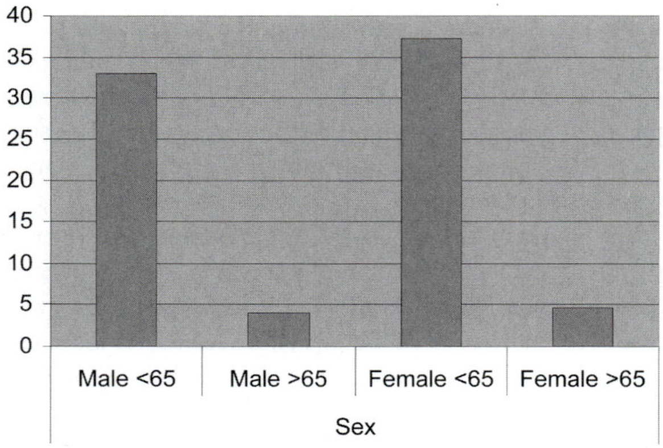

Fig. 3.4. Sex associated with 5-year relative survival: USA 1996–2003 [6].

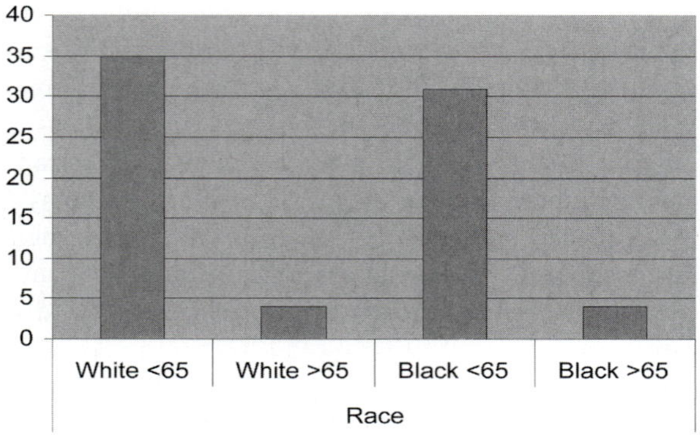

Fig. 3.5. Race associated with 5-year relative survival: USA 1996–2003 [6].

median survival was 4 months and this, notably, was regardless of the type of therapeutic effort [18]. Age has further been shown to be inversely associated with (1) referral to a treatment center [24], and/or inclusion into a clinical trial [25], (2) tolerance to induction treatment (early death or death during the immediate postchemotherapy phase) [26], and (3) the ability to achieve remission [27, 28]. In older patients (> 60 years), standard induction therapy achieves complete remission in only 30–50% of treated individuals [29].

Even though results of major clinical studies report higher rates of disease-free survival (e.g., 4-year survival rates of up to 42%) [30], data can differ considerably. The differences in survival results seen among various trials using similar chemotherapy may be explained by the prevalence of negative prognostic characteristics within a study population [31]. To understand clinical features and outcomes of that significant number of patients not meeting inclusion criteria for clinical studies, population-based evaluations have found increasing attention. Some results on age distribution, treatment decisions, remission rates, and survival in AML do show quite significant variability to some of the large clinical investigations. In one report, of a total of 170 AML patients, 55% were treated outside a study protocol. Non-study patients differed significantly from patients included in clinical trials with respect to age and performance status at clinical presentation, comorbidity, and type of AML. Patients who participated in a clinical trial had a median age of 46 years (16–73 years), whereas those not included were significantly older (median age 63 years; 21–83 years). Survival was significantly better in patients treated in a clinical protocol (median OS: 15 vs. 3.4 months) [25]. For survival results in population-based studies see Table 3.1. It can be assumed that

Table 3.1. Selected population-based studies of myeloid neoplasias in various populations: survival irrespective of treatment strategy [94]

Population	Median age	Median survival (weeks)
Northern Sweden (24)	63	7
Northern England (93)	71	8
Italy (18)	69	28

part of the increase in median survival in the last years may be attributed to improved supportive care over past decades.

3.1.7 Survivorship II

At St. Jude Children's Hospital, the incidence of and risk factors for the development of late sequelae of treatment in patients who survived for more than 10 years (median: 15 years) after diagnosis of childhood AML have been evaluated. The most common late effects in adulthood consisted in growth abnormalities (51%). Depending on the treatment modality (chemotherapy only; combined chemo-, radiotherapy; or combined chemo-, radiotherapy with consecutive bone marrow or peripheral stem cell transplantation), endocrine abnormalities, cataracts, cardiac abnormalities, academic difficulties, and secondary malignancies resulted in 14–51%. Besides physical late effects, psychosocial complications were observed in long-term survivors [32].

Patients that survived AML and treatment have also been monitored in a long-term follow-up at the University of Texas M.D. Anderson Cancer Center [33]. Some very relevant conclusions have been drawn in this report: Only 10% of all 1892 patients entered the potentially cured cohort, which was defined as the patient population in complete remission after a follow-up of 3 years. Those patients in the potentially cured cohort were most likely to be able to return to work, suggesting that the major threat to patients with newly diagnosed AML is the disease and not the treatment.

3.2 Etiology

The development of AML has been associated with several risk factors. Remarkably though, as of yet defined risk factors account for only a small number of observed cases [34]. These include age, antecedent hematological disease, genetic disorders as well as exposures to viruses, radiation, chemical or other occupational hazards, and previous chemotherapy [9, 35–37] (see Table 3.2).

The development of leukemia is a process consisting of multiple single steps that requires the susceptibility of a hematopoietic progenitor cell to inductive agents at multiple stages. The different subtypes of AML may have distinct mechanisms, suggesting a functional link between a particular molecular abnormality or mutation and the causal agent [38]. In most cases of AML the malignancy arises de novo and no leukemogenic exposure can be deciphered.

Table 3.2. Selected risk factors associated with AML

Genetic disorders	Down syndrome Klinefelter's syndrome Patau's syndrome Ataxia telangiectasia Schwachman syndrome Kostman syndrome Neurofibromatosis Fanconi anemia Li-Fraumeni syndrome
Physical and chemical exposures	Benzene Drugs as Pipobroman Pesticides Cigarette smoking Embalming fluids Herbicides Drugs as Pipobroman
Chemotherapy	Alkylating agents Topoisomerase II inhibitors Anthracyclines
Radiation exposure	Nontherapeutic, therapeutic radiation

3.2.1 Genetics

3.2.1.1 Genetic Factors

Genetic disorders and constitutional genetic defects are important risk factors associated with AML in children [37]. Children with Down syndrome have a 10- to 20-fold increased likelihood of developing acute leukemia [39, 40]. Other inherited diseases associated with AML include Klinefelter's syndrome, Li-Fraumeni syndrome [41], Fanconi anemia, and neurofibromatosis [9]. Furthermore, risk factors for developing AML in children were identified and include race/ethnicity, the father's age at time of conception, and time since the mother's last live birth [35]. Specifically, Asian/Pacific

Islander children had a higher risk than non-Hispanic white infants; children born to fathers older than 35, compared to those aged 20–34, had an increased risk; and longer time since the last live birth (at least 7 years) resulted in an increased risk.

In this context, acute promyelocytic leukemia (APL) has been investigated in more detail. Representing an example of a unique AML subtype (FAB M3) with a characteristic morphology associated with distinct chromosomal and gene-rearrangement aberrations, it has been shown to also have separate epidemiological features. For yet unknown reasons, an increased incidence of APL has been recognized in adult patients originating in Latin America and in children in Southern Europe. Of interest, the APL-specific gene rearrangement is different in patients of Latin American decent, with the majority of breakpoints in the RARα gene in the PML/RARα transcript in intron 6 (called bcr1). It is therefore speculated that this particular breakpoint site may be determined genetically [42–45].

3.2.1.2 Acquired Genetic Abnormalities

Acquired ("somatic") clonal chromosomal abnormalities are found in 50–80% of AML [24, 46–49] with rising incidences in patients with secondary leukemia [50] or older age [13, 51, 52]. Frequently found abnormalities include loss or deletion of chromosome 5, 7, Y, and 9, translocations such as t(8;21)(q22;q22); t(15;17)(q22;q11), trisomy 8 and 21, and other abnormalities involving chromosomes 16, 9, and 11.

Cytogenetic abnormalities constitute at present the most important predictors of short- [53–55] and long-term [33] outcome. To name selected examples, patients with a good prognosis are those with functional inactivation of the core binding factors (CBFs): AML1 and CBFβ. These cases include patients with AML and t(8;21) (q22;q22) or inv(16) (p13;q22), two of the most frequent recurrent cytogenetic abnormalities in de novo AML in younger patients [56].

Poor-risk cytogenetics have a loss of all or part of chromosome 5 or 7, translocations involving 11q23, or abnormalities of chromosome 3 [57].

A model of a "two-hit-hypothesis" for the AML phenotype by so-called class I and II mutations has been established. It describes the cooperativity of activating mutations in FLT3 (Fms-like tyrosine kinase 3) (=class I) and gene rearrangements involving hematopoietic transcription factors (=class II). The expression of both classes may result in the AML phenotype. FLT3 mutations can appear in all subtypes of AML and with the majority of known chromosomal translocations associated with AML. In this hypothesis, FLT3 mutations serve as exemplary of class I mutations that, alone, confer a proliferative and survival advantage to hematopoietic progenitors but do not affect cell differentiation. Further examples of class I mutations are activating mutations in N-RAS or K-RAS in AML. In contrast, class II mutations would be exemplified by AML1/ETO, CBFβ/SMMHC, PML/RARα, and MLL-related fusion genes. They appear to impair hematopoietic differentiation, but are not solely sufficient to cause leukemia. This new hypothesis may have important implications to novel treatment approaches (e.g., molecular targeting of both, FLT-3 and fusion proteins) [58].

Data has been published showing that individuals with certain polymorphisms in genes metabolizing carcinogens have an increased risk of developing AML [59]. NAD(P)H:quinone oxidoreductase 1 (NQO1), for example, is a carcinogen-metabolizing enzyme that detoxifies quinones and reduces oxidative stress. A polymorphism at nucleotide 609 of the NQO1 complementary DNA results in a lowering of the enzymes' activity. This polymorphic variant is associated with a predisposition to therapy-related AML [60] and selected cytogenetic subgroups of de novo AML [61].

3.2.2 Physical and Chemical Factors

A variety of environmental and chemical exposures are assumed to be associated with a variably elevated risk of developing AML in adults. A selection of hazards will be mentioned here.

Exposure to ionizing radiation is linked to AML [62]. Among survivors of the atomic bomb explosions in Japan, an increased incidence of AML was observed with a peak at 5–7 years after exposure. Also, therapeutic radiation has been found to increase the risk of secondary AML [63].

Chemotherapeutic agents, such as alkylating agents and topoisomerase II inhibitors, have been reported to increase the incidence of AML [64, 65] and will be discussed in detail below. A number of other substances (therapeutic [66] and occupational [9]) have been linked to an increased risk of AML. Chronic exposure to certain chemicals clearly shows an increased risk for the development of AML. Benzene is the best studied and widely used potentially leukemogenic agent [67]. Persons exposed to embalming fluids, ethylene oxides, and herbicides also appear to be at increased risk [68]. Furthermore, smoking has been discussed to be associated with an increased risk of developing AML (particularly of FAB subtype M2), especially in those aged 60–75 [69]. For summary see Table 3.2.

3.2.3 Viruses

Viruses – particularly RNA retroviruses – have been found to cause many neoplasms in experimental animal models, including leukemia [70]. As of now, a clear retroviral cause for AML in humans has not been identified even though an association between the exposure to certain viruses and the development of AML has been suggested. Parvovirus B19 could thus play a role in the pathogenesis of AML [71]. It has so far not been demonstrated, however, that simple infection with either a RNA- or DNA-based virus alone is a cause of AML.

3.2.4 Secondary AML

As mentioned, the cause of the disease is unknown for most patients with acute myeloid leukemia. "The true secondary AML" has been recommended to be referred to patients who have a clear clinical history of prior myelodysplastic syndrome (MDS), myeloproliferative disorder, or exposure to potentially leukemogenic therapies or agents; it is thus a rather broad category [56]. Secondary leukemias are in more than 90% of myeloid origin. Patients have a particularly poor outcome, with a lower incidence of achieving complete remission and shorter duration of survival than for patients with de novo AML [72–74].

Treatment-related secondary leukemia was first observed in survivors of successfully treated Hodgkin's disease [75]. Later on, survivors of ALL [76] and other disease entities such as ovarian or breast cancer and multiple myeloma [77] were included. The development of secondary AML shows a maximum in the 5–10 years following therapy. The distinct pattern of cytogenetic and genetic abnormalities in secondary or treatment-related AML is worthy of notice [78]. AML arises after previous therapy for other malignancies in a subset of 10–20% of patients. The risk of therapy-related AML after intensive chemotherapy may be increased to more than 100 times [79].

Specific cytogenetic abnormalities currently serve as the most important factor in distinguishing differences in AML biology, response to treatment and prognosis [49]. The different abnormalities result in gene rearrangements that may reflect the etiology and pathogenesis of the disease [80]. Treatment-related or secondary leukemias are examples in which genetic aberrations provide information on its specific etiology. In understanding the mechanisms associated with the development of secondary AML, general facts about the possible etiology of leukemia can been elucidated.

In this context, genetic pathways with different etiology and biologic characteristics have been proposed for cytogenetic changes that can be related to previous exposure to different chemically well-defined cytostatic agents with a known mechanism of action [81]. Among those are for alkylating agents: deletions or loss of 7q or monosomy 7 with normal chromosome 5 [82–84], and deletions or loss of 5q or monosomy 5 [85]. For epipodophyllotoxins, balanced translocations to chromosome bands 11q23, primarily in children, have been described [76]. Topoisomerase II inhibitors have been linked to t(8;21), inv(16) [86]. Topoisomerase II inhibitors, anthracyclines, mitoxantrone [87], as well as radiotherapy [88] may be associated with therapy-related acute prolymphocytic leukemia with t(15;17) and chimeric rearrangements between PML and RARA genes as well as different translocations to chromosome bands 11q15 and chimeric rearrangement between the NUP98 gene and its partner genes [89].

Another subgroup includes 10–15% of all patients with secondary AML, with normal karyotype or various chromosome aberrations uncharacteristic of t-AML or at least not identified as such as of now [90].

It is to be expected that in the future, many more genetic and epigenetic changes may be discovered. As of now, methylation of the p15 promoter is the only abnormality observed in a high percentage of patients with AML, especially in patients with secondary AML [91].

In current times there is a rapid gain in insight regarding epi-/genetic changes associated with the development of hematological malignancies like AML. It can be hoped for that many epidemiological and etiological findings may be explained and the development of new specific treatment strategies can further be enhanced on this basis.

References

1. Redaelli A, Lee JM, Stephens JM, Pashos CL (2003) Acute myeloid leukemia: Epidemiology and clinical burden. Expert Rev Anticancer Ther 3(5):695–710
2. Sandler DP, Ross JA (1997) Epidemiology of acute leukemia in children and adults. Semin Oncol 24(1):3–16
3. Greenlee RT, Hill-Harmon MB, Murray T, Thun M (2001) Cancer statistics 2001. CA Cancer J Clin 51:15–36
4. Hernández JA, Land KJ, McKenna RW (1995) Leukemia, myeloma, and other lymphoreticular neoplasms. Cancer 75:381
5. Wingo PA, Tong T, Bolden S (1995) Cancer statistics 1995. CA Cancer J Clin 45:8
6. Ries LAG, Eisner MP, Kosary CL, Hankey BF, Miller BA, Clegg L, Mariotto A, Fay MP, Feuer EJ, Edwards BK (eds) (2004) SEER cancer statistics review, 1975–2004, National Cancer Institute. Bethesda, MD, http://seer.cancer.gov/csr/1975–2004 based on November 2006 SEER data submission, posted to SEER web site, 2007
7. Jemal A, Thomas A, Murray T, Thun M (2002) Cancer statistics 2002. CA Cancer J Clin 52:23–47
8. Ries LAG, Miller BA, Hankey BF, et al. (eds) (1994) SEER cancer statistics review, 1972–1991: Tables and graphs, National Cancer Institute. NIH Pub. No. 94–2789. Bethesda, MD
9. Aquino VM (2002) Acute myelogenous leukemia. Curr Probl Pediatr Adolesc Health Care 32(2):50–58
10. Gurney JG, Severson RK, Davis S, et al. (1995) Incidence of cancer in children in the USA. Sex-, race-, and 1-year age-specific rates by histologic type. Cancer 75:2186–2195
11. Forman D, Stockton D, Moller H, Quinn M, Babb P, De Angelis R, Micheli A (2003) Cancer prevalence in the UK: Results from the EUROPREVAL study. Ann Oncol 14:648–654
12. Sekeres MA, Stone RM (2002) The challenge of acute myeloid leukemia in older patients. Curr Opin Oncol 14(1):24–30
13. Head DR (1996) Revised classification of acute myeloid leukemia. Leukemia 10:1826–1831
14. Xie Y, Davies SM, Xiang Y, Robinson LL, Ross JA (2003) Trends in leukemia incidence and survival in the United States (1973–1998). Cancer 97(9):2229–2235. Erratum in: Cancer 2003; 98(3):659
15. Gurney JG, Severson RK, Davis S, et al. (1995) Incidence of cancer in children in the United States. Sex-, race-, and 1-year age-specific rates by histologic type. Cancer 75:2186–2195
16. Lowenberg B, Zittoun R, Kerkhofs H, et al. (1989) on the value of intensive remission-induction chemotherapy in elderly patients of 65+ years with acute myeloid leukemia: A randomized phase III study of the European Organization for Research and Treatment of Cancer Leukemia Group. J Clin Oncol 7:1268–1274
17. Pulsoni A, Pagano L, Latagliata R, et al. (2004) Acute myelogenous leukemia in elderly patients: Survival of a large population irrespectively of treatment protocol enrollment, role of aggressive versus non-aggressive treatment. A retrospective survival analysis on 1005 patients. Haematologica 89(3):434–440
18. Estey E (2000) How I treat older patients with AML. Blood 96:1670–1673
19. Deschler B, deWitte T, Mertelsmann R, Lübbert M (2006) Treatment decision-making for older patients with high-risk MDS and AML: Problems and approaches Haematologica, 91(11): 1515-1524
20. Wingo PA, Cardinez CJ, Landis SH, Greenlee RT, Ries LA, Anderson RN, Thun MJ (2003) Long-term trends in cancer mortality in the United States, 1930–1998. Cancer 97(12 Suppl):3133–3275
21. Levi F, Lucchini F, Negri E, La Vecchia C (2002) Cancer mortality in the European Union, 1988–1997: The fall may approach 80000 deaths a year. Int J Cancer 98(4):636–637
22. American Cancer Society (2003) Cancer Facts & Figures 2003. www.cancer.org
23. Groves FD, Linet MS, Devesa SS (1995) Patterns of occurence of leukaemias. Eur J Cancer 31A:941–949
24. Wahlin A, Hörnsten P, Jonsson H (1991) Remission rate and survival in acute myeloid leukemia: Impact of selection and chemotherapy. Eur J Haematol 46:240–247
25. Mengis C, Aebi S, Tobler A, Dähler W, Fey M (2003) Assessment of differences in patient populations selected for or excluded from participation in clinical phase III acute myelogenous leukemia trials. J Clin Oncol 21:3933–3939
26. Dillmann RO, Davis RB, Green MR, et al. (1991) A comparative study of two different doses of cytarabine for acute myeloid leukemia: A phase III trial of Cancer and Leukemia Group B. Blood 78:2520–2526
27. Yates J, Gildewell O, Wienik P, et al. (1982) Cytosine arabinoside with daunorubicin or adriamycin for therapy of acute myelocytic leukemia: A CALGB study. Blood 60:454
28. Rai KR, Holland JF, Glidewell OJ, et al. (1981) Treatment of acute myelocytic leukemia: A study by Cancer and Leukemia Group B. Blood 58:1203
29. Hiddemann W, Kern W, Schoch C, Fonatsch C, Heinecke A, Wörmann B, Büchner T (1999) Management of acute myeloid leukemia in elderly patients. J Clin Oncol 17:3569–3576
30. Löwenberg B, van Putten W, Theobald M, Gmür J, Verdonck L, Sonneveld P, Fey M, Schouten H, de Greef G, Ferrant A, et al. for the Dutch-Belgian Hemato-Oncology (HOVON) Cooperative Group and the Swiss Group for Clinical Cancer Research (2003) Effect of priming with granulocyte colony-stimulating factor on the outcome of chemotherapy for acute myeloid leukemia. N Engl J Med 349(8):743–752
31. Keating A, Baker MA (1990) Effect of exclusion criteria on interpretation of clinical outcome in AML. In: Gale RP (ed) Acute myelogenous leukemia: Progress and controversies. Wiley-Liss, New York, p 235
32. Leung W, Hudson MM, Strickland DK, Phipps S, Srivastava DK, Ribeiro RC, Rubnitz JE, Sandlund JT, Kun LE, Bowman LC, et al. (2000) Late effects of treatment in survivors of childhood acute myeloid leukemia. J Clin Oncol 18:3273–3279
33. Estey E, deLima M, Strom S, Pierce S, Freireich EJ, Keating MJ (1997) Long-term follow-up of patients with newly diagnosed acute myeloid leukemia treated at the University of Texas M.D. Anderson Cancer Center. Cancer 80(11):2176–2180
34. Sandler DP, Collman GW (1987) Cytogenetic and environmental factors in the etiology of the acute leukemias in adults. Am J Epidemiol 126:1017–1032
35. Reynolds P, Von Behren J, Elkin EP (2002) Birth characteristics and leukemia in young children. Am J Epidemiol 155(7):603–613
36. Pogoda JM, Preston-Martin S, Nichols PW, Ross RK (2002) Smoking and risk of acute myeloid leukemia: Results from a Los Angeles County case-control study. Am J Epidemiol 155(6):546–553
37. Pui CH (1995) Childhood leukemias. N Engl J Med 332:1618–1630

38. Crane MM, Stom SS, Halabi S, et al. (1996) Correlation between selected environmental exposures and karyotype in acute myelocytic leukemia. Cancer Epidemiol Biomarkers Preven 5(8):639–644
39. Fong CT, Brodeur GM (1987) Down's syndrome and leukemia: Epidemiology, genetics, cytogenetics and mechanisms of leukemogenesis. Cancer Genet Cytogenet 28(1):55–76
40. Bhatia S, Neglia JP (1995) Epidemiology of childhood acute myelogenous leukemia. J Pediatr Hematol Oncol 17(2):94–100
41. Pötzsch C, Voigtlander T, Lübbert M (2002) p53 Germline mutation in a patient with Li-Fraumeni Syndrome and three metachronous malignancies. J Cancer Res Clin Oncol 128(8):456–460
42. Douer D, Preston-Martin S, Chang E, Nichols PW, Watkins KJ, Levin AM (1996) High frequency of acute promyelocytic leukemia among latinos with acute myeloid leukemia. Blood 87(1):308–313
43. Estey E, Thall P, Kantarjian H, Pierce S, Kornblau S, Keating M (1997) Association between increased body mass index and a diagnosis of acute promyelocytic leukemia in patients with acute myeloid leukemia. Leukemia 11(10):1661–1664
44. Douer D (2003) The epidemiology of acute promyelocytic leukemia. Best Pract Res Clin Haematol 16(3):357–367
45. Douer D, Santimillana S, Ramezani L, Samanez C, Slovak ML, Lee MS, Watkins K, Williams T, Vallejos C (2003) Acute promyelocytic leukemia in patients originating in Latin America is associated with an increased frequency of the bcr1 subtype of the PML/RARα fusion gene. Br J Haematol 122:563–570
46. Heim S, Mitelman F (1992) Cytogenetic analysis in the diagnosis of acute myeloid leukemia. Cancer 70:1701–1709
47. Moorman AV, Roman E, Willett EV, Dovey GJ, Cartwright RA, Morgan GJ (2001) Karyotype and age in acute myeloid leukemia. Are they linked? Cancer Genet Cytogenet 126(2):155–161
48. Bloomfield CD, Lawrence C, Byrd JC, et al. (1998) Frequency of prolonged remission duration after high-dose cytarabine intensification in acute myeloid leukemia varies by cytogenetic subtype. Cancer Res 58:4173–4179
49. Grimwade D, Walker H, Oliver F, et al. (1998) The importance of diagnostic cytogenetics on outcome in AML: Analysis of 1612 patients entered into MCR AML 10 trial. Blood 92:2322–2333
50. Sanderson RN, Johnson PR, Maguire C, Moorman AV, Roman E, Willett E, Bown N, Taylor P, Proctor SJ, Bowen DT (2003) Population-based study of unselected acute myeloid leukemia cases reveals distinct cytogenetic pathways analogous to therapy-related AML/MDS. Blood 102(11)
51. Mauritzson N, Johansson B, Albin N, Billström R, et al. (1999) A single-center population-based consecutive series of 1500 cytogenetically investigated adult hematological malignancies: Karyotypic features in relation to morphology, age and gender. Eur J Haematol 62:95–102
52. Rossi G, Pelizzari AM, Bellotti D, Tonelli M, Barlati S (2000) Cytogenetic analogy between myelodysplastic syndrome and acute myeloid leukemia of elderly patients. Leukemia 14(4):636–641
53. Keating MJ, Smith TL, Kantarjian H, et al. (1988) Cytogenetic pattern in acute myelogenous leukemia: A major reproducible determinant of outcome. Leukemia 2:403
54. Schiffer CA, Lee EJ, Tomiyasu T, Wiernik PH, Testa JR (1989) Prognostic impact of cytogenetic abnormalities in patients with de novo acute nonlymphcytic leukemia. Blood 73:263
55. Ferrant A, Lapopin M, Frassoni F, et al. (1997) Karyotype in acute myeloblastic leukemia: Prognostic significance for bone marrow transplantation in first remission: A European Group for Blood and Marrow Transplantation Study. Blood 76:2931
56. Cheson BD, Bennett JM, Kopecky KJ, Büchner T, Willman CL, Estey EH, Schiffer CA, Doehner H, Tallman MS, Lister TA, et al. (2003) Revised recommendations of the international working group for diagnosis, standardization of response criteria, treatment outcomes, and reporting standards for therapeutic trials in acute myeloid leukemia. J Clin Oncol 21:4642–4649
57. Grimwade, Walker H, Harrison G, Oliver F, Chatters S, Harrison CJ, Wheatley K, Burnett AK, Goldstone AH; Medical Research Council Adult Leukemia Working Party (2001) The predictive value of hierarchical cytogenetic classification in older adults with acute myeloid leukemia (AML): Analysis of 1065 patients entered into the United Kingdom Medical Research Council AML11 trial. Blood 98(5):1312–1320
58. Gilliland DG, Griffin JD (1999) The role of FLT3 in hematopoiesis and leukemia. Blood 100(5):1532–1542
59. Bowen D, Frew ME, Rollinson S, Roddam PL, Dring A, Smith MT, Langabeer SE, Morgan GJ (2003) CYP1A1*2B (Val) allele is overrepresented in a subgroup of acute myeloid leukemia patients with poor-risk karyotype associated with NRAS mutation, but nor associated with FLT3 internal tandem duplication. Blood 101(7):2770–2774
60. Larson RA, Wang Y, Banerjee M, Wiemels J, Hartford C, Le Beau MM, Smith MT (1999) Prevalence of inactivating $^{609}C \rightarrow T$ polymorphism in the NAD(P)H:Quinone oxidoreductase (NQO1) gene in patients with primary and therapy-related myeloid leukemia. Blood 94(2):803–807
61. Smith MT, Wang Y, Kane E, Rollinson S, Wiemels JL, Roman E, Roddam P, Cartwright R, Morgan G (2001) Low NAD(P)H.quinone oxidoreductase 1 activity is associated with increased risk of acute leukemia in adults. Blood 91(5):1422–1426
62. Preston DL, Kusumi S, Tomonaga M, et al. (1994) Cancer incidence in atomic bomb survivors. Part III. Leukemia, lymphoma and multiple myeloma, 1950–1987. Radiat Res 137(2 Suppl): 68–97
63. Kossman SE, Weiss MA (2000) Acute myelogenous leukemia after exposure to strontium-89 for the treatment of adenocarcinoma of the prostate. Cancer 88(3):620–624
64. Le Beau MM, Albain KS, Larson RA, et al. (1986) Clinical and cytogenetic correlations in 63 patients with therapy-related myelodysplastic syndromes and acute nonlymphocytic leukemia: Further evidence for characteristic abnormalities of chromosomes no. 5 and 7. J Clin Oncol 4(3):325–345
65. Pui CH, Ribeiro RC, Hancock ML, et al. (1991) Acute myeloid leukemia in children treated with epipodophyllotoxins for acute lymphoblastic leukemia. N Engl J Med 325(24):1682–1687
66. De Sactis V, Mazzucconi MG, Spadea A, Mancini AM, Bizzoni L, Peraino M, Mandelli (2003) Long-term evaluation of 164 patients with essential thrombocythaemia treated with pipobroman: Occurence of leukaemic evolution. Br J Haematol 123:517–521
67. Savitz DA, Andrews KW (1997) Review of epidemiology evidence on benzene and lymphatic and hematopoietic cancers. Am J Int Med 31:287
68. Flodin U, Anderson L, Anjou CG, et al. (1981) A case-referral study on acute myeloid leukemia, background radiation and exposure to solvents and other agents. Scand J Work Environ Health 7:169

69. Pogoda JM, Preston-Martin S, Nichols PW, Ross RK (2002) Smoking and risk of acute myeloid leukemia: Results from a Los Angeles County case-control study. Am J Epidemiol 155(6):546–553
70. Ben-David Y, Bernstein A (1991) Friend virus-induced erythroleukemia and the multistage nature of cancer. Cell 66:831
71. Kerr JR, Barah F, Cunniffe VS, Smith J, Vallely PJ, Will AM, Wynn RF, Stevens RF, Taylor GM, Cleator GM, et al. (2003) Association of acute parvovirus B19 infection with new onset of acute lymphoblastic and myeloblastic leukemia. J Clin Pathol 56(11):873–875
72. Gajewski JL, Ho WG, Nimer SD, et al. (1989) Efficacy of intensive chemotherapy for acute myelogenous leukemia associated with preleukemic syndrome. J Clin Oncol 7:1637
73. Neugut AI, Robinson E, Nieves J, Murray T, Tsai WY (1990) Poor survival of treatment-related acute nonlymphocytic leukemia. JAMA 264:1006
74. Kantarjian HM, Keating MJ (1987) Therapy-related leukemia and myelodysplastic syndrome. Semin Oncol 14:435
75. Arseneau JC, Sponzo RW, Levin DL, et al. (1972) Nonlymphomatous malignant tumors complicating Hodgkin's disease. N Engl J Med 287:1119
76. Pui CH, Behm FG, Raimondi SC, et al. (1989) Secondary acute myeloid leukemia in children treated for acute lymphoid leukemia. N Engl J Med 321:136
77. van Leeuwen FE (1996) Risk of acute myelogenous leukaemia and myelodysplasia following cancer treatment. Baillieres Clin Haematol 9(1):57–85
78. Gojo I, Karp JE (2001) The impact of biology on the treatment of secondary AML. Cancer Treat Res 108:231–255
79. Pedersen-Bjergaard J, Philip P, Larsen SO, et al. (1993) Therapy-related myelodysplasia and acute myeloid leukemia: Cytogenetic characteristics of 115 consecutive cases and risk in seven cohorts of patients treated intensively for malignant diseases in the Copenhagen series. Leukemia 7:1975–1986
80. Lowenberg B, Downing JR, Burnett A (1999) Acute myeloid leukemia. New Engl J Med 341:1951–1962
81. Pedersen-Bjergaard J, Andersen MK, Christiansen DH, Nerlov C (2002) Genetic pathways in therapy-related myelodysplasias and acute myeloid leukemia. Blood 99(6):1909–1912
82. Le Beau MM, Albain KS, Larson RA, et al. (1986) Clinical and cytogenetic correlations in 63 patients with therapy-related myelodysplastic syndromes and acute nonlymphocytic leukemia: Further evidence for characteristic abnormalities of chromosomes no. 5 and 7. J Clin Oncol 4:325–345
83. Johansson B, Mertens F, Heim S, et al. (1991) Cytogenetics of secondary myelodysplasia (sMDS) and acute nonlymphocytic leukemia (sANLL). Eur J Haematol 47:17–27
84. Pedersen-Bjergaard J, Pedersen M, Roulston D, et al. (1995) Different genetic pathways in leukemogenesis for patients presenting with therapy-related myelodysplasia and therapy-related acute myeloid leukemia. Blood 86:3542–3552
85. Odero MD, Carlson KM, Calasanz MJ, Rowley JD (2001) Further characterization of complex chromosomal rearrangements in myeloid malignancies: Spectral karyotyping adds precision in defining abnormalities associated with poor prognosis. Leukemia 15:1133–1145
86. Quesnel B, Katarjian H, Pedersen-Bjergaard J, et al. (1993) Therapy-related acute myeloid leukemia with t(8;21): inv(16): and t(8;16): A report on 25 cases and review of the literature. J Clin Oncol 11:2370–2379
87. Carli PM, Sgro C, Parchin-Geneste N, et al. (2000) Increase therapy-related leukemia secondary to breast cancer. Leukemia 14:1014–1017
88. Andersen MK, Johansson B, Larsen SO, Pedersen-Bjergaard J (1998) Chromosomal abnormalities in secondary MDS and AML. Relationship to drugs and radiation with specific emphasis on the balanced rearrangements. Haematologica 83:483–488
89. Ahuja HG, Felix CA, Aplan PD (1999) The t(11;20)(p15q11) chromosomal translocation associated with therapy-related myelodysplastic syndrome results in an NUP)(-TOP1 fusion. Blood 94: 741–747
90. Pedersen-Bjergaard J, Andersen MK, Christiansen DH, Nerlov C (2002) Genetic pathways in therapy-related myelodysplasias and acute myeloid leukemia. Blood 99(6):1909–1912
91. Christiansen DH, Andersen MK, Pedersen-Bjergaard J (2003) Methylation of p15INK4B is common, is associated with deletion of genes on chromosome arm 7q and predicts a poor prognosis in therapy-related myelodysplasia and acute myeloid leukemia. Leukemia 17(9):1813–1819
92. Parkin DM, Whelan SL, Ferlay J, Raymond L, Young J (eds) (1997) Cancer incidence in five continents (vol VII). IARC Scientific publications No. 143. IARC, Lyon
93. Taylor PR, Reid MM, Stark AN, Bown N, Hamilton PJ, Proctor SJ (1995) De novo acute myeloid leukaemia in patients over 55-years-old: A population-based study of incidence, treatment and outcome. Northern Region Haematology Group. Leukemia 9(2):231–237
94. Deschler B, Lübbert M (2006) Acute myeloid leukaemia: Epidemiology and etiology. Cancer 107(9):2099–2107

Relapsed and Refractory Acute Myeloid Leukemia

Syed Abutalib, Martin S. Tallman

Contents

4.1 Introduction

Despite effective initial therapy, the majority of adults with acute myeloid leukemia (AML) who achieve a complete remission (CR) eventually relapse and usually within 2 years. Furthermore, approximately 20% of patients never achieve first complete remission (CR1). In these settings, alternative treatment strategies have limited efficacy and allogeneic hematopoietic stem cell transplantation (HSCT), with generation of the potent immunologic reaction graft-vs.-leukemia (GVL) effect, is considered the best curative strategy. However, many patients do not have a suitable donor or are not candidates for transplantation. Therefore, the treatment of patients who relapse or are refractory to conventional initial therapy is challenging. The definition of refractory AML includes patients who fail conventional induction chemotherapy, those with a short (less than 6–12 months) CR1 duration, and patients who have relapsed twice or more [1]. This definition has been useful in defining relatively uniform populations of patients for clinical trials.

In general, younger (< 60 years) patients have initial CR rates of 60–80% with conventional induction chemotherapy [2–4]. Older (> 60 years) adults, representing the majority of the AML population, have lower initial CR rates of 40–60% [5, 6]. The rate of CR in patients with recurrent AML with reinduction chemotherapy is typically lower than that achieved with initial induction therapy and most patients have a shorter duration of CR2 compared to CR1 [7]. If a CR2 is achieved, the median duration of remission and disease-free survival (DFS) are generally short (< 12 months).

During the past several decades, extraordinary insights have been made in deciphering the molecular genetics of AML. The remarkable efficacy of all-trans retinoic acid (ATRA) in acute promyelocytic leukemia (APL), and of the tyrosine kinase inhibitor, Imatinib, in patients with chronic myeloid leukemia (CML) highlight the potential clinical benefits of developing molecularly targeted therapies in leukemia and reflect the exciting shift in clinical research from conventional cytotoxic chemotherapy to targeted drug development. A second major area of promising innovative research focuses on HSCT with the development of reduced-intensity conditioning (RIC) regimens with allogeneic HSCT and refinements in the identification of alternative donor sources such as umbilical cord stem cells. The ability to harness GVL effect has made it possible to extend the curative potential of allogeneic HSCT to patients for whom such an intensive approach historically has been contraindicated because of age or comorbidities.

4.2 Prognostic Factors in Patients with Relapsed or Refractory AML

With the exception of patients with relapsed APL, the prognosis for the majority of adults with relapsed or refractory AML whose initial CR duration is less than 12 months is very poor whether treatment includes conventional cytotoxic chemotherapy such as high-dose ara-C (HiDAC) or investigational agents [8] (Fig. 4.1). Patients whose CR1 duration is between 1–2 years fare better with HiDAC rather than investigational strategies. The identification of factors which predict for a favorable or unfavorable outcome with salvage chemotherapy can guide therapeutic strategies.

In a seminal study, advancing age, abnormal liver function, elevated serum lactate dehydrogenase level, abnormal karyotype, the proportion of blasts plus promyelocytes, and a shorter (< 1 year) CR1 duration were inversely associated with response and survival after salvage chemotherapy [9]. In two recent studies, the outcomes of approximately 1200 younger patients with AML in first relapse based on four clinical parameters (length of relapse-free interval after CR1, cytogenetics at diagnosis, age at relapse and whether HSCT had been performed), known as European Prognostic Index (EPI), were reported [10, 11]. Prognostic scores ranged from 0 to 14 points based on strictly defined criteria, with higher scores predicting for a worse prognosis. Using this stratification system, three risk groups were defined: a favorable prognostic group (0–6), an intermediate risk group (7–9), and a poor risk group (10–14). Both studies showed comparable 1-year overall

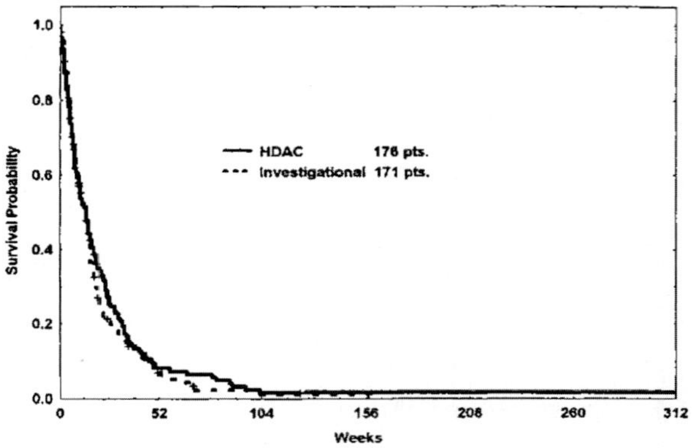

Fig. 4.1. Survival probability by type of salvage regimen (HDAC-based vs. investigational) in patients whose initial CR was < 1 year [8].

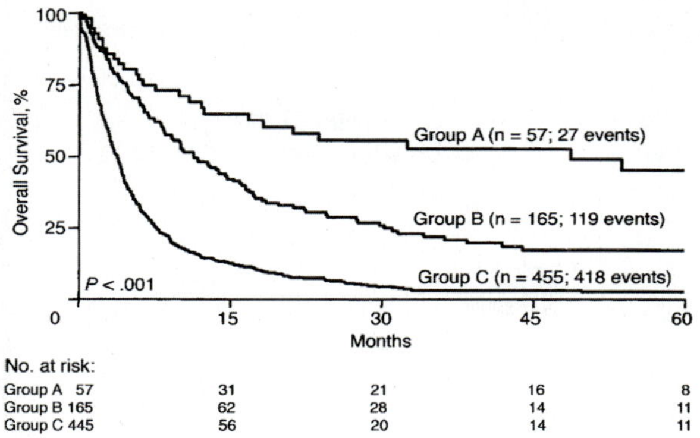

Fig. 4.2. Cumulative rates of overall survival among acute myeloid leukemia patients in first relapse according to prognostic group. Favorable risk group **A** contains patients with score of 1 to 6 points, intermediate group **B:** 7 to 9 points, poor group **C:** 10 to 14 points. P value was calculated with use of the log-rank test [10].

survival (OS) rates of 70% and 64% for the favorable prognostic group, 49% and 38% for the intermediate risk group, and 16% and 17% for the poor risk group. Results from the Dutch-Belgian Hemato-Oncology Group (HOVON) are shown in Fig. 4.2. The reproducibility and simplicity of this stratification schema may facilitate therapeutic decisions and the assessment of novel treatment strategies for first salvage therapy.

In addition to improving outcomes in patients with relapsed and refractory AML, efforts have been undertaken to identify quantitative methods that predict for relapse in patients who are in apparent morphologic CR. For example, early intervention in this setting has been beneficial in patients with APL where treatment at the time of molecular relapse may be associated with a better outcome than that observed with treatment only after overt relapse demonstrated by morphology of the bone marrow [12]. Furthermore, such efforts have provided important clues into the mechanisms by which chemoresistance is mediated and may influence the design of strategies for the prevention of relapsed disease. As an example, a persistently abnormal karyotype in patients in apparent CR by morphologic criteria predicts for relapse [13].

4.2.1 Age

In virtually every study conducted to date, the CR rate with conventional cytotoxic salvage chemotherapy is inversely related to age (Table 4.1) [1, 9, 14–16]. In a retrospective study by Rees and colleagues, which included a large number of patients in each age subgroup, the CR2 rate among 375 patients was 33% for younger patients compared to 19% among older patients [16]. Furthermore, an analysis by the Eastern Cooperative Oncology Group (ECOG) of the outcome of approximately 3000 newly diagnosed AML patients, demonstrated a poorer 5-year OS rate among 1000 older (>55 years) patients compared to 2000 younger (<55 years) patients [17]. In addition, several cooperative groups have shown an improvement in CR1 rates, but not in OS in older adults during the last two decades [17, 18]. Since AML is generally a disease of older adults, with a median age of approximately 68 years, this observation carries important implications. Patients with relapsed and refractory AML, particularly older adults, are frequently encountered and there is an urgent need for more effective and less toxic therapy.

4.2.2 Duration of CR1 and Cytogenetics

The most important predictor of achieving a CR2 with salvage chemotherapy appears to be the duration of

Table 4.1. Selected studies demonstrating the impact of age on achieving a second complete response

Study	Age <60 years		Age >60 years	
	CR2/total patients	CR2 (%)	CR2/total patients	CR2 (%)
Rees, et al. 1986 [16]	124/375	33	21/110	19
Keating, et al. 1989 [9]	75/208	36	5/35	14
Hiddemann, et al. 1990 [1]	56/104	54	14/32	44
Kern, et al. 1998 [15]	67/138	49	21/48	44
Sternberg, et al. 2000 [14]	10/22	45	19/25	76

Table 4.2. Selected studies demonstrating the impact of initial complete response duration on achieving a second complete response

Study	Age <1 years		Age >1 years	
	CR2/total patients	CR2 (%)	CR2/total patients	CR2 (%)
Rees, et al. 1986 [16]	32/251	13	113/234	48
Keating, et al. 1989 [9]	20/105	19	51/82	62
Hiddemann, et al. 1990 [1]	40/87	46	29/49	60
Estey, et al. 1993 [19]	6/24	25	9/10	90
Thalhammer, et al. 1996 [20]	40/121	33	26/47	55

Table 4.3. Impact of diagnostic cytogenetics on second complete response rate and survival in patients with first relapse AML

Risk groups	Weltermann, et al. 2004 [26]		Kern, et al. 2002 [27]	Wheatley, et al. 1999 [24]	
	CR rate (%)	3-year survival (%)	CR rate (%)	CR rate (%)	5-year survival (%)
*Good	88	43	80	90	72
**Intermediate	64	18	49	54	43
***Poor	36	0	30	45	17

* Good risk = Presence of t(15;17), t(8;21) or inv (16)

** Intermediate risk = Presence of a normal karyotype or cytogenetic abnormalities not included in favorable or poor risk groups

*** Poor risk = Presence of a complex karyotype or abnormalities of chromosome 3, 5, or 7.

the CR1 [1, 9, 16, 19–21]. For reasons of convenience, patients with relapsed AML are usually categorized into two groups, those with a CR1 > or <1 year (Table 4.2). The explanation for the apparent recovery of sensitivity and tolerance to cytotoxic chemotherapy with time is unknown. However, many of the factors present in newly diagnosed patients such as performance status may play a role [22].

Pretreatment cytogenetics have important prognostic implications in patients with relapsed and refractory AML [23–26]. A favorable karyotype is more frequent in patients whose first remissions were at least 12 months in duration, while the opposite was found in patients with an unfavorable karyotype [23]. Other investigators have provided similar observations concerning the prognostic significance of pretreatment cytogenetics on patients with relapsed and refractory AML (Table 4.3) [24–26]. Kern and colleagues reported that unfavorable cytogenetics were associated with a lower rate of CR2 and were a poor prognostic factor with regard to survival after first relapse [25]. The independent prognostic impact of genomic instability at relapse remains unclear. Kern and colleagues have also suggested that cytogenetics at relapse tend to relate to outcome more strongly than cytogenetics at diagnosis [27]. However, other studies found that a change in the cytogenetic pattern at first relapse did not influence the prognosis of therapy for first relapse in the majority of patients [28].

4.3 Treatment of Relapsed and Refractory AML

4.3.1 Introduction

Despite the success of initial treatment in inducing CR in many patients, most patients with AML eventually die of their disease. Relapse is likely to become a more important cause for treatment failure as improvements in supportive care favorably influence the early death rate [29]. New, less toxic antifungal agents such as itraconazole have replaced amphotericin in neutropenic patients with hematologic malignancies and can prevent invasive fungal infections, reduce mortality from these infections, and decrease the rate of invasive Aspergillus infections [30].

A number of chemotherapeutic agents have activity when used alone or in combination in patients with relapsed or refractory AML. The management of patients with relapsed and refractory AML is highly individualized and based on multiple prognostic factors described above. Importantly, published data should be interpreted with caution since response rates may not only reflect the therapy used, but also patient selection. The practical challenges in recruiting patients with previously untreated AML to clinical trials are formidable [31].

Furthermore, it is likely that even more barriers exist for accrual of patients with relapsed and refractory AML related to performance status and prior therapy.

4.3.2 Conventional Cytotoxic Chemotherapy

During the past three decades, a wide variety of salvage cytotoxic chemotherapy regimens has been studied in patients with relapsed or refractory AML which result in modest success. There is no standard chemotherapy regimen that provides a durable second or greater CR. One of the most active and the most studied agents is ara-C. Doses range from 500 mg/m^2 to 3 gm/m^2 every 12 h for up to 6 days given either alone or in combination with other active agents including anthracyclines, asparaginase, etoposide, mitoxantrone, or amsacrine [15, 32–38]. In general, variable second CR rates in the range of 30 to 65% have been observed with associated reinduction mortality rates of 12–25%. It is not clear that the higher doses of ara-C are more effective. A German AML Cooperative group trial has compared cytarabine 3 g/m^2 with 1 g/m^2 administered twice daily on days 1, 2, 7, and 8 in patients younger than age 60 years [15]. All patients received mitoxantrone. There was no substantial difference in the CR rate (approximately 47%) or OS rate. Therefore, although dose-intense cytarabine is viewed as an essential component of many conventional salvage programs, dose escalation to 3 g/m^2 may not be justified in many patients given the potential for increased toxicity. It is desirable to select a salvage chemotherapy regimen with minimal toxicity since many suitable patients are subsequently offered HSCT.

Similarly, there is no definitive evidence that additional agents given with intermediate- or HiDAC improves OS. A large randomized trial conducted by Southwest Oncology Group (SWOG) failed to demonstrate a benefit in OS with the addition of mitoxantrone to HiDAC every 12 h for total of 6 days [37]. Similarly, nonstatistically significant results were obtained when etoposide was combined with HiDAC. A CR rate of 45% with combination compared to CR rate of 40% with HiDAC [39]. Novel regimens with cytotoxic chemotherapy such as mitoxantrone and etoposide, or purine analogs, have also been explored, but there is no evidence that they represent any substantial improvement over intermediate- or HiDAC-containing regimens [40–44].

4.3.3 Novel Agents Combined with Conventional Cytotoxic Chemotherapy

Several novel therapies have been combined with conventional chemotherapy to improve outcome. These include so-called targeted therapies (discussed in detail below), many of which are small molecules which inhibit or perturb signal transduction pathways. Another strategy has been to promote intracellular drug retention by inhibiting the efflux pump- p-glycoprotein (P-gp), a product of the multidrug resistance (MDR)-1 gene. The latter is possible by administration of cyclosporine (CsA) [45, 46] or its analog PSC-833 [47, 48]. Other novel inhibitors such as Zosuquidar, with pharmacokinetic properties such that concomitant chemotherapy doses do not have to be reduced as with other MDR inhibitors, are currently being investigated [49]. Despite strong preclinical data, trials utilizing these agents alone or in combination with chemotherapy and gemtuzumab ozogamicin (GO) [50, 51] have shown variable and generally disappointing results. However, a Phase III trial conducted by the SWOG demonstrated significant improvements in relapse-free-survival (RFS) and OS when CsA was combined with infusional daunorubicin and HiDAC [45], but these results are not validated by other studies using a similar strategy [46]. In addition, the exact mechanism by which CsA resulted in a benefit in RFS and OS in the SWOG trial was not clear.

4.4 Hematopoietic Stem Cell Transplantation

4.4.1 Myeloablative Allogeneic Hematopoietic Stem Cell Transplantation

4.4.1.1 In Relapsed AML

Allogeneic HSCT remains the only known curative treatment for patients with relapsed or refractory AML. However, only a minority of patients benefit from this strategy. Gale and colleagues demonstrated significantly better leukemia-free survival (LFS) with matched sibling donor (MSD) HSCT compared to chemotherapy in adults younger than or equal to 30 years and CR1 longer than 1 year (41% vs. 17%; P = 0.017) or adults older than 30 years and CR1 shorter than 1 year (18% vs. 7%) [52]. Three-year probabilities of TRM with chemotherapy and transplantation were 7% vs. 56%, respectively. It is reasonable to consider HSCT in early first relapse in younger (< 60 years) adults if a suitable MSD is readily available. Clift and colleagues demonstrated a 5-year DFS of 28% and a cure rate of 25–30% among 126 patients transplanted for AML in first untreated relapse [53]. These results are comparable when MSD-HSCT is carried out in CR2 [54, 55]. Reiffers and colleagues demonstrated a 3-year DFS of 35% among 459 patients. Moreover, approximately 50% of patients in first relapse successfully achieved CR2 and 15–20% died during reinduction chemotherapy [55].

A widely adopted strategy is to induce CR2 with salvage chemotherapy followed by allogeneic HSCT. There is no standard chemotherapy regimen for this clinical setting. The selection of one regimen over the other is based on CR1 duration and age. The FLAG +/– idarubicin regimen (fludarabine, ara-C, G-CSF) had been used for cytoreduction, followed by either matched sibling or MUD-HSCT with some success [56]. Promising results have been reported with either autologous or allogeneic HSCT using a preparative regimen which includes increased radiation dose delivered by ^{131}I-labeled anti-CD45 antibody [57, 58]. Generally, younger patients proceed to HSCT. A MSD may be preferred compared to a matched-unrelated donor (MUD) to avoid potentially prohibitive TRM, but the best choice between either of these strategies and auto-HSCT has not been prospectively studied. The role of autologous HSCT in younger patients with CR1 > 1 year is unclear, since there are no randomized trials comparing this approach with MUD-HSCT. Finally, patients between the ages of 30 to 60 and CR1 duration of < 1 year are also candidates for MSD-HSCT. All other adult patient subgroups may be best approached with investigational agents in the context of a well-design clinical trial.

It is important to emphasize that interpretation of data comparing HSCT and chemotherapy as consolidation therapy should be viewed with caution. Differing results are likely, in part, due to patient selection bias and difficulties in defining duration of response in chemotherapy arm because most patients proceed to other therapies including HSCT. Lastly, the superiority of any particular treatment modality should account for the prognostic factors and associated treatment-related morbidity and mortality.

4.4.1.2 Relapse After Transplantation

Relapse following allo-HSCT in CR2 is the major cause of treatment failure. The optimal management of patients relapsing after allo-HSCT is controversial. Without further therapy, the median survival of patients relapsing after an allo-HSCT is approximately 3–4 months. Options such as immunotherapy, donor lymphocyte infusion (DLI), or a second allo-HSCT after a fully myeloablative conditioning have been explored, but result in limited success. Choi and colleagues treated 16 patients who relapsed after allo-HSCT with cytoreductive chemotherapy followed immediately by G-CSF-primed DLI [59]. Ten of the 16 patients achieved CR, of whom 4 remained in CR at the time of publication. The OS at 2 years was 31%. The duration of CR after HSCT (> or < 6 months) was the only significant prognostic factor for OS. Interestingly, all five patients who relapsed after the chemotherapy followed by DLI strategy did so in extramedullary sites. This observation has been previously made [60]. Retrospective data indicate that response rates to DLI for relapsed AML range from 15 to 30%. However, CRs are durable in a minority of patients [61]. Associated toxicities of DLI include acute GVHD (> grade II in 30%) and a TRM rates are estimated to be up to 20%. In younger patients refractory to DLI, or among those with a longer CR duration after allo-HSCT, it is still important to consider a second allo-HSCT [62]. However, both relapse and mortality rates associated with second transplants are higher, 42% and 30%, respectively in the series from the Center For International Blood and Marrow Transplant Research (CIBMTR) [63] and reduced-intensity conditioning (RIC) transplantation is frequently required.

Further investigation and development of new approaches for this clinical setting to maximize the effects of GVL and minimize GVHD and toxicity are underway (discussed below). Umbilical cord blood-derived stem cells are yet an alternative source for transplantation for those patients who lack a suitable MSD or MUD [64, 65]. To increase the graft cell dose present in a single umbilical cord unit, double cord units have been evaluated with some success [66]. Although promising none of these transplant approaches from alternative donor stem cell sources can be considered standard of care and remain investigational.

4.4.1.3 In Refractory AML

Allogeneic HSCT offers the best chance for achieving sustained CR in primary refractory AML (PR-AML) patients. The outcome appears to be better among patients without peripheral blood blasts and in patients with less than 30% blasts in the bone marrow prior to conditioning [67]. Data from the City of Hope showed a cumulative probability of DFS of 43% at 10 years in 21 young (<41 years) AML (n=16) and ALL (n=5) patients after MSD-HSCT [68]. Another study by Biggs and colleagues reported 88 AML patients (<52 years) who were refractory to at least two courses of cytotoxic chemotherapy and subsequently proceeded to MSD-HSCT. The 3-year probability of LFS in these patients was 21% (14–31%) with a 3-year TRM of 44% [69]. Cook and coworkers showed that allo-HSCT can cure a small proportion of patients refractory to induction chemotherapy [70].

Similar to MUD-HSCT, the use of partially mismatched related donors (PMRD) extends access to allo-HSCT in PR-AML. This novel strategy is a reasonable alternative in patients with no MSD available, and may result in a similar outcome [71]. In a retrospective trial by Singhal and colleagues, the outcome of 24 MSD (median age 24 years) and 19 partially HLA-mismatched related donors (PMRD) (median age 34 years; P=0.04) allogeneic HSCT recipients with primary refractory AML and other hematological malignancies were compared. All PMRD patients and 90% of the MSD patients achieved CR2 [72]. The advantage of PMRD transplantation over MUD-HSCT is the ready and rapid potential availability of the donor – a factor that is of critical importance in patients with refractory progressive acute leukemia. Haploidentical stem cell transplantation is another alternative strategy which has met with success [73–75].

4.4.2 Non-Myeloablative Allogeneic Hematopoietic Stem Cell Transplantation

During remission, selected patients who are precluded from receiving full ablative HSCT may benefit from RIC or nonmyeloablative ("mini") HSCT [76–78]. RIC allows patients to benefit from GVL effect without incurring the toxicities of myeloablative conditioning regimens used in fully ablative HSCT. However, the GVL effect usually requires several months to be maximally therapeutic [79, 80]. Therefore, leukemia relapse prior to the establishment of donor chimerism remains a major limitation of RIC. The precise role of this modality as consolidation therapy awaits trials assessing refinements in preparative and immunosuppressive regimens, in the selection of subpopulations of infused effector cells [81] and in the identification of appropriate patients. In addition, RIC followed by haploidentical HSCT is a novel strategy which has also been explored [82, 83].

4.4.3 Autologous Hematopoietic Stem Cell Transplantation

The exact role of autologous HSCT in younger patients with relapsed AML without an HLA matched donor for allo-HSCT remains to be defined. With lack of randomized studies, the data are unclear and demonstrate variable results. Results from the European Group for Blood and Marrow Transplantation (EBMT) registry show DFS probabilities in the range of 30 to 35% for those undergoing autologous HSCT in CR2 [84, 85]. However, autologous HSCT when compared with chemotherapy has not shown statistically significantly improved survival [86]. Moreover, for the majority of AML patients who receive autologous HSCT in CR1 and relapse, a second autologous HSCT is rarely feasible. The EBMT data demonstrate that only 56 of 1579 AML patients (3.5%) were eligible for a second autologous HSCT after failure of the first autologous HSCT in CR1 [87].

A recent analysis by Lazarus and colleagues for the IBMTR (1989–1996) showed superior outcomes with autologous HSCT (n=668) when compared with MUD-HSCT (n=476) in both CR1 (n=692) and CR2 (n=452) [88] (Fig. 4.3). However, multiple confounding factors may have favored autologous HSCT including limitations in defining the degree of genetic disparity between unrelated donors–recipient pairs, accrual of

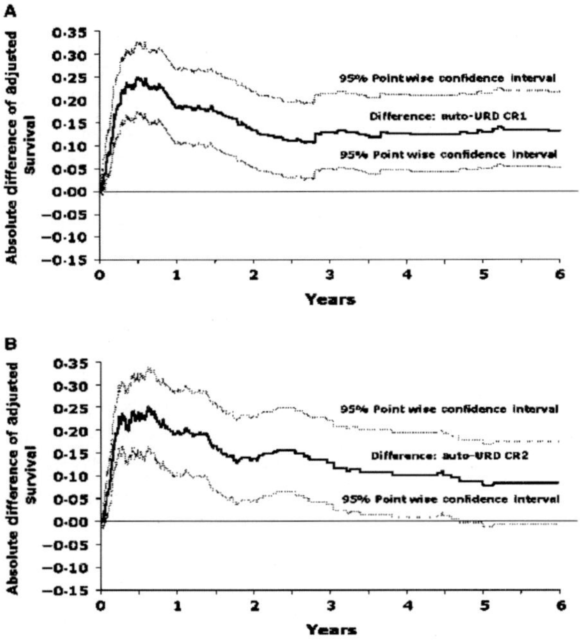

Fig. 4.3. Absolute difference of adjusted survival probabilities with 95% confidence interval (CI) for patients transplanted in (**A**) first (CR1) or (**B**) second complete remission (CR2) for acute myeloid leukemia (AML; Difference = Survival with autotransplant Survival with URD transplant) [88].

older patients, and patients with adverse cytogenetics to MUD-HSCT.

4.5 Investigational Agents in Relapsed and Refractory Acute Myeloid Leukemia

4.5.1 New Purine Analogs

Clofarabine (2-chloro-2′-fluoro-deoxy-9-β-D-arabinofuranosyladenine) is a newer second generation adenosine nucleoside analog with less toxicity than earlier described purine analogs [41]. The drug is highly resistant to cleavage by bacterial purine nucleoside phosphorylase and is resistant to deamination by adenosine deaminase (ADA). Clofarabine acts by inhibiting ribonucleotide reductase and DNA polymerase, depleting the amount of intracellular dNTPs available for DNA replication and also resulting in premature DNA chain termination. In a phase II trial in relapsed and refractory patients with AML and other hematologic malignancies, an overall response rate of 48% was achieved, including a CR rate of 32% [89]. In a subsequent phase I–II trial in relapsed and refractory leukemias, predominantly AML, clofarabine was combined with cytarabine in an effort to modulate cytarabine triphosphase accumulation [90]. The overall response rate was 38% with a CR rate of 22%. Dose-limiting toxicities include reversible hepatotoxicity and rash, but no neurotoxicity. Other cytotoxic agents have been introduced. Phase I/II trials with these novel agents have demonstrated some therapeutic efficacy and currently are under further investigation in combination regimens (Table 4.4). Troxacitabine is a novel L-nucleoside analog with activity in refractory AML both as a single agent as well as when combined with cytotoxic chemotherapy [91, 92].

4.6 Gemtuzumab Ozogamicin

Gemtuzumab ozogamicin (GO) (Mylotarg) is an immunoconjugate composed of an humanized and CD33 monoclonal antibody chemically linked to a potent cytotoxic antitumor antibiotic, calicheamicin [93]. The immunoconjugate is internalized into the leukemia cell expressing CD33 and the calicheamicin is liberated intracellularly after the acid environment of the cell results in hydrolysis of the chemical linker [94]. A compilation of three phase II trials show an overall response rate of approximately 30% (15% CR by conventional criteria and another 15% CRp defined as CR, but with incomplete recovery of the platelet count) among patients in first relapse who had a relatively favorable prognosis since they had a relatively long CR1 duration and could not have had secondary AML or AML which had evolved from an antecedent hematologic disorder [95].

These results led to the approval of GO by the US FDA for older adults in first relapse who are not candidates for intensive chemotherapy [96]. In a final analysis of 277 patients in first relapse treated with GO, 26% achieved remission (13% CR and 13% CRp) with a median recurrence-free survival of 6.4 months for patients who achieved CR [96, 97]. The unique toxicity veno-occlusive disease (VOD) or sinusoidal obstructive syndrome (SOS), has been observed rarely (<1%), but the incidence is higher among patients who undergo allo-HSCT within 3.5 months from exposure to GO [98, 99]. Given the limited effectiveness of this agent as monotherapy, phase II studies exploring combinations of GO with chemotherapy have been carried out. These trials showed encouraging results. Therefore, GO has

Table 4.4. Novel agents in relapsed/refractory AML

Agent	Class	Mechanism of action	Comments
Clofarabine	Nucleoside analogue	Inhibits RNR	CR in 18% in first salvage patient with short CR1 and 75% with long CR1, 38% and 50% in second or greater salvage Phase II trials as single agent or in combination with Ara-C, particularly in older adults underway [90, 91] Randomized trials of clofarabine compared to conventional chemotherapy are ongoing
Gemtuzumab ozogamicin	Immuno-conjugates	Antitumor Antibiotic Calicheamicin	OR 30% in older adults in late first relapse [93–97] Randomized trials of conventional chemotherapy +/– GO and as in vivo purge prior to autologous HSCT underway
Troxacitabine	Nucleoside analogue	Inhibits RNR	OR 18% in refractory AML, combination studies show anti-leukemia activity; causes unique hand–foot syndrome [91, 92]
Cloretazine	Alkylating agent	DNA damage	Very modest activity in relapsed AML with short CR1 duration Phase III trials underway evaluating chemotherapy +/– cloretazine [100, 101]
FLT3 inhibitor	Small molecule inhibitor	Inhibits TK	Reduction in blasts in blood and marrow, but rare CR Phase III trials evaluating chemotherapy +/– inhibitor planned [102]
SU5416	Small molecule inhibitor	Inhibits VEGF receptor	Modest clinical efficacy as a single agent [103]
FTI	Nonpeptidometric enzyme-specific linked inhibitor	Inhibits farnesyl protein transferase	Modest clinical activity, but with some CRs [104] Phase III trial in older adults in CR1 or any age in CR2 after consolidation as maintenance underway
Oblimersen	Antisense	Inhibits bcl-2	Can be combined with chemotherapy [105]
Decitabine	Nucleoside analog hypomethylating agent	Removes methyl groups from DNA	Induces some CRs [106]

CR, complete remission; ara-C, cytosine arabinoside; RNR, ribonucleotide reductase; FLT3, fms-like tyrosine kinase3: TK, tyrosine kinase; VEGF, vascular endothelial growth factor; OR, overall response; FTI, farnesyltransferase inhibitor.

been incorporated in ongoing randomized trials in untreated patients with AML evaluating its benefit when combined with induction chemotherapy and as an in vivo purging agent prior to autologous HSCT.

4.6.1 Novel Alkylating Agents

Cloretazine is a sulfonylhydrazine alkylating agent which has specificity for alkylation at the O^6 position of guanine distinguishing it from other alkylating agents [100, 101]. Very modest activity in high-risk relapsed AML patients (CR1 duration <6 months), has been demonstrated with a CR2 rate of 4% [101]. This agent may prove more effective when combined with other agents. In a phase I trial of patients with generally advanced AML of cloretazine combined with intermediate-dose ara-C, a CR rate of 10% and CRp rate of 15% were observed [100]. A prospective randomized trial for patients in first relapse comparing conventional chemotherapy with or without cloretazine is underway.

4.6.2 Targeted Agents

A myriad of other agents with novel mechanisms of action are now being investigated in patients with relapsed or refractory AML (Table 4.4). These include FLT3 inhibitors [102], receptor tyrosine kinase inhibitors such as SU5416 [103], farnesyltransferase inhibitors (FTI), which appear to interfere with Ras signaling, such as Zarnestra [104], apoptosis inhibitors such as the bcl-2 antisense oligonucleotide which down regulates bcl-2 [105], and methyltransferase inhibitors which induce hypomethylation of CpG-containing parts of the genome such as 5-aza-2-deoxycytidine (Decitabine) [106]. FLT3 inhibitors such as CEP-701 have quite modest antileukemic activity as single agents as demonstrated by reductions in peripheral blood and occasionally bone marrow blasts, but few, if any, patients achieve CR. Recent data suggest that combining these agents with cytotoxic chemotherapy may be a fruitful avenue of research to pursue [107, 108]. Stone and colleagues tested the FLT3 inhibitor PKC-412 combined with daunorubicin and ara-C in newly diagnosed patients. Ninety-one percent of patients with FLT3 mutations achieved CR compared to 53% of those without FLT3 mutations. In a trial of another FLT3 inhibitor, CEP-701 (Lestaurtinib), restricted to first relapse, there was a greater than 85% inhibition of FLT3 in the plasma in 76% of patients [107].

4.7 Relapsed and Refractory Acute Promyelocytic Leukemia

4.7.1 Introduction

Acute promyelocytic leukemia (APL) is the only subtype of adult AML in which treatment of relapsed and refractory disease is highly successful. Therefore, a separate discussion is warranted. Acute promyelocytic leukemia accounts for approximately 5–10% of patients with AML and is now highly curable in most patients. This subtype is characterized by unique genetic features including the t(15;17) (q22;q12–21) translocation and the formation of the PML-RARα fusion transcript. The t(15;17) translocation fuses the promyelocytic leukemia (PML) gene on chromosome 15 to the retinoic acid receptor (RARα) gene on chromosome 17 resulting in the chimeric gene encoding PML-RARα fusion protein. The fusion transcript-PML-RARα permits precise diagnosis and provides a marker for the identification of minimal residual disease [109–111].

4.7.2 Treatment of Relapsed and Refractory APL

The outcome of patients with APL has dramatically improved following the combined use of ATRA and anthracycline-based induction, anthracycline-based consolidation and maintenance, but relapse still occurs in 10–25% of the patients, generally those classified as high-risk based on the presenting high white blood cell (WBC) count requiring salvage therapy [112].

Arsenic trioxide is highly effective in patients with relapsed or refractory APL and has emerged as the standard therapy [113, 114]. Patients with an ATRA-free period longer than 12 months can be retreated with ATRA and many will achieve another CR [115]. Moreover, arsenic trioxide does not require the addition of anthracyclines, is well tolerated, and, most importantly, induces a high rate of molecular remission. Interestingly, Kwong and colleagues showed successful combination of arsenic trioxide with Idarubicin to induce molecular remission (MR) in eight relapsed APL patients [116] (Table 4.4); but combination of arsenic with ATRA has a limited role [117]. Monotherapy with GO in relapsed APL patients has also been effective [118], but its role is mainly reserved for patients who, for whatever reason, cannot receive arsenic trioxide therapy (discussed in detail below).

Once patients achieve CR2, the best postremission strategy is not known. There are few data addressing the duration of remission and PCR negativity with arsenic trioxide alone in patients with relapsed APL. One study of a small number of patients suggested that the DFS might be better when patients in a CR2 following arsenic trioxide therapy are treated with arsenic trioxide plus chemotherapy compared to arsenic trioxide alone (2/11 relapses versus 12/18 relapses; $P<0.01$, respectively) [119]. However, for the majority of patients, a sustained remission can best be induced with autologous HSCT. Therefore, patients should be considered for either autologous or allo-HSCT depending primarily on RT-PCR analysis for PML-RARα after at least two courses of arsenic trioxide prior to HSCT.

4.7.3 Studies with Arsenic Trioxide

Arsenic trioxide has shown substantial efficacy in treating both newly diagnosed and relapsed patients with APL. As a single agent, it induces prolonged CRs, with few adverse effects and minimal myelosuppression. Arsenic trioxide is a highly useful agent in relapsed APL and studies are underway to establish its role as initial therapy in combination with ATRA and anthracyclines.

Arsenic trioxide acts on APL cells through a variety of mechanisms, influencing numerous signal transduction pathways and resulting in a wide range of cellular effects. In vitro studies indicate that arsenic trioxide may exert two effects on APL cells; triggering apoptosis at relatively high concentrations (1.0–2.0 µmol/L) with collapse of mitochondrial transmembrane potentials in a thiol-dependent manner and inducing partial differentiation at low concentration (0.1–0.5 µmol/L) (Fig. 4.4) [120, 121].

In 1996, investigators in China reported that 73% of the 30 patients with previously untreated APL and 52% of 42 patients with relapsed or refractory disease achieved CR with arsenic trioxide [122]. Additional studies conducted in the USA and elsewhere confirmed that arsenic trioxide can induce CR in relapsed APL patients [116, 119, 123–125] (Table 4.5). In the US trial 11 of 12 patients with relapsed disease who received 12 to 39 days (median 33 days) of arsenic trioxide at a dose of 0.06–0.2 mg/kg of body weight achieved CR after extensive prior therapy [123]. Moreover, eight of these 11 patients in CR also tested negative molecularly by RT-PCR for the PML-RARα transcript. In a subsequent multicenter phase II trial 34 of 40 patients (85%) with relapsed or refractory disease who were treated with arsenic trioxide at a dose of 0.15 mg/kg/day achieved CR

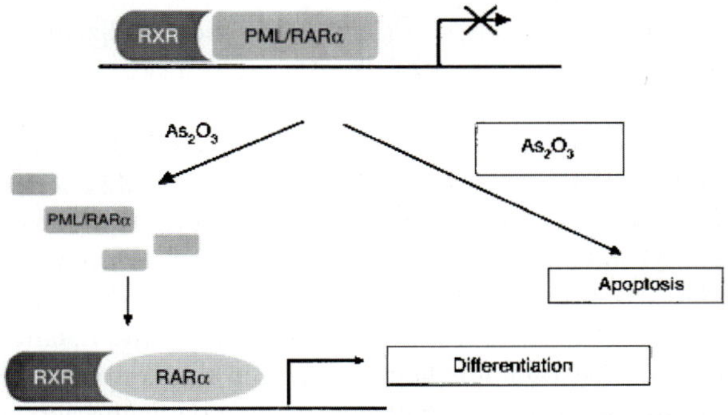

Fig. 4.4. At low concentrations, arsenic trioxide induces differentiation of malignant promyelocytes through degradation of the fusion protein PML-RARα; at high concentrations, arsenic trioxide induces apoptosis of malignant promyelocytes through PML-RARα-dependent and -independent mechanisms. PML, promyelocytic leukemia; RARα, retinoic acid receptor alpha; RXR, retinoic X receptor [33].

Table 4.5. Studies with arsenic trioxide in relapsed and refractory acute promyelocytic leukemia (APL)

Study	N	CR rate (%)	Comments
Zhang, et al. 1996 [122]	42	22 (52)	73% of the 30 previously untreated patients achieved CR
Shen, et al. 1997 [125]	10	9 (90)	Duration of As_2O_3 treatment for CR between 28 and 44 days (median, 38 days)
Soignet, et al. 1998 [123]	12	11 (92)	8 of 11 patients in CR also tested negative molecularly by RT-PCR for the PML-RARα transcript
Niu, et al. 1999 [119]	47	30 (85.1)	31 patients were treated with arsenic trioxide alone: CR rate 84% 11 patients with combination of arsenic trioxide and chemotherapy; CR rate 82% 5 patients with arsenic trioxide and ATRA: CR rate 100.0%
Soignet, et al. 2001 [124]	40	34 (85)	Using a 10-4 sensitivity level 78% of patients exhibited molecular conversion form positive to negative by RT-PCR for the PML-RARα transcript
Kwong, et al. 2001 [116]	8	8 (100)	All patients achieved morphological but not molecular remission after arsenic trioxide, but all patients attained molecular remission after subsequent idarubicin treatment

at a median of 53 days (range 28 to 35) [124]. An important observation was that 78% of patients exhibited molecular conversion from positive to negative by RT-PCR for the PML-RARα transcript. Patients who had failed multiple chemotherapy regimens and HSCT responded equally well. The 2-year RFS rate was 50%. Patients who achieved CR were able to tolerate subsequent HSCT.

Arsenic trioxide is well tolerated and has unique adverse reactions. These include leukocytosis and the APL differentiation syndrome (in 25% of patients), dizziness, hyperglycemia, musculoskeletal pain, and skin rash (in 20% of patients). The differentiation syndrome is similar to the retinoic acid syndrome and responds readily to dexamethasone. Neuropathy is generally mild and reversible. The most important toxicity is prolongation of the QT interval on the EKG, presenting a risk of ventricular arrhythmias. The EKG and electrolytes should be monitored at frequent intervals. Potassium and magnesium levels should be kept well within the normal limit range, because hypokalemia and hypomagnesaemia may contribute to the QT prolongation and predispose to ventricular arrhythmias. Other medications which may prolong the QT interval by inducing hypokalemia, such as amphotericin and diuretics, should be avoided. In the clinical trials reported from China, severe hepatotoxicity, sometimes fatal, has been observed. However, in clinical trials in other countries hepatic toxicity has not been a significant problem [119, 122, 124].

4.7.4 Studies with Hematopoietic Stem Cell Transplantation in Relapsed Acute Promyelocytic Leukemia

Once a patient has achieved CR2, it is appropriate to consider transplantation. The result of autologous HSCT in CR2 depends on the presence of minimal residual disease established by molecular techniques in the collected stem cells prior to transplantation [126]. In contrast, molecular remission at the time of allo-HSCT may be less important. Allogeneic HSCT is also capable of producing long-term remissions in patients who have achieved a second CR, although high rates of treatment-related and nonrelapse mortality have been problematic. In one series, for example, treatment-related mortality was 39%, while nonrelapse mortality was 32% in another [127]. However in both studies, only three of 12 PCR-positive patients relapsed following allogeneic HSCT.

Meloni and colleagues have reported that RT-PCR negativity at the 10^{-4} level seems to be associated with a favorable posttransplant outcome [126]. These investigators reported a very small study of 15 consecutive patients with relapsed APL who underwent autologous HSCT with unpurged marrow. Thirteen patients received anthracycline-based chemotherapy as initial treatment, and two were treated by combined ATRA and idarubicin. All patients received three cycles of consolidation therapy. The CR1 duration ranged from 6 to 40 months. Second CR was achieved in all patients with oral ATRA. All but three patients received consolidation therapy with intravenous cytarabine at 1 g/m^2 days 1 through 4 and intravenous mitoxantrone at 6 mg/m^2 days 1 through 4. In this study, six (45%) of the 15 patients remain alive and well and in molecular remission. All seven patients who underwent autologous HSCT with persistent PCR-detectable MRD in the transfused cells relapsed within 9 months after transplant, which confirms the value of PCR positivity during remission as a predictor of relapse in APL. Only one of eight patients with a negative PCR relapsed, and one developed secondary leukemia.

In a recent study by European Acute Promyelocytic Leukemia Group, the outcome of 73 relapsed APL patients, initially treated with ATRA and chemotherapy and received auto or allo-HSCT after achievement of hematological CR2, was retrospectively analyzed [127] (Table 4.5). RT-PCR analysis was performed before auto or allo-HSCT in 53% of the patients undergoing transplantation, including 30 of the 50 autologous HSCT patients and nine of the 23 allogeneic HSCT patients. None of the patients received arsenic trioxide as salvage chemotherapy. The outcome among those patients undergoing allogeneic HSCT was less favorable, due mainly to high incidence of TRM (Fig. 4.5). However, patients with persistently molecularly positive disease had fewer relapses following allogeneic HSCT when compared to autologous HSCT.

Sanz and colleagues [128] on behalf of the EBMT have also reported an OS, LFS, relapse rate and TRM for patients in CR1 undergoing allogeneic HSCT of 77%, 70%, 15%, and 20%, respectively, and for autologous HSCT, 73%, 70%, 24%, and 12%, respectively. For patients in CR2, the results for allogeneic HSCT were 58%, 57%, 15%, and 33%, respectively compared to 40%, 45%, 44%, and 25%, for autologous HSCT. These

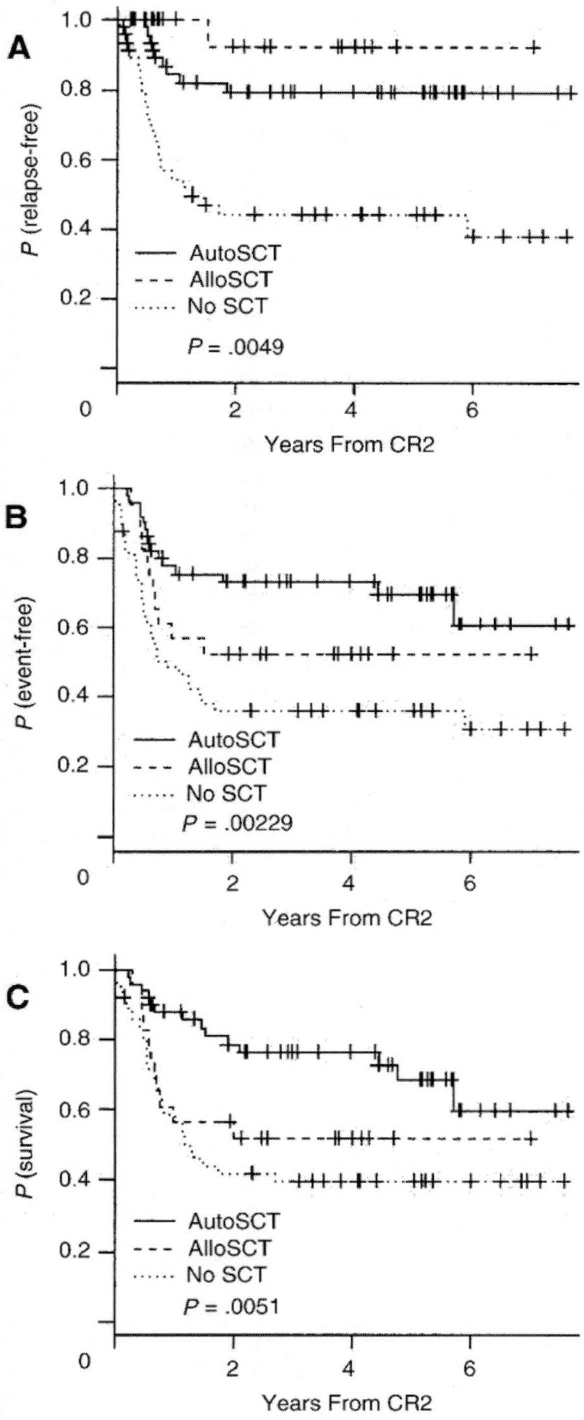

Fig. 4.5. Outcome of the 122 APL patients in second hematological complete remission according to postremission therapy. (**A**) Relapse-free survival; (**B**) event-free survival; (**C**) overall survival [127].

studies demonstrate that patients with negative PCR after achieving CR2 will fare well with autologous HSCT and patients with positive PCR should not routinely be offered an autologous HSCT.

4.7.5 Gemtuzumab Ozogamicin in Relapsed Acute Promyelocytic Leukemia

Gemtuzumab ozogamicin offers a highly attractive approach for treatment of APL for several reasons. Firstly, compared to other AML subtypes, CD33 antigen is detectable in virtually all cells with a highly homogeneous expression pattern [129, 130]. Secondly, P-gp, a mediator of MDR which acts as an efflux pump to extrude chemotherapy, is minimally expressed on APL blasts, which accounts for the striking sensitivity of APL to anti-CD33 strategies [131]. Finally, calicheamicin is a potent intercalator, similar to anthracyclines, which are known to be highly effective in APL [132].

GO monotherapy in molecularly relapsed APL has been well tolerated and is effective [118, 133]. Lo Cocco and colleagues [118] demonstrated this in 16 such patients. All patients were treated with two doses of GO (6 mg/m^2), and a third dose was given to patients who tested negative for PML-RARα fusion transcript. Molecular response was obtained in nine (91%) of 11 patients after two doses and in 13 (100%) of 13 patients after the third dose. Of the three remaining patients, one patient developed hepatic toxicity after a single dose of GO and therefore received no further therapy, and remaining two patients progressed while on treatment. Quantitative RT-PCR demonstrated that patients who responded had a dramatic decline (at least 2 logs) of the PML-RARα transcript following first GO dose. Of 14 responders, seven remained in sustained molecular remission for a median of 15 months (range, 7 to 31 months) while seven relapsed at 3–15 months later. GO was readministered in two patients in relapse, and both achieved a molecular remission. Since a high proportion of patients relapsed, the authors suggested that patients should be given further treatment (consolidation/maintenance) after achieving molecular remission to improve long-term outcome.

4.7.6 Central Nervous System (CNS) Relapse in Acute Promyelocytic Leukemia

Extramedullary disease (EMD) occurs in approximately 5–10% of adults with AML, most commonly in the myelomonocytic, monocytic, and possibly high-risk APL subtypes [134–136]. Over the last few decades, the incidence of EMD in APL appears to have been increased possibly due to more long-term survivors. Several investigators have attributed an increased incidence of CNS relapse to ATRA exposure and suggested that ATRA induces neural adhesion molecules such as CD11c, CD13, and CD56 facilitating CNS infiltration by APL cells [129, 137, 138]. However, the Italian cooperative group GIMEMA found that APL patients receiving ATRA do not have an increased risk of developing extramedullary relapse as compared with those treated with chemotherapy alone [139]. Since relapses in the auditory canal are noteworthy and rarely reported previously [140] it is quite possible that ATRA itself may contribute to these extramedullary relapses or that the therapeutic concentration of ATRA may not reach leukemia cells in these sanctuaries. Whether or not ATRA plays a role in the development of EMD remains a matter for further study.

4.7.7 Treatment of CNS Relapse

Treatment of CNS relapse likely is best treated with systemic reinduction with arsenic trioxide or another systemic approach along with multiple courses of intrathecal methotrexate possibly alternating with ara-C until the spinal fluid is free of leukemic cells. Then autologous HSCT can be considered if molecularly negative cells can be harvested. Mobilization with intermediate-dose ara-C or HiDAC, depending on the age of the patient, has the advantage of providing additional treatment of CNS disease. To date, there is no specific risk factor identified to predict CNS relapse. However, relapse appears to occur more frequently among younger patients, in patients with WBC counts ≥10 000/mm^3, and patients with the bcr-3 (short isoform) PML-RARα breakpoint [141]. Whether CNS prophylaxis by intrathecal chemotherapy and/or systemic HiDAC should be routinely performed in patients with any these risk factors, particularly patients with a WBC ≥10 000/mm^3 remains to be established. Two recent studies have suggested that intermediate-dose ara-C or HiDAC either in induction or in consolidation may decrease the risk of CNS relapse [142, 143].

4.7.8 Strategies to Detect Early Relapse in AML

Current remission criteria have low sensitivity to detect minimal residual disease (MRD). Therefore, there is interest in investigating more sensitive methods such as cytogenetics, flow cytometry, and RT-PCR. These methods when combined with morphological remission criteria may decrease relapses, provide insight into the clinical efficacy of different therapeutic strategies and could improve overall prognostic stratification in AML patients. Marcucci and colleagues [13] evaluated 118 AML patients with abnormal cytogenetics at diagnosis. Patients converting to normal cytogenetics at CR1 (NCR1; n = 103) were compared with those with abnormal cytogenetics both at diagnosis and at CR1 (ACR1; n = 15). ACR1 patients had significantly shorter OS (P = 0.006) and DFS (P = 0.0001), and higher cumulative incidence of relapse (CIR) (P = 0.0001). In multivariable models, the NCR1 and ACR1 groups were predictors for OS (P = 0.03), DFS (P = 0.02), and CIR (P = 0.05) (Fig. 4.6). The relative risk of relapse or death was 2.1 times higher for ACR1 patients than for NCR1 patients (95% CI, 1.1–3.9). Notably, there was no significant difference in time of attaining CR1 between the NCR1 and ACR1 groups. At 3 years, all patients in the ACR1 group had relapsed compared to 61% in the NCR1 group.

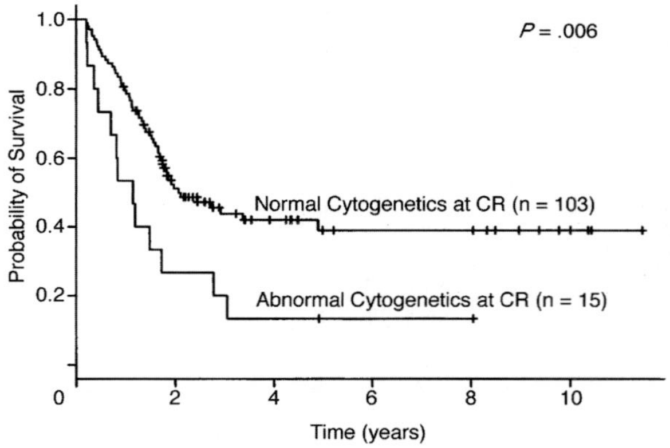

Fig. 4.6. Overall survival according to the presence or absence of cytogenetic abnormalities on the first day of complete (CR) following induction chemotherapy in acute myeloid leukemia patients with abnormal cytogenetics at diagnosis [13].

The ability of immunophenotyping, using 4-color FACS technology, to identify a leukemia-associated phenotype (LAP) has significantly increased the sensitivity of MRD detection in patients with AML. An Italian study by Buccisano and colleague [144] used this technique to evaluate MRD at two time points, at the end of induction and following consolidation, in a total of 92 patients. The threshold discriminating MRD- from MRD+ cases was set at $3.5\times10(-4)$ residual leukemic cells. The results showed that the MRD status at the end of consolidation was the most significant predictor of outcome with 5-year actuarial probability of RFS and OS at 5 years of 71% and 64%, respectively, for MRD– patients, compared to 13% and 16%, respectively, for those in the MRD+ patients. Interestingly, the majority of patients with MRD+ status at the end of consolidation relapsed following autologous HSCT.

Controversy exists as to the prognostic significance of FMS-like receptor tyrosine kinase (FLT3) mutations. Although the exact mechanism by which FLT3 mutation exerts increased relapse risk remains to be defined, it appears to relate to an increased regrowth potential caused by a cytokine-independent phenotype rather than resistance to conventional chemotherapy, making it another possible therapeutic target. Recent data from Del Poeta and colleagues [145] suggest that the bax/bcl-2 ratio is a predictor of both OS and time to relapse. However, the value of this index in risk stratifying AML patients remains to be defined. In patients with APL, more sensitive techniques such as RT-PCR to detect PML-RAR*α* transcript, especially when rises in transcript quantity are seen serially, correlate with increased probability of hematological relapse [110] and such data are now used to identify patients who require early salvage therapy with arsenic trioxide and subsequent HSCT. All these approaches are of value in detecting patients at a high risk of relapse in whom early intervention could be justified.

4.8 Summary

The treatment of patients with relapsed or refractory AML is generally disappointing and remains a major challenge. Depending on a number of prognostic factors, particularly the duration of CR1, many patients can achieve a CR2 with salvage chemotherapy. However, most of such patients are unlikely to be cured without some form of allogeneic HSCT. Many new antileukemic agents with a variety of novel mechanisms of action are now available and are undergoing rigorous study in the context of clinical trials as single agents and in combination with chemotherapy. Many of these new agents are directed towards specific genetic mutations, which may perturb specific signal transduction pathways upon which leukemia cells depend for growth and proliferation. New transplant strategies hold promise to provide more patients with the potentially potent GVL effect. Future directions include the identification of more sensitive prognostic factors, the development of therapy, directed at specific molecular targets based on the biology of the specific subtype of AML, the identification of more sophisticated and sensitive methods to detect MRD, the exploitation of GVL with RIC allo-HSCT and alternative donors. Gene expression profiling will likely facilitate the identification and classification of specific genetic subtypes of AML and direct future therapy [146].

References

1. Hiddemann W, Martin WR, Sauerland CM, et al. (1990) Definition of refractoriness against conventional chemotherapy in acute myeloid leukemia: A proposal based on the results of retreatment by thioguanine, cytosine arabinoside, and daunorubicin (TAD 9) in 150 patients with relapse after standardized first line therapy. Leukemia 4(3):184–188
2. Slovak ML, Kopecky KJ, Cassileth PA, et al. (2000) Karyotypic analysis predicts outcome of preremission and postremission therapy in adult acute myeloid leukemia: A Southwest Oncology Group/Eastern Cooperative Oncology Group Study. Blood 96(13):4075–4083
3. Buchner T, Hiddemann W, Berdel WE, et al. (2003) 6-Thioguanine, cytarabine, and daunorubicin (TAD) and high-dose cytarabine and mitoxantrone (HAM) for induction, TAD for consolidation, and either prolonged maintenance by reduced monthly TAD or TAD-HAM-TAD and one course of intensive consolidation by sequential HAM in adult patients at all ages with de novo acute myeloid leukemia (AML): A randomized trial of the German AML Cooperative Group. J Clin Oncol 21(24):4496–4504
4. Moore JO, George SL, Dodge RK, et al. (2005) Sequential multiagent chemotherapy is not superior to high-dose cytarabine alone as postremission intensification therapy for acute myeloid leukemia in adults under 60 years of age: Cancer and Leukemia Group B Study 9222. Blood 105(9):3420–3427
5. Rowe JM, Neuberg D, Friedenberg W, et al. (2004) A phase 3 study of three induction regimens and of priming with GM-CSF in older adults with acute myeloid leukemia: A trial by the Eastern Cooperative Oncology Group. Blood 103(2):479–485
6. Goldstone AH, Burnett AK, Wheatley K, et al. (2001) Attempts to improve treatment outcomes in acute myeloid leukemia (AML) in

older patients: The results of the United Kingdom Medical Research Council AML11 trial. Blood 98(5):1302–1311
7. Lee S, Tallman MS, Oken MM, et al. (2000) Duration of second complete remission compared with first complete remission in patients with acute myeloid leukemia. Eastern Cooperative Oncology Group. Leukemia 14(8):1345–1348
8. Estey EH (2000) Treatment of relapsed and refractory acute myelogenous leukemia. Leukemia 14(3):476–479
9. Keating MJ, Kantarjian H, Smith TL, et al. (1989) Response to salvage therapy and survival after relapse in acute myelogenous leukemia. J Clin Oncol 7(8):1071–1080
10. Breems DA, Van Putten WL, Huijgens PC, et al. (2005) Prognostic index for adult patients with acute myeloid leukemia in first relapse. J Clin Oncol 23(9):1969–1978
11. Giles F, Verstovsek S, Garcia-Manero G, et al. (2006) Validation of the European Prognostic Index for younger adult patients with acute myeloid leukaemia in first relapse. Br J Haematol 134(1):58–60
12. Lo Coco F, Diverio D, Avvisati G, et al. (1999) Therapy of molecular relapse in acute promyelocytic leukemia. Blood 94(7):2225–2229
13. Marcucci G, Mrozek K, Ruppert AS, et al. (2004) Abnormal cytogenetics at date of morphologic complete remission predicts short overall and disease-free survival, and higher relapse rate in adult acute myeloid leukemia: Results from cancer and leukemia group B study 8461. J Clin Oncol 22(12):2410–2418
14. Sternberg DW, Aird W, Neuberg D, et al. (2000) Treatment of patients with recurrent and primary refractory acute myelogenous leukemia using mitoxantrone and intermediate-dose cytarabine: A pharmacologically based regimen. Cancer 88(9):2037–2041
15. Kern W, Aul C, Maschmeyer G, et al. (1998) Superiority of high-dose over intermediate-dose cytosine arabinoside in the treatment of patients with high-risk acute myeloid leukemia: Results of an age-adjusted prospective randomized comparison. Leukemia 12(7):1049–1055
16. Rees JK, Gray RG, Swirsky D, et al. (1986) Principal results of the Medical Research Council's 8th acute myeloid leukaemia trial. Lancet 2(8518):1236–1241
17. Appelbaum FR, Rowe JM, Radich J, et al. (2001) Acute myeloid leukemia hematology. Am Soc Hematol Educ Program, pp 62–86
18. Burnett AK, Mohite U (2006) Treatment of older patients with acute myeloid leukemia—New agents. Semin Hematol 43(2): 96–106
19. Estey E, Plunkett W, Gandhi V, et al. (1993) Fludarabine and arabinosylcytosine therapy of refractory and relapsed acute myelogenous leukemia. Leuk Lymphoma 9(4–5):343–350
20. Thalhammer F, Geissler K, Jager U, et al. (1996) Duration of second complete remission in patients with acute myeloid leukemia treated with chemotherapy: A retrospective single-center study. Ann Hematol 72(4):216–222
21. Estey E (1996) Treatment of refractory AML. Leukemia 10(6):932–936
22. Appelbaum FR, Gundacker H, Head DR, et al. (2006) Age and acute myeloid leukemia. Blood 107(9):3481–3485
23. Kantarjian HM, Keating MJ, Walters RS, et al. (1988) The characteristics and outcome of patients with late relapse acute myelogenous leukemia. J Clin Oncol 6(2):232–238
24. Wheatley K, Burnett AK, Goldstone AH, et al. (1999) A simple, robust, validated and highly predictive index for the determination of risk-directed therapy in acute myeloid leukaemia derived from the MRC AML 10 trial. United Kingdom Medical Research Council's Adult and Childhood Leukaemia Working Parties. Br J Haematol 107(1):69–79
25. Kern W, Haferlach T, Schoch C, et al. (2003) Early blast clearance by remission induction therapy is a major independent prognostic factor for both achievement of complete remission and long-term outcome in acute myeloid leukemia: Data from the German AML Cooperative Group (AMLCG) 1992 Trial. Blood 101(1):64–70
26. Weltermann A, Fonatsch C, Haas OA, et al. (2004) Impact of cytogenetics on the prognosis of adults with de novo AML in first relapse. Leukemia 18(2):293–302
27. Kern W, Haferlach T, Schnittger S, et al. (2002) Karyotype instability between diagnosis and relapse in 117 patients with acute myeloid leukemia: Implications for resistance against therapy. Leukemia 16(10):2084–2091
28. Estey E, Keating MJ, Pierce S, et al. (1995) Change in karyotype between diagnosis and first relapse in acute myelogenous leukemia. Leukemia 9(6):972–976
29. Anderlini P, Luna M, Kantarjian HM, et al. (1996) Causes of initial remission induction failure in patients with acute myeloid leukemia and myelodysplastic syndromes. Leukemia 10(4):600–608
30. Glasmacher A, Prentice A, Gorschluter M, et al. (2003) Itraconazole prevents invasive fungal infections in neutropenic patients treated for hematologic malignancies: Evidence from a meta-analysis of 3597 patients. J Clin Oncol 21(24):4615–4626
31. Mengis C, Aebi S, Tobler A, et al. (2003) Assessment of differences in patient populations selected for excluded from participation in clinical phase III acute myelogenous leukemia trials. J Clin Oncol 21(21):3933–3939
32. van Prooijen HC, Dekker AW, Punt K (1984) The use of intermediate dose cytosine arabinoside (ID Ara-C) in the treatment of acute non-lymphocytic leukaemia in relapse. Br J Haematol 57(2):291–299
33. Herzig RH, Lazarus HM, Wolff SN, et al. (1985) High-dose cytosine arabinoside therapy with and without anthracycline antibiotics for remission reinduction of acute nonlymphoblastic leukemia. J Clin Oncol 3(7):992–997
34. Capizzi RL, Powell BL (1987) Sequential high-dose ara-C and asparaginase versus high-dose ara-C alone in the treatment of patients with relapsed and refractory acute leukemias. Semin Oncol 14(2 Suppl 1):40–50
35. Capizzi RL, Davis R, Powell B, et al. (1988) Synergy between high-dose cytarabine and asparaginase in the treatment of adults with refractory and relapsed acute myelogenous leukemia—A Cancer and Leukemia Group B Study. J Clin Oncol 6(3):499–508
36. Carella AM, Carlier P, Pungolino E, et al. (1993) Idarubicin in combination with intermediate-dose cytarabine and VP-16 in the treatment of refractory or rapidly relapsed patients with acute myeloid leukemia. The GIMEMA Cooperative Group. Leukemia 7(2):196–199
37. Karanes C, Kopecky KJ, Head DR, et al. (1999) A phase III comparison of high dose ARA-C (HIDAC) versus HIDAC plus mitoxantrone in the treatment of first relapsed or refractory acute myeloid leukemia Southwest Oncology Group Study. Leuk Res 23(9):787–794
38. Tavernier E, Le QH, Elhamri M, et al. (2003) Salvage therapy in refractory acute myeloid leukemia: Prediction of outcome based on analysis of prognostic factors. Leuk Res 27(3):205–214

39. Vogler WR, McCarley DL, Stagg M, et al. (1994) A phase III trial of high-dose cytosine arabinoside with or without etoposide in relapsed and refractory acute myelogenous leukemia. A Southeastern Cancer Study Group trial. Leukemia 8(11):1847–1853
40. Daenen S, Lowenberg B, Sonneveld P, et al. (1994) Efficacy of etoposide and mitoxantrone in patients with acute myelogenous leukemia refractory to standard induction therapy and intermediate-dose cytarabine with amsidine. Dutch Hematology-Oncology Working Group for Adults (HOVON). Leukemia 8(1):6–10
41. Gandhi V, Estey E, Keating MJ, et al. (1996) Chlorodeoxyadenosine and arabinosylcytosine in patients with acute myelogenous leukemia: Pharmacokinetic, pharmacodynamic, and molecular interactions. Blood 87(1):256–264
42. Kornblau SM, Gandhi V, Andreeff HM, et al. (1996) Clinical and laboratory studies of 2-chlorodeoxyadenosine +/− cytosine arabinoside for relapsed or refractory acute myelogenous leukemia in adults. Leukemia 10(10):1563–1569
43. Lee EJ, George SL, Amrein PC, et al. (1998) An evaluation of combinations of diaziquone, etoposide and mitoxantrone in the treatment of adults with relapsed or refractory acute myeloid leukemia: Results of 8722, a randomized phase II study conducted by Cancer and Leukemia Group B. Leukemia 12(2): 139–143
44. Robak T, Wrzesien-Kus A, Lech-Maranda E, et al. (2000) Combination regimen of cladribine (2-chlorodeoxyadenosine), cytarabine and G-CSF (CLAG) as induction therapy for patients with relapsed or refractory acute myeloid leukemia. Leuk Lymphoma 39(1–2):121–129
45. List AF, Kopecky KJ, Willman CL, et al. (2001) Benefit of cyclosporine modulation of drug resistance in patients with poor-risk acute myeloid leukemia: A Southwest Oncology Group study. Blood 98(12):3212–3220
46. Yin J, Wheatley K, Rees JK, et al. (2001) Comparison of "sequential" versus "standard" chemotherapy as re-induction treatment, with or without cyclosporine, in refractory/relapsed acute myeloid leukaemia (AML): Results of the UK Medical Research Council AML-R trial. Br J Haematol 122:164–165
47. Advani R, Saba HI, Tallman MS, et al. (1999) Treatment of refractory and relapsed acute myelogenous leukemia with combination chemotherapy plus the multidrug resistance modulator PSC 833 (Valspodar). Blood 93(3):787–795
48. Greenberg PL, Lee SJ, Advani R, et al. (2004) Mitoxantrone, etoposide, and cytarabine with or without valspodar in patients with relapsed or refractory acute myeloid leukemia and high-risk myelodysplastic syndrome: A phase III trial (E2995). J Clin Oncol 22(6):1078–1086
49. Dantzig AH, Shepard RL, Cao J, et al. (1996) Reversal of P-glycoprotein-mediated multidrug resistance by a potent cyclopropyldibenzosuberane modulator, LY335979. Cancer Res 56(18): 4171–4179
50. Tsimberidou A, Cortes J, Thomas D, et al. (2003) Gemtuzumab ozogamicin, fludarabine, cytarabine and cyclosporine combination regimen in patients with CD33+ primary resistant or relapsed acute myeloid leukemia. Leuk Res 27(10):893–897
51. Apostolidou E, Cortes J, Tsimberidou A, et al. (2003) Pilot study of gemtuzumab ozogamicin, liposomal daunorubicin, cytarabine and cyclosporine regimen in patients with refractory acute myelogenous leukemia. Leuk Res 27(10):887–891
52. Gale RP, Horowitz MM, Rees JK, et al. (1996) Chemotherapy versus transplants for acute myelogenous leukemia in second remission. Leukemia 10(1):13–19
53. Clift RA, Buckner CD, Appelbaum FR, et al. (1992) Allogeneic marrow transplantation during untreated first relapse of acute myeloid leukemia. J Clin Oncol 10(11):1723–1729
54. Appelbaum FR, Clift RA, Buckner CD, et al. (1983) Allogeneic marrow transplantation for acute nonlymphoblastic leukemia after first relapse. Blood 61(5):949–953
55. Reiffers J (2000) In: Atkinson K (ed) Clinical bone marrow and blood stem cell transplantation. Cambridge University Press, Cambridge, pp 433–445
56. Byrne JL, Dasgupta E, Pallis M, et al. (1999) Early allogeneic transplantation for refractory or relapsed acute leukaemia following remission induction with FLAG. Leukemia 13(5):786–791
57. Matthews DC, Appelbaum FR, Eary JF, et al. (1995) Development of a marrow transplant regimen for acute leukemia using targeted hematopoietic irradiation delivered by 131I-labeled anti-CD45 antibody, combined with cyclophosphamide and total body irradiation. Blood 85(4):1122–1131
58. Matthews D, Appelbaum FR, Eary JF, et al. (1999) Phase I Study of (131) I-anti-CD45 antibody plus cyclophosphamide and total body irradiation for advanced acute leukemia and myelodysplastic syndrome. Blood 94:1237–1247
59. Choi SJ, Lee JH, Lee JH, et al. (2004) Treatment of relapsed acute myeloid leukemia after allogeneic bone marrow transplantation with chemotherapy followed by G-CSF-primed donor leukocyte infusion: A high incidence of isolated extramedullary relapse. Leukemia 18(11):1789–1797
60. Seo S, Kami M, Honda H, et al. (2000) Extramedullary relapse in the so-called "sanctuary" sites for chemotherapy after donor lymphocyte infusion. Bone Marrow Transplant 25(2):226–227
61. Porter DL (2003) Donor leukocyte infusions in acute myelogenous leukemia. Leukemia 17(6):1035–1037
62. Bosi A, Bacci S, Miniero R, et al. (1997) Second allogeneic bone marrow transplantation in acute leukemia: A multicenter study from the Gruppo Italiano Trapianto Di Midollo Osseo (GITMO). Leukemia 11(3):420–424
63. Eapen M, Giralt SA, Horowitz MM, et al. (2004) Second transplant for acute and chronic leukemia relapsing after first HLA-identical sibling transplant. Bone Marrow Transplant 34(8):721–727
64. Barker JN, Weisdorf DJ, DeFor TE, et al. (2003) Rapid and complete donor chimerism in adult recipients of unrelated donor umbilical cord blood transplantation after reduced-intensity conditioning. Blood 102(5):1915–1919
65. Rocha V, Labopin M, Sanz G, et al. (2004) Transplants of umbilical-cord blood or bone marrow from unrelated donors in adults with acute leukemia. N Engl J Med 351(22):2276–2285
66. Majhail NS, Brunstein CG, Wagner JE (2006) Double umbilical cord blood transplantation. Curr Opin Immunol 18(5):571–575
67. Sierra J, Storer B, Hansen JA, et al. (1997) Transplantation of marrow cells from unrelated donors for treatment of high-risk acute leukemia: The effect of leukemic burden, donor HLA-matching, and marrow cell dose. Blood 89(11):4226–4235
68. Forman SJ, Schmidt GM, Nademanee AP, et al. (1991) Allogeneic bone marrow transplantation as therapy for primary induction failure for patients with acute leukemia. J Clin Oncol 9(9):1570–1574

69. Biggs JC, Horowitz MM, Gale RP, et al. (1992) Bone marrow transplants may cure patients with acute leukemia never achieving remission with chemotherapy. Blood 80(4):1090–1093
70. Cook G, Clark RE, Crawley C, et al. (2006) The outcome of sibling and unrelated donor allogeneic stem cell transplantation in adult patients with acute myeloid leukemia in first remission who were initially refractory to first induction chemotherapy. Biol Blood Marrow Transplant 12(3):293–300
71. Henslee-Downey PJ, Abhyankar SH, Parrish RS, et al. (1997) Use of partially mismatched related donors extends access to allogeneic marrow transplant. Blood 89(10):3864–3872
72. Singhal S, Powles R, Henslee-Downey PJ, et al. (2002) Allogeneic transplantation from HLA-matched sibling or partially HLA-mismatched related donors for primary refractory acute leukemia. Bone Marrow Transplant 29(4):291–295
73. Aversa F, Terenzi A, Felicini R, et al. (2002) Haploidentical stem cell transplantation for acute leukemia. Int J Hematol 76 (Suppl 1): 165–168
74. Singhal S, Henslee-Downey PJ, Powles R, et al. (2003) Haploidentical vs autologous hematopoietic stem cell transplantation in patients with acute leukemia beyond first remission. Bone Marrow Transplant 31(10):889–895
75. Spitzer TR (2005) Haploidentical stem cell transplantation: The always present but overlooked donor. Hematology (Am Soc Hematol Educ Program), pp 390–395
76. Gorin NC, Labopin M, Boiron JM, et al. (2006) Results of genoidentical hemopoietic stem cell transplantation with reduced intensity conditioning for acute myelocytic leukemia: Higher doses of stem cells infused benefit patients receiving transplants in second remission or beyond – The Acute Leukemia Working Party of the European Cooperative Group for Blood and Marrow Transplantation. J Clin Oncol 24(24):3959–3966
77. de Lima M, Anagnostopoulos A, Munsell M, et al. (2004) Nonablative versus reduced-intensity conditioning regimens in the treatment of acute myeloid leukemia and high-risk myelodysplastic syndrome: Dose is relevant for long-term disease control after allogeneic hematopoietic stem cell transplantation. Blood 104(3): 865–872
78. Sayer HG, Kroger M, Beyer J, et al. (2003) Reduced intensity conditioning for allogeneic hematopoietic stem cell transplantation in patients with acute myeloid leukemia: Disease status by marrow blasts is the strongest prognostic factor. Bone Marrow Transplant 31(12):1089–1095
79. Dey BR, McAfee S, Colby C, et al. (2003) Impact of prophylactic donor leukocyte infusions on mixed chimerism, graft-versus-host disease, and antitumor response in patients with advanced hematologic malignancies treated with nonmyeloablative conditioning and allogeneic bone marrow transplantation. Biol Blood Marrow Transplant 9(5):320–329
80. Hegenbart U, Niederwieser D, Sandmaier BM, et al. (2006) Treatment for acute myelogenous leukemia by low-dose, total-body, irradiation-based conditioning and hematopoietic cell transplantation from related and unrelated donors. J Clin Oncol 24(3):444–453
81. Ermann J, Hoffmann P, Edinger M, et al. (2005) Only the CD62L+ subpopulation of CD4+CD25+ regulatory T cells protects from lethal acute GVHD. Blood 105(5):2220–2226
82. Spitzer TR, McAfee SL, Dey BR, et al. (2003) Nonmyeloablative haploidentical stem-cell transplantation using anti-CD2 monoclonal antibody (MEDI-507)-based conditioning for refractory hematologic malignancies. Transplantation 75(10):1748–1751
83. Ogawa H, Ikegame K, Kawakami M, et al. (2004) Powerful graft-versus-leukemia effects exerted by HLA-haploidentical grafts engrafted with a reduced-intensity regimen for relapse following myeloablative HLA-matched transplantation. Transplantation 78(3):488–489
84. Gorin NC, Labopin M, Meloni G, et al. (1991) Autologous bone marrow transplantation for acute myeloblastic leukemia in Europe: Further evidence of the role of marrow purging by mafosfamide. European Co-operative Group for Bone Marrow Transplantation (EBMT). Leukemia 5(10):896–904
85. Gorin NC, Labopin M, Fouillard L, et al. (1996) Retrospective evaluation of autologous bone marrow transplantation vs allogeneic bone marrow transplantation from an HLA identical related donor in acute myelocytic leukemia. A study of the European Cooperative Group for Blood and Marrow Transplantation (EBMT). Bone Marrow Transplant 18(1):111–117
86. Burnett AK, Hills R, Goldstone AH, et al. (2004) The impact of transplant in AML in 2nd CR: A prospective study of 741 in the MRC AML 10 and 12 trials. Blood 104:179a (abstr)
87. Ringden O, Labopin M, Gorin NC, et al. (2000) The dismal outcome in patients with acute leukaemia who relapse after an autograft is improved if a second autograft or a matched allograft is performed. Acute Leukaemia Working Party of the European Group for Blood and Marrow Transplantation (EBMT). Bone Marrow Transplant 25(10):1053–1058
88. Lazarus HM, Perez WS, Klein JP, et al. (2006) Autotransplantation versus HLA-matched unrelated donor transplantation for acute myeloid leukaemia: A retrospective analysis from the Center for International Blood and Marrow Transplant Research. Br J Haematol 132(6):755–769
89. Kantarjian H, Gandhi V, Cortes J, et al. (2003) Phase 2 clinical and pharmacologic study of clofarabine in patients with refractory or relapsed acute leukemia. Blood 102(7):2379–2386
90. Faderl S, Verstovsek S, Cortes J, et al. (2006) Clofarabine and cytarabine combination as induction therapy for acute myeloid leukemia (AML) in patients 50 years of age or older. Blood 108(1):45–51
91. Giles FJ, Garcia-Manero G, Cortes JE, et al. (2002) Phase II study of troxacitabine, a novel dioxolane nucleoside analog, in patients with refractory leukemia. J Clin Oncol 20(3):656–664
92. Giles FJ, Faderl S, Thomas DA, et al. (2003) Randomized phase I/II study of troxacitabine combined with cytarabine, idarubicin, or topotecan in patients with refractory myeloid leukemias. J Clin Oncol 21(6):1050–1056
93. Sievers EL, Appelbaum FR, Spielberger RT, et al. (1999) Selective ablation of acute myeloid leukemia using antibody-targeted chemotherapy: A phase I study of an anti-CD33 calicheamicin immunoconjugate. Blood 93(11):3678–3684
94. van Der Velden VH, te Marvelde JG, Hoogeveen PG, et al. (2001) Targeting of the CD33-calicheamicin immunoconjugate Mylotarg (CMA-676) in acute myeloid leukemia: In vivo and in vitro saturation and internalization by leukemic and normal myeloid cells. Blood 97(10):3197–3204

95. Sievers EL, Larson RA, Stadtmauer EA, et al. (2001) Efficacy and safety of gemtuzumab ozogamicin in patients with CD33-positive acute myeloid leukemia in first relapse. J Clin Oncol 19(13):3244–3254
96. Bross PF, Beitz J, Chen G, et al. (2001) Approval summary: Gemtuzumab ozogamicin in relapsed acute myeloid leukemia. Clin Cancer Res 7(6):1490–1496
97. Larson RA, Sievers EL, Stadtmauer EA, et al. (2005) Final report of the efficacy and safety of gemtuzumab ozogamicin (Mylotarg) in patients with CD33-positive acute myeloid leukemia in first recurrence. Cancer 104(7):1442–1452
98. Rajvanshi P, Shulman HM, Sievers EL, et al. (2002) Hepatic sinusoidal obstruction after gemtuzumab ozogamicin (Mylotarg) therapy. Blood 99(7):2310–2314
99. Wadleigh M, Richardson PG, Zahrieh D, et al. (2003) Prior gemtuzumab ozogamicin exposure significantly increases the risk of veno-occlusive disease in patients who undergo myeloablative allogeneic stem cell transplantation. Blood 102(5):1578–1582
100. Giles F, Verstovsek S, Thomas D, et al. (2005) Phase I study of cloretazine (VNP40101M), a novel sulfonylhydrazine alkylating agent, combined with cytarabine in patients with refractory leukemia. Clin Cancer Res 11(21):7817–7824
101. Giles F, Verstovsek S, Faderl S, et al. (2006) A phase II study of cloretazine (VNP40101M), a novel sulfonylhydrazine alkylating agent, in patients with very high risk relapsed acute myeloid leukemia. Leuk Res 30(12):1591–1595
102. Smith BD, Levis M, Beran M, et al. (2004) Single-agent CEP-701, a novel FLT3 inhibitor, shows biologic and clinical activity in patients with relapsed or refractory acute myeloid leukemia. Blood 103(10):3669–3676
103. Giles FJ, Stopeck AT, Silverman LR, et al. (2003) SU5416, a small molecule tyrosine kinase receptor inhibitor, has biologic activity in patients with refractory acute myeloid leukemia or myelodysplastic syndromes. Blood 102(3):795–801
104. Karp JE, Lancet JE, Kaufmann SH, et al. (2001) Clinical and biologic activity of the farnesyltransferase inhibitor R115777 in adults with refractory and relapsed acute leukemias: A phase 1 clinical-laboratory correlative trial. Blood 97(11):3361–3369
105. Marcucci G, Stock W, Swiebe J, et al. (2003) Clinical activity of Genasense (GNS, Oblimersen Sodium), in combination with daunorubicin and cytarabine: A phase I study in previously untreated elderly acute myeloid leukemia. Blood 385a (abstr)
106. Lubbert M, Minden M (2005) Decitabine in acute myeloid leukemia. Semin Hematol 42(3 Suppl 2):S38–42
107. Levis M, Smith B. D., Beran M B, MR, et al. (2005) A randomized, open-label study of Lestaurtinib (CEP-701), an oral FLT3 inhibitor, administered in sequence with chemotherapy in patients with relapse AML harboring FLT3 activating mutations: Clinical response correlates with successful FLT3 inhibition. Blood 106(11):121a (abstr)
108. Stone RM, Fischer T, Paquette R, et al. (2005) Phase IB study of PKC412, and oral FLT3 kinase inhibitor, in sequential and simultaneous combinations with daunorubicin and cytarabine (DA) induction and high-dose cytarabine consolidation in newly diagnosed patients with AML. Blood 106(11):121a (abstr)
109. Melnick A, Licht JD (1999) Deconstructing a disease: RARalpha, its fusion partners, and their roles in the pathogenesis of acute promyelocytic leukemia. Blood 93(10):3167–3215
110. Diverio D, Rossi V, Avvisati G, et al. (1998) Early detection of relapse by prospective reverse transcriptase-polymerase chain reaction analysis of the PML/RARalpha fusion gene in patients with acute promyelocytic leukemia enrolled in the GIMEMA-AIEOP multicenter "AIDA" trial. GIMEMA-AIEOP Multicenter "AIDA" Trial. Blood 92(3):784–789
111. Ikeda K, Sasaki K, Tasaka T, et al. (1993) Reverse transcription-polymerase chain reaction for PML-RAR alpha fusion transcripts in acute promyelocytic leukemia and its application to minimal residual leukemia detection. Leukemia 7(4):544–548
112. Tallman MS, Nabhan C, Feusner JH, et al. (2002) Acute promyelocytic leukemia: Evolving therapeutic strategies. Blood 99(3): 759–767
113. Douer D (2002) New advances in the treatment of acute promyelocytic leukemia. Int J Hematol 76(Suppl 2):179–187
114. Ohno R, Asou N, Ohnishi K (2003) Treatment of acute promyelocytic leukemia: Strategy toward further increase of cure rate. Leukemia 17(8):1454–1463
115. Fenaux P, Chomienne C, Degos L (2001) All-trans retinoic acid and chemotherapy in the treatment of acute promyelocytic leukemia. Semin Hematol 38(1):13–25
116. Kwong YL, Au WY, Chim CS, et al. (2001) Arsenic trioxide- and idarubicin-induced remissions in relapsed acute promyelocytic leukaemia: Clinicopathological and molecular features of a pilot study. Am J Hematol 66(4):274–279
117. Raffoux E, Rousselot P, Poupon J, et al. (2003) Combined treatment with arsenic trioxide and all-trans-retinoic acid in patients with relapsed acute promyelocytic leukemia. J Clin Oncol 21(12):2326–2334
118. Lo-Coco F, Cimino G, Breccia M, et al. (2004) Gemtuzumab ozogamicin (Mylotarg) as a single agent for molecularly relapsed acute promyelocytic leukemia. Blood 104(7):1995–1999
119. Niu C, Yan H, Yu T, et al. (1999) Studies on treatment of acute promyelocytic leukemia with arsenic trioxide: Remission induction, follow-up, and molecular monitoring in 11 newly diagnosed and 47 relapsed acute promyelocytic leukemia patients. Blood 94(10):3315–3324
120. Chen GQ, Shi XG, Tang W, et al. (1997) Use of arsenic trioxide (As2O3) in the treatment of acute promyelocytic leukemia (APL): I. As2O3 exerts dose-dependent dual effects on APL cells. Blood 89(9):3345–3353
121. Miller WH, Jr (2002) Molecular targets of arsenic trioxide in malignant cells. Oncologist 7(Suppl 1):14–19
122. Zang P, Wang S, Hu XH (1996) Arsenic trioxide treated 72 cases of acute promeylocytic leukemia. Clin J Hematol 17:58–62
123. Soignet SL, Maslak P, Wang ZG, et al. (1998) Complete remission after treatment of acute promyelocytic leukemia with arsenic trioxide. N Engl J Med 339(19):1341–1348
124. Soignet SL, Frankel SR, Douer D, et al. (2001) United States multicenter study of arsenic trioxide in relapsed acute promyelocytic leukemia. J Clin Oncol 19(18):3852–3860
125. Shen ZX, Chen GQ, Ni JH, et al. (1997) Use of arsenic trioxide (As2O3) in the treatment of acute promyelocytic leukemia (APL): II. Clinical efficacy and pharmacokinetics in relapsed patients. Blood 89(9):3354–3360
126. Meloni G, Diverio D, Vignetti M, et al. (1997) Autologous bone marrow transplantation for acute promyelocytic leukemia in second remission: Prognostic relevance of pretransplant minimal re-

sidual disease assessment by reverse-transcription polymerase chain reaction of the PML/RAR alpha fusion gene. Blood 90(3):1321–1325
127. de Botton S, Fawaz A, Chevret S, et al. (2005) Autologous and allogeneic stem-cell transplantation as salvage treatment of acute promyelocytic leukemia initially treated with all-trans-retinoic acid: A retrospective analysis of the European acute promyelocytic leukemia group. J Clin Oncol 23(1):120–126
128. Sanz M, Arcese W, de la Rubia J, et al. (2000) Stem cell transplantation (SCT) for acute promyelocytic leukemia (APL) in the ATRA era: A survey of the European. Blood and Marrow Transplantation Group (EBMT). Blood 96:2246 (abstr)
129. Guglielmi C, Martelli MP, Diverio D, et al. (1998) Immunophenotype of adult and childhood acute promyelocytic leukaemia: Correlation with morphology, type of PML gene breakpoint and clinical outcome. A cooperative Italian study on 196 cases. Br J Haematol 102(4):1035–1041
130. Paietta E (2003) Expression of cell-surface antigens in acute promyelocytic leukaemia. Best Pract Res Clin Haematol 16(3):369–385
131. Paietta E, Andersen J, Gallagher R, et al. (1994) The immunophenotype of acute promyelocytic leukemia (APL): An ECOG study. Leukemia 8(7):1108–1112
132. Bernard J, Weil M, Boiron M, et al. (1973) Acute promyelocytic leukemia: Results of treatment by daunorubicin. Blood 41(4): 489–496
133. Petti MC, Pinazzi MB, Diverio D, et al. (2001) Prolonged molecular remission in advanced acute promyelocytic leukaemia after treatment with gemtuzumab ozogamicin (Mylotarg CMA-676). Br J Haematol 115(1):63–65
134. Liso V, Specchia G, Pogliani EM, et al. (1998) Extramedullary involvement in patients with acute promyelocytic leukemia: A report of seven cases. Cancer 83(8):1522–1528
135. Byrd JC, Edenfield WJ, Shields DJ, et al. (1995) Extramedullary myeloid cell tumors in acute nonlymphocytic leukemia: A clinical review. J Clin Oncol 13(7):1800–1816
136. Evans GD, Grimwade DJ (1999) Extramedullary disease in acute promyelocytic leukemia. Leuk Lymphoma 33(3–4):219–229
137. Hickstein DD, Hickey MJ, Collins SJ (1988) Transcriptional regulation of the leukocyte adherence protein beta subunit during human myeloid cell differentiation. J Biol Chem 263(27):13863–13867
138. Ravandi F, Cortes J, Estrov Z, et al. (2002) CD56 expression predicts occurrence of CNS disease in acute lymphoblastic leukemia. Leuk Res 26(7):643–649
139. Specchia G, Lo Coco F, Vignetti M, et al. (2001) Extramedullary involvement at relapse in acute promyelocytic leukemia patients treated or not with all-trans retinoic acid: A report by the Gruppo Italiano Malattie Ematologiche dell'Adulto. J Clin Oncol 19(20):4023–4028
140. Breccia M, Petti MC, Testi AM, et al. (2002) Ear involvement in acute promyelocytic leukemia at relapse: A disease-associated "sanctuary"? Leukemia 16(6):1127–1130
141. de Botton S, Sanz MA, Chevret S, et al. (2006) Extramedullary relapse in acute promyelocytic leukemia treated with all-trans retinoic acid and chemotherapy. Leukemia 20(1):35–41
142. Lengfelder E, Reichert A, Schoch C, et al. (2000) Double induction strategy including high dose cytarabine in combination with all-trans retinoic acid: Effects in patients with newly diagnosed acute promyelocytic leukemia. German AML Cooperative Group. Leukemia 14(8):1362–1370
143. Lo Coco F, Avvisati G, Vignetti M, et al. (2004) Front-line treatment of acuate promyelocytic leukemia with aIDA induction followed by risk-adapted consolidation: Results of the AIDA-2000 trial of the Italian GIMEMA Group. Blood 104(11):115a
144. Buccisano F, Maurillo L, Gattei V, et al. (2006) The kinetics of reduction of minimal residual disease impacts on duration of response and survival of patients with acute myeloid leukemia. Leukemia 20:1783–1789
145. Del Poeta G, Venditti A, Del Principe MI, et al. (2003) Amount of spontaneous apoptosis detected by Bax/Bcl-2 ratio predicts outcome in acute myeloid leukemia (AML). Blood 101(6):2125–2131
146. Wilson CS, Davidson GS, Martin SB, et al. (2006) Gene expression profiling of adult acute myeloid leukemia identifies novel biologic clusters for risk classification and outcome prediction. Blood 108(2):685–696

Part II – Acute Lymphoblastic Leukemia

Acute Lymphoblastic Leukemia: Epidemiology and Etiology

Daniel Wartenberg, Frank D. Groves, Aaron S. Adelman

Contents

5.1 Introduction

Acute lymphoblastic leukemia (ALL), also known as acute lymphocytic leukemia, is a malignant neoplasm of the lymphocyte precursor cells, or lymphoblasts, that occurs annually in nearly 4000 people in the US [51]. Leukemic lymphoblasts have exaggerated and uncontrolled growth, fail to mount a normal immune response, and cause a drop in production of normal bone marrow cells that leads to a deficiency of circulating red cells (anemia), platelets (thrombocytopenia), and white cells other than lymphocytes (especially neutrophils, or neutropenia) [146]. Both T-cell and B-cell precursors can give rise to ALL; B-cell ALL represents about 88% of all cases.

ALL afflicts whites more than blacks, males more than females, and those in Western, affluent countries more than those in the developing world. It often occurs in clusters, or small geographic aggregations of cases, has been studied extensively, and yet we still know surprisingly little about what causes it. It appears that chromosomal alterations and mutations that are associated with the disease may be inherited from pregnancy or develop through infancy and childhood, and these alterations and mutations then interact with certain environmental exposures which can lead to at least some types of ALL.

In this review, we present first the descriptive epidemiology of ALL (Table 5.1), mainly using incidence and survival data from the US National Cancer Institute's Surveillance, Epidemiology and End Results (SEER) Program (http://seer.cancer.gov), and mortality data from the US National Center for Health Statistics (http://www.cdc.gov/nchs/deaths.htm), followed by a brief discussion of parental and sociodemographic characteristics of ALL cases. Where possible, in our discussion of the descriptive epidemiology, we report patterns for race and gender specific subgroups. However, when looking at trends or individual years, subgroup data often are not reported due to small numbers of events.

We then review the published literature on biological, physical, and chemical risk factors for ALL. Because the incidence of ALL peaks around the third birthday, our discussion of the etiology of ALL will focus more on the pediatric population. Our review is neither exhaustive nor comprehensive, but rather summarizes our view of key findings in understanding the patterns and etiology of this disease.

5.2 Demographic Patterns

5.2.1 Incidence

ALL represents approximately less than 1% of adult cancers, and 25% of all childhood cancers. In the USA, among all ages, it represents less than 0.4% of all cancers, 13.6% of all leukemias, and 29.6% of all lymphocytic leukemias. Age-adjusted incidence rates for ALL vary several-fold, internationally, with the highest rates occurring in Spain, among Hispanics in Los Angeles, and in Caucasians in Quebec and Ontario, Canada, and in New Zealand. The lowest rates are found in developing countries, among US blacks, Israeli Jews, and Chinese and Asian Indians, whose rates may be many times lower than those in more affluent, developed countries [42, 75].

Among children under age 20, ALL is the most common malignancy, except in Africa and the Middle East. The highest rates of childhood ALL occur in Costa Rica and among Hispanics in Los Angeles, and the lowest rates among US blacks, in the Middle East, and in India [38, 75]. In the US, it represents almost 25% of all childhood cancers and 79.5% of all childhood leukemias, and 99% of all lymphocytic leukemias (Table 5.1). Despite being the most common type of cancer in children, it remains a relatively rare disease in both children and the total population (3.6 and 1.4 cases per 100 000 per year, respectively).

When we compare the secular trends of ALL to those of all leukemias, we see some marked differences. Secular trends in leukemia for the entire US population show that incidence rates from 1975 to 2001 decreased slightly for white males and increased slightly for white females (–0.1%, 0.2% per year, respectively), but from 2001 to 2003 rates for white females decreased rapidly (–6% per year). For black males and females from 1975 to 2003 the rates for leukemia decreased (–0.7%, –0.6% per year, respectively). In males, for whites and blacks combined, ALL incidence rates increased from 1975 to about 1990, and then declined through 2002, while female ALL incidence rates showed a very slight increase until the late 1990s, when they also began to decline.

In children of both genders and races, total leukemia incidence rates increased at a rate of about 1.0% per year from 1975 to the late 1980s, apparently driven by ALL, which increased at about 1.8% per year during this same period [117]. Some have suggested that this greater increase in ALL is due to improved characterization of leukemia subtypes, information that was obtained to help physicians specify appropriate treatment agents [77, 117]. From the late 1980s on, incidence rates both for total leukemia and for ALL increased at a rate of about 0.3% per year [117].

5.2.2 Survival

Less than half of all adult leukemias survive 5 years after diagnosis, but nearly two-thirds of all adult ALL cases survive at least 5 years after diagnosis. Childhood leukemia survival is much better than that for adults, with more than three-quarters of all children with leukemias and more than four-fifths of ALL cases surviving at least 5 years past diagnosis [117]. Childhood ALL survival is one of the most dramatic success stories in the history of chemotherapy, showing a remarkable improvement due to innovative treatments, with the 5-year survival rate in 1964 being only 3% [162], rising to 57% in 1975–1977 and 87% in 1996–2002 (Fig. 5.1) [117].

Table 5.1. Age-adjusted incidence and mortality rates per 100 000 persons, and 5-year relative survival rates

Gender	Race	Incidence			Mortality			5-year survival		
		All cancers	All leukemias	Acute lymphoblastic leukemia	All cancers	All leukemias	Acute lymphoblastic leukemia	All cancers	All leukemias	Acute lymphoblastic leukemia
All ages										
Total	All	480.4	12.4	1.4	197.8	7.6	2.2	66.3	47.1	62.9
	White	489.1	13.1	1.5	195.3	7.8	0.5	67.8	48.9	64.9
	Black	519.3	9.6	0.7	248.1	6.8	0.4	57.2	35.5	48.8
Males	All	567.0	16.3	1.6	247.5	10.2	3.1	66.6	47.8	62.5
	White	569.7	17.1	1.7	242.5	10.4	0.6	68.2	49.6	64.7
	Black	692.5	12.4	0.8	339.4	8.9	0.5	60.1	35.0	46.7
Females	All	421.9	9.6	1.2	165.5	5.8	1.6	66.1	46.2	63.6
	White	435.6	10.1	1.3	164.5	6.0	0.4	67.3	47.8	65.2
	Black	404.1	7.8	0.7	194.3	5.4	0.3	54.0	36.0	52.0
Ages 0–14										
Total	All	15.0	4.6	3.6	2.5	0.8	0.4	78.6	80.2	86.4
	White	16.1	–*	–	2.5	–	–	–	–	–
	Black	10.7	–	–	2.4	–	–	–	–	–
Males	All	15.6	4.9	3.9	2.7	0.8	0.4	79.9	–	–
	White	16.7	–	–	2.7	–	–	–	–	–
	Black	10.7	–	–	2.6	–	–	–	–	–
Females	All	14.3	4.2	3.4	2.3	0.7	0.3	73.0	–	–
	White	15.5	–	–	2.4	–	–	–	–	–
	Black	10.6	–	–	2.2	–	–	–	–	–

All ages
Incidence: 1998–2002 (SEER 9 areas); All Cancers: Table II-2; Leukemia: Table XIII-2; ALL: Table XIII-3
Mortality: 1998–2002 (NCHS public use US data file); All Cancers: Table II-3; Leukemia: Table XIII-8; ALL: Tables I-4, I-5, I-6
Survival: 1995–2001 (SEER 9 areas); All Cancers: Table II-4; Leukemia: Table XIII-8; ALL: Table XIII-9
Ages 0–14
Incidence 1998–2002 (SEER 9 Areas) Table XXVIII-7
Mortality 1998–2002 (NCHS public use US data file for entire US) Table XXVII-7
Survival 1995–2001 (SEER 9 Areas) Table XXVII-8
*not reported
Source: SEER Cancer Statistics Reviews 1975–2002

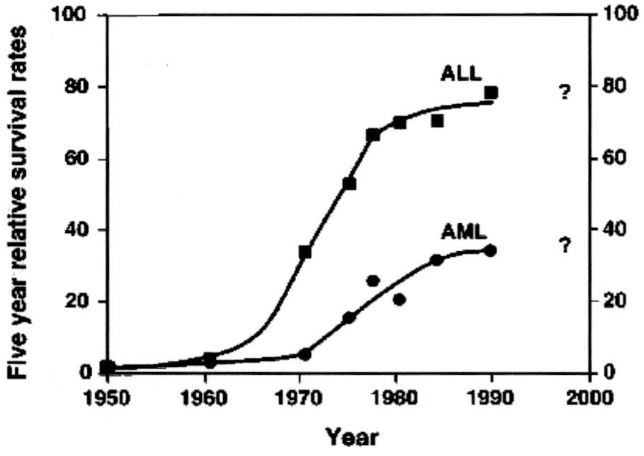

Fig. 5.1. Survival rates for childhood ALL. Five-year relative survival rates for ALL and AML: End Results Group National Cancer Institute Surveillance, Epidemiology and End Results Program, 1996. *Squares*: ALL; *circles*: AML represent defined time periods. The "best fit" curve was drawn by the author (from Kersey [54]).

5.2.3 Mortality

ALL represents less than 1.1% of total US cancer related deaths and 28.9% of all leukemia deaths. In US children, however, ALL represents almost 16% of total cancer mortality and 50% of all leukemia deaths. Total leukemia mortality rates in whites of both sexes decreased from the 1980s through 2002. In blacks of both sexes, however, total leukemia mortality rates increased after 1975, peaking in 1983 among females and in 1991 among males, then decreasing through 2002. For all children considered together, the mortality rates both for total leukemia and for ALL declined from 1975 to 2002, but the rate of decrease was greater in the 1990s [117].

5.2.4 Sex Differences

Incidence rates for total leukemia, and to a lesser extent for ALL, are higher among males than among females, and this gender difference is considerably more pronounced among whites (70% more leukemia in males and 60% more ALL in males) than among blacks (30% and 15%, respectively). In children, the incidence rates for all leukemias, and for ALL, are slightly higher in males than in females, up to about a 30% excess [77]. Similar patterns are seen in the mortality data for all leukemias, but for ALL male rates show an even greater excess [117].

5.2.5 Race Differences

Overall differences in incidence and mortality rates by race are also noteworthy. In the USA, for leukemia, for males, females, and all combined, whites have higher incidence rates than blacks (30–40% excess), and this same pattern is seen even more strongly for ALL (85–215% excess). A similar pattern is seen for mortality [117].

In children, SEER summaries provide tabulations of race-specific data only for all cancers [117]. For those data, whites have about a 45–55% excess in incidence rates, depending on gender, and similarly for mortality rates, whites have a 5–10% excess depending on gender. Other studies suggest that the rate of ALL in white children is double that in black children in the USA [43, 77].

5.2.6 Age Differences

Leukemia incidence increases from birth through age 3, then decreases until about age 50, when rates begin to increase slowly. ALL incidence rates increase more dramatically from birth to age 3 (up to more than 9 cases per 100 000 per year), drop off to lower levels until about age 50 (less than 1 per 100 000 per year), and then increase slightly, but never approach the rates observed between ages 1 and 14 (Fig. 5.2). The peak incidence period is from age 2–5 [145] with a smaller, secondary peak after age 60 (Fig. 5.3). It is interesting to note that the age 2–5 peak in ALL was noted first in Western countries between 1920 and 1945, thereafter in Japan and China, and the incidence rate in affluent countries continues to increase at a rate of about 1% per year [38]. Understanding the mechanism of this unexplained difference between Western, affluent, developed countries and those in the developing world might help unlock the etiologic secret of what causes the leukemias and ALL.

5.2.7 Parental and Birth Characteristics

Researchers have noted a variety of patterns among parental and birth characteristics of leukemia and ALL cases. For example, first-born babies have a higher risk of ALL, as do high-birth-weight babies [124], babies whose mothers are over 35 years of age, and mothers who have had a prior fetal loss [120]. Maternal cigarette

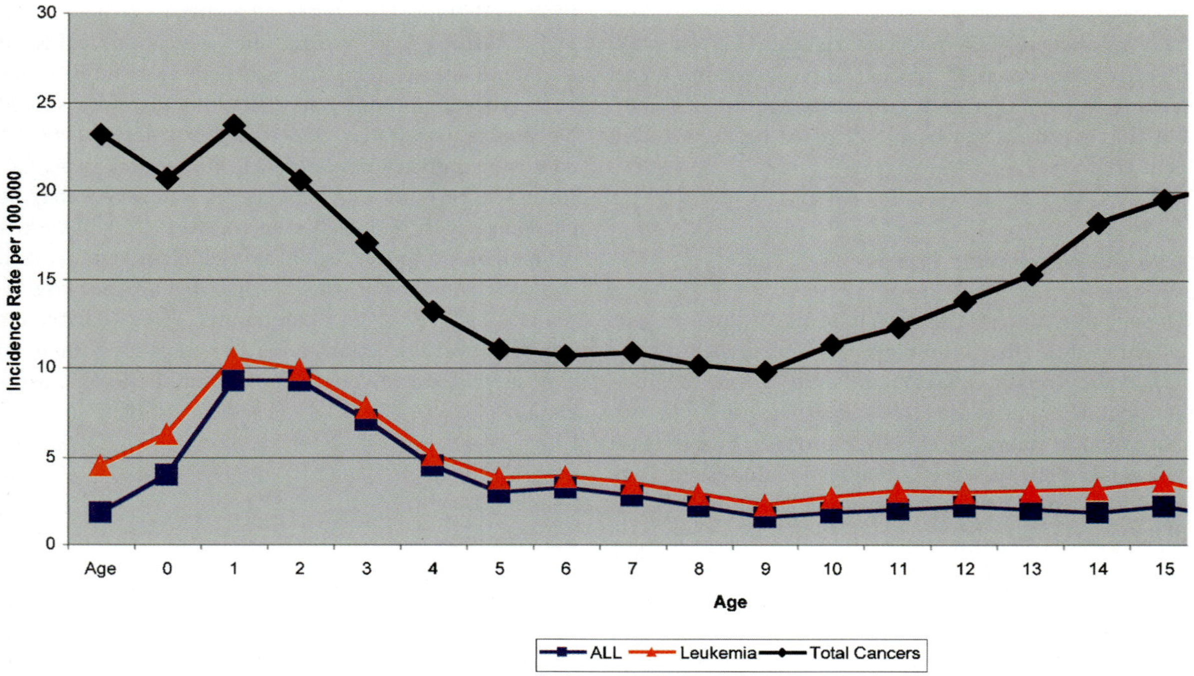

Fig. 5.2. Age adjusted incidence rates per 100 000 by age (data from Ries [117]).

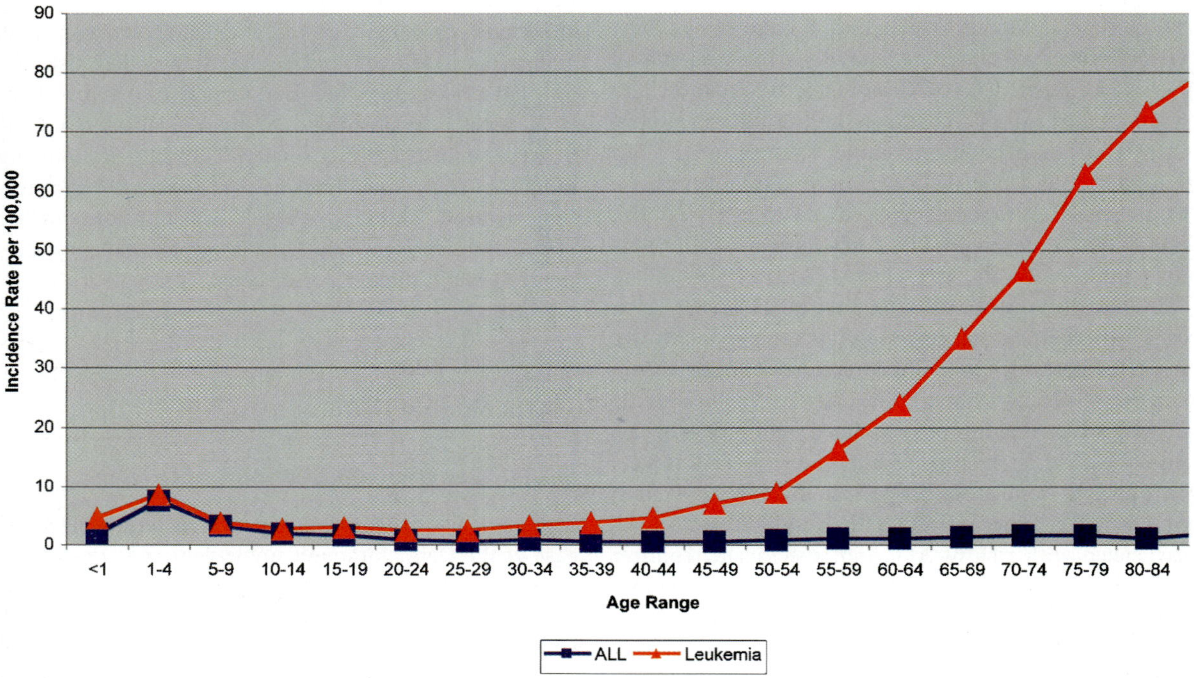

Fig. 5.3. Age adjusted incidence rates per 100 000 by age (data from Ries [117]).

smoking and certain parental dietary constituents have been associated with increased risk of ALL, although there are no accepted mechanisms of action. Breast feeding was thought to be protective against ALL [36], but this effect has not been supported by more recent data [74].

5.2.8 Socioeconomic Status

The apparent excess observed in several studies of ALL in whites and other ethnic groups compared to blacks has led several investigators to suggest that the incidence of ALL may be directly associated with higher socioeconomic status (SES). While probably not a direct cause, SES may be a useful marker for underlying risk factors that may help us better understand the etiology of ALL.

One must be specific in what one means by SES. SES can be inferred from data on individuals (e.g., head of household or family), or aggregate data (e.g., averages from census regions, such as tracts, communities, or zip codes). In addition, there is a wide variety of metrics used, such as mean income, median income, per capita income, percent below poverty line. While related, each can give somewhat different results [63, 106].

In general, studies of SES and childhood ALL have yielded mixed results. A review of six pre-1983 studies reported a positive association between SES and childhood ALL in five of six studies [40]. Studies using residential neighborhood or community measures of SES generally found that ALL was more common in areas of higher SES, although some critics suggested that this was due to a diagnostic bias, such as in a recent Canadian study (OR = 0.9, 95% CI 0.8–1.0) [12], possibly attributable to greater access to good medical care. A recent Danish study that reviewed this issue reported that in previous studies individual measures of SES gave inconsistent results while SES measures of a child's residential area tended to be associated with higher leukemia rates, although some recent studies were less clear or found the opposite effect [111]. In their own data, they found that community rather than individual SES was associated with risk of ALL and, specifically, children born into poorer regions were at a statistically significant greater risk (RR = 2.2, 95% CI 1.1–4.6). No association was found with SES at diagnosis. The most recent review, by Poole and colleagues, reported that associations between childhood leukemia and SES varied with place and time [106]. They also suggest that different SES measures (e.g., income and education) collected at different scales (e.g., individual or community) may be surrogates for different risks and therefore should be reported separately. SES remains an interesting but confusing marker for risk of ALL. One complicating factor noted by Buffler and colleagues is that SES may be correlated with and even a surrogate for various environmental exposures, such as pesticides, traffic, and diet [13]. Since many studies adjust for SES because often it is believed to be a confounder, these adjustments may remove any associations between environmental exposures and ALL, obscuring potential etiologic associations.

5.3 Etiology

It is somewhat surprising how little is known about the causes of ALL. It occurs more commonly among whites and in Western, affluent countries, reaches peak incidence among children, a population of great concern, and often is reported in concentrated clusters (high local incidences), a situation that one might think would be particularly amenable to etiologic study. Among childhood, only ionizing radiation and certain genetic disorders are known risk factors. Many other risk factors have been suggested but remain under investigation, such as exposure to pesticides, automobile exhaust, certain chemicals such as benzene, nonionizing radiation (e.g., magnetic fields), parental exposures (e.g., cigarette smoking, alcohol consumption and use of some pharmaceuticals), and even parental consumption of certain dietary constituents.

5.3.1 Biological Factors

5.3.1.1 Genetics of Childhood ALL

Leukemia, like other forms of cancer, is ultimately a disease of the DNA. Although single-gene mutations (e.g., BRCA1 and BRCA2) are known to predispose to solid tumors (e.g., carcinomas of breast and ovary), no such single-gene mutations have been linked to childhood ALL, which tends instead to be associated with chromosomal anomalies.

5.3.1.2 Cytogenetic Abnormalities

Cytogenetic abnormalities frequently found in ALL cases include germ-line karyotypic abnormalities, somatic karotypic abnormalities, translocations, and deletions. The germ-line abnormalities associated with childhood leukemia include Down syndrome (trisomy 21) [64, 118, 144], Bloom syndrome [64], Fanconi anemia, Klinefelter syndrome, and ataxia-telangiectasia [37]. The somatic abnormalities associated with childhood leukemia include aneuploidy (in one form or another in 92% of childhood ALL cases), pseudodiploidy (in 41.5% of ALL cases) and hyperdiploidy (in 20–30% of pre-B ALL and about 90% of early pre-B ALL) [108, 127].

Translocations frequently found in ALL cases include the *TEL-AML1* translocation (found in about 20–25% of B-lineage childhood ALLs) [11, 34, 91, 95, 125]; MLL translocations (found in about 70–80% of infant leukemias [16, 53, 94, 109, 126], but less commonly in other leukemias, both childhood and adult); *MLL-AF4* gene fusion (very common in infant ALL and also found in ALL of older children); and other translocations occurring in childhood ALL including t(9, 11)(p22;q23) [16, 53] and t(11, 19) [46], and *CDK6-MLL* [112]. TEL-AML1 is found in about 1% of cord blood specimens, yet only about 1% of those with this translocation will develop ALL in childhood.

Deletion of 6q occurs in 11% of childhood ALL cases [108]. Among childhood ALL cases with t(12, 21), 77% also have 12p12–13 deletions [15].

In short, the chromosomes that are known to be involved in karyotypic abnormalities found in childhood ALL are 1, 4, 6–9, 11, 12, 14, 19, 21, and 22. Neither X nor Y is known to be involved with childhood ALL. Translocations are especially common in childhood ALL.

Triggers for molecular anomalies may be inherited during pregnancy, and may develop during infancy or early childhood [13].

5.3.1.3 Infectious Etiology

The most widely accepted current theory of causation of childhood ALL is based on an infectious etiology associated with decreased immune function. Three variations on this theme of the "infection" that have been put forward are (1) exposure to a specific infectious agent postnatally, proposed by Kinlen [56], (2) exposure to a specific infectious agent prenatally or around the time of birth, proposed by Smith [137], or (3) a delay in the initial exposure to infectious agents in general beyond the first year of life, proposed by Greaves [39]. A recent review of this topic is provided by McNally and Eden [88], but does not resolve the controversy. We provide a brief review of some of the literature supporting each of these hypotheses.

5.3.1.4 Postnatal Infection by a Specific Leukemogenic Pathogen

According to Kinlen's hypothesis [56, 57], "outbreaks" of ALL follow epidemics of some common (and perhaps subclinical) infection, of which ALL is a rare outcome. These outbreaks tend to occur when infectious and susceptible populations come into close proximity or intermingle ("population mixing"), thus facilitating the spread of the pathogen. In relatively rural, isolated populations it is more likely that a sizeable portion of the population has not previously been exposed to the infectious agent, and thus is susceptible.

Kinlen and colleagues have published many studies that are consistent with this theory. For example, he has documented high rates of leukemia mortality among preschool children in Kirkcaldy, following a rapid population increase due to the construction of the new town of Glenrothes [56], and excess leukemia mortality in five rural British New Towns founded between 1946 and 1950, which brought together new residents from a variety of isolated (i.e., low-density) rural settings. The statistically significant excess leukemia mortality was seen in rural towns for the time period 1946–1965 but not 1966–1985, consistent with the population mixing hypothesis. The excess leukemia mortality was not seen in overspill towns, which were less rural and had smaller rates of in-migration, also supporting the population mixing hypothesis. The relationship between population influx and childhood ALL received further support from a Cumbria-based study of children of "incomers" (both parents born outside Cumbria), who were at higher risk of common ALL than children of "local residents" (at least one parent born inside Cumbria) [21]. Studies in other countries found similar effects, such as extraordinarily high childhood leukemia mortality rates in Italy and Greece during 1958–1987, which have been attributed to high levels of population mixing associated with massive rural-to-urban migration in the years following World War II [59]; a study in Hong Kong that showed evidence of statistically significant clustering of ALL in preschool children in small geographic regions (TPUs) in the highest decile of population growth during 1981–1991 [5]; a Canadian study in which leukemia incidence among children under 5 years of age was higher than expected in rural areas where the population grew, and lower than expected in growing urban areas [62]; and a US study using data from the SEER program that showed that rural counties with the greatest increase in population from 1980–1989 had the highest childhood leukemia incidence rates [153]. In contrast, in a study conducted in France, leukemia mortality rates were average among preschool children who resided in 43 rapidly-growing French administrative units (communes) [69].

5.3.1.5 Prenatal Infection by a Specific Leukemogenic Pathogen

According to Smith's hypothesis [136, 137], high rates of ALL are attributable to in utero exposures to infections that result mainly in cases of precursor B-cell ALL. To investigate this hypothesis, several studies have compared ALL rates among children of mothers who reported infections during pregnancy to children of mothers who did not report infections during pregnancy. Early studies have been reviewed by Little [78] and show equivocal results. For example, the Oxford Survey of Childhood Cancers, a matched case-control study in England and Wales, found that children of mothers ill with an infective disease during pregnancy had increased rates of childhood malignancies (13 cases among mothers with infections during pregnancy versus 1 case among control mothers) [144]. However, in a more recent and more focused matched case-control study in Scotland, infection (any, respiratory tract, viral, genitourinary, or fungal) during pregnancy did not statistically significantly affect the risk of ALL in children ages 0 to 14 [85]. Similarly, a study by Infante-Rivard et al. looking at recurrent maternal infections did not find a statistically significant association with ALL in children [47]. However, a study of maternal lower genital tract infection reported a statistically significant association [99], as did a study of mothers with Epstein-Barr virus (EBV) [72].

5.3.1.6 Delayed Exposure to Pathogens in General

Greaves' hypothesis is that secondary mutations and/or proliferation due to early exposure to general infectious agents transmitted from parents, siblings, and other contacts early in life will tend to reduce the risk of childhood ALL. This is because he believes that ALL is a consequence of two independent mutations: the first occurring in utero or shortly after birth, and the second occurring between 2 and 6 years of age that may be triggered by infection [35, 38]. Supporting this theory is the observation that the majority of childhood ALL cases diagnosed between ages 2 and 6 have the TEL/AML1 mutation. For example, in one study, eight of 12 children ages 2 to 5 recently diagnosed with *TEL-AML1*-positive ALL, including a pair of twins, were found to have *TEL-AML1* fusion in the neonatal blood spots on their Guthrie cards, and the twins shared the same *TEL-AML1* sequence (Wiemels et al. 1999a). This is interpreted to be the first of the two mutations in Greaves' theory.

His theory supposes that a second mutation occurs in early childhood, causing ALL. The second mutation may be promoted by common infections. Further, relative isolation, as in Kinlen's hypothesis, may delay exposures to common infections, enabling the susceptible preleukemic cells to multiply, increases the likelihood of occurrence of the second mutation.

Various sources of childhood infection, or protection from infection, have been considered in light of this hypothesis. Breast feeding, an opportunity for infectious exposure after birth, tends to show decreased risk of ALL, although this effect may be confounded by SES, according to McNally [88], as cases in these studies tended to have lower SES. As a counter example, researchers have shown that attendance at a day care facility increases a child's risk of infection, and thus should increase their risk of ALL according to this theory, but was found to be protective. However, as with breast feeding, SES may be a confounder as cases tended to have lower SES. Other sources of infectious exposures, such as older siblings, parents with occupations that bring them into contact with many people, and migration, also tend to be protective [88]. Studies have also found associations of allergies and asthma with ALL [139, 154].

Finally, seasonality may suggest an infectious etiology. Various authors have examined the seasonal pattern of ALL diagnosis or symptoms. Karimi and Yarmohammadi found a late fall, early winter peak in Iran, Sorensen et al. [138] a fall peak in Denmark, Higgins et al. [44], Westerbeek et al. [157] and Badrinath et al. [7] summer peaks in Europe, and Ross and colleagues [123] a summer peak in the northern USA, with approximately a 7.5% excess over the mean in July and August. This suggests a possible link to allergic and infections processes in the summer that may trigger the ALL disease process, although further research is needed to more precisely define this effect.

5.3.2 Physical Factors

5.3.2.1 Ionizing Radiation

The importance of ionizing radiation as an etiologic agent for leukemia and other lymphohematopoeitic cancers has been known since the early 1900s from studies of radiologists [8]. However, the most compelling evidence for this association has come from studies of survivors of the atomic bomb blasts in Hiroshima and Nagasaki [107] and patients treated for ankylosing spondylitis [20]. For both of these types of exposures, leukemias (other than chronic lymphocytic) were noted as early as 3 years after exposure, with peak incidence occurring 5–10 years after exposure, and additional cases were diagnosed even 30 years after exposure [60]. For ankylosing spondylitis, the strongest effect was for AML rather than ALL.

There also is evidence for leukemia risk associated with occupational exposure to ionizing radiation among those involved with the nuclear industry [75]. Studies of military personnel on maneuvers at a nuclear bomb test showed statistically elevated leukemia incidence and mortality [96], as do the most recent studies of workers at other nuclear facilities. A review and pooled analysis of nuclear worker studies conducted by the International Agency for Research on Cancer (IARC) found statistically significant excess relative risks for leukemia excluding chronic lymphocytic leukemia [14]. The leukemia exposure-response effect was consistent with but smaller than the values estimated from the studies atomic bomb survivors reported in the BEIR V report from the National Research Council [97]. Studies of workers at naval nuclear shipyards are inconsistent, while studies of fallout from bomb testing showed small increases in cases of leukemia [33], particularly acute leukemias among children, although the interpretations of these data vary [67, 82, 84, 143].

Prenatal exposures are also a concern. In the 1950s, a British study showed that radiography of a pregnant woman's abdomen increased the child's risk of leukemia by about 50% [144]. While this relationship is believed to be causal, few women today undergo this type of diagnostic testing, making this a nonissue, at least in terms of public health impact. Studies of prenatal exposure from atomic bomb blasts did not show increased risk, nor did studies of children of atomic bomb survivors who were not exposed prenatally [160]. However, those exposed prenatally may have higher risks as adults [159, 161].

Concern about leukemia risk from ionizing radiation also arose in the early 1980s from an apparent cluster among children living in close proximity to the Sellafield nuclear fuels reprocessing plant in Seascale, England. Initial studies suggested that residential proximity to the plant, and paternal employment at the plant were risk factors [30–32]. Further studies, however, did not confirm either risk factor [10, 50, 70, 86, 149]. Kinlen suggested that this situation supports his population mixing theory [58].

Another suggested physical environmental cause of leukemia is radionuclides in water and air. For example, ingestion of radium-containing groundwater in an ecologic study conducted in Florida showed an association with leukemia [80]. Subsequent studies seeking to clarify this issue provided limited support [6, 17, 29]. Studies examining inhaled radon found an increased risk of leukemia, through the hypothesized mechanism of irradiation to the bone marrow. This association was shown in ecologic studies but not other studies, and thus is unlikely to be etiologic [71].

5.3.2.2 Nonionizing Radiation

Concern also has been raised over the apparent elevated leukemia incidence among children and workers exposed to electric and magnetic fields (EMF) [49, 98, 100]. The risk was first documented in a case-control study of children who had lived in homes with high magnetic fields [156], and the results were replicated in many subsequent population-based studies [22, 79, 131]. Some studies did not show this association [28, 76, 148]. As yet, no mechanism for this risk has been established. Prompted by positive results in these studies, a series of occupational mortality studies were undertaken of workers in electrical, electronic, and telecommunications occupations and ham radio operators and showed increased risks for ALL, AML, CML, and CLL occurring inconsistently across studies [24, 92, 93, 130, 147]. The interpretation of these studies remains controversial. Because no viable mechanism has been postulated for nonionizing radiation to cause leukemia, there is much controversy over the definition of relevant exposure and interpretation of results, although only magnetic fields rather than electrical fields are implicated. Exposure metrics under consideration include peak, average, time-weighted average, and variability measures, although the data from different studies are contradictory.

Many weight-of-evidence reviews have been conducted to summarize subjectively the available data. Two recent expert panel reviews of the EMF issue were conducted in the USA [98, 100] and one in Europe [49]. While the first [98], under the sponsorship of the National Academy of Sciences, using a consensus process, reported that "no *conclusive and consistent* evidence shows that exposures to residential electric and magnetic fields produce cancer [our emphasis]," they also asserted that "an association between residential wiring configurations ... and childhood leukemia persists in multiple studies ..." The second panel [100], convened by the National Institute of Environmental Health Sciences (NIEHS), using a majority rule process, concluded that "ELF EMF are possibly carcinogenic to humans (Group 2B)." This was based principally on "the results of studies on childhood leukemia in residential environments and on CLL [chronic lymphocytic leukemia] in adults in occupational settings." In addition, the participants stated that the in vitro and mechanistic data provide weak support based on studies at very high levels of exposures (>100 μT). The third expert panel [49], convened by IARC, also using a majority rule process, also concluded that ELF EMF exposures are possibly carcinogenic to humans (Group 2B).

In addition to those data-based, albeit subjective, reviews, a variety of meta-analyses and pooled analyses were conducted to summarize this body of literature analytically. In a meta-analysis, the investigator extracts results from published papers and combines them statistically to provide an average risk estimate for the set of studies as a whole. In a pooled analysis, the investigator obtains the original, individual subject data for a set of studies and then combines them statistically to provide an average risk estimate for the set of studies as a whole while adjusting for confounding variables for individual subjects and differences among the study characteristics. Pooled analyses are believed to be more reliable than meta-analyses.

A meta-analysis of occupational studies [55] did not find consistent results regarding the risk of leukemia. The most recent meta-analyses for residential exposures to children [151] reported that the risk for leukemia was elevated and marginally statistically significant, particularly at the higher exposure cutpoints. There was some evidence that supported an exposure-response gradient. Two pooled analyses of childhood leukemia reported statistically significant elevated risks at the highest exposure categories [3, 41].

There still is much controversy over exposure to EMFs as a cause of cancer, with the excess risk suggested by the combined studies for exposures 4 times greater than background being in the range of 50–100%. However, there is added concern because exposures are ubiquitous, there are no truly unexposed comparison groups, and residential exposures rarely can be greater than 50 times background, while occupational exposures, although typically only short-term, on rare occasion can reach 1000 to 40 000 times background.

A study of children with ALL found that event-free survival varied across different levels of EMF exposure (events were defined as incomplete remission following therapy, leukemia relapse, secondary cancers, or deaths from any cause) [25]. After adjusting for risk group and socioeconomic status, the authors reported elevated risks of any event (Hazard Ratio = 1.9) including mortality (Hazard Ratio = 4.5) among those exposed to higher magnetic fields (>0.3 μT vs. <0.1 μT). The robustness of the study results was limited by small sample sizes.

5.3.3 Chemical Factors

5.3.3.1 Solvents

Workers in a variety of occupations, such as the leather, shoe, rubber, and printing industries, are exposed to benzene, and studies have reported increased risks of leukemia. Although exposure to benzene has been shown to cause leukemia, most studies have reported excesses of AML rather than ALL [60], with one exception [4]. There also has been concern that exposure to other solvents may cause leukemia, although most data are inconclusive and may not be specific to ALL [1, 73, 81, 87]. For example, in studies of the health effects of trichloroethylene, there have been some suggestions of excess leukemia and other lymphohematopoeitic malignancies [152], although these data are not compelling, and leukemia subtypes typically were not reported. Concerns have also been raised about exposures to petroleum workers, although recent updates do not implicate ALL [45, 158].

A few studies have suggested an association between parental exposures to solvents and childhood ALL. In one review, direct toxic exposures including solvents, paints and pigments, and motor vehicle related occupations were associated with leukemia but not ALL [18]. A subsequent case-control study reported that mothers of ALL cases were more likely to report occupational exposure to solvents (OR = 1.6; 95% CI = 1.1–2.3) and paints or thinners (OR = 1.7; 95% CI = 1.2–2.3) during pregnancy [135]. A subsequent case-control study in Germany also found an increased risk of ALL among children whose mothers were exposed to paints or lacquers but not solvents or plastics, prior to conception (OR = 1.6; 95% CI = 1.1–2.4) and during pregnancy (OR = 2.0; 95% CI = 1.2–3.3), but not during the postnatal period [132]. Paternal exposures to industrials dusts also showed a small elevation of risk for ALL. Elevated risks for children were also found for exposure to artwork solvents [135] and, in another study, for those living in homes that had been painted just prior to or during occupancy [26]. It was noted that solvents, paints, and thinners are all likely to cross the placental barrier, suggesting a mechanism of action [135]. However, post pregnancy, neither maternal exposure to solvents nor parental exposure to plastic materials was associated with childhood ALL.

An overriding concern with studies of the risks of parental exposures is the possibility of recall bias in the self-reported exposure assessment [18, 89, 133].

5.3.3.2 Pesticides

Numerous studies have examined the association between lymphohematopoeitic cancers, pesticides and farming, and they report limited evidence to suggest an association with ALL. Some recent studies, however, have suggested a link specifically to childhood leukemia and ALL. For example, Infante-Rivard and colleagues found indoor and garden use of pesticides was associated with increased rates of childhood ALL, and some of these associations were increased among carriers of the CYP1A1m1 and CYP1A1m2 mutations [48].

In the Northern California Childhood Leukemia Study, the use of professional pest control services any time from 1 year before to 3 years after birth was associated with a significantly increased risk of childhood leukemia (OR = 2.8; 95% CI = 1.4–5.7), with the highest risk associated with exposure during the second year (OR = 3.6; 95% CI = 1.6–8.3). Children with the most frequent exposure to insecticides had the highest risk of leukemia (OR = 2.4; 95% CI = 1.2–5.1), and leukemia risk was elevated for exposure to indoor insecticides (OR = 1.6; 95% CI = 1.0–2.7); exposures to outdoor insecticides or herbicides were not associated with leukemia risk [83]. A subsequent California case control study found small but statistically significant elevations of ALL risk for maternal residential proximity to areas of use of certain agricultural pesticides [115]. Most recently, Menegaux and colleagues reported that childhood ALL was statistically significantly associated with maternal indoor use of pesticides during pregnancy and childhood and garden use of pesticides during childhood [90].

5.3.3.3 Outdoor Air Pollution

Some researchers have suggested that outdoor air pollution may be a risk factor for leukemia. Various hypotheses exist, most notably that the risk is attributable to benzene, a component of automobile exhaust. To investigate this, investigators have conducted more than a dozen studies in the USA and Europe, assessing the possible association between leukemia incidence or mortality and various measures of traffic density, a crude surrogate for air pollution [19, 23, 61, 68, 101, 103, 110, 113, 114, 129, 142, 150]. Some specifically analyzed ALL risk. Of these studies, eight reported a positive association for childhood leukemia; five did not. It is difficult to draw a conclusion as studies varied by design, exposure measure and adjustments for confounding.

A California study using modeled concentrations of 25 potentially carcinogenic hazardous air pollutants (HAPs) provided by the US Environmental Protection Agency at the census tract level, reported an association of HAPs with childhood leukemia [116]. Their analysis showed elevated rate ratios and a statistically significant trend in the tracts ranked highest for the combined 25

HAPs (RR = 1.21; 95% confidence interval, 1.03, 1.42) and in tracts ranked highest for point source HAP exposure (RR = 1.32; 95% confidence interval, 1.11, 1.57). The authors suggest that more comprehensive exposure assessments and individual level data are needed to better understand the observed relationships.

5.3.3.4 Tobacco Smoke

The association of tobacco smoke and lymphohematopoietic cancers has been assessed in several studies. In general, the most consistent findings are for non-Hodgkin lymphoma, and those for leukemia are not statistically significant [2, 141]. However, several studies, including more than a dozen case control studies and two large cohort studies, have looked at the association between passive smoke exposure and childhood leukemia, and have reported inconsistent results [13]. Limitations of these studies include imprecise exposure estimates and limited adjustment for potentially confounding variables. A meta-analysis reported no statistically significant association between maternal smoking during pregnancy and all leukemias or ALL [9]. More recently, the large United Kingdom Childhood Cancer Study examined this issue and also did not find any statistically significant associations of parental tobacco smoking and either leukemia or ALL [102].

5.3.3.5 Diet

There have been only a limited number of studies investigating the role of diet in the occurrence of leukemia among adults. In one study, Kwiatkowski reported a decreased risk of ALL with increased consumption of vegetables, and an increased risk with consumption of milk, poultry, and soft water [66]. In another study, as part of the Iowa Women's Health Study, Ross and colleagues reported that a diet rich in vegetables had a protective effect against adult leukemia, although only 3 of the 138 leukemia cases were ALL [121]. A Canadian population-based case-control study, reported by Fritschi and colleagues, found that greater fish consumption was associated with a lower risk of leukemia [27]. Unfortunately, cancer subtypes were not presented.

It has been suggested that both maternal and childhood diets may affect the risk of childhood leukemia. A Chinese case-control study found a reduced risk of childhood leukemia associated with a child's consumption of cod liver oil, which contains high levels of vitamin A and D [134].

Parental diets may also affect childhood leukemia risks. Some concern was raised by two case control studies, in the early 1990s, investigating the possible association of processed meat consumption by child and/or parents with risk of childhood leukemia [104] and ALL [128], suggesting that *N*-nitroso precursors used as preservatives might be converted into *N*-nitroso carcinogens. The only statistically significant results found had to do with hot dog consumption, which may have been due to confounding by socioeconomic status [13].

As part of the Northern California Childhood Leukemia Study, Jensen and colleagues report that maternal consumption of vegetables, protein sources, and fruits were associated with a lower risk of ALL, as did maternal consumption of provitamin A carotenoids and the antioxidant glutathione [52]. In the same study, Kwan and colleagues reported a protective effect from child consumption of bananas, oranges, and orange juice [65]. In a nationwide study in Greece, Petridou and colleagues found that a diet rich in fruits and vegetables during pregnancy decreases the child's risk of leukemia, while one with sugar, syrups, meats, and meat products increases the risk [105].

Following a specific mechanistic hypothesis regarding diet, Ross and colleagues have examined the role of dietary inhibitors of DNA topoisomerase II, an enzyme necessary for gene transcription, DNA recombination and replication, and acute childhood leukemia [119, 122, 140]. They report that maternal consumption of foods containing DNA topoisomerase II inhibitors may increase the risk of AML but does not appear to affect the risk of ALL. Maternal consumption of fruits and vegetables, on the other hand, decreases the risk of ALL.

5.3.3.6 Maternal Pharmaceutical Use

There are limited data on the possible association between maternal use of pharmaceuticals and the risk of ALL. A study by Wen and colleagues found that maternal use of vitamins and iron during pregnancy was associated with a decreased the risk of childhood ALL, while parental use of amphetamines or diet pills and mind-altering drugs before and during the index pregnancy was associated with an increased the risk of childhood ALL, especially if both parents used the drugs [155]. They also reported that maternal use of antihistamines and allergy remedies was associated with an increased risk of ALL.

5.4 Summary

ALL is a complex, heterogeneous disease that is difficult to study. It is rare, comprehensive exposure assessments are complicated to conduct, and most studies are potentially plagued by possible reporting biases, for example by parents; selection biases, for example in selection of control and comparison populations; and substantial confounding, for example by SES. Nonetheless, as the most common childhood cancer, it has a substantial public health impact and is of great concern to parents and the public, in general, and demands prompt, thorough, and reliable research.

Studies have shown associations of ALL with several risk factors, such as maternal exposure to solvents, residential proximity to electric power lines, and pesticides, but none save ionizing radiation are thorough and convincing. These studies provide numerous leads and suggestions for further study.

One topic of investigation that has sparked considerable research, particularly in the UK, is the role of infection and immune response in the occurrence of childhood leukemia. This set of etiologic hypotheses includes consideration of biological, genetic, physical, and chemical risk factors in conjunction with the molecular basis of this dreaded disease. And yet, here, too, after more than 25 years of study and investigation, while numerous patterns and associations have been detected and documented, the underlying debate of what causes childhood leukemia remains largely unresolved.

We hope that with the recent gains in understanding the genetic basis and variation of ALL, and the many advances in molecular and genetic technology, exposure assessment, and study design and implementations, will provide additional clues and avenues for future investigation.

References

1. Acquavella JF, Leonard RC (2001) A review of the epidemiology of 1,3-butadiene and chloroprene. Chem Biol Interact 135–136:43–52
2. Adami J, Nyren O, Bergstrom R, Ekbom A, Engholm G, Englund A, et al. (1998) Smoking and the risk of leukemia, lymphoma, and multiple myeloma. Cancer Causes Control 9:49–56
3. Ahlbom A, Day N, Feychting M, Roman E, Skinner J, Dockerty J, et al. (2000) A pooled analysis of magnetic fields and childhood leukemia. Br J Cancer 83:692–698
4. Aksoy M, Erdem S, Dincol G (1976) Types of leukemia in a chronic benzene poisoning: A study in thirty-four patients. Acta Haematologica 55:65–72
5. Alexander FE, Chan LC, Lam TH, Yuen P, Leung NK, Ha SY, et al. (1997) Clustering of childhood leukaemia in Hong Kong: Association with the childhood peak and common acute lymphoblastic leukaemia and with population mixing. Br J Cancer 75:457–463
6. Auvinen A, Kurttio P, Pekkanen J, Pukkala E, Ilus T, Salonen L (2002) Uranium and other natural radionuclides in drinking water and risk of leukemia: A case-cohort study in Finland. Cancer Causes Control 13:825–829
7. Badrinath P, Day NE, Stockton D (1997) Seasonality in the diagnosis of acute lymphocytic leukaemia. Br J Cancer 75:1711–1713
8. Berrington A, Darby SC, Weiss HA, Doll R (2001) 100 years of observation on British radiologists: Mortality from cancer and other causes 1897–1997. Br J Radiol 74:507–519
9. Boffetta P, Tredaniel J, Greco A (2000) Risk of childhood cancer and adult lung cancer after childhood exposure to passive smoke: A meta-analysis. Environ Health Perspect 108:73–82
10. Boice JD, Jr, Bigbee WL, Mumma MT, Blot WJ (2003) Cancer mortality in counties near two former nuclear materials processing facilities in Pennsylvania, 1950–1995. Health Physics 85:691–700
11. Borkhardt A, Cazzaniga G, Viehmann S, Valesecchi MG, Ludwig WD, Burci L, et al. (1977) Incidence and clinical relevance of TEL/AML1 fusion genes in children with acute lymphoblastic leukemia enrolled in the German and Italian multicenter therapy trials. Blood 90:571–577
12. Borugian MJ, Spinelli JJ, Mezei G, Wilkins R, Abanto Z, McBride ML (2005) Childhood leukemia and socioeconomic status in Canada. Epidemiology 16:526–531
13. Buffler PA, Kwan MI, Reynolds P, Urayama KY (2005) Environmental and genetic risk factors for childhood leukemia: Appraising the evidence. Cancer Invest 1:60–75
14. Cardis E, Vrijheid M, Blettner M, Gilbert E, Hakama M, Hill C, et al. (2005) Risk of cancer after low doses of ionizing radiation: Retrospective cohort study in 15 countries. Br Med J 331:77–82
15. Cave H, Cacheux V, Raynaud S, Brunie G, Bakkus M, Cochaux P, et al. (1997) ETV6 is the target of chromosome 12p deletions in t(12;21) childhood acute lymphocytic leukemia. Leukemia 11:1459–1464
16. Cimino G, Lo Coco F, Biondi A, Elia L, Luciano A, Croce CM, et al. (1993) ALL-1 gene at chromosome 11q23 is consistently altered in acute leukemia of early infancy. Blood 82:544–546
17. Collman G, Loomis D, Sandler D (1991) Childhood cancer mortality and radon concentration in drinking water in North Carolina. Br J Cancer 63:626–629

18. Colt JS, Blair S (1998) Parental occupational exposures and risk of childhood cancers. Environ Health Perspect 106(Suppl):909–925
19. Crosignani P, Tittarelli A, Borgini A, Codazzi T, Rovelli A, Porro E, et al. (2004) Childhood leukemia and road traffic: A population-based case-control study. Int J Cancer 108(4):596–599
20. Darby SC, Doll R, Gill SK, Smith PG (1987) Long term mortality after a single treatment course with X-rays in patients treated for ankylosing spondylitis. Br J Cancer 55:179–190
21. Dickinson HO, Parker L (1999) Quantifying the effect of population mixing on childhood leukemia risk: The Seascale cluster. Br J Cancer 81:144–151
22. Feychting M, Ahlbom A (1993) Magnetic fields and cancer in children residing near Swedish high-voltage power lines. Am J Epidemiol 138:467–481
23. Feychting M, Svensson D, Ahlbom A (1998) Exposure to motor vehicle exhaust and childhood cancer. Scand J Work Env Health 24:8–11
24. Floderus B, Persson T, Stenlund C, Wennberg A, Ost A, Knave B (1993) Occupational exposure to electromagnetic fields in relation to leukemia and brain tumors: A case-control study in Sweden. Cancer Causes Control 4:465–476
25. Foliart DE, Pollock BH, Mezei G, Iriye R, Silva JM, Ebi KL, et al. (2006) Magnetic field exposure and long-term survival among children with leukemia. Br J Cancer 94:161–164
26. Freedman DM, Stewart P, Kleinerman RA, Wacholder S, Hatch EE, Tarone R, et al. (2001) Household solvent exposures and childhood acute lymphoblastic leukemia. Am J Public Health 91: 564–567
27. Fritschi L, Ambrosini GL, Kliewer EV, Johnson KC, Canadian Cancer Registries Epidemiologic Research Group (2004) Dietary fish intake and risk of leukaemia, multiple myeloma, and non-Hodgkin lymphoma. Cancer Epidemiol Biomarkers Prev 13(4):532–537
28. Fulton J, Cobb S, Preble L, Leone L, Forman E (1980) Electrical wiring configurations and childhood leukemia in Rhode Island. Am J Epidemiol 111:292–296
29. Fuortes L (1990) Leukemia incidence and radioactivity in drinking water in 59 Iowa towns. Am J Public Health 80:1261–1262
30. Gardner MJ (1991) Childhood cancer and nuclear installations. Public Health 105:277–285
31. Gardner MJ, Hall AJ, Downes S, Terrell JD (1987) Follow up study of children born elsewhere but attending schools in Seascale, West Cumbria (schools cohort). Br Med J 295:819–827
32. Gardner MJ, Snee MP, Hall AJ, Powell CA, Downes S, Terrell JD (1990) Results of case-control study of leukaemia and lymphoma among young people near Sellafield nuclear plant in West Cumbria. Br Med J 300:423–429
33. Gilbert ES, Land CE, Simon SL (2002) Health effects from fallout. Health Physics 82:726–735
34. Golub TR, Barker GF, Bohlander SK, Hiebert SW, Ward DC, Bray-Ward P, et al. (1995) Fusion of the TEL gene on 12p13 to the AML1 gene on 21q22 in acute lymphoblastic leukemia. Proc Natl Acad Sci 92:4917–4921
35. Greaves MF (1988) Speculations on the cause of childhood acute lymphoblastic leukemia. Leukemia 2:120–125
36. Greaves MF (1997) Aetiology of acute leukemia. Lancet 349:344–349
37. Greaves MF (1999) Molecular genetics, natural history and the demise of childhood leukemia. Eur J Cancer 35:1941–1953
38. Greaves MF (2006) Infection, immune responses and the aetiology of childhood leukemia. Nat Rev Cancer 6:193–203
39. Greaves MF, Alexander FE (1993) An infectious etiology for common acute lymphoblastic leukemia in childhood? Leukemia 7:349–360
40. Greenberg RS, Shuster JL, Jr (1985) Epidemiology of cancer in children. Epidemiology Rev 7:22–48
41. Greenland S, Sheppard AR, Kaune WT, Poole C, Kelsh MA (2000) A pooled analysis of magnetic fields, wire codes and childhood leukemia. Epidemiology 11:624–634
42. Groves FD, Linet MS, Devesa SS (1995) Patterns of occurrence of the leukemias. Eur J Cancer 31A:941–949
43. Gurney JG, Severson RK, Davis S, Robison LL (1995) Incidence of cancer in children in the United States. Cancer 75:2186–2195
44. Higgins CD, dos-Santos-Silva I, Stiller CA, Swerdlow AJ (2001) Season of birth and diagnosis of children with leukaemia: An analysis of over 15000 UK cases occurring from 1953–1995. Br J Cancer 84:406–412
45. Huebner WW, Wojcik NC, Roamilia K, Jorgensen G, Milano CA (2004) Mortality updates (1970–1997) of two refinery/petrochemical plant cohorts at Baton Rouge, Louisiana and Baytown, Texas. J Occup Environ Med 46:1229–1245
46. Huret JL, Brizard A, Slater R, Charrin C, Bertheas MF, Guilhot F, et al. (1993) Cytogenetic heterogeneity in t(11;19) acute leukemia: Clinical, hematological and cytogenetic analyses of 48 patients – Updated published cases and 16 new observations. Leukemia 7:152–160
47. Infante-Rivard C, Fortier I, Olson E (2000) Markers of infection, breast-feeding and childhood acute lymphoblastic leukaemia. Br J Cancer 83:1559–1564
48. Infante-Rivard C, Labuda D, Krajinovic M, Sinnett D (1999) Risk of childhood leukemia associated with exposure to pesticides and with gene polymorphisms. Epidemiology 10:481–487
49. International Agency for Research on Cancer (2005) IARC Monographs on the Evaluation of Carcinogenic Risks to Humans. IARC Press, Lyon
50. Jablon S, Hrubec Z, Boice JD Jr (1991) Cancer in populations living near nuclear facilities. JAMA 265:1403–1408
51. Jemal A, Siegel R, Ward E, Murray T, Xu J, Smigal C, et al. (2006) Cancer statistics, 2006. CA Cancer J Clin 56:106–130
52. Jensen CD, Block G, Buffler P, Ma X, Selvin S, Month S (2004) Maternal dietary risk factors in childhood acute lymphoblastic leukemia (United States). Cancer Causes Control 15(6):559–570
53. Katz F, Ball S, Gibbons B (1990) Acute lymphoblastic leukaemia in infancy: Clinical and biological features. Leuk Lymph 2:259
54. Kersey JH (1997) Fifty years of studies of the biology and therapy of childhood leukemia. Blood 90:4243–4251
55. Kheifets L, Afifi AA, Buffler PA, Zhang Z, Matkin C (1997) Occupational electric and magnetic field exposure and leukemia. J Occup Environ Med 39:1074–1091
56. Kinlen LJ (1988) Evidence for an infective cause of childhood leukemia: Comparison of a Scottish new town with nuclear reprocessing sites in Britain. Lancet ii:1323–1327
57. Kinlen LJ (1995) Epidemiological evidence for an infective basis in childhood leukemia [editorial]. Br J Cancer 71:1–5
58. Kinlen LJ (2000) Infection, childhood leukemia and the Seascale cluster. Radiological Protection Bulletin 226:9–18

59. Kinlen LJ, Petridou E (1995) Childhood leukemia and rural population movements: Greece, Italy, and other countries. Cancer Causes Control. 6:445–450
60. Kipen HM, Wartenberg D (2005) Lymphohematopoietic malignancies. In: Rosenstock L, Cullen MR, Brodkin CA, Redlich CA, (eds) Textbook of clinical occupational and environmental medicine. Elsevier Saunders, New York, pp 744–756
61. Knox EG, Gilman EA (1997) Hazard proximities of childhood cancers in Great Britain from 1953–1980. J Epidemiol Community Health 51:151–159
62. Koushik A, King WD, McLaughlin JR (2001) An ecologic study of childhood leukemia and population mixing in Ontario, Canada. Cancer Causes Control 12:483–490
63. Krieger N, Chen JT, Waterman P, Soobader M-J, Subramanian SV, Carson R (2002) Geocoding and monitoring of US socioeconomic inequalities in mortality and cancer incidence: Does the choice of area-based measure and geographic level matter? Am J Epidemiol 156:471–482
64. Krivit W, Good RA (1957) Simultaneous occurrence of mongolism and leukemia. Am J Dis Children 94:289–293
65. Kwan ML, Block G, Selvin S, Month S, Buffler PA (2004) Food consumption by children and the risk of childhood acute leukemia. Am J Epidemiol 160:1098–1107
66. Kwiatkowski A (1993) Dietary and other environmental risk factors in acute leukemias: A case-control study of 119 patients. Eur J Cancer Prev 2:139–146
67. Land CE, McKay FW, Machado SG (1984) Childhood leukemia and fallout from the Nevada nuclear tests. Science 223:139–144
68. Langholz B, Ebi K, Thomas C, Peters J, London S (2002) Traffic density and the risk of childhood leukemia in a Los Angeles case control study. Annals Epidemiol 12:482–487
69. Laplanche A, de Vathaire F (1994) Leukaemia mortality in French communes (administrative units) with a large and rapid population increase. Br J Cancer 69:110–113
70. Laurier D, Grosche B, Hall P (2002) Risk of childhood leukaemia in the vicinity of nuclear installations–findings and recent controversies [Review]. [118 refs]. Acta Oncologica 41:14–24
71. Laurier D, Valenty M, Tirmarche M (2001) Radon exposure and the risk of leukemia: A review of epidemiologic studies. Health Physics 81:272–288
72. Lehtinen M, Koskela P, Ogmundsdottir HM, Bloigu A, Dillner J, Gudnadottir M, et al. (2003) Maternal herpes virus infection and risk of acute lymphoblastic leukemia in the offspring. Am J Epidemiol 158:207–213
73. Lemen RA, Meinhardt TJ, Carndall MS, et al. (1990) Environmental epidemiologic investigations in the styrene-butadiene rubber production industry. Environ Health Perspect 86:103–106
74. Lightfoot TJ, Roman E (2004) Causes of childhood leukemia and lymphoma. Toxicol Appl Pharmacol 199:104–117
75. Linet MS, Cartwright R (1996) The Leukemias. In: Schottenfeld D, Fraumeni J, (eds) Cancer epidemiology and prevention. Oxford University Press, New York, pp 841–892
76. Linet MS, Hatch EE, Kleinerman RA, Robison LL, Kaune WT, Friedman DR, et al. (1997) Residential exposure to magnetic fields and acute lymphoblastic leukemia in children. N Engl J Med 337:1–7
77. Linet MS, Wacholder S, Zahm SH (2003) Interpreting epidemiologic research: Lessons from studies of childhood cancer. Pediatrics 112:218–232
78. Little J (1999) Epidemiology of childhood cancer. (No. 149). IARC. IARC Scientific Publications, Lyon, France
79. London S, Thomas D, Bowman JD, Sobel E, Cheng T-C, Peters J (1991) Exposure to residential electric and magnetic fields and risk of childhood leukemia. Am J Epidemiol 134:923–937
80. Lyman G, Lyman C, Johnson W (1985) Association of leukemia with radium groundwater contamination. JAMA 254:621–626
81. Lynge E, Anttila A, Hemminki K (1997) Organic solvents and cancer. Cancer Causes Control 8:406–419
82. Lyon JL, Klauber MR, Gardner JW, Udall KS (1979) Childhood leukemias associated with fallout from nuclear testing. N Engl J Med 300:397–402
83. Ma X, Buffler PA, Selvin S, Matthay KK, Wiencke JK, Wiemels JL, et al. (2002) Daycare attendance and risk of childhood acute lymphocytic leukaemia. Br J Cancer 86:1419–1424
84. Machado SG, Land CE, McKay FW (1987) Cancer mortality and radioactive fallout in southwestern Utah. Am J Epidemiol 125: 44–61
85. McKinney PA, Juszczak E, Findlay E, Smith K, Thomson CS (1999) Pre- and perinatal risk factors for childhood leukemia and other malignancies: A Scottish case control study. Br J Cancer 80: 1844–1851
86. McLaughlin JR, King WD, Anderson TW, Clarke EA, Ashmore JP (1993) Paternal radiation exposure and leukemia in offspring: The Ontario case-control study. Br Med J 307:959–966
87. McMichael A, Spirtas R (1975) Solvent exposure and leukemia among rubber workers: An epidemiologic study. J Occup Med 17:234–239
88. McNally RJQ, Eden TOB (2004) An infectious aetiology for childhood acute leukaemia: A review of the evidence. Br J Haematol 127:243–263
89. Meinert R, Schuz J, Kaletsch U, Kaatsch P, Michaelis J (2000) Leukemia and non-Hodgkin's lymphoma in childhood and exposure to pesticides: Results of a register-based case-control study in Germany. Am J Epidemiol 151:639–648
90. Menegaux F, Baruchel A, Betrand Y, Lescoeur B, Leverger G, Nelken B, et al. (2006) Household exposure to pesticides and risk of childhood acute leukemia. Occup Environ Med 63:131–134
91. Mikhail FM, Serry KA, Hatem N, Mourad ZI, Farawela HM, El Kaffash DM, et al. (2002) A new translocation that rearranges the AML1 gene in a patient with T-cell acute lymphoblastic leukemia. Cancer Genet Cytogenet 135:96–100
92. Milham S (1982) Mortality from leukemia in workers exposed to electrical and magnetic fields. N Engl J Med 307:249
93. Milham S (1985) Silent keys: Leukemia mortality in amateur radio operators. Lancet 1:812
94. Morgan GJ, Cotter F, Katz FE, Ridge SA, Domer P, Korsmeyer S, et al. (1992) Breakpoints at 11q23 in infant leukemias with the t(11;19)(q23;p13) are clusters. Blood 80:2172–2175
95. Mori H, Colman SM, Xiao Z, Ford AM, Healy LE, Donaldson C, et al. (2002) Chromosome translocations and covert leukemic clones are generated during normal fetal development. Proc Natl Acad Sci 99:8242–8247
96. Muirhead CR, Kendall GM, Darby SC, Doll R, Haylock RG, O'Hagen JA, et al. (2004) Epidemiologic studies of UK test veterans: II. Mortality and cancer incidence. J Radiation Protection 24: 219–341

97. National Research Council (1990) Health effects of exposure to low levels of ionizing radiation. BEIR V. National Research Council Committee on the Biological Effects of Ionizing Radiation (eds) National Academy Press, Washington, DC
98. National Research Council (1997) Possible health effects of exposure to residential electric and magnetic fields. Committee on the Possible Effects of Electromagnetic Fields on Biologic Systems (eds) National Academy Press, Washington, DC
99. Naumberg E, Bellocco R, Cnattingius S, Honzon A, Ekbom A (2002) Perinatal exposure to infection and risk of childhood leukemia. Med Pediatr Oncol 38:391–397
100. NIEHS Working Group (1998) Assessment of health effects from exposure to power-line frequency electric and magnetic fields. Portier CJ, Wolfe MS. NIH Publication No. 98-3981, -508. Research Triangle Park, NC, National Institute of Environmental Health Sciences, National Institutes of Health, US Department of Health and Human Services, Public Health Service
101. Nordlinder R, Jarvholm B (1997) Environmental exposure to gasoline and leukemia in children and young adults – An ecologic study. Int Arch Occup Environ Health 70:57–60
102. Pang D, McNally RJQ, Birch JM, United Kingdom childhood cancer study (2003) Parental smoking and childhood cancer: Results from the United Kingdom childhood cancer study. Br J Cancer 88:373–381
103. Pearson RL, Wachtel H, Ebi KL (2000) Distance-weighted traffic density in proximity to a home is a risk factor for leukemia and other childhood cancers. J Air Waste Manage Assoc 50:175–180
104. Peters JM, Preston-Martin S, London SJ, Bowman JD, Buckley JD, Thomas DC (1994) Processed meats and risk of childhood leukemia. Cancer Causes Control 5:195–202
105. Petridou E, Ntouvelis E, Dessypris N, Terzidis A, Trichopoulos D, the Childhood Hematology-Oncology Group (2005) Maternal diet and acute lymphoblastic leukemia in young children. Cancer Epidemiol Biomark Prev 14(8):1935–1939
106. Poole C, Greenland S, Luetters C, Kelsey JL, Mezei G (2006) Socioeconomic status and childhood leukemia: A review. Int J Epidemiol 35:370–384
107. Preston DL, Kusumi S, Tomonaga M, Izumi S, Ron E, Kuramoto A, et al. (1994) Cancer incidence in atomic bomb survivors. Part III: Leukemia, lymphoma and multiple myeloma, 1950–1987. Radiat Res 137:S68–S97
108. Pui CH, Crist WM, Look AT (1990) Biological and clinical significance of cytogenetic abnormalities in childhood acute lymphoblastic leukemia. Blood 76:1149–1163
109. Pui CH, Kane JR, Crist WM (1995) Biology and treatment of infant leukemias. Leukemia 9:762–769
110. Raaschou-Nielsen O, Hertel O, Thomsen BL, Olsen JH (2001) Air pollution from traffic at the residence of children with cancer. Am J Epidemiol 153:433–443
111. Raaschou-Nielsen O, Obel J, Dalton S, TjOnneland A, Hansen J (2004) Socioeconomic status and risk of childhood leukemia in Denmark. Scand J Public Health 32:279–286
112. Raffini LJ, Slater DJ, Rappaport EF, Lo Nigro L, Cheung NK, Biegel JA, et al. (2002) Panhandle and reverse-panhandle PCR enable cloning of der(11) and der(other) genomic breakpoint junctions of MLL translocations and identify complex translocation of MLL, AF-4, and CDK6. Proc Natl Acad Sci 99:4568–4573
113. Reynolds P, Elkin E, Scalf R, Von Behren J, Neutra RR (2001) A case-control pilot study of traffic exposures and early childhood leukemia using a geographic information systems. Bioelectromagnetics 5(Suppl):S58–S68
114. Reynolds P, Gunier RB, Goldberg DE, Hertz A (2004) Residential exposure to traffic in California and childhood cancer. Epidemiology 15:6–12
115. Reynolds P, Von Behren J, Gunier RB, Goldberg DE, Harnly ME, Hertz A (2005) Agricultural pesticide use and childhood cancer in California. Epidemiology 16:93–100
116. Reynolds P, Von Behren J, Gunier RB, Goldberg DE, Hertz A, Smith DF (2003) Childhood cancer incidence rates and hazardous air pollutants in California: An exploratory analysis. Environ Health Perspect 111:663–668
117. Ries LAG, Harkins D, Krapcho M, Mariotto A, Miller BA, Feuer EJ, Clegg L, Eisner MP, Horner MJ, Howlader N, et al. (2006) SEER Cancer Statistics Review, 1975–2003. Bethesda, MD, National Cancer Institute (http://seer.cancer.gov/csr/1975_2003)
118. Robison LL, Mertens A, Neglia JP (1991) Epidemiology and etiology of childhood cancer. In: Fernbach D, Vietti TJ, (eds) Clinical pediatric oncology. Mosby, St. Louis, pp 13–15
119. Ross JA (1998) Maternal diet and infant leukemia: A role for DNA topoisomerase II inhibitors? Int J Cancer 11(Suppl):26–28
120. Ross JA, Davies SM, Potter JD, Robison LL (1994) Epidemiology of childhood leukemia, with a focus on infants. Epidemiology Rev 16:243–272
121. Ross JA, Kasum CM, Davies SM, Jacobs DR, Folsom AR, Potter JD (2002) Diet and risk of leukemia in the Iowa Women's Health Study. Cancer Epidemiol Biomark Prev 11:777–781
122. Ross JA, Potter JD, Reaman GH, Pendergrass TW, Robison LL (1996) Maternal exposure to potential inhibitors of DNA topoisomerase II and infant leukemia (United States): A report from the Children's Cancer Group. Cancer Causes Control 7(6): 581–590
123. Ross JA, Severson RK, Swensen AR, Pollock BH, Gurney JG, Robison LL (1999) Seasonal variations in the diagnosis of childhood cancer in the United States. Br J Cancer 81:549–553
124. Ross JA, Spector LG, Davies SM (2005) Biological basis of cancer and blood disorder. Etiology of childhood cancer: Recent reports. Pediatr Blood Cancer 45:239–241
125. Rubnitz JE, Downing JR, Pui CH, Shurtleff SA, Raimondi SC, Evans WE, et al. (1997) TEL gene rearrangement in acute lymphoblastic leukemia: A new genetic marker with prognostic significance. Clin Oncol 15:1150–1157
126. Sandler DP, Ross JA (1997) Epidemiology of acute leukemia in children and adults. Semin Oncol 24:3–16
127. Sandler DP, Ross JA (1997) Epidemiology of acute leukemia in children and adults. [Review] [223 refs]. Semin Oncol 24(1): 3–16
128. Sarasua S, Savitz DA (1994) Cured and broiled meat consumption in relation to childhood cancer. Cancer Causes Control 5:141–148
129. Savitz DA, Feingold L (1989) Association of childhood cancer with residential traffic density. Scand J Work Env Health 15: 360–363
130. Savitz DA, Loomis DP (1995) Magnetic field exposure in relation to leukemia and brain cancer mortality among electric utility workers. Am J Epidemiol 141:123–134

131. Savitz DA, Wachtel H, Barnes FA, John EM, Tvrdik JG (1988) Case-control study of childhood cancer and exposure to 60-Hertz magnetic fields. Am J Epidemiol 128:21–38
132. Schuz J, Kaletsch U, Meinert R, Kaatsch P, Michaelis J (2000) Risk of childhood leukemia and parental self-reported occupational exposure to chemicals, dusts, and fumes: Results from pooled analyses of German population-based case-control studies. Cancer Epidemiol Biomark Prev 9:835–838
133. Schuz J, Spector LG, Ross JA (2003) Bias in studies of parental self-reported occupational exposure and childhood cancer. Am J Epidemiol 158:710–716
134. Shu XO, Gao Y-T, Brinton LA, et al. (1988) A population-based case-control study of childhood leukemia in Shanghai. Cancer 62:934–937
135. Shu XO, Stewart P, Wen W-Q, Han D, Potter J, Buckley JD, et al. (1999) Parental occupational exposure to hydrocarbons and risk of acute lymphocytic leukemia in offspring. Cancer Epidem Biomark Prev 8:783–791
136. Smith M (1997) Considerations on a possible viral etiology for B-precursor acute lymphoblastic leukemia of childhood. J Immunother 20:89–100
137. Smith MA, Simon R, Strickler HD, McQuillan G, Ries LAG, Linet MS (1998) Evidence that childhood acute lymphoblastic leukemia is associated with an infectious agent linked to hygiene conditions. Cancer Causes Control 9:285–298
138. Sorensen HT, Pedersen L, Olsen J, Rothman K (2001) Seasonal variation in month of birth and diagnosis of early childhood acute lymphoblastic leukaemia. JAMA 285:168–169
139. Spector LG, Groves FD, DeStefano F, Liff J, Klein M, Mullooly J, et al. (2004) Medically recorded allergies and the risk of childhood acute lymphoblastic leukemia. Eur J Cancer 40:579–584
140. Spector LG, Xie Y, Robison LL, Heerema NA, Hilden JM, Lange B, et al. (2005) Maternal diet and infant leukemia: The DNA topoisomerase II inhibitor hypothesis: A report from the children's oncology group. Cancer Epidemiol Biomark Prev 14(3):651–655
141. Stagnaro E, Ramazzotti V, Crosignani P, Fontana A, Masala G, Miligi L, et al. (2001) Smoking and hematolymphopoietic malignancies. Cancer Causes Control 12:325–334
142. Steffen C, Auclerc MF, Auvrignon A, Baruchel A, Kebaili K, Lambilliotte A, et al. (2004) Acute childhood leukaemia and environmental exposure to potential sources of benzene and other hydrocarbons; a case-control study. Occup Env Med 61(9):773–778
143. Stevens W, Thomas DC, Lyon JL, Till JE, Kerber RA, Simon SL, et al. (1990) Leukemia in Utah and radioactive fallout from the Nevada test site. JAMA 264:585–591
144. Stewart A, Webb J, Hewitt D (1958) A survey of childhood malignancies. Br Med J 28:1497–1507
145. Swensen AR, Ross JA, Severson RK, Pollock BH, Robison LL (1997) The age peak in childhood acute lymphoblastic leukemia. Cancer 79:2045–2051
146. The Leukemia and Lymphoma Society (2005) Acute lymphocytic leukemia. The Leukemia and Lymphoma Society, White Plains, NY
147. Theriault GP, Goldberg M, Miller AB, Armstrong B, Guenel P, Deadman J, et al. (1994) Cancer risks associated with occupational exposure to magnetic fields among electric utility workers in Ontario and Quebec, Canada, and France: 1970–1989. Am J Epidemiol 139:550–572
148. Tomenius L (1986) 50-Hz electromagnetic environment and the incidence of childhood tumors in Stockholm County. Bioelectromagnetics 7:191–207
149. Viel J-E, Richardson S, Danel P, Boutard P, Malet M, Barrelier P, et al. (1993) Childhood leukemia incidence in the vicinity of La Hague nuclear waste reprocessing facility (France). Cancer Causes Control 4:341–343
150. Visser O, van Wijnen JH, van Leeuwen FE (2004) Residential traffic density and cancer incidence in Amsterdam, 1989–1997. Cancer Causes Control 15(4):331–339
151. Wartenberg D (2001) Residential EMF exposure and childhood leukemia: Meta-analysis and population attributable risk. Bioelectromagnetics 5(Suppl):S86–S104
152. Wartenberg D, Reyner D, Scott CS (2000) Trichloroethylene and cancer: The epidemiologic evidence. Environ Health Perspect 108(Suppl 2):161–176
153. Wartenberg D, Schneider D, Brown S (2004) Childhood leukemia incidence and the population mixing hypothesis in US SEER data. Br J Cancer 90:1771–1776
154. Wen W, Shu XO, Linet MS, Neglia JP, Potter JD, Trigg ME, et al. (2000) Allergic disorders and the risk of childhood acute lymphoblastic leukemia (United States). Cancer Causes Control 11(4): 303–307
155. Wen W, Shu XO, Potter JD, Severson RK, Buckley JD, Reaman GH, et al. (2002) Parental medication use and risk of childhood acute lymphoblastic leukemia. Cancer 95(8):1786–1794
156. Wertheimer N, Leeper E (1979) Electrical wiring configurations and childhood cancer. Am J Epidemiol 109:273–284
157. Westerbeek RMC, Blair V, Eden OB, Kelsey AM, Stevens RF, Will AM, et al. (1998) Seasonal variations in the onset of childhood leukaemia and lymphoma. Br J Cancer 78:119–124
158. Wong O, Harris F, Rosamilia K, Raabe GK (2001) Updated mortality study of workers at a petroleum refinery in Torrance, California, 1959–1997. J Occup Environ Med 43:1089–1102
159. Yoshimoto Y (1990) Cancer risk among children of atomic bomb survivors: A review of RERF epidemiologic studies. JAMA 264: 596–600
160. Yoshimoto Y, Kato H, Schull WJ (1988) Risk of cancer among children exposed in utero to A-bomb radiations, 1950–1984. Lancet 2:665–669
161. Yoshimoto Y, Neel JV, Schull WJ, et al. (1990) Malignant tumors during the first 2 decades of life in the offspring of atomic bomb survivors. Am J Hum Genet 46:1040–1052
162. Zuelzer WW (1964) Implications of long-term survivals in acute stem cell leukemia of childhood treated with composite cyclic therapy. Blood 24:477–494 (as cited by The Leukemia and Lymphoma Society 2005)

Molecular Biology and Genetics

Meir Wetzler, Mrózek Kryzstof

Contents

6.1 Introduction

Acute lymphoblastic leukemia (ALL) is characterized by distinctive morphologic, cytogenetic, and molecular genetic features, some of which have important clinical implications for both diagnosis and predicting response to specific treatment regimens, while the role of others is yet to be defined. This chapter will describe the cytogenetic and molecular aberrations in ALL.

6.2 Cytogenetic Aberrations

Cytogenetic aberrations can be structural, e.g., reciprocal and unbalanced translocations, deletions, dicentric chromosomes, or inversions; or numerical, e.g., gain of a whole chromosome (trisomy) or loss of a whole chromosome (monosomy). In many instances, molecular dissection of structural chromosome abnormalities, especially reciprocal translocations, identified specific genes associated with leukemogenesis. The most common structural cytogenetic aberrations and their affected genes are shown in Table 6.1.

Table 6.1. Most frequent cytogenetic aberrations and their corresponding genes

Cytogenetic aberration	Genes involved*	Frequency (%)
t(9;22)(q34;q11.2)	*BCR/ABL*	11–34
t(4;11)(q21;q23)	*MLL/AF4*	3–7
del(9p) or t(9p)	*CDKN2A* and *CDKN2B*	5–15
del(12p) or t(12p)	*ETV6*	4–5
t(14q11-q13)†	*TCR* α and δ	4–6
t(14q32) not t(8;14)(q24;q32)	*IGH, BCL11A, TCL-1BCL11B*	5
del(6q)	?	2–6
t(1;19)(q23;p13)	*E2A/PBX1*	3
Extrachromosome 9q	*NUP214/ABL*	4

*, please refer to text for abbreviations;

†, please refer to Table 6.2 for 14q11 partner genes.

6.3 Structural Aberrations

6.3.1 t(9;22)(q34;q11.2)

The t(9;22)(q34;q11.2) is the single most frequent chromosome abnormality in adult ALL, being detected in 11–34% of patients with ALL, and is associated with an unfavorable prognosis [1–9]. It rarely occurs in therapy-related ALL [10]. The reciprocal translocation between chromosomes 9 and 22 results in the head-to-tail fusion of variable numbers of 5′ breakpoint cluster region (*BCR*) exons on chromosome band 22q11.2 with the exon 2 of the *ABL* gene (named after the Abelson murine leukemia virus) located on chromosome band 9q34 [11]. The protein product of the fusion gene resulting from the t(9;22) plays a central role in the development of this form of ALL. Two main types of fusion proteins, $p190^{BCR/ABL}$ and $p210^{BCR/ABL}$, each containing NH2-terminal domains of Bcr and COOH-terminal domains of Abl, are produced depending on the location of the breakpoint within the *BCR* gene. The $p190^{BCR/ABL}$ product contains the first exon of *BCR* and occurs in 50–78% of the ALL cases with t(9;22) [12–15]. The $p210^{BCR/ABL}$ product contains either exon 13 or exon 14 of *BCR* and is less frequent in ALL. However, $p190^{BCR/ABL}$ transcripts are frequently detected at a low level in $p210^{BCR/ABL}$-positive ALL [16]. Clinically, there is no clear distinction between the two molecular variants of the disease [17–19], except for one report showing that the $p210^{BCR/ABL}$ product is associated with patients' older age [20] and another report demonstrating a higher risk of relapse in $p190^{BCR/ABL}$ ALL following allogeneic transplantation [21]. Of interest, imatinib-containing treatment did not reveal any outcome difference between the two disease types [22].

Secondary chromosomal aberrations accompanying t(9;22) occur in 41–86% of adult ALL patients [18, 19, 23–26]. The most common additional aberrations in CALGB series [26] were, in order of decreasing frequency, +der(22)t(9;22), 9p rearrangements, hyperdiploidy (>50 chromosomes), +8, and −7. In this study, the presence of +der(22)t(9;22) was associated with a higher cumulative incidence of relapse while the presence of −7 as a sole secondary abnormality was associated with a lower complete remission rate [26].

At the molecular level, *BCR/ABL* has recently been shown to activate the Src kinases Lyn, Hck, and Fgr in ALL cells [27]. These kinases have not been activated in CML, suggesting a unique downstream signaling pathway in *BCR/ABL*-positive ALL. Further, application of DNA microarray gene expression profiling assay revealed that *BCR/ABL*-positive pediatric ALL is characterized by gene expression profiles distinct from other prognostically relevant leukemia subtypes [28]. These results were recently partially confirmed and validated in samples from adult ALL patients [29]. While adult *BCR/ABL*-positive ALL patients could be clearly distinguished from patients with T-cell ALL and patients with 11q23 rearrangements, their expression signatures were similar to those observed in a heterogeneous group of patients with B-precursor ALL who did not carry t(9;22) or t(11q23) chromosomal aberrations. It is hoped that microarray gene expression analyses will lead to identification of genes that can be targeted with individualized therapies and that this will increase response rates.

6.3.2 MLL Gene Rearrangements

The mixed lineage leukemia (*MLL* gene, also known as *ALL-1*, *HTRX*, or *HRX*) gene, located at chromosome band 11q23 [30], encodes a putative transcriptional regulator. It is involved in reciprocal translocations with several gene partners, localized on different chromosomes, both in ALL and acute myeloid leukemia (AML) [31]. While the *MLL* gene can be amplified in a subset of AML patients, its amplification is very rare in ALL [32]. The distribution of 11q23/*MLL* translocation partners differs between ALL and AML, with t(4;11)(q21;q23) being by far the most frequent 11q23 translocation in ALL (see below). The breaks in *MLL* in most translocations occur in the 8.3 kb BCR, between exons 8 and 12. Fusion of a COOH-terminal partner is essential for leukemogenesis, as expression of the NH2-terminus alone was not sufficient to immortalize cells [33]. Partial tandem duplication, described in AML [34], has not been thus far detected in ALL. *MLL* translocations have been described in both de novo and therapy-related disease [35].

MLL-positive ALL also has a unique gene expression profile [29, 36]. Specifically, some *HOX* (homeobox) genes are expressed at higher levels in *MLL*-positive ALL than in *MLL*-negative ALL [37]. Furthermore, gene expression profiles predictive of relapse were recently identified in pediatric *MLL*-positive ALL in one study [38] but did not reach statistical significance in the other [28]. Further work in this area is ongoing.

6.3.3 t(4;11)(q21;q23)

The t(4;11)(q21;q23) is the most frequent chromosomal rearrangement involving the *MLL* gene in adult ALL, being detected in 3–7% of ALL patients, and is associated with an unfavorable outcome [1–5, 7, 8]. It results in two reciprocal fusion products coding for chimeric proteins derived from *MLL* and from a serine/proline-rich protein encoded by the *AF4* (*ALL1* fused gene from chromosome 4) gene [39]. Studies have revealed different fusion sequences documenting variable *MLL* and *AF4* exon involvement in t(4;11) [40–42]. To our knowledge, the different fusion sequences affect neither disease characteristics nor outcome.

Griesinger et al. [43] have demonstrated the presence of *MLL-AF4* gene fusions in adult ALL patients without cytogenetically detectable t(4;11). Another study analyzed the clinical significance of molecularly detected *MLL-AF4* gene without karyotypic evidence of t(4;11), and established that patients whose blasts were *MLL-AF4*-positive in the absence of t(4;11) had outcome similar to patients whose blasts were *MLL-AF4*-negative [44]. This study suggests that additional treatment is not needed for patients whose blasts are *MLL-AF4*-positive but t(4;11)-negative. Furthermore, the finding of MLL-AF4 transcripts by nested reverse-transcriptase (RT) polymerase chain reaction (PCR) in four of 16 fetal bone marrow samples, five of 13 fetal livers, and one of six normal infant marrows shows that healthy individuals carry rare nonmalignant cells with the *MLL-AF4* gene fusion and indicates that the presence of *MLL-AF4* is not sufficient for leukemogenesis [44]. Therefore, to be clinically relevant, the presence of *MLL-AF4* should not be detected solely by nested RT-PCR but confirmed using another technique such as cytogenetic, Southern blot, and/or FISH analyses.

Secondary cytogenetic aberrations in addition to t(4;11) are found in approximately 40% of patients [4, 45, 46]. The most common additional changes were i(7)(q10) and +6 in one series [45] and +X, i(7)(q10), and +8 in another [46]. With treatment carried out according to modern risk-adapted therapy, no difference in outcome was observed between patients with and without clonal chromosome aberrations in addition to t(4;11) at diagnosis [46], although this series was relatively small thus warranting further study of a larger number of patients with t(4;11) ALL.

Other recurrent, albeit rare in ALL, translocations include t(6;11)(q27;q23), t(9;11)(p22;q23), t(10;11)(p12;q23), and t(11;19)(q23;p13.3) [47]. The respective fusion partners of the *MLL* gene are *AF6*, *AF9*, *AF10*, and *ENL* (eleven-nineteen leukemia). Other less common *MLL* partners were also described [48].

6.3.4 del(9p) or t(9p)

Deletions or translocations involving the short arm of chromosome 9 occur in 5–15% of adult ALL patients [4, 5, 7, 8]. Most of the breakpoints are located at 9p21, although other breaksites have also been reported. Anomalies of 9p are most often associated with other clonal aberrations (in up to 90% of patients), that in almost one third of the cases include t(9;22) [8]. These data suggest that del(9p) likely represent secondary cytogenetic abnormalities.

The genes most commonly involved in del(9p) are *CDKN2A* (cyclin-dependent kinase inhibitor 2A, also known as *MTS1* and $p16^{INK4A}$) and *CDKN2B* (also known as *MTS2* and $p15^{INK4B}$), both located at 9p21 [49, 50] adjacent to each other, with *CDKN2B* centromeric to *CDKN2A* [51]. One report describes these aberrations to occur frequently in T-lineage ALL [52], while another does not [49]. Interestingly, in some cases both genes are deleted and in others only one of them is [52]. In addition to deletion, loss of function of these genes in ALL can occur through methylation [53, 54]. Finally, in pediatric ALL, loss of 9p occurred preferentially on the maternally derived allele [55]; no such data are available for adult ALL.

Other recurrent aberrations involving the short arm of chromosome 9 are dicentric chromosomes: dic(9;12)(p11-13;p11-13) and dic(9;20)(p11;q11); these aberrations are associated with a favorable clinical outcome [56–58]. The former has been recently shown to result in a fusion of the *ETV6* (*ETS* variant gene 6, also known as *TEL*) gene at 12p13 with the *PAX5* (paired box gene 5) at 9p13 [59]. This finding has allowed refinement of cytogenetic description of the dic(9;12) to dic(9;12)(p13;p13). The molecular consequences of dic(9;20) are currently unknown. dic(9;12) is frequently associated with additional structural chromosomal aberrations or trisomy 8 [56], whereas trisomy 21 is a nonrandom secondary aberration in patients with dic(9;20) [57, 58].

6.3.5 del(12p) or t(12p)

Abnormalities of the short arm of chromosome 12 have been described in 4–5% of adult ALL patients [4, 5, 7, 8]. In one series, 20 of 23 cases with abnormal 12p had net loss of 12p material, eight caused by deletions and 12 by unbalanced translocations [4]. It is believed that a putative tumor suppressor gene is located in chromosome band 12p12.3 [60, 61]. The outcome of patients with abnormalities of the short arm of chromosome 12, who did not have t(9;22) was favorable in two adult ALL series [5, 8]. A cryptic t(12;21)(p12;q22), commonly found in pediatric ALL, and also associated with a favorable outcome, is rare in adult ALL [62–64]. The genes involved in this translocation include *ETV6* [65] and *RUNX1* (runt-related transcription factor 1, also known as *AML1* and *CBFA2*) [66]. An intriguing explanation for the favorable outcome of pediatric patients with t(12;21) may lie in the finding that the ETV6/RUNX1 protein can overcome drug resistance through transcriptional repression of the multidrug resistance-1 gene expression [67]. Further, t(12;21) ALL is associated with a lower expression of genes involved in purine metabolism and lower de novo purine synthesis [68]. Taken together, these data may explain the favorable outcome of pediatric t(12;21) ALL.

6.3.6 t(14q11-q13)

Abnormalities of the proximal part of the long arm of chromosome 14 have been described in 4–6% of adult ALL patients [4, 8]. The genes involved in t(14q11-q13) are T-cell receptor (TCR) α and δ [4]. Many partner chromosomes have been described to participate in translocations involving bands 14q11-q13 including the following chromosomal loci: 1q32, 1q34, 5q34, 8q24, 9p21-p22, 10q24, 11p13, 11p15, 11q23, 12p13, 14q32, and Xq28 [48]. Please refer to Table 6.2 for the corresponding genes. The most frequent 14q11 abnormality is t(10;14)(q24;q11), detected in 13 of 25 patients with 14q11-q13 translocations in one series [4] and four of 11 in another [8]. Translocation (10;14) results in a fusion between T-cell receptor δ and the *TLX1* (tailless, also known as *HOX11*) gene [69–71]. The t(10;14)(q24;q11) appears to be a primary cytogenetic abnormality in adult ALL and to confer favorable outcome.

Table 6.2. 14q11 partner genes

Karyotypic breakpoint	Gene	Reference
1q32	TAL1	[142–144]
1q34	TAL1	[145–148]
5q33-34	*RanBP17/ HOX11L2*	[149]
8q24	*MYC, ReHF-1*	[150, 151]
9p21-p22	*CDKN2A*	[152]
10q24	*TLX1/HOX11/ TCL3*	[69, 71, 153–156]
11p13	*TTG2/RBTN2*	[157, 158]
11p15	*LMO1*	[159]
11q23	*MLL*	[160]
12p13	?	[161]
14q32	Immuno-globulin heavy chain locus	[162, 163]
Xq28	*MTCP1*	[164, 165]

6.3.7 Translocations Involving Band (14q32) Other than t(8;14)(q24;q32)

Abnormalities of the distal part of the long arm of chromosome 14 have been described in approximately 5% of adult ALL patients [8]. The genes involved in t(14q32) are the immunoglobulin heavy chain locus [72] and the krüeppel zinc-finger gene (BCL11A) [73] on chromosome 14q32.3, both in B-lineage ALL, the TCL1 (T-cell leukemia) gene on chromosome 14q32.1 [74] and the distal region of a krüeppel-like zinc-finger transcription factor BCL11B (also called CTIP2) on chromosome 14q32.2 [75, 76], both in T-lineage ALL. Many partner chromosomes involved in translocations affecting 14q32 have been identified. In B-lineage ALL, the loci rearranged with 14q32 include 1q21, 1q25, 2p13, 5q31, 8q11, 11q23, 18q21 and 19q13.1, and in T-lineage ALL, 5q35, and 14q11 [48].

6.3.8 del(6q)

Deletions of the long arm of chromosome 6 were reported in 2–6% of adult ALL patients [1, 4–7, 77]. In one large series, most deletions encompassed band 6q21 (in 20 of 23 patients), with del(6)(q12q16) being present in three remaining patients [4]. In most patients, del(6q) is found together with additional chromosome abnormalities [8]. It is unclear, from data presented, whether del(6q) represents a primary or secondary cytogenetic abnormality. The outcome of patients with del(6q) was somewhat better than that of patients with a normal karyotype [4]. The genes involved in this aberration are not identified to date. It seems clear that *MYB* is not involved [78] but there may be a role for the estrogen receptor located on 6q25.1 [79] or *GRIK2* (glutamate receptor, ionotropic, kainate 2) located on 6q16 [80].

6.3.9 t(1;19)(q23;p13)

This aberration is significantly less common in adult than in pediatric ALL. It was recognized as a separate entity in adult ALL in only one series where it was found in 3% of the patients [4]. The genes involved in this translocation are *E2A* (early region of adenovirus type 2 encoding helix-loop-helix proteins E12/E47) on chromosome band 19p13.3 [81, 82] and *PBX1* (Pre-B cell leukemia transcription factor 1) on chromosome band 1q23 [83, 84]. Rare ALL cases with t(1;19)(q23;p13.3) lack *E2A/PBX1* fusion gene [85]. A recent study of a t(1;19)-positive cell line with pre-B cell phenotype identified a novel gene fusion between the *MEFD2D* (myocyte enhancer factor 2D) gene at 1q22 and *DAZAP1* (deleted in azoospermia associated protein 1) gene at 19p13.3 [86]. It is currently unknown how frequent the *MEF2D/DAZAP1* fusion is among adults with ALL.

At the molecular level, *ENA/PBX1* ALL has a unique gene expression pattern [28]. In addition to the potential of this pattern to serve for diagnostic purposes, some of the genes identified can provide insights into the biology of this disease. For example, gene profiling of pediatric *ENA/PBX1* ALL led to the identification of high expression levels of the *c-MER* gene in pretreatment samples [28]. c-MER is a receptor tyrosine kinase [87] with known transforming abilities [88]. Targeting c-MER may be a potential future therapeutic approach for this disease.

6.3.10 Extrachromosomal Amplification of the NUP214/ABL Fusion Gene in T-Cell ALL

Two recent studies revealed a novel genetic phenomenon in T-cell ALL, namely cryptic extrachromosomal amplification of a segment from chromosome 9 containing the *ABL* gene. Barber et al. [89] were the first to report that amplification involving the *ABL* gene occurred in five of 210 (2.3%) children and three of 70 (4.3%) adults with T-cell ALL, even though there was no cytogenetic evidence of amplification such as double minutes. The authors suggested that amplified *ABL* sequences were located on submicroscopic circular extrachromosomal DNA molecules called episomes. No amplification was detected among over 1600 pediatric and 300 adult patients with B-cell ALL screened with the same probe set [89]. A subsequent study [90] confirmed the episomal localization of the amplified material, and extended these observations by demonstrating that amplified sequences on episomes contained a fusion between *ABL* and *NUP214* (nucleoporin), a gene also located at 9q34. Notably, further analyses have revealed that *NUP214/ABL* is a constitutively activated tyrosine kinase activating similar pathways as *BCR/ABL* and is sensitive to inhibition with imatinib. While creation and amplification of *NUP214/ABL* fusion gene likely represents a genetic event of primary significance, most patients had also concurrent rearrangements, that is hemi- or homozygous deletions of tumor-suppressor genes *CDKN2A* and *CDKN2B*, and mutually exclusive overexpression of either the *TLX1* or *TLX3* (also called *HOX11L2*) gene, thus supporting the notion of a multistep pathogenesis of T-cell ALL [90].

6.4 Numerical Aberrations

6.4.1 High Hyperdiploidy

A high hyperdiploid karyotype, defined by the presence of >50 chromosomes, is detected in 2–9% of adult ALL patients [1, 2, 4–8]. The most common extra chromosomes in 30 patients with high hyperdiploidy (range 51 to 65 chromosomes) were (in decreasing order) 21, 4, 6, 14, 8, 10, and 17 [4]. In pediatric ALL, gain of X chromosome appears to be the most common chromosome abnormality being detected in nearly all children with a high hyperdiploid karyotype and up to one third of the patients with low hyperdiploid karyotype (i.e., 47–50) chromosomes [91]. Interestingly, chromosomes 6, 8, and 10 were also the most common chromosomes lost in the hypodiploid group, along with chromosome 21. The reason for the involvement of these specific chromosomes in both types of aberrations is unclear. Translocation (9;22) is common as a structural aberration in patients with high hyperdiploidy; it was present in 11 of 30 (37%) patients in one series [4] and seven of 11 (64%) in another [25]. Patients with hyperdiploidy and t(9;22) were older and had shorter DFS than those without t(9;22) [4].

The mechanism leading to hyperdiploidy is unknown. Several possibilities were suggested including polyploidization with subsequent losses of chromosomes, successive gains of individual chromosomes in consecutive cell divisions, and a simultaneous occurrence of trisomies in a single abnormal mitosis [92]. Paulsson et al. [93] studied samples from 10 pediatric ALL patients with hyperdiploidy and demonstrated an equal allele dosage for tetrasomy 21 suggesting that hyperdiploidy originated in a single aberrant mitosis. They further showed that trisomy 8 was of paternal origin in four of four patients and trisomy 14 was of maternal origin in seven of eight patients [93]. However, imprinting was not pathogenetically important in all other chromosomes. Similar studies are needed in adult ALL with hyperdiploidy.

The clinical outcome of adult patients with hyperdiploid karyotypes varies in different series. In two studies, the outcome of patients with hyperdiploid karyotypes was better than that of other adult ALL patients [1, 5, 7] while the other studies [2, 4, 8, 25] showed poor outcome for these patients except for those with near tetraploidy [4]. The reason for this discrepancy is unclear. In two studies [5, 8], the analysis was restricted to patients with hyperdiploidy without structural abnormalities. The other studies [1, 2, 4, 7, 25] did not provide information regarding structural abnormalities. It may be that T-cell lineage, known to be characterized by longer DFS and overall survival [94], confers a more important effect on treatment outcome than does chromosome number. A study of a larger cohort of adult ALL patients analyzing the effect of hyperdiploid karyotype without structural abnormalities as an independent prognostic factor is warranted.

At the molecular level, high hyperdiploidy in pediatric patients has a unique gene expression profile [28], with almost 70% of the genes that defined this group localized to either chromosome X or 21. The class-defining genes on chromosome X were overexpressed irrespective of whether the leukemic blasts had an extra copy of this chromosome [28]. It is unclear what mechanism leads to this pattern.

6.4.2 Hypodiploidy

Hypodiploidy is defined by the presence of <46 chromosomes. This karyotype is found in 4–9% of adult ALL patients [1, 4, 5, 7, 95]. These patients tend to be somewhat younger than patients with a normal karyotype [4, 5]. Most of these patients have a B-cell lineage immunophenotype [4, 5, 95], and B-lineage is characterized by shorter DFS and overall survival than T-lineage disease [94]. A recent analysis subgrouped patients with hypodiploidy into those with near-haploidy (23–29 chromosomes), low hypodiploidy (33–39 chromosomes), and high hypodiploidy (42–45 chromosomes) [95]. There were only six adult patients in that series, five of them in the low hypodiploidy group and one in the high hypodiploidy group. The most common losses in seven patients with hypodiploidy ranging from 30 to 39 chromosomes involved chromosomes 1, 5, 6, 8, 10, 11, 15, 18, 19, 21, 22, and the sex chromosomes [4]. Only one study reported specifically on hypodiploidy without structural abnormalities [5]. The impact of structural abnormalities in patients with hypodiploid karyotypes in the other series is unknown. Patients with hypodiploidy have a DFS between 2 to 4 months and therefore the abnormality is classified as unfavorable.

6.4.3 Trisomy 8

Trisomy 8 in ALL is most often associated with other karyotypic abnormalities; it is rare as a sole abnormality [96]. Furthermore, most previous reports have used karyotype prioritization designs [1–5] to compare the prognosis of different cytogenetic groups. In these designs, patients with trisomy 8 were combined with patients with other cytogenetic aberrations. Only one series defined patients with trisomy 8 as a separate group [8]. Twelve of 23 (52%) patients with trisomy 8 also had t(9;22). However, patients with trisomy 8 without t(9;22) but with miscellaneous other abnormalities fared as poorly as those with trisomy 8 and t(9;22) [8]. It is unclear whether the adverse outcome is due to the other primary abnormalities or associated with the presence of trisomy 8. A study of a larger cohort of patients is warranted in order to analyze the effect of trisomy 8 as an independent prognostic factor in adult ALL patients.

6.4.4 Monosomy 7

As with trisomy 8, monosomy 7 is most often associated with other karyotypic abnormalities; monosomy 7 as a sole abnormality is rare in ALL. Only one series defined patients with monosomy 7 as a separate group [8]. Nine of 14 (64%) patients with monosomy 7 had t(9;22). Patients with monosomy 7 without t(9;22) but with miscellaneous other abnormalities fared as poorly as those with monosomy 7 and t(9;22) [8]. It is unclear whether the adverse outcome is due to the other primary abnormalities or is associated with the presence of monosomy 7. A study of a larger cohort of adult ALL patients is warranted in order to analyze the independent effect of monosomy 7 on prognosis.

6.5 Molecular Aberrations

Molecular aberrations are divided into those that emerge from gene profiling, specific aberrations, and polymorphism.

6.5.1 Relapse-Classifying Gene Sets

Several groups have identified distinctive gene sets in diagnostic samples from patients whose disease relapsed [28, 29, 97–100]. In spite of the different age groups studied (pediatric [28, 97, 98] vs. adult [29, 99, 100]), assortment of array platforms, and diverse treatment protocols, all Affymetrix ALL array data and two sets of cDNA arrays validated the predictability of these gene sets to delineate the known cytogenetic prognostic groups [101]. Further, in at least two comparison analyses, a correlation between the relapse-classifying gene sets ([97, 100] and [28, 29]) was detected. Utilization of these gene sets to predict relapse risk and adjust treatment is awaiting validation in prospective trials. Nevertheless, some of these genes, such as *c-MER*, are being targeted for therapy.

6.5.2 Resistance-Classifying Gene Sets

A different analysis was completed when leukemia cells were tested for in vitro sensitivity to the four most commonly used drugs in ALL, i.e., prednisolone, vincristine, asparaginase, and daunorubicin [102]. Interestingly, only three genes for which results were significant in these analyses, *RPL6*, *ARHA*, and *SLC2A14*, have previously been associated with resistance to doxorubicin. Gene expression profiles that differed according to sensitivity or resistance to the four drugs were compared with treatment outcome. These two gene sets were significantly and independently predictive of outcome. They are now being analyzed in prospective studies to tailor treatment according to patterns of resistance.

6.5.3 Smad3

Smad [Sma and Mad (Mothers against Decapentaplegic)] 3 is involved in signal transduction from the transforming growth factor (TGF)-β superfamily of receptors to the nucleus [103]. Smad3 protein was recently shown to be absent in T-cell ALL but present in B-cell ALL and AML [104]. The *Smad3* transcript was intact in all leukemia subtypes. These data suggest that Smad3 is functioning as a tumor-suppressor gene in T-cell ALL. In mice, loss of one allele for *Smad3* works in tandem with homozygous inactivation of $p27^{Kip1}$ to promote T-cell leukemogenesis [104]. It will be of interest to understand the mechanism leading to the downregulation of Smad3 in this disease.

6.5.4 FLT3

FLT3 activating mutations are in general rare in ALL but have been detected in approximately 20% of ALL with rearrangement of the *MLL* gene [38, 105, 106], 25% of hyperdiploid ALL [106, 107], and in the rare subset of CD117/KIT-positive, CD3-positive ALL [108]. Interestingly, the internal tandem duplication of the *FLT3* gene, commonly detected in AML, has thus far not been seen in ALL. Flt3 inhibitors (e.g., PKC412, CEP-701) can suppress *FLT3*-positive ALL and therefore warrant clinical trials [105, 109].

6.5.5 TLX1

Gene expression profiles in T-cell ALL revealed five different signature patterns: *TLX1* (*HOX11*), *TLX3* (*HOX11L2*), *TAL1* plus *LMO1/2*, *LYL1* plus *LMO2*, and *MLL-ENL* [110]. Only the *TLX1*-expressing samples were associated with a favorable outlook in children [111] and adults [112] with T-cell ALL. Interestingly, these results were not reproduced by another group [100] and therefore will require further validation prior to implementing treatment strategies according to the presence or absence of *TLX1* gene expression.

6.5.6 Cryptic t(5;14)(q35;q32) and the Overexpression of the TLX3 Gene

TLX3 gene expression was shown to represent one of the five signature patterns in T-cell ALL [110]. This gene is located on chromosome 5q35 and was found to be transcriptionally activated as a result of a translocation between chromosome 5 and 14, t(5;14)(q35;q32) [113]. Studying samples from 23 childhood T-cell ALL patients revealed that this translocation was cryptic in five of them [113]. Larger studies [114, 115] have confirmed the cryptic nature of this translocation. Further, in a few cases, *TLX3* was overexpressed without the presence of the translocation by either conventional cytogenetic or FISH analyses, suggesting a different mechanism leading to the gene overexpression. Finally, overexpression of *TLX3* was reported by one group [116] to be associated with poor prognosis but this has not been confirmed by other larger studies [114, 115].

6.5.7 NOTCH1

NOTCH1 point mutations, insertions and deletions producing aberrant increases in NOTCH1 signaling are frequently present in T-cell ALL [117–119]. Further, NOTCH1 signaling was shown to be required for sustained growth and, in a subset of cell lines, for survival. Finally, experiments with small molecule inhibitors of γ-secretase, a protease required for normal NOTCH signal transduction and the activity of the mutated forms of NOTCH1, found inhibitory activity in T-cell ALL with NOTCH1 mutations. These results provide a rationale for clinical trials with NOTCH1 inhibitors, such as γ-secretase antagonists [118, 119].

6.5.8 Pharmacogenetics

Pharmacogenetics is the study of genetic variations in drug-processing genes and individual responses to drugs [120]. It enables the improved identification of patients at higher risk for either disease relapse or chemotherapy-associated side effects. In pharmacogenetic studies, single nucleotide polymorphisms and rarely haplotypes, that is, larger variations across a gene, are usually analyzed. To our knowledge, these studies have been performed only in pediatric ALL and studies in adult ALL are warranted.

It was recognized, more than 20 years ago, by measuring enzyme activity, that the activity of thiopurine-S-methyltransferase (TPMT), the enzyme involved in the metabolism of 6-mercaptopurine and 6-thioguanine, differs among patients and that approximately one in 300 individuals demonstrates reduced enzyme activity [121–125]. Molecular testing to identify this polymorphism was developed shortly thereafter [126, 127] and depicted good correlation with the enzymatic activity. Based on the molecular testing it has become clear that homozygous carriers for one of the three *TPMT* mutant alleles experience severe myelotoxicity and increased risk of relapse due to treatment delays [128, 129]. Interestingly, patients with the mutated *TPMT* alleles have a significantly higher risk of developing secondary brain tumors if treated with whole-brain radiation [130]. Similarly, there was a trend towards increased risk of secondary AML in patients with decreased enzymatic activity [131].

Similarly, single nucleotide polymorphism involving four of the enzymes involved in methotrexate metabolism have been implicated in increased relapse risk or toxicity in pediatric ALL patients: methylenetetrahydrofolate reductase [132–136], reduced folate carrier [137–139], thymidylate synthetase [140, 141], and methylenetetrahydrofolate dehydrogenase [136]. The results of these analyses are not always statistically significant; the discrepancies may be due to different patient populations, an assortment of treatment protocols and/or small patient numbers.

6.6 Future Directions

We believe that progress in cytogenetic and genetic dissection of ALL will lead to risk-adapted treatment in adult ALL as is already being accomplished for pediatric ALL. Currently, allogeneic transplantation in first remission is offered to adults with unfavorable karyotypes. The future promises a more refined approach, based on the information from genetic analyses, that will hopefully lead to improved outcome in adult ALL.

References

1. Bloomfield CD, Secker-Walker LM, Goldman AI, et al. (1989) Six-year follow-up of the clinical significance of karyotype in acute lymphoblastic leukemia. Cancer Genet Cytogenet 40(2):171–185
2. Fenaux P, Lai JL, Morel P, et al. (1989) Cytogenetics and their prognostic value in childhood and adult acute lymphoblastic leukemia (ALL) excluding L3. Hematol Oncol 7(4):307–317
3. Walters R, Kantarjian HM, Keating MJ, et al. (1990) The importance of cytogenetic studies in adult acute lymphocytic leukemia. Am J Med 89(5):579–587
4. Hématologique GFdC (1996) Cytogenetic abnormalities in adult acute lymphoblastic leukemia: Correlations with hematologic findings outcome. A Collaborative Study of the Group Francais de Cytogenetique Hematologique. Blood 88(7):3135–3142
5. Secker-Walker LM, Prentice HG, Durrant J, Richards S, Hall E, Harrison G (1997) Cytogenetics adds independent prognostic information in adults with acute lymphoblastic leukaemia on MRC trial UKALL XA. MRC Adult Leukaemia Working Party. Br J Haematol 96(3):601–610
6. Faderl S, Kantarjian HM, Talpaz M, Estrov Z (1998) Clinical significance of cytogenetic abnormalities in adult acute lymphoblastic leukemia. Blood 91(11):3995–4019
7. Chessells JM, Hall E, Prentice HG, Durrant J, Bailey CC, Richards SM (1998) The impact of age on outcome in lymphoblastic leukaemia; MRC UKALL X and XA compared: A report from the MRC Paediatric and Adult Working Parties. Leukemia 12(4):463–473
8. Wetzler M, Dodge RK, Mrozek K, et al. (1999) Prospective karyotype analysis in adult acute lymphoblastic leukemia: The cancer and leukemia Group B experience. Blood 93(11):3983–3993
9. Gleissner B, Rieder H, Thiel E, et al. (2001) Prospective BCR-ABL analysis by polymerase chain reaction (RT-PCR) in adult acute B-lineage lymphoblastic leukemia: Reliability of RT-nested-PCR and comparison to cytogenetic data. Leukemia 15(12):1834–1840
10. Block AW, Carroll AJ, Hagemeijer A, et al. (2002) Rare recurring balanced chromosome abnormalities in therapy-related myelodysplastic syndromes and acute leukemia: Report from an international workshop. Genes Chromosomes Cancer 33(4):401–412
11. Faderl S, Talpaz M, Estrov Z, O'Brien S, Kurzrock R, Kantarjian HM (1999) The biology of chronic myeloid leukemia. N Engl J Med 341(3):164–172
12. Kantarjian HM, Talpaz M, Dhingra K, et al. (1991) Significance of the P210 versus P190 molecular abnormalities in adults with Philadelphia chromosome-positive acute leukemia. Blood 78(9): 2411–2418
13. Westbrook CA, Hooberman AL, Spino C, et al. (1992) Clinical significance of the BCR-ABL fusion gene in adult acute lymphoblastic leukemia: A Cancer and Leukemia Group B Study (8762). Blood 80(12):2983–2990
14. Melo JV, Gordon DE, Tuszynski A, Dhut S, Young BD, Goldman JM (1993) Expression of the ABL-BCR fusion gene in Philadelphia-positive acute lymphoblastic leukemia. Blood 81(10): 2488–2491
15. Lim LC, Heng KK, Vellupillai M, et al. (1999) Molecular and phenotypic spectrum of de novo Philadelphia positive acute leukemia. Int J Mol Med 4(6):665–667
16. van Rhee F, Hochhaus A, Lin F, Melo JV, Goldman JM, Cross NC (1996) p190 BCR-ABL mRNA is expressed at low levels in p210-positive chronic myeloid and acute lymphoblastic leukemias. Blood 87(12):5213–5217
17. Secker-Walker LM, Craig JM, Hawkins JM, Hoffbrand AV (1991) Philadelphia positive acute lymphoblastic leukemia in adults: Age distribution, BCR breakpoint and prognostic significance. Leukemia 5(3):196–199
18. Rieder H, Ludwig WD, Gassmann W, et al. (1996) Prognostic significance of additional chromosome abnormalities in adult patients with Philadelphia chromosome positive acute lymphoblastic leukaemia. Br J Haematol 95(4):678–691
19. Ko BS, Tang JL, Lee FY, et al. (2002) Additional chromosomal abnormalities and variability of BCR breakpoints in Philadelphia chromosome/BCR-ABL-positive acute lymphoblastic leukemia in Taiwan. Am J Hematol 71(4):291–299
20. Gleissner B, Gokbuget N, Bartram CR, et al. (2002) Leading prognostic relevance of the BCR-ABL translocation in adult acute B-lineage lymphoblastic leukemia: A prospective study of the Ger-

man Multicenter Trial Group and confirmed polymerase chain reaction analysis. Blood 99(5):1536–543
21. Radich J, Gehly G, Lee A, et al. (1997) Detection of bcr-abl transcripts in Philadelphia chromosome-positive acute lymphoblastic leukemia after marrow transplantation. Blood 89(7):2602–2609
22. Thomas DA, Faderl S, Cortes J, et al. (2004) Treatment of Philadelphia chromosome-positive acute lymphocytic leukemia with hyper-CVAD and imatinib mesylate. Blood 103(12):4396–4407
23. Preti HA, O'Brien S, Giralt S, Beran M, Pierce S, Kantarjian HM (1994) Philadelphia-chromosome-positive adult acute lymphocytic leukemia: Characteristics, treatment results, and prognosis in 41 patients. Am J Med 97(1):60–65
24. Thomas X, Thiebaut A, Olteanu N, et al. (1998) Philadelphia chromosome positive adult acute lymphoblastic leukemia: Characteristics, prognostic factors and treatment outcome. Hematol Cell Ther 40(3):119–128
25. Faderl S, Kantarjian HM, Thomas DA, et al. (2000) Outcome of Philadelphia chromosome-positive adult acute lymphoblastic leukemia. Leuk Lymphoma 36(3–4):263–273
26. Wetzler M, Dodge RK, Mrozek K, et al. (2004) Additional cytogenetic abnormalities in adults with Philadelphia chromosome-positive acute lymphoblastic leukaemia: A study of the Cancer and Leukaemia Group B. Br J Haematol 124(3):275–288
27. Hu Y, Liu Y, Pelletier S, et al. (2004) Requirement of Src kinases Lyn, Hck and Fgr for BCR-ABL1-induced B-lymphoblastic leukemia but not chronic myeloid leukemia. Nat Genet 36(5):453–461
28. Yeoh EJ, Ross ME, Shurtleff SA, et al. (2002) Classification, subtype discovery, and prediction of outcome in pediatric acute lymphoblastic leukemia by gene expression profiling. Cancer Cell 1(2):133–143
29. Kohlmann A, Schoch C, Schnittger S, et al. (2004) Pediatric acute lymphoblastic leukemia (ALL) gene expression signatures classify an independent cohort of adult ALL patients. Leukemia 18(1):63–71
30. Tkachuk DC, Kohler S, Cleary ML (1992) Involvement of a homolog of Drosophila trithorax by 11q23 chromosomal translocations in acute leukemias. Cell 71(4):691–700
31. Harrison CJ, Cuneo A, Clark R, et al. (1998) Ten novel 11q23 chromosomal partner sites. European 11q23 Workshop participants. Leukemia 12(5):811–822
32. Cuthbert G, Thompson K, McCullough S, et al. (2000) MLL amplification in acute leukaemia: A United Kingdom Cancer Cytogenetics Group (UKCCG) study. Leukemia 14(11):1885–1891
33. Ayton PM, Cleary ML (2001) Molecular mechanisms of leukemogenesis mediated by MLL fusion proteins. Oncogene 20(40): 5695–5707
34. Strout MP, Marcucci G, Caligiuri MA, Bloomfield CD (1999) Core-binding factor (CBF) and MLL-associated primary acute myeloid leukemia: Biology and clinical implications. Ann Hematol 78(6): 251–264
35. Bloomfield CD, Archer KJ, Mrozek K, et al. (2002) 11q23 balanced chromosome aberrations in treatment-related myelodysplastic syndromes and acute leukemia: Report from an international workshop. Genes Chromosomes Cancer 33(4):362–378
36. Rozovskaia T, Ravid-Amir O, Tillib S, et al. (2003) Expression profiles of acute lymphoblastic and myeloblastic leukemias with ALL-1 rearrangements. Proc Natl Acad Sci 100(13):7853–7858
37. Armstrong SA, Staunton JE, Silverman LB, et al. (2002) MLL translocations specify a distinct gene expression profile that distinguishes a unique leukemia. Nat Genet 30(1):41–47
38. Tsutsumi S, Taketani T, Nishimura K, et al. (2003) Two distinct gene expression signatures in pediatric acute lymphoblastic leukemia with MLL rearrangements. Cancer Res 63(16):4882–4887
39. Gu Y, Nakamura T, Alder H, et al. (1992) The t(4;11) chromosome translocation of human acute leukemias fuses the ALL-1 gene, related to Drosophila trithorax, to the AF-4 gene. Cell 71(4):701–708
40. Hilden JM, Chen CS, Moore R, Frestedt J, Kersey JH (1993) Heterogeneity in MLL/AF-4 fusion messenger RNA detected by the polymerase chain reaction in t(4;11) acute leukemia. Cancer Res 53(17):3853–3856
41. Biondi A, Rambaldi A, Rossi V, et al. (1993) Detection of ALL-1/AF4 fusion transcript by reverse transcription-polymerase chain reaction for diagnosis and monitoring of acute leukemias with the t(4;11) translocation. Blood 82(10):2943–2947
42. Yamamoto K, Seto M, Iida S, et al. (1994) A reverse transcriptase-polymerase chain reaction detects heterogeneous chimeric mRNAs in leukemias with 11q23 abnormalities. Blood 83(10): 2912–2921
43. Griesinger F, Elfers H, Ludwig WD, et al. (1994) Detection of HRX-FEL fusion transcripts in pre-pre-B-ALL with and without cytogenetic demonstration of t(4;11). Leukemia 8(4):542–548
44. Uckun FM, Herman-Hatten K, Crotty ML, et al. (1998) Clinical significance of MLL-AF4 fusion transcript expression in the absence of a cytogenetically detectable t(4;11)(q21;q23) chromosomal translocation. Blood 92(3):810–821
45. Pui CH (1992) Acute leukemias with the t(4;11)(q21;q23). Leuk Lymphoma 7(3):173–179
46. Schoch C, Rieder H, Freund M, Hoelzer D, Riehm H, Fonatsch C (1995) Twenty-three cases of acute lymphoblastic leukemia with translocation t(4;11)(q21;q23): The implication of additional chromosomal aberrations. Ann Hematol 70(4):195–201
47. Secker-Walker LM (1998) General Report on the European Union Concerted Action Workshop on 11q23, London, UK, May 1997. Leukemia 12(5):776–778
48. Mitelman F, Johansson B, Mertens F (2003) Mitelman database of chromosome aberrations in cancer. http://cgap nci nih gov/Chromosomes/Mitelman
49. Otsuki T, Clark HM, Wellmann A, Jaffe ES, Raffeld M (1995) Involvement of CDKN2 (p16INK4A/MTS1) and p15INK4B/MTS2 in human leukemias and lymphomas. Cancer Res 55(7):1436–440
50. Cayuela JM, Madani A, Sanhes L, Stern MH, Sigaux F (1996) Multiple tumor-suppressor gene 1 inactivation is the most frequent genetic alteration in T-cell acute lymphoblastic leukemia. Blood 87(6):2180–2186
51. Dreyling MH, Bohlander SK, Le Beau MM, Olopade O (1995) Refined mapping of genomic rearrangements involving the short arm of chromosome 9 in acute lymphoblastic leukemias and other hematologic malignancies. Blood 86(5):1931–1938
52. Hebert J, Cayuela JM, Berkeley J, Sigaux F (1994) Candidate tumor-suppressor genes MTS1 (p16INK4A) and MTS2 (p15INK4B) display frequent homozygous deletions in primary cells from T- but not from B-cell lineage acute lymphoblastic leukemias. Blood 84(12): 4038–4044

53. Chim CS, Tam CY, Liang R, Kwong YL (2001) Methylation of p15 and p16 genes in adult acute leukemia: Lack of prognostic significance. Cancer 91(12):2222–2229
54. Hoshino K, Asou N, Okubo T, et al. (2002) The absence of the p15INK4B gene alterations in adult patients with precursor B-cell acute lymphoblastic leukaemia is a favourable prognostic factor. Br J Haematol 117(3):531–540
55. Morison IM, Ellis LM, Teague LR, Reeve AE (2002) Preferential loss of maternal 9p alleles in childhood acute lymphoblastic leukemia. Blood 99(1):375–377
56. Behrendt H, Charrin C, Gibbons B, et al. (1995) Dicentric (9;12) in acute lymphocytic leukemia and other hematological malignancies: Report from a dic(9;12) study group. Leukemia 9(1): 102–106
57. Rieder H, Schnittger S, Bodenstein H, et al. (1995) dic(9;20): A new recurrent chromosome abnormality in adult acute lymphoblastic leukemia. Genes Chromosomes Cancer 13(1):54–61
58. Clark R, Byatt SA, Bennett CF, et al. (2000) Monosomy 20 as a pointer to dicentric (9;20) in acute lymphoblastic leukemia. Leukemia 14(2):241–246
59. Strehl S, Konig M, Dworzak MN, Kalwak K, Haas OA (2003) PAX5/ETV6 fusion defines cytogenetic entity dic(9;12)(p13;p13). Leukemia 17(6):1121–1123
60. Aissani B, Bonan C, Baccichet A, Sinnett D (1999) Childhood acute lymphoblastic leukemia: Is there a tumor suppressor gene in chromosome 12p12.3? Leuk Lymphoma 34(3–4):231–239
61. Montpetit A, Larose J, Boily G, Langlois S, Trudel N, Sinnett D (2004) Mutational and expression analysis of the chromosome 12p candidate tumor suppressor genes in pre-B acute lymphoblastic leukemia. Leukemia 18(9):1499–1504
62. Aguiar RC, Sohal J, van Rhee F, et al. (1996) TEL-AML1 fusion in acute lymphoblastic leukaemia of adults. M.R.C. Adult Leukaemia Working Party. Br J Haematol 95(4):673–677
63. Raynaud S, Mauvieux L, Cayuela JM, et al. (1996) TEL/AML1 fusion gene is a rare event in adult acute lymphoblastic leukemia. Leukemia 10(9):1529–1530
64. Kwong YL, Wong KF (1997) Low frequency of TEL/AML1 in adult acute lymphoblastic leukemia. Cancer Genet Cytogenet 98(2): 137–138
65. Golub TR, Barker GF, Lovett M, Gilliland DG (1994) Fusion of PDGF receptor beta to a novel ets-like gene, tel, in chronic myelomonocytic leukemia with t(5;12) chromosomal translocation. Cell 77(2):307–316
66. Romana SP, Le Coniat M, Berger R (1994) t(12;21): A new recurrent translocation in acute lymphoblastic leukemia. Genes Chromosomes Cancer 9(3):186–191
67. Asakura K, Uchida H, Miyachi H, et al. (2004) TEL/AML1 overcomes drug resistance through transcriptional repression of multidrug resistance-1 gene expression. Mol Cancer Res 2(6): 339–347
68. Zaza G, Yang W, Kager L, et al. (2004) Acute lymphoblastic leukemia with TEL-AML1 fusion has lower expression of genes involved in purine metabolism and lower de novo purine synthesis. Blood 104(5):1435–441
69. Dube ID, Kamel-Reid S, Yuan CC, et al. (1991) A novel human homeobox gene lies at the chromosome 10 breakpoint in lymphoid neoplasias with chromosomal translocation t(10;14). Leukemia 78(11):2996–3003
70. Hatano M, Roberts CW, Minden M, Crist WM, Korsmeyer SJ (1991) Deregulation of a homeobox gene, HOX11, by the t(10;14) in T-cell leukemia. Science 253(5015):79–82
71. Kennedy MA, Gonzalez-Sarmiento R, Kees UR, et al. (1991) HOX11, a homeobox-containing T-cell oncogene on human chromosome 10q24. Proc Natl Acad Sci 88(20):8900–8904
72. Willis TG, Dyer MJ (2000) The role of immunoglobulin translocations in the pathogenesis of B-cell malignancies. Blood 96(3): 808–822
73. Satterwhite E, Sonoki T, Willis TG, et al. (2001) The BCL11 gene family: Involvement of BCL11A in lymphoid malignancies. Blood 98(12):3413–3420
74. Fu TB, Virgilio L, Narducci MG, Facchiano A, Russo G, Croce CM (1994) Characterization and localization of the TCL-1 oncogene product. Cancer Res 54(24):6297–6301
75. MacLeod RA, Nagel S, Kaufmann M, Janssen JW, Drexler HG (2003) Activation of HOX11L2 by juxtaposition with 3′-BCL11B in an acute lymphoblastic leukemia cell line (HPB-ALL) with t(5;14)(q35;q32.2). Genes Chromosomes Cancer 37(1):84–91
76. Bernard OA, Busson-LeConiat M, Ballerini P, et al. (2001) A new recurrent and specific cryptic translocation, t(5;14)(q35;q32), is associated with expression of the Hox11L2 gene in T acute lymphoblastic leukemia. Leukemia 15(10):1495–1504
77. Mancini M, Vegna ML, Castoldi GL, et al. (2002) Partial deletions of long arm of chromosome 6: Biologic and clinical implications in adult acute lymphoblastic leukemia. Leukemia 16(10):2055–2061
78. Park JG, Reddy EP (1992) Large-scale molecular mapping of human c-myb locus: c-myb proto-oncogene is not involved in 6q-abnormalities of lymphoid tumors. Oncogene 7(8):1603–1609
79. Issa JP, Zehnbauer BA, Civin CI, et al. (1996) The estrogen receptor CpG island is methylated in most hematopoietic neoplasms. Cancer Res 56(5):973–977
80. Sinclair PB, Sorour A, Martineau M, et al. (2004) A fluorescence in situ hybridization map of 6q deletions in acute lymphocytic leukemia: Identification and analysis of a candidate tumor suppressor gene. Cancer Res 64(12):4089–4098
81. Mellentin JD, Murre C, Donlon TA, et al. (1989) The gene for enhancer binding proteins E12/E47 lies at the t(1;19) breakpoint in acute leukemias. Science 246(4928):379–382
82. Murre C, McCaw PS, Baltimore D (1989) A new DNA binding and dimerization motif in immunoglobulin enhancer binding, daughterless, MyoD, and myc proteins. Cell 56(5):777–783
83. Nourse J, Mellentin JD, Galili N, et al. (1990) Chromosomal translocation t(1;19) results in synthesis of a homeobox fusion mRNA that codes for a potential chimeric transcription factor. Cell 60(4):535–545
84. Kamps MP, Murre C, Sun XH, Baltimore D (1990) A new homeobox gene contributes the DNA binding domain of the t(1;19) translocation protein in pre-B ALL. Cell 60(4):547–555
85. Troussard X, Rimokh R, Valensi F, et al. (1995) Heterogeneity of t(1;19)(q23;p13) acute leukaemias. French Haematological Cytology Group. Br J Haematol 89(3):516–526
86. Yuki Y, Imoto I, Imaizumi M, et al. (2004) Identification of a novel fusion gene in a pre-B acute lymphoblastic leukemia with t(1;19)(q23;p13). Cancer Sci 95(6):503–507
87. Graham DK, Dawson TL, Mullaney DL, Snodgrass HR, Earp HS (1994) Cloning and mRNA expression analysis of a novel human protooncogene, c-mer. Cell Growth Differ 5(6):647–657

88. Georgescu MM, Kirsch KH, Shishido T, Zong C, Hanafusa H (1999) Biological effects of c-Mer receptor tyrosine kinase in hematopoietic cells depend on the Grb2 binding site in the receptor and activation of NF-kappaB. Mol Cell Biol 19(2):1171–1181
89. Barber KE, Martineau M, Harewood L, et al. (2004) Amplification of the ABL gene in T-cell acute lymphoblastic leukemia. Leukemia 18(6):1153–1156
90. Graux C, Cools J, Melotte C, et al. (2004) Fusion of NUP214 to ABL1 on amplified episomes in T-cell acute lymphoblastic leukemia. Nat Genet 36(10):1084–1089
91. Heinonen K, Mahlamaki E, Riikonen P, Meltoranta RL, Rahiala J, Perkkio M (1999) Acquired X-chromosome aneuploidy in children with acute lymphoblastic leukemia. Med Pediatr Oncol 32(5):360–365
92. Onodera N, McCabe NR, Rubin CM (1992) Formation of a hyperdiploid karyotype in childhood acute lymphoblastic leukemia. Blood 80(1):203–208
93. Paulsson K, Panagopoulos I, Knuutila S, et al. (2003) Formation of trisomies and their parental origin in hyperdiploid childhood acute lymphoblastic leukemia. Blood 102(8):3010–3015
94. Czuczman MS, Dodge RK, Stewart CC, et al. (1999) Value of immunophenotype in intensively treated adult acute lymphoblastic leukemia: Cancer and leukemia Group B study 8364. Blood 93(11):3931–3939
95. Harrison CJ, Moorman AV, Broadfield ZJ, et al. (2004) Three distinct subgroups of hypodiploidy in acute lymphoblastic leukaemia. Br J Haematol 125(5):552–559
96. Garipidou V, Yamada T, Prentice HG, Secker-Walker LM (1990) Trisomy 8 in acute lymphoblastic leukemia (ALL): A case report and update of the literature. Leukemia 4(10):717–719
97. Cario G, Stanulla M, Fine BM, et al. (2004) Distinct gene expression profiles determine molecular treatment response in childhood acute lymphoblastic leukemia. Blood 105(2):821–826
98. Willenbrock H, Juncker AS, Schmiegelow K, Knudsen S, Ryder LP (2004) Prediction of immunophenotype, treatment response, and relapse in childhood acute lymphoblastic leukemia using DNA microarrays. Leukemia 18(7):1270–1277
99. Tsukasaki K, Tanosaki S, DeVos S, et al. (2004) Identifying progression-associated genes in adult T-cell leukemia/lymphoma by using oligonucleotide microarrays. Int J Cancer 109(6):875–881
100. Chiaretti S, Li X, Gentleman R, et al. (2004) Gene expression profile of adult T-cell acute lymphocytic leukemia identifies distinct subsets of patients with different response to therapy and survival. Blood 103(7):2771–2778
101. Mitchell SA, Brown KM, Henry MM, et al. (2004) Inter-platform comparability of microarrays in acute lymphoblastic leukemia. BMC Genomics 5(1):71
102. Holleman A, Cheok MH, den Boer ML, et al. (2004) Gene-expression patterns in drug-resistant acute lymphoblastic leukemia cells and response to treatment. N Engl J Med 351(6):533–542
103. Derynck R, Zhang YE (2003) Smad-dependent and Smad-independent pathways in TGF-beta family signalling. Nature 425(6958):577–584
104. Wolfraim LA, Fernandez TM, Mamura M, et al. (2004) Loss of Smad3 in acute T-cell lymphoblastic leukemia. N Engl J Med 351(6):552–559
105. Armstrong SA, Kung AL, Mabon ME, et al. (2003) Inhibition of FLT3 in MLL. Validation of a therapeutic target identified by gene expression based classification. Cancer Cell 3(2):173–183
106. Taketani T, Taki T, Sugita K, et al. (2004) FLT3 mutations in the activation loop of tyrosine kinase domain are frequently found in infant ALL with MLL rearrangements and pediatric ALL with hyperdiploidy. Blood 103(3):1085–1088
107. Armstrong SA, Mabon ME, Silverman LB, et al. (2004) FLT3 mutations in childhood acute lymphoblastic leukemia. Blood 103(9):3544–3546
108. Paietta E, Ferrando AA, Neuberg D, et al. (2004) Activating FLT3 mutations in CD117/Klt(+) T-cell acute lymphoblastic leukemias. Blood 104(2):558–560
109. Brown P, Levis M, Shurtleff S, Campana D, Downing J, Small D (2004) FLT3 inhibition selectively kills childhood acute lymphoblastic leukemia cells with high levels of FLT3 expression. Blood 105(2):812–820
110. Ferrando AA, Look AT (2003) Gene expression profiling in T-cell acute lymphoblastic leukemia. Semin Hematol 40(4):274–280
111. Ferrando AA, Neuberg DS, Staunton J, et al. (2002) Gene expression signatures define novel oncogenic pathways in T-cell acute lymphoblastic leukemia. Cancer Cell 1(1):75–87
112. Ferrando AA, Neuberg DS, Dodge RK, et al. (2004) Prognostic importance of TLX1 (HOX11) oncogene expression in adults with T-cell acute lymphoblastic leukaemia. Lancet 363(9408): 535–536
113. Bernard OA, Busson-LeConiat M, Ballerini P, et al. (2001) A new recurrent and specific cryptic translocation, t(5;14)(q35;q32), is associated with expression of the Hox11L2 gene in T acute lymphoblastic leukemia. Leukemia 15(10):1495–1504
114. Berger R, Dastugue N, Busson M, et al. (2003) t(5;14)/HOX11L2-positive T-cell acute lymphoblastic leukemia. A collaborative study of the Groupe Francais de Cytogenetique Hematologique (GFCH). Leukemia 17(9):1851–1857
115. Cave H, Suciu S, Preudhomme C, et al. (2004) Clinical significance of HOX11L2 expression linked to t(5;14)(q35;q32), of HOX11 expression, and of SIL-TAL fusion in childhood T-cell malignancies: Results of EORTC studies 58881 and 58951. Blood 103(2):442–450
116. Ballerini P, Blaise A, Busson-Le Coniat M, et al. (2002) HOX11L2 expression defines a clinical subtype of pediatric T-ALL associated with poor prognosis. Blood 100(3):991–997
117. Weng AP, Ferrando AA, Lee W, et al. (2004) Activating mutations of NOTCH1 in human T-cell acute lymphoblastic leukemia. Science 306(5694):269–271
118. Pear WS, Aster JC (2004) T-cell acute lymphoblastic leukemia/lymphoma: A human cancer commonly associated with aberrant NOTCH1 signaling. Curr Opin Hematol 11(6):426–433
119. Beverly LJ, Capobianco AJ (2004) Targeting promiscuous signaling pathways in cancer: Another Notch in the bedpost. Trends Mol Med 10(12):591–598
120. Aplenc R, Lange B (2004) Pharmacogenetic determinants of outcome in acute lymphoblastic leukaemia. Br J Haematol 125(4):421–434
121. Weinshilboum RM, Sladek SL (1980) Mercaptopurine pharmacogenetics: Monogenic inheritance of erythrocyte thiopurine methyltransferase activity. Am J Hum Genet 32(5):651–662

122. Lennard L, Lilleyman JS (1987) Are children with lymphoblastic leukaemia given enough 6-mercaptopurine? Lancet 2(8562): 785–787
123. Lennard L, Van Loon JA, Lilleyman JS, Weinshilboum RM (1987) Thiopurine pharmacogenetics in leukemia: Correlation of erythrocyte thiopurine methyltransferase activity and 6-thioguanine nucleotide concentrations. Clin Pharmacol Ther 41(1):18–25
124. Koren G, Ferrazini G, Sulh H, et al. (1990) Systemic exposure to mercaptopurine as a prognostic factor in acute lymphocytic leukemia in children. N Engl J Med 323(1):17–21
125. Schmiegelow K, Schroder H, Gustafsson G, et al. (1995) Risk of relapse in childhood acute lymphoblastic leukemia is related to RBC methotrexate and mercaptopurine metabolites during maintenance chemotherapy. Nordic Society for Pediatric Hematology and Oncology. J Clin Oncol 13(2):345–351
126. Krynetski EY, Schuetz JD, Galpin AJ, Pui CH, Relling MV, Evans WE (1995) A single point mutation leading to loss of catalytic activity in human thiopurine S-methyltransferase. Proc Natl Acad Sci 92(4):949–953
127. Yates CR, Krynetski EY, Loennechen T, et al. (1997) Molecular diagnosis of thiopurine S-methyltransferase deficiency: Genetic basis for azathioprine and mercaptopurine intolerance. Ann Intern Med 126(8):608–614
128. McLeod HL, Krynetski EY, Relling MV, Evans WE (2000) Genetic polymorphism of thiopurine methyltransferase and its clinical relevance for childhood acute lymphoblastic leukemia. Leukemia 14(4):567–572
129. Relling MV, Hancock ML, Boyett JM, Pui CH, Evans WE (1999) Prognostic importance of 6-mercaptopurine dose intensity in acute lymphoblastic leukemia. Blood 93(9):2817–2823
130. Relling MV, Rubnitz JE, Rivera GK, et al. (1999) High incidence of secondary brain tumours after radiotherapy and antimetabolites. Lancet 354(9172):34–39
131. Relling MV, Yanishevski Y, Nemec J, et al. (1998) Etoposide and antimetabolite pharmacology in patients who develop secondary acute myeloid leukemia. Leukemia 12(3):346–352
132. Chiusolo P, Reddiconto G, Casorelli I, et al. (2002) Preponderance of methylenetetrahydrofolate reductase C677T homozygosity among leukemia patients intolerant to methotrexate. Ann Oncol 13(12):1915–1918
133. Taub JW, Matherly LH, Ravindranath Y, Kaspers GJ, Rots MG, Zantwijk CH (2002) Polymorphisms in methylenetetrahydrofolate reductase and methotrexate sensitivity in childhood acute lymphoblastic leukemia. Leukemia 16(4):764–765
134. Bernbeck B, Mauz-Korholz C, Zotz RB, Gobel U (2003) Methylenetetrahydrofolate reductase gene polymorphism and glucocorticoid intake in children with ALL and aseptic osteonecrosis. Klin Padiatr 215(6):327–331
135. Kishi S, Griener J, Cheng C, et al. (2003) Homocysteine, pharmacogenetics, and neurotoxicity in children with leukemia. J Clin Oncol 21(16):3084–3091
136. Krajinovic M, Lemieux-Blanchard E, Chiasson S, Primeau M, Costea I, Moghrabi A (2004) Role of polymorphisms in MTHFR and MTHFD1 genes in the outcome of childhood acute lymphoblastic leukemia. Pharmacogenomics J 4(1):66–72
137. Gorlick R, Cole P, Banerjee D, et al. (1999) Mechanisms of methotrexate resistance in acute leukemia. Decreased transport and polyglutamylation. Adv Exp Med Biol 457:543–550
138. Belkov VM, Krynetski EY, Schuetz JD, et al. (1999) Reduced folate carrier expression in acute lymphoblastic leukemia: A mechanism for ploidy but not lineage differences in methotrexate accumulation. Blood 93(5):1643–1650
139. Laverdiere C, Chiasson S, Costea I, Moghrabi A, Krajinovic M (2002) Polymorphism G80A in the reduced folate carrier gene and its relationship to methotrexate plasma levels and outcome of childhood acute lymphoblastic leukemia. Blood 100(10): 3832–3834
140. Krajinovic M, Costea I, Chiasson S (2002) Polymorphism of the thymidylate synthase gene and outcome of acute lymphoblastic leukaemia. Lancet 359(9311):1033–1034
141. Lauten M, Matthias T, Stanulla M, Beger C, Welte K, Schrappe M (2002) Association of initial response to prednisone treatment in childhood acute lymphoblastic leukaemia and polymorphisms within the tumour necrosis factor and the interleukin-10 genes. Leukemia 16(8):1437–1442
142. Brown L, Cheng JT, Chen Q, et al. (1990) Site-specific recombination of the tal-1 gene is a common occurrence in human T-cell leukemia. EMBO J 9(10):3343–3351
143. Bernard O, Lecointe N, Jonveaux P, et al. (1991) Two site-specific deletions and t(1;14) translocation restricted to human T-cell acute leukemias disrupt the 5′ part of the tal-1 gene. Oncogene 6(8):1477–1488
144. Bernard O, Barin C, Charrin C, Mathieu-Mahul D, Berger R (1993) Characterization of translocation t(1;14)(p32;q11) in a T and in a B acute leukemia. Leukemia 7(10):1509–1513
145. Chen Q, Yang CY, Tsan JT, et al. (1990) Coding sequences of the tal-1 gene are disrupted by chromosome translocation in human T-cell leukemia. J Exp Med 172(5):1403–1408
146. Carroll AJ, Crist WM, Link MP, et al. (1990) The t(1;14)(p34;q11) is nonrandom and restricted to T-cell acute lymphoblastic leukemia: A Pediatric Oncology Group study. Blood 76(6):1220–1224
147. Xia Y, Brown L, Tsan JT, et al. (1992) The translocation (1;14) (p34;q11) in human T-cell leukemia: Chromosome breakage 25 kilobase pairs downstream of the TAL1 protooncogene. Genes Chromosomes Cancer 4(3):211–216
148. Martin-Henao GA, Sureda A (1995) Translocation (1;14)(p34;q11) and trisomy 8 in a T-cell acute lymphoblastic leukemia patient. Cancer Genet Cytogenet 79(2):177–181
149. Hansen-Hagge TE, Schafer M, Kiyoi H, et al. (2002) Disruption of the RanBP17/Hox11L2 region by recombination with the TCRdelta locus in acute lymphoblastic leukemias with t(5;14) (q34;q11). Leukemia 16(11):2205–2212
150. Inaba T, Murakami S, Oku N, et al. (1990) Translocation between chromosomes 8q24 and 14q11 in T-cell acute lymphoblastic leukemia. Cancer Genet Cytogenet 49(1):69–74
151. Kasai M, Aoki K, Matsuo Y, Minowada J, Maziarz RT, Strominger JL (1994) Recombination hotspot associated factors specifically recognize novel target sequences at the site of interchromosomal rearrangements in T-ALL patients with t(8;14)(q24;q11) and t(1;14)(p32;q11). Int Immunol 6(7):1017–1025
152. Duro D, Bernard O, Della Valle V, Berger R, Larsen CJ (1995) A new type of p16INK4/MTS1 gene transcript expressed in B-cell malignancies. Oncogene 11(1):21–29
153. Zutter M, Hockett RD, Roberts CW, et al. (1990) The t(10;14) (q24;q11) of T-cell acute lymphoblastic leukemia juxtaposes

the delta T-cell receptor with TCL3, a conserved and activated locus at 10q24. Proc Natl Acad Sci 87(8):3161–3165
154. Lu M, Gong ZY, Shen WF, Ho AD (1991) The tcl-3 proto-oncogene altered by chromosomal translocation in T-cell leukemia codes for a homeobox protein. EMBO J 10(10):2905–2910
155. Park JK, Le Beau MM, Shows TB, Rowley JD, Diaz MO (1992) A complex genetic rearrangement in a t(10;14)(q24;q11) associated with T-cell acute lymphoblastic leukemia. Genes Chromosomes Cancer 4(1):32–40
156. Salvati PD, Watt PM, Thomas WR, Kees UR (1999) Molecular characterization of a complex chromosomal translocation breakpoint t(10;14) including the HOX11 oncogene locus. Leukemia 13(6):975–979
157. Royer-Pokora B, Loos U, Ludwig WD (1991) TTG-2, a new gene encoding a cysteine-rich protein with the LIM motif, is overexpressed in acute T-cell leukaemia with the t(11;14)(p13;q11). Oncogene 6(10):1887–1893
158. Fizzotti M, Chen EY, Link MP, et al. (1994) Simultaneous expression of RBTN-2 and BCR-ABL oncogenes in a T-ALL with a t(11;14)(p13;q11) and a late-appearing Philadelphia chromosome. Leukemia 8(7):1124–1130
159. Valge-Archer V, Forster A, Rabbitts TH (1998) The LMO1 AND LDB1 proteins interact in human T-cell acute leukaemia with the chromosomal translocation t(11;14)(p15;q11). Oncogene 17(24):3199–3202
160. Ziemin-van der Poel S, McCabe NR, Gill HJ, et al. (1991) Identification of a gene, MLL, that spans the breakpoint in 11q23 translocations associated with human leukemias. Proc Natl Acad Sci 88(23):10735–10739
161. Le Coniat M, Della Valle V, Marynen P, Berger R (1997) A new breakpoint, telomeric to TEL/ETV6, on the short arm of chromosome 12 in T-cell acute lymphoblastic leukemia. Leukemia 11(8):1360–1363
162. Bertness VL, Felix CA, McBride OW, et al. (1990) Characterization of the breakpoint of a t(14;14)(q11.2;q32) from the leukemic cells of a patient with T-cell acute lymphoblastic leukemia. Cancer Genet Cytogenet 44(1):47–54
163. Chervinsky DS, Grossi M, Kakati S, Block AW, Aplan PD (1995) Concurrent presence of inv(14)(q11q32) and t(4;11)(q21;q23) in pre-B acute lymphoblastic leukemia. Genes Chromosomes Cancer 12(3):229–236
164. Fisch P, Forster A, Sherrington PD, Dyer MJ, Rabbitts TH (1993) The chromosomal translocation t(X;14)(q28;q11) in T-cell prolymphocytic leukaemia breaks within one gene and activates another. Oncogene 8(12):3271–3276
165. Stern MH, Soulier J, Rosenzwajg M, et al. (1993) MTCP-1: A novel gene on the human chromosome Xq28 translocated to the T-cell receptor alpha/delta locus in mature T-cell proliferations. Oncogene 8(9):2475–2483

Acute Lymphoblastic Leukemia: Clinical Presentation, Diagnosis, and Classification

Richard A. Larson, John Anastasi

Contents

7.1 Introduction

Acute lymphoblastic leukemia (ALL) is a malignant neoplasm of lymphocytes characterized by the clonal accumulation of immature blood cells in the bone marrow. These abnormal cells are arrested in the lymphoblast stage of the normal maturation pathway. Aberrations in proliferation and differentiation of these cells are common, and normal hematopoiesis is suppressed. Symptoms result from varying degrees of anemia, neutropenia, and thrombocytopenia or from infiltration of ALL cells into tissues. Although virtually any organ system may become involved, once leukemia cells enter the peripheral blood, the lymph nodes, spleen, liver, central nervous system (CNS), and skin are the most common sites detected clinically.

ALL is a heterogeneous disease with distinct biologic and prognostic groupings. Treatment strategies tailored to specific prognostic groups have already yielded dramatic improvements in the outcomes for children with ALL, and similar risk-adapted strategies based on the biological heterogeneity of the disease are now being applied to adults with ALL. Increasing knowledge of the cytogenetic classification of this disease plays an important role in the prognostic groupings, and thus, cytogenetics will be emphasized in this review.

7.2 Clinical Presentation

7.2.1 Epidemiology

ALL is the most common malignant disease in childhood, peaking in incidence between ages 2 to 5. In contrast, ALL only accounts for approximately 20% of acute leukemias in adults. Although the median age for adults with ALL who are entered onto clinical trials is 30–35 years, it is very likely that older patients are underrepresented in these reports. Registry data suggest that the incidence of ALL increases steadily above the age of 50 years [1].

The incidence of ALL is more common in Caucasians compared with African-Americans; the age-adjusted overall incidence in the USA is 1.5/100 000 in whites and 0.8/100 000 in blacks [1, 2]. Geographic variations, with higher incidence rates in Spain and among Latin Americans, are likely related to a number of factors including socioeconomics, ethnicity, and an urban or rural setting [3]. A higher frequency of ALL has been reported in industrialized countries and urban areas.

ALL is slightly more common among males than females (1.3:1) [2].

7.2.2 Presentation

The clinical presentation of ALL is most often sudden. Patients commonly present with a short history of fatigue, or spontaneous bleeding. Malaise, lethargy, weight loss, fevers, and night sweats are often present but typically are not severe. Compared to AML, patients with ALL experience more bone and joint pain. Rarely, they may present with asymmetric arthritis, low back pain, diffuse osteopenia, or lytic bone lesions [4]. Children experience these symptoms more frequently than adults. Young children may have difficulty walking due to bone pain [2]. Lymphadenopathy, splenomegaly, and hepatomegaly are more common than in AML and affect half of adults with ALL. CNS involvement is also more common in ALL compared to AML. Patients may present with cranial neuropathies (most often involving the 6th and 7th cranial nerves). Nausea, vomiting, headache, or papilledema may result from meningeal infiltration and obstruction of the outflow of cerebrospinal fluid (CSF) leading to raised intracranial pressure. Testicular involvement, presenting as a painless, unilateral mass, is noted at diagnosis in approximately 2% of boys. It is associated with infant or adolescent age, hyperleukocytosis, splenomegaly, and mediastinal mass [2]. The diagnosis of testicular involvement is made by wedge biopsies. Bilateral biopsies are necessary due to the high incidence of contralateral testicular disease [5].

The physical exam is often notable for pallor, generalized lymphadenopathy, signs associated with thrombocytopenia, such as gingival bleeding, epistaxis, petechiae/ecchymoses, or fundal hemorrhages, and hepatosplenomegaly. Dermal involvement by leukemia cutis may be noted.

7.3 Diagnosis

7.3.1 Initial Laboratory Evaluation

The morphologic recognition of lymphoblasts in the blood and bone marrow and their phenotypic characterization are of major importance to the correct diagnosis and classification of ALL. These require careful evaluation of well-prepared peripheral blood and bone marrow aspirate smears, and phenotypic analysis of the blasts by cytochemical studies and by flow cytometry or immunohistochemistry with an appropriate panel of surface and cytoplasmic markers.

The setting in which lymphoblasts are seen in the peripheral blood and bone marrow aspirate can vary significantly. In the majority of cases, the counts and cellularity are high, but in some there can be pancytopenia, and hypocellularity, which make the recognition of the blasts more critical. A leukoerythroblastic picture can be seen in some cases, and in rare T-ALL cases there may be dysplasia in the granulocytic elements. One particular unusual morphologic presentation of ALL is that of precursor-B ALL with eosinophilia. The entity can show eosinophilia proceeding, concurrent with, or following ALL at either diagnosis or relapse. Sometimes the eosinophilia can be so extreme as to obscure the blasts. This entity is associated with the specific cytogenetic abnormality, t(5;14)(q31;q32) [6]. Another unique presentation is that of precursor-T ALL with a mediastinal mass associated with eosinophilia and immature myeloid precursors. This is also associated with a recurring chromosomal abnormality, t(8;13)(p11;q12) [6].

The evaluation of cytospin slides made from the cerebrospinal fluid (CSF) may indicate CNS involvement. The definition of CNS involvement used by the Children's Cancer Group (CCG) is >5 WBC/μL of CSF plus unequivocal blasts identified on the cytospin [7]. However, there is much debate regarding this definition, and difficulties in interpretation arise when there are <5 WBC/μL of CSF, but blasts present. One approach has been to classify CNS leukemia into three groups: CNS 1 (<5 WBC/μL of CSF and no blasts), CNS 2 (<5 WBC/μL of CSF and blasts), and CNS 3 (>5 WBC/μL of CSF and blasts, or cranial nerve findings) [8]. Additionally, some studies advocate using immunocytochemistry in addition to cytology to identify blasts in the CSF more accurately [9].

In cases with a high cell turnover (e.g., mature-B ALL or ALL-L3), the evaluation of blood chemistries may reflect evidence of tumor lysis, with hypocalcemia, hyperkalemia, hyperphosphatemia, elevated LDH, hyperuricemia, and elevated creatinine.

7.3.2 Cytomorphology

The cytomorphologic characteristics of lymphoblasts are varied, but are usually sufficient to suggest a blastic or neoplastic process for which phenotyping can confirm and further characterize the process. The most typical lymphoblast is a small- to intermediate-sized cell with round or oval nucleus that has a smudgy nuclear chromatin, absent or small nucleoli, and scanty cytoplasm. Comparison to normal-appearing "mature" lymphocytes in the blood or marrow aspirate is useful for the assessment of size and degree of chromatin condensation. The scant cytoplasm is quite dramatic in many cells as the nucleus has an appearance of bulging out of the cell cytoplasm. The cytoplasm is pale blue and not intensely stained. Lymphoblasts with these typical features have been considered "L1" lymphoblasts according to the French American British (FAB) classification scheme [10, 11], and are particularly common in pediatric cases.

In some cases, lymphoblasts exhibit significant morphologic variation. Such lymphoblasts are larger than the typical "L1" lymphoblast, and have oval or irregular nuclear outlines and less homogeneous chromatin. Nuclei are variable but frequently prominent, and sometimes multiple. The cytoplasm is more abundant but still pale blue. Cases with these more variable lymphoblasts usually contain at least some typical "L1" lymphoblasts, which are helpful to note, as they are less likely to be confused with myeloblasts. Cases with the morphologic varied lymphoblasts were referred to as "L2" ALL by the FAB [10, 11], but this classification is now believed to have little significance, and the terminology is used here only for descriptive purposes. Other than being more common in children and adults, respectively, "L1" and "L2" ALL do not define specific disease entities, show no consistent correlation with phenotypic or cytogenetic features, and have not been adopted in the WHO classification of ALL, which is based on immunophenotype and genotype [12].

Compared to the blasts described above, blasts in cases of Burkitt lymphoma/leukemia ("L3" blasts by the FAB scheme [10, 11], referred to as Burkitt leukemia for the remainder of this review) are usually quite distinctive. The blasts are large and homogeneous and have distinctive deep blue cytoplasm, which commonly contains sharply defined vacuoles. The nuclei of Burkitt cells are large and round or oval. They have a finely stippled chromatin, and variable nucleoli, which sometimes are quite prominent. The larger size and intense cytoplasmic basophilia with vacuolization are decidedly the most distinctive features but are not entirely specific. Vacuoles can be seen in monoblastic and erythroid leukemia, and, together with the deep blue cytoplasm, can be seen in other cases of ALL as well as in some cases of AML [13, 14]. Conversely, some cases of Burkitt leukemia with the associated chromosomal translocations lack the usual "L3" morphology [15].

A number of additional cytologic variants of lymphoblasts deserve mention. Although there are no particular clinical, phenotypic, or genetic correlates with these variant blasts, their recognition will help avoid exclusion of ALL from diagnostic consideration in cases where they are seen.

Small lymphoblasts can be seen in rare cases of ALL [16]. These blasts are closer in size to small "mature" lymphocytes, making them difficult to distinguish from the small lymphoid cells of chronic lymphocytic leukemia (CLL). The small lymphoblasts also have more condensed chromatin, making the distinction still more difficult. Lymphoblasts with cytoplasmic granulation can be seen in a small percentage of ALL cases [17, 18]. The granules are usually present in the larger blasts rather than in the small "L1" type. They are azurophilic and usually not numerous. Nuclear clefts can be seen in lymphoblasts and are present as deep nuclear groves. The so-called hand mirror cell is probably not a defining characteristic for a certain entity [19]. Whether such cells are due to an artifact of the preparation is debatable. The different lymphoblasts are illustrated in Fig. 7.1.

7.3.3 Histology

Evaluation of the histology of ALL from biopsy sections becomes important when there are few circulating blasts in the blood and when the bone marrow is inaspirable. It is also critical in evaluating extramedullary sites of involvement such as lymph nodes, testes or skin. Whether bone marrow biopsies are necessary in the typical patient with a high number of blasts in the circulation and bone marrow aspirate is disputable. However, the biopsy may provide a baseline for cellularity, degree of residual normal hematopoiesis, and the presence of necrosis or other associated features.

In typical cases, the marrow cellularity is markedly increased due to the infiltration by the densely packed blastic elements with no particular pattern of involvement. Rare cases have a predilection for paratrabecular growth, but this is very unusual. On H&E stained sections, the blastic morphology is not easily distinguishable from myeloblasts, and the distinction between the

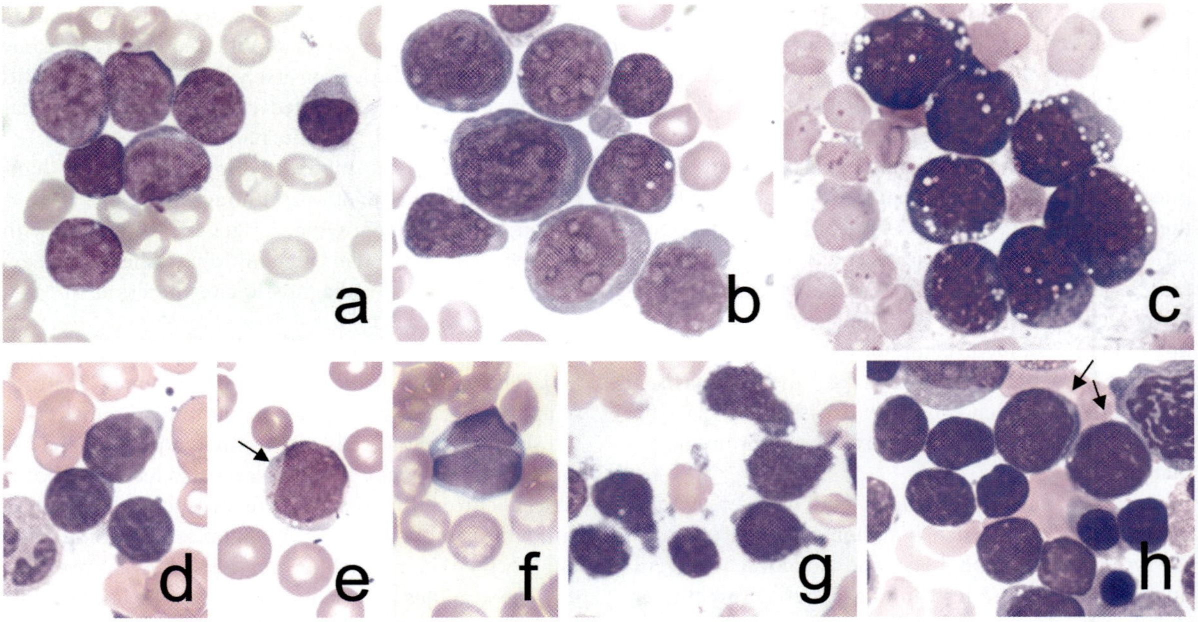

Fig. 7.1. Varied cytomorphology of lymphoblasts in comparison to Burkitt leukemia cells and hematogones (Wright-stained blood and bone marrow aspirate smears). (**a**) Small uniform blasts, previously called "L1" type, are about two times the size of erythrocytes, and have a smudgy homogenous chromatin without prominent nucleoli. Comparison to small lymphocyte (*right*) is always helpful. (**b**) Varied lymphoblasts, including numerous larger blasts with more open chromatin, prominent nucleoli and abundant cytoplasm (previously considered "L-2 " type). The presence of a few small "L1" blasts in the background is always helpful in considering ALL. (**c**) Burkitt leukemia cells (previously called "L3" blasts) are usually distinctive with homogeneous large size, and deep blue cytoplasm with prominent vacuoles. Vacuoles can, however, be seen in some cases of AML and ALL. (**d**) Some lymphoblasts can be small with more clumped chromatin, and can be difficult to distinguish morphologically from CLL cells. (**e**) Granular lymphoblast (*arrow*). These blasts may resemble myeloblasts, but the granules are myeloperoxidase negative. (**f**) Lymphoblast with nuclear cleft, (**g**) So-called "hand-mirror" cells are sometimes an artifact of poor preparations, as they are not equally distributed on the slide. (**h**) Hematogones (*arrows*) resemble lymphoblasts. They can be distinguished by flow immunophenotyping, and due to the associated background of small lymphocytes and regenerating bone marrow.

"L1" and "L2" blasts, recognized in Wright-stained material, is also usually not possible. Burkitt leukemia does, however, have a particular histologic pattern. The features are similar to the lymph node involvement by Burkitt lymphoma. These features are illustrated in Fig. 7.2.

Hypocellular presentations of ALL are relatively rare, but can present a diagnostic challenge due to the paucity of cells and limited material for immunophenotyping [20]. Some cases of ALL can present with frank fibrosis [21], but increased reticulin is more common. Some cases are inaspirable due to the fibrosis or to the dense packing of the marrow by lymphoblasts. Necrosis is present in a small number of cases and can complicate the diagnosis, due to the lack of viable cells for either morphologic evaluation or for immunophenotyping [22]. Necrosis can be focal or widespread, and can recur with relapsed disease. Occasional cases can show bone changes, which include osteoporosis or osteopenia [23].

In some cases of ALL the principle manifestation of disease is extramedullary [24]. This is not uncommon in precursor-T-cell ALL/lymphoma which can present with a mediastinal mass and lymphadenopathy. Other sites that may be identified prior to blood and bone marrow disease include lymph node, skin, testes, and CNS. Whenever there is concern of a lymphoblastic process in an extramedullary location, careful review of the blood and evaluation of the marrow is imperative.

Differential diagnostic considerations based on the cytomorphologic and histologic features of blasts in the peripheral blood and marrow depend in part on

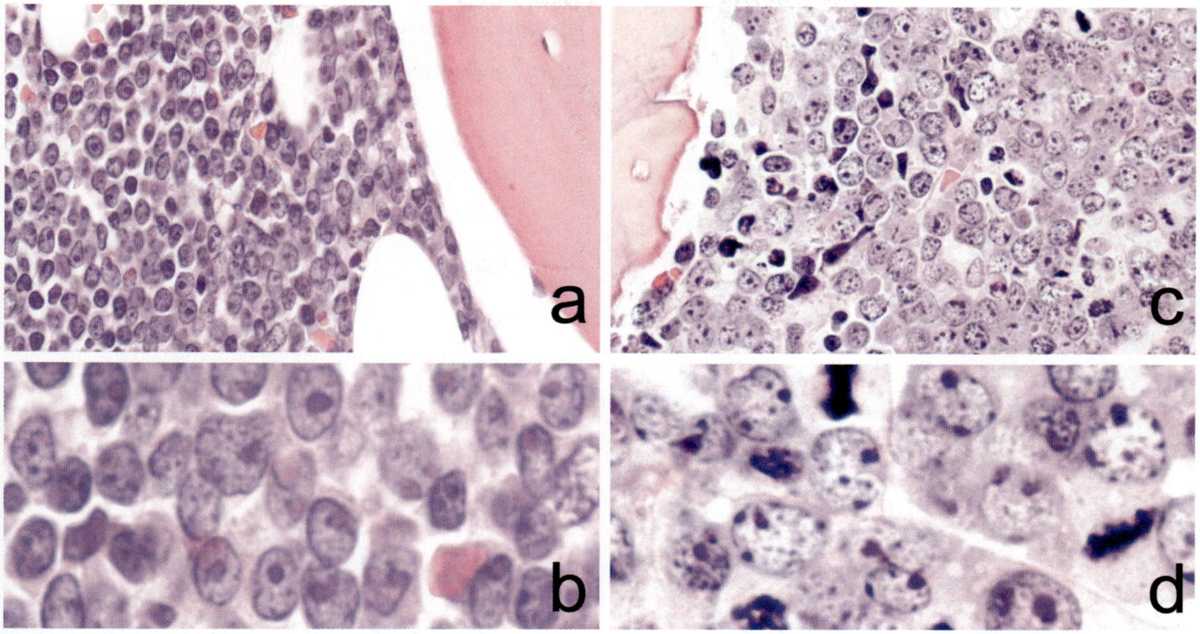

Fig. 7.2. Histologic features of "L1/L2" ALL vs. Burkitt leukemia (H&E-stained bone marrow biopsy sections). (**a, b**) "L1/L2" blasts are equally distributed and have a fine, "blastic" chromatin and variable nucleoli. (**c, d**) Burkitt leukemia shows a syncytial appearance. The cells are larger, have a punctate chromatin, numerous smaller nucleoli, and indistinct cytoplasm. The mitotic rate is markedly elevated.

the patient's age. In pediatric patients with high peripheral blood counts, pertussis must be considered. Pertussis can result in lymphocytosis of 20000–30000/μl, and the lymphocytes can sometimes appear atypical, although they should have mature-appearing chromatin. In the bone marrow, hematogones or normal immature lymphoid elements can be increased in number in regenerative situations. These require careful evaluation, as they closely resemble malignant lymphoblasts [25]. Evaluation of the clinical history and careful interpretation of flow immunophenotyping is critical to rule out ALL (see below). Small round blue cell tumors seen in pediatric patients can also mimic ALL in the marrow, but immunohistochemical studies can usually resolve any diagnostic concerns. In adults, CLL and leukemic manifestations of lymphoma, particularly the blastic variant of mantle cell lymphoma [26], can mimic ALL. Although these can usually be distinguished by morphologic features, it is not uncommon to see an initial misinterpretation due to poorly prepared peripheral blood smears. Immunophenotyping is needed to resolve the diagnosis in such cases. A blastic type of plasma cell myeloma in the marrow might also provide some initial diagnostic difficulty in adults, but this should be resolved with immunohistochemistry for kappa and lambda. In both children and adults, the differential also includes AML, biphenotypic leukemia, and CML presenting in lymphoid blast phase. In all except the latter, immunophenotyping by flow or by immunohistochemistry can resolve the diagnostic dilemma. These differential diagnostic considerations, as well as a list of nonhematologic processes that may resemble ALL, are summarized in Table 7.1.

7.3.4 Phenotype

Phenotypic evaluation begins with cytochemical studies, and specifically with a myeloperoxidase or Sudan black B reaction, as well as nonspecific esterase reactions (ANA, ANB) to quickly exclude most cases of AML. AML with minimal differentiation (FAB: M0), erythroleukemia, and megakaryoblastic leukemia are the exceptions, as these require additional studies for exclusion. Additional cytochemistry such as PAS, and oil red O are being used less commonly due to the reliance on

Table 7.1. Differential diagnosis of ALL
Non-hematologic processes:
Tuberculosis
Heavy metals
Human immunodeficiency virus (HIV)
Infectious mononucleosis
Autoimmune diseases
Juvenile rheumatoid arthritis
Osteomyelitis
Hematologic processes:
Differential diagnostic considerations from cytomorphology and histology
In children
Pertussis
Hematogones
Small round blue cell tumors
In adults
Chronic lymphocytic leukemia (CLL)
Prolymphocytic leukemia (PLL)
Lymphoma, especially blastic variant of mantle cell
Plasmablastic myeloma
In children and adults
Reactive lymphocytosis (mononucleosis)
Thymoma
AML with minimal differentiation (M0) and without maturation (M1)
Acute biphenotypic leukemia
CML presenting in lymphoid blast phase

Table 7.2. Immunophenotype
A. Pertinent markers available for immunohistochemical studies
General: TdT, CD34
B-cell: CD20, CD79A
T-cell: CD3, CD4, CD8, CD5, CD45RO
Myeloid: MPO, CD68, lysozyme, glycophorin A, Factor VIII, CD61
Other: keratin, NSE, myogenin, CD99
B. Commonly used markers for flow immunophenotyping in acute leukemia
General: CD34, HLA-DR, TdT, CD45
B-cell markers: CD10, CD19, cCD22, CD20, cCD79A, CD24, cμ, sIg
T-cell markers: CD1a, CD2, cCD3, CD4, CD8, CD5, CD7
Myeloid: cMPO, CD117, CD13, CD33, CD11c, CD14, CD15
C. B-lineage ALL phenotypes:
Pro-B: TdT+, CD19/22/79A+, CD10–, cμ–, sIg–
Common precursor-B: TdT+, CD19/22/79A+, CD10+, cμ–, sIg–
Pre-B: TdT+, CD19/22/79A+, CD10+, cμ+, sIg–
Burkitt: TdT–, CD19/22/79A+, CD10+, sIg+
D. T-lineage ALL phenotypes
Pro/immature Thymocyte: TdT+, cCD3+, CD2/5/7+/–
Common thymocyte: TdT+, cCD3+, CD2/5/7+, CD4+/CD8+, CD1a+
Mature thymocyte: TdT+/-, CD3+, CD2/5/7+, CD4+ or CD8+, CD1a–

surface and cytoplasmic markers evaluated by flow cytometry and immunohistochemistry.

Immunophenotypic analysis is critical to confirm a morphologic diagnosis of ALL [27], to resolve a difficult differential diagnosis and to further subclassify cases into precursor-B and precursor-T lineage types. However, a specific immunophenotype identified at diagnosis might also be useful for evaluating residual disease by flow cytometry. Most immunophenotyping studies are performed from blood or marrow aspirates with surface and cytoplasmic markers by flow cytometry, but a growing number of markers are now available for immunophenotyping on tissue sections by immunohistochemical techniques. This is of importance especially in cases which have low peripheral blast counts and in which bone marrow material is insufficient for flow analysis or in which a diagnosis is being made from an extramedullary site. Currently, there are many markers available for tissue immunophenotyping in acute leukemia [28], and a list of pertinent markers is given in Table 7.2 A. There are various recommendations concerning which antibodies to include in a routine flow cytometric panel for the work-up of an acute leukemia [29, 30], but there is no uniformly accepted panel. Commonly used markers are listed in Table 7.2 B.

The vast majority of cases of ALL (~85%) are of B lineage. These have been grouped into further subtypes, which may correspond to different levels of maturation in normal B-cell development. However, such differentiation schemes are not universally agreed upon and the terminology for the different subtypes is also not uniform. In fact, due to the lack of conformity, and the questionable significance of the further subclassification, the WHO classification scheme simply classifies cases as "precursor-B" and "precursor-T" ALL without additional categorization. The most common B-lineage ALL is the precursor-B phenotype with B-cell markers (CD19, CD22), TdT, cytoplasmic CD79A, CD34, CD10 (CALLA), and lack of cytoplasmic μ (cμ) and of surface immunoglobulin (sIg) expression. This type has variably been called "common precursor B" ALL, or "early precursor-B" ALL. A less common type lacks CALLA and may be at an earlier level of maturation that has been termed "pro-B" ALL. This type has a worse prognosis. A type with more maturation than common precursor-B ALL is characterized by the presence of cμ, and is referred to as "Pre-B"ALL. Reports are conflicting, but this may be more commonly associated with t(1;19)(q23;p13). Burkitt leukemia has the immunophenotype of mature B cells with sIg expression. Whether rare cases of non-Burkitt ALL also exhibit a mature B phenotype (sIg+) is questionable, although such cases have been reported on [31]. B-lineage ALL phenotypes are listed in Table 7.2 C.

T lineage ALL accounts for only 15–20% of cases and can also be separated into phenotypic groups which may correspond to different stages of thymic T-cell development [32]. As in B-lineage ALL, a type with intermediate differentiation is the most common. This "common thymocyte" type shows expression of the pan T-cell markers, CD2, cytoplasmic CD3 (cCD3), CD7, and CD5 and distinctively shows coexpression of CD4 and CD8, and expression of CD1a. A more primitive type called "prothymocyte" or "immature thymocyte" type has TdT, cCD3, and variable expression of CD5, CD2, and CD7, but lacks CD4, CD8, and CD1a. A more mature phenotype than the "common thymocyte" type has variable TdT, the pan T-cell markers, CD4 or CD8 but lacks CD1a. Again, because of lack of conformity and variability of marker expression, the WHO classification recognizes only the "precursor-T" group without further immunophenotypic categorization [12]. T-lineage ALL phenotypes are listed in Table 7.2 D.

Table 7.3. Scoring system for biphenotypic leukemia

Score	Lineage B-lymphoid	T-lymphoid	Myeloid
2	cCD79A cμ cCD22	cCD3 anti-TCR	MPO
1	CD19 CD20 CD10	CD2 CD5 CD8 CD10	CD117 CD13 CD33 CD65
0.5	TdT CD24	TdT CD7 CD1a	CD14 CD15 CD64

Greater than 2 points are needed to consider a lineage involved [36]

Coexpression of other nonlymphoid markers is common on the lymphoblasts in both precursor-B and precursor-T ALL, and does not necessarily indicate bilineal potential. The myeloid markers, CD13 and CD33, are the most frequently expressed [33]. In the past, these have erroneously been interpreted as indicating a biphenotypic process and a worse prognosis, but more recently, this has not been found [34, 35]. Recently, more strict criteria with a uniform grading system have been instituted to help define the "biphenotypic" entity, illustrated in Table 7.3 [36]. Cytoplasmic expression of myeloperoxidase in ALL has also been reported by flow cytometric analysis. However, this does not correspond to the cytochemical detection of enzyme reactivity, and when identified with a polyclonal antibody, it is of only questionable significance [37].

Differential diagnostic considerations that have to be considered in immunophenotyping include hematogones, thymoma, biphenotypic leukemia, and CML presenting in lymphoid blast phase. Hematogones have the same immunophenotype as common precursor B ALL cells, but the hematogones exhibit a spectrum of maturation with a continuum of cells from immature to mature showing loss of CD34, and gain of CD20 and sIg [38, 39].

Thymoma cells have the phenotype of common thymocytes, and cannot be distinguished from common T ALL/lymphoblastic lymphoma by immunophenotype alone. Correlation with clinical presentation and histology are important for the correct interpretation. When

CML presents in lymphoid blast crisis, distinction from Philadelphia chromosome positive ALL cannot be made based on immunophenotype, as the blasts are frequently precursor B lymphoblasts. In most cases the presence of a concurrent myeloid component to the leukemia will alert one to the correct diagnosis. If this were not present, lineage analysis showing the BCR/ABL fusion in myeloid as well as lymphoid cells has been suggested as a means to differentiate the stem cell process, CML, from the lymphoid-restricted process, ALL [40]. In some cases, only the emergence of a myeloid component after treatment can indicate the correct diagnosis.

7.3.5 Cytogenetic Evaluation

Cytogenetic analysis of each patient's ALL cells has become an essential component of diagnosis prior to treatment. It has furthered our understanding of leukemogenesis at a molecular level. Specific and well-characterized recurring chromosomal abnormalities facilitate diagnosis, confirm subtype classification, and have major prognostic value for treatment planning. Abnormalities in chromosome number or structure are found in approximately 90% of children and 70% of adult ALL patients [41]. These cytogenetic abnormalities are acquired somatic (rather than germline) mutations that frequently result from translocations of chromosomal DNA, resulting in new (abnormal) protein products from the resultant fusion genes. It is assumed that the protein products from these fusion genes are responsible for the cellular dysregulation that leads to the malignant state. Deletions or loss of DNA may eliminate genes that have tumor suppressor functions. Gains of additional chromosomes may lead to gene dosage effects that provide transformed cells with survival advantages.

Conventional cytogenetic analysis requires dividing cells, is technically difficult, and can be time consuming due to the presence of multiple abnormal cell lines and complex chromosomal banding patterns. Therefore, alternative diagnostic methods have been sought, including fluorescence in situ hybridization (FISH), in which labeled probes are hybridized to either metaphase chromosomes or interphase nuclei and then detected with fluorochromes. This method of analysis is more rapid, and in some cases more sensitive, than conventional cytogenetic analysis. Additionally, FISH can be used to study differentiated or nondividing cells.

7.3.6 Molecular Evaluation

Polymerase chain reaction (PCR) is an enzyme assay that provides a more sensitive and rapid method to detect clonal gene rearrangements. Translocations that result in fusion genes are especially suited for analysis with reverse transcriptase PCR (RT-PCR), a technique in which the fusion mRNA is reverse transcribed into cDNA, and then amplified by PCR using gene-specific primers. Quantitative RT-PCR allows for quantification of minimal residual disease (MRD). A number of large prospective studies in pediatric ALL have demonstrated the independent prognostic significance of MRD detection [42, 43]; less is known about the significance of MRD detection in adult ALL.

7.4 Conclusion

In summary, the initial approach to the diagnosis of ALL still involves evaluation of the peripheral blood smear and bone marrow specimens with cytomorphology, immunohistochemistry, and cytogenetic analysis. Cytogenetic analysis is used to establish prognostically distinct subgroups of ALL. Through enhanced knowledge of the leukemogenic pathways involved in the different ALL subgroups, one can anticipate improved accuracy in diagnosis and prognosis, and ultimately, improved disease outcome for these patients.

References

1. Hoelzer D, Gokbuget N (2000) Recent approaches in acute lymphoblastic leukemia in adults. Crit Rev Oncol Hematol 36(1):49–58
2. Farhi DC, Rosenthal NS (2000) Acute lymphoblastic leukemia. Clin Lab Med 20(1):17–28, vii
3. Groves FD, Linet MS, Devesa SS (1995) Patterns of occurrence of the leukaemias. Eur J Cancer 31A(6):941–949
4. Gur H, Koren V, Ehrenfeld M, Ben-Bassat I, Sidi Y (1999) Rheumatic manifestations preceding adult acute leukemia: Characteristics and implication in course and prognosis. Acta Haematol 101(1):1–6
5. Stoffel TJ, Nesbit ME, Levitt SH (1975) Extramedullary involvement of the testes in childhood leukemia. Cancer 35(4):1203–1211
6. Ferrando AA, Look AT (2000) Clinical implications of recurring chromosomal and associated molecular abnormalities in acute lymphoblastic leukemia. Semin Hematol 37(4):381–395
7. Mastrangelo R, Poplack D, Bleyer A, Riccardi R, Sather H, D'Angio G (1986) Report and recommendations of the Rome workshop concerning poor- prognosis acute lymphoblastic leukemia in chil-

dren: Biologic bases for staging, stratification, and treatment. Med Pediatr Oncol 14(3):191–194
8. Mahmoud HH, Rivera GK, Jancock ML, Krance RA, Kun LE, Behm FG, Ribeiro RC, Sandlund JT, Crist WM, Pui CH (1993) Low leukocyte counts with blast cells in cerebrospinal fluid of children with newly diagnosed acute lymphoblastic leukemia. N Engl J Med 329:314–319
9. Tani E, Costa I, Svedmyr E, Skoog L (1995) Diagnosis of lymphoma, leukemia, and metastatic tumor involvement of the cerebrospinal fluid by cytology and immunocytochemistry. Diagn Cytopathol 12(1):14–22
10. Bennett JM, Catovsky D, Daniel MT, Flandrin G, Galton DA, Gralnick HR, et al. (1976) Proposals for the classification of the acute leukaemias. French-American-British (FAB) Co-operative Group. Br J Haematol 33(4):451–458
11. Bennett JM, Catovsky D, Daniel MT, Flandrin G, Galton DA, Gralnick HR, et al. (1981) The morphological classification of acute lymphoblastic leukaemia: Concordance among observers and clinical correlations. Br J Haematol 47(4):553–561
12. World Health Organization classification of tumours (2001) Pathology and genetics of tumours of haematopoietic and lymphoid tissues. IARC Press, Lyon
13. Lilleyman JS, Hann IM, Stevens RF, Richards SM, Eden OB (1988) Blast cell vacuoles in childhood lymphoblastic leukaemia. Br J Haematol 70(2):183–186
14. Al-Rubei K, Rose PE, Hill FG (1984) Morphological heterogeneity in childhood B cell acute lymphoblastic leukaemia. J Clin Pathol 37(12):1348–1352
15. Khalidi HS, Chang KL, Medeiros LJ, Brynes RK, Slovak ML, Murata-Collins JL, et al. (1999) Acute lymphoblastic leukemia. Survey of immunophenotype, French-American-British classification, frequency of myeloid antigen expression, and karyotypic abnormalities in 210 pediatric and adult cases. Am J Clin Pathol 111(4):467–476
16. Kim Y, Kang CS, Lee EJ, Kim WI, Shim SI, Kim SM, et al. (1998) Acute lymphoblastic leukemia with maturation – A new entity with clinical significance. Leukemia 12(6):875–881
17. Darbyshire PJ, Lilleyman JS (1987) Granular acute lymphoblastic leukaemia of childhood: A morphological phenomenon. J Clin Pathol 40(3):251–253
18. Schwarzinger I, Fodinger M, Scherrer R, Wolzt M, Mannhalter C, Speiser W (1993) Hypergranular acute lymphoblastic leukemia (ALL). Report of a case and review of the literature. Ann Hematol 67(6):301–303
19. Schumacher HR, Desai SN, McClain KL, Domenico DR, Dizikes GJ, Bird ML (1989) Acute lymphoblastic leukemia-hand mirror variant. Analysis for endogenous retroviral antibodies in bone marrow plasma. Am J Clin Pathol 91(4):410–416
20. Wegelius R (1986) Preleukaemic states in children. Scand J Haematol 45(Suppl):133–139
21. Wallis JP, Reid MM (1989) Bone marrow fibrosis in childhood acute lymphoblastic leukaemia. J Clin Pathol 42(12):1253–1254
22. Macfarlane SD, Tauro GP (1986) Acute lymphocytic leukemia in children presenting with bone marrow necrosis. Am J Hematol 22(4):341–346
23. Ribeiro RC, Pui CH, Schell MJ (1988) Vertebral compression fracture as a presenting feature of acute lymphoblastic leukemia in children. Cancer 61(3):589–592
24. Steinherz PG, Siegel SE, Bleyer WA, Kersey J, Chard R Jr, Coccia P, et al. (1991) Lymphomatous presentation of childhood acute lymphoblastic leukemia. A subgroup at high risk of early treatment failure. Cancer 68(4):751–758
25. Longacre TA, Foucar K, Crago S, Chen IM, Griffith B, Dressler L, et al. (1989) Hematogones: A multiparameter analysis of bone marrow precursor cells. Blood 73(2):543–552
26. Ott G, Kalla J, Ott MM, Schryen B, Katzenberger T, Muller JG, et al. (1997) Blastoid variants of mantle cell lymphoma: Frequent bcl-1 rearrangements at the major translocation cluster region and tetraploid chromosome clones. Blood 89(4):1421–1429
27. Huh YO, Ibrahim S (2000) Immunophenotypes in adult acute lymphocytic leukemia. Role of flow cytometry in diagnosis and monitoring of disease. Hematol Oncol Clin North Am 14(6): 1251–1265
28. Pileri SA, Ascani S, Milani M, Visani G, Piccioli M, Orcioni GF, et al. (1999) Acute leukaemia immunophenotyping in bone-marrow routine sections. Br J Haematol 105(2):394–401
29. Braylan RC, Orfao A, Borowitz MJ, Davis BH (2001) Optimal number of reagents required to evaluate hematolymphoid neoplasias: Results of an international consensus meeting. Cytometry 46(1): 23–27
30. Bain BJ, Barnett D, Linch D, Matutes E, Reilly JT (2002) Revised guideline on immunophenotyping in acute leukaemias and chronic lymphoproliferative disorders. Clin Lab Haematol 24(1): 1–13
31. Vasef MA, Brynes RK, Murata-Collins JL, Arber DA, Medeiros LJ (1998) Surface immunoglobulin light chain-positive acute lymphoblastic leukemia of FAB L1 or L2 type: A report of 6 cases in adults. Am J Clin Pathol 110(2):143–149
32. Gassmann W, Loffler H, Thiel E, Ludwig WD, Schwartz S, Haferlach T, et al. (1997) Morphological and cytochemical findings in 150 cases of T-lineage acute lymphoblastic leukaemia in adults. German Multicentre ALL Study Group (GMALL). Br J Haematol 97(2): 372–382
33. Czuczman MS, Dodge RK, Stewart CC, Frankel SR, Davey FR, Powell BL, et al. (1999) Value of immunophenotype in intensively treated adult acute lymphoblastic leukemia: Cancer and leukemia Group B study 8364. Blood 93(11):3931–3939
34. Hann IM, Richards SM, Eden OB, Hill FG (1998) Analysis of the immunophenotype of children treated on the Medical Research Council United Kingdom Acute Lymphoblastic Leukaemia Trial XI (MRC UKALLXI). Medical Research Council Childhood Leukaemia Working Party. Leukemia 12(8):1249–1255
35. Larson RA, Dodge RK, Burns CP, Lee EJ, Stone RM, Schulman P, et al. (1995) A five-drug remission induction regimen with intensive consolidation for adults with acute lymphoblastic leukemia: Cancer and leukemia group B study 8811. Blood 85(8):2025–2037
36. Matutes E, Morilla R, Farahat N, Carbonell F, Swansbury J, Dyer M, et al. (1997) Definition of acute biphenotypic leukemia. Haematologica 82(1):64–66
37. Arber DA, Snyder DS, Fine M, Dagis A, Niland J, Slovak ML (2001) Myeloperoxidase immunoreactivity in adult acute lymphoblastic leukemia. Am J Clin Pathol 116(1):25–33
38. Rimsza LM, Larson RS, Winter SS, Foucar K, Chong YY, Garner KW, et al. (2000) Benign hematogone-rich lymphoid proliferations can be distinguished from B-lineage acute lymphoblastic leukemia by integration of morphology, immunophenotype, adhesion mole-

cule expression, and architectural features. Am J Clin Pathol 114(1):66–75

39. van Wering ER, van der Linden-Schrever BE, Szczepanski T, Willemse MJ, Baars EA, van Wijngaarde-Schmitz HM, et al. (2000) Regenerating normal B-cell precursors during and after treatment of acute lymphoblastic leukaemia: Implications for monitoring of minimal residual disease. Br J Haematol 110(1):139–146
40. Anastasi J, Feng J, Dickstein JI, Le Beau MM, Rubin CM, Larson RA, et al. (1996) Lineage involvement by BCR/ABL in Ph+ lymphoblastic leukemias: Chronic myelogenous leukemia presenting in lymphoid blast vs. Ph+ acute lymphoblastic leukemia. Leukemia 10(5):795–802
41. Le Beau MM, Larson RA (2000) Cytogenetics and Neoplasia. In: Hoffman R BJE, Shattil SJ, et al. (eds) Hematology: Basic principles and practice, 3rd edn. Churchill Livingstone, Philadelphia, pp 848–869
42. van Dongen JJ, Seriu T, Panzer-Grumayer ER, Biondi A, Pongers-Willemse MJ, Corral L, et al. (1998) Prognostic value of minimal residual disease in acute lymphoblastic leukaemia in childhood. Lancet 352(9142):1731–1738
43. Cave H, van der Werff ten Bosch J, Suciu S, Guidal C, Waterkeyn C, Otten J, et al. (1998) Clinical significance of minimal residual disease in childhood acute lymphoblastic leukemia. European Organization for Research and Treatment of Cancer – Childhood Leukemia Cooperative Group. N Engl J Med 339(9):591–598

Diagnosis of Acute Lymphoblastic Leukemia

Maher Albitar, Francis J. Giles, Hagop Kantarjian

Contents

8.1 Introduction

The diagnosis of acute lymphoblastic leukemia (ALL) is dependent on the identification and characterization of blast cells in peripheral blood or bone marrow. Although it is not clear why blasts have a tendency to circulate in some patients and not in others, ALL can be reliably diagnosed using peripheral blood or bone marrow blasts when blasts are in circulation [79]. However, distinguishing blasts from activated lymphocytes is difficult in some patients, particularly children. Standard care and thorough evaluation of patients with ALL thus require good bone marrow aspiration, with high-quality smears and bone marrow biopsy specimens. When bone marrow biopsy specimens are available, touch imprints should be made [1].

Diagnosis and classification are generally based on the morphologic, cytochemical, and immunologic features of the blasts. However, cytogenetic and molecular studies are frequently needed to confirm the diagnosis, predict clinical behavior, and stratify patients for therapy [14, 27, 36, 45, 65]. The French, American, and British (FAB) classification of ALL, which recognizes three subclasses of ALL (L1, L2, and L3), is based strictly on blast morphology and cytochemistry [5], whereas the World Health Organization (WHO) classification scheme also incorporates immunophenotyping and cytogenetics [36].

Clinically and biologically, ALL and lymphoblastic lymphoma are considered a single entity and the terms are often used interchangeably [58]. However, the term "lymphoma" is preferred when the bulk of the disease is in the lymph nodes or soft tissues, whereas "leukemia" should be used when the bulk of the disease is in the bone marrow and blood [21, 53]. Approximately 80% of patients with ALL have enlarged lymph nodes, most likely due to involvement with the leukemic process [21].

In this chapter we present diagnostic criteria for ALL and its subtypes and discuss the importance of cytogenetic and molecular abnormalities for diagnosis, classification, and determining clinical management.

8.2 Morphology

Lymphoblasts in patients with ALL tend to be heterogeneous in size and shape. Unlike the recent WHO classification, which takes cytogenetic and immunologic features into account, the FAB classification of ALL emphasizes the presence of subgroups of precursor lymphoblasts: L1, which is more common in children than in adults (85% vs. 30%) and L2, which is more common in adults than in children (60% vs. 15%). The FAB and WHO classifications both recognize the more mature subtypes of B-cells as Burkitt L3 cells [5, 80].

L1 precursor lymphoblasts are small with scant cytoplasm, fine chromatin, and indistinct nucleoli (>90% of total blasts) (Fig. 8.1). L2 precursor lymphoblasts, on the other hand, are typically medium-to-large cells with high nucleus-to-cytoplasm ratios, prominent nucleoli, and irregular or folded nuclear membrane outlines (Fig. 8.1). Morphologic heterogeneity is almost always seen in L2 and, to a lesser degree, L1 precursor lymphoblasts. Occasional cells with vacuoles can be seen in L2-type precursor lymphoblasts, especially after relapse or therapy [64]. Although the reproducibility of classifying L1 and L2 precursor lymphoblasts is poor, distinguishing L1 from L2 morphology remains useful for diagnosis and for its descriptive value. Several studies suggest that patients with the L1 cell type have better response to therapy, with better disease-free survival than patients with the L2 cell morphology [2, 5, 44, 56, 77].

L3 (Burkitt) blasts have distinct morphology, with medium-sized and more uniformly rounded nuclei and finely clumped chromatin. The diagnostic feature of this cell subtype is a deeply basophilic and vacuolated cytoplasm (Fig. 8.2). The vacuoles in L3-type cells contain lipids and stain positively with oil-red O stain. Nucleoli are seen but are not dominant [5]. The cells of Burkitt leukemia have a very high rate of turnover (proliferation and apoptosis). This phenomenon manifests morphologically as the starry-sky appearance frequently seen in bone marrow biopsy specimens or tissue sections (Fig. 8.1), and biochemically with extremely high levels of lactate dehydrogenase [7, 72].

In addition to morphology, ALL is classified according to the B-cell or T-cell status. B-cell precursor ALL accounts for about 85% of ALL cases, with T-cell ALL accounting for about 15%. Although T-cell ALL lymphoblasts occasionally demonstrate conspicuous folded or cerebriform nuclei, T-cell precursor lymphoblasts cannot be reliably distinguished from B-cell lymphoblasts based on morphology alone [80]; immunophenotyping is always needed for confirmation.

8.3 Cytochemistry and Immunophenotyping

The key diagnostic cytochemical feature of ALL is the lack of myeloperoxidase (MPO) activity and negativity for nonspecific esterase (NSE) [5, 71]. The functional MPO test using cytochemistry remains the gold standard for assessing MPO activity, but laboratories are increasingly using the chloroacetate esterase stain and immunostain, especially for detection by flow cytometry [62]. To distinguish ALL from increased peripheral blood or bone marrow blasts, fewer than 3% of blasts should express MPO activity [5]. However, it is not unusual to detect slightly greater than 3% MPO-positive blasts in patients with chronic myeloid leukemia (CML) in lymphoid blast crisis, with overwhelming lymphoid surface markers. Most likely these few MPO-positive blasts reflect the active chronic cell population that coexists along with the lymphoid blasts. Sudan black B (SBB) can also be used to confirm the presence of MPO granules in these cells [71]. However, some cases of ALL exhibit fine SBB-positive granules rather than large, dark positive granules. Periodic acid-Schiff (PAS) staining is also positive in ALL lymphoblasts, showing a large, globular pattern. This PAS pattern is

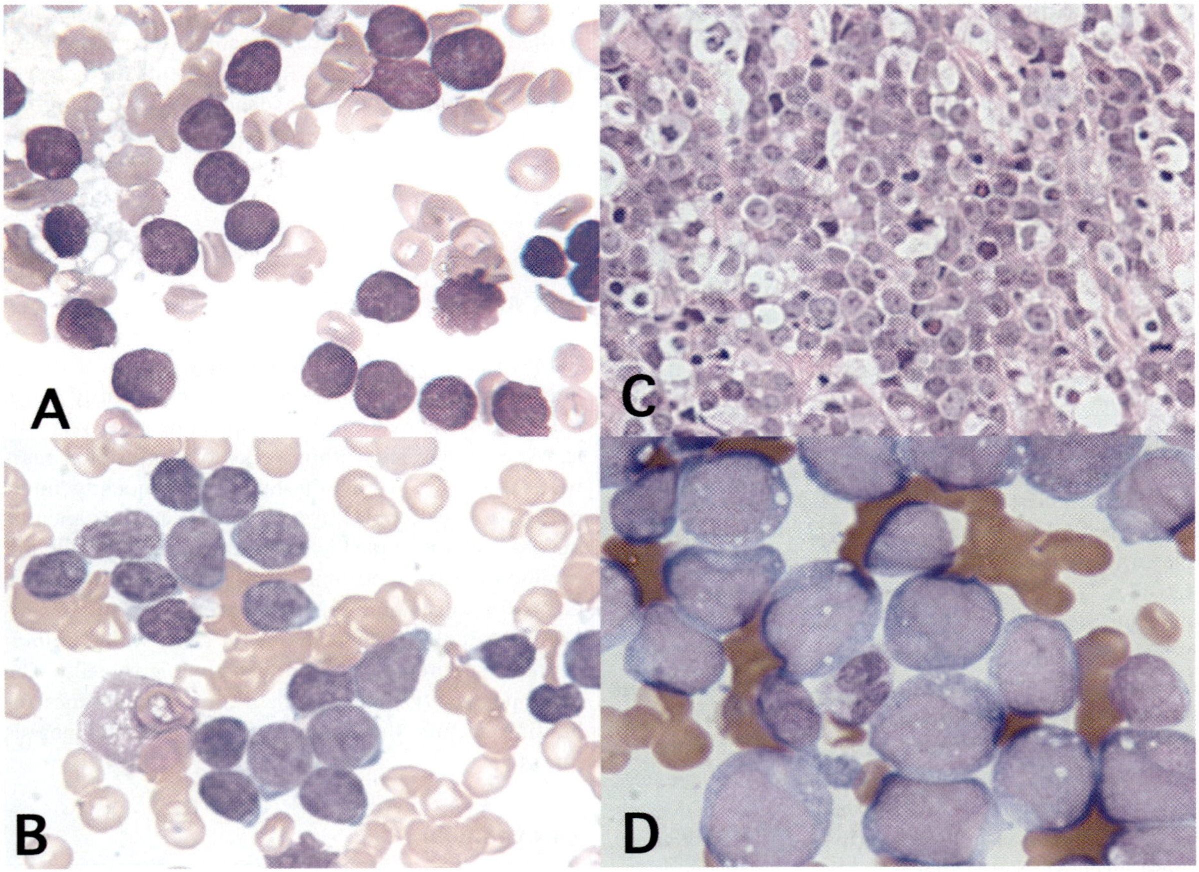

Fig. 8.1. Morphology of blasts in acute lymphoblastic leukemia. (**A**) L1 blasts; (**B**) L2 blasts; (**C**) "Starry sky" morphology on bone marrow biopsy in a case with L3 leukemia; (**D**) L3 blasts.

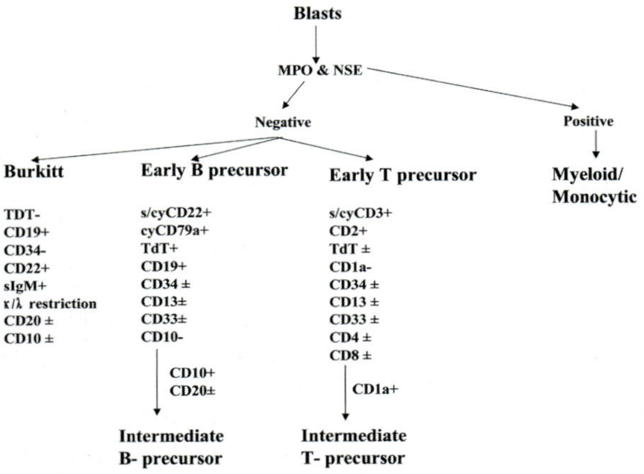

Fig. 8.2. Schematic approach for the diagnosis of blasts that are negative for myeloperoxidase and nonspecific esterase.

not specific and can be seen in erythroleukemia and other leukemia subtypes [71].

Negativity for MPO and NSE should raise the possibility of an ALL diagnosis, but further flow cytometric evaluation is necessary as illustrated in Fig. 8.2. Generally, the following markers are useful and used by most laboratories: CD34, TdT, CD1a, CD2, CD19, CD3, CD7, CD4, CD8, CD10, CD13, CD14, CD22, CD33, CD64, CD117, cCD79a, and surface immunoglobulin (Ig)M. MPO should be evaluated by flow cytometry if it was not assessed with cytochemical staining. Other cytoplasmic stains are useful when the lineage of the leukemic cells cannot be determined with these markers. Cytoplasmic CD3 (cyCD3), cyIgM, and cyCD22 are usually helpful.

Terminal deoxynucleotidyltransferase (TdT) expression along with CD19+ or cyCD79a and surface or cytoplasmic CD22+ are diagnostic for early precursor B-cell involvement, irrespective of CD13 and CD33 expression. The expression of CD10 (common ALL antigen, CALLA) in addition to the above markers is diagnostic for more mature (intermediate) precursor ALL. Although CD19 protein expression is diagnostic for B-cell lineage, it is detected in 80% of acute myeloid leukemia (AML) cases that carry the t(8;21) chromosomal abnormality [46]; however, these cases are MPO positive and easily distinguished from ALL. CD20 is expressed in approximately 55% of patients with precursor B-cell ALL and more frequently in Burkitt leukemia patients. In most but not all cases, precursor B-cell cells are surface IgM-negative. Blast cells that lack TdT expression are classified as Burkitt (L3) if they show L3-type morphology (vacuolated, deeply basophilic cytoplasm); otherwise, they should be classified as "Burkitt-like." Most importantly, these cells must show blast morphology (Fig. 8.1).

The diagnosis of precursor T-cell ALL is based on lack of expression of B-cell markers and expression of surface CD3 (sCD3) or cytoplasmic CD3 (cyCD3) in MPO-negative/NSE-negative blasts. However, approximately 10% of precursor T-cell ALL cases are TdT negative [25] and many coexpress CD4, CD8, and CD2. Lack of CD1a expression indicates early-stage differentiation; these T-cell ALL cases appear to be especially aggressive [71].

8.4 Atypical Acute Lymphoblastic Leukemia

8.4.1 Burkitt-Like (Atypical Burkitt) ALL

Rare cases of ALL show blasts with only mature B-cell markers (TdT–, CD19+, and surface IgM+) that are morphologically similar to the L2 rather than L3 cell type (lack deep blue cytoplasm with vacuoles). These cases are classified as Burkitt-like and are treated as Burkitt leukemia [24, 25].

8.4.2 ALL with Eosinophilia

Some cases of ALL demonstrate significant eosinophilia, which appears to be stimulated by the secretion of IL-5 and IL-3. The eosinophils have normal morphology and are reactive, not leukemic. In some of these patients, the IL-3 gene on chromosome 5q31 is translocated to the IgH gene locus on chromosome 14 (translocation t(5;14) (q31;q32) [9, 71, 83]. Rarely, patients may present with eosinophilia without evidence of ALL, raising the question of hypereosinophilic syndrome, which converts to ALL within weeks to months. The eosinophilia disappears with remission and may come back as an early sign of relapse [9, 71, 83].

8.4.3 Aplastic and Hypoplastic ALL

Rarely, young patients with ALL may present with hypoplastic or aplastic bone marrow. In the early stage, leukemic blasts may not be conspicuous and overt leukemia may manifest within weeks to months after marrow recovery. This manifestation is frequently interpreted as myelodysplastic syndrome or aplastic anemia, but the lack of dysplastic changes should help rule out myelodysplastic syndrome. This phenomenon may be due to an unusual immune response attempting to suppress the leukemic hematopoietic cells, which coincidentally suppresses normal hematopoietic cells. The other possibility is that the leukemic cells produce inhibiting factors that suppress normal hematopoiesis [71, 55].

8.4.4 Granular ALL

Rare cases of ALL show significant numbers of blasts with large (0.25-micron) basophilic granules. These granules are believed to be either abnormal mitochondria or cytoplasmic organelles, but their clinical significance is not known. Although the granules are MPO negative, they are more common in ALL cases that coexpress myeloid markers [37, 42, 71]. The blasts should not be confused with those of acute basophilic leukemia, which is more frequently seen in patients with acute-phase CML.

8.4.5 Hand Mirror ALL

Blasts in some cases of leukemia show uropod (handle) morphology with elongated cytoplasm, which may represent an attachment or endocytotic process. This morphology can be seen in reactive lymphoid and monocytoid cells as well as blasts. Once thought to be specific for ALL or mixed-lineage leukemia, this morphology can also be seen in AML [81].

8.4.6 Natural Killer ALL (Blastic NK)

Rare cases of ALL have been reported in which the blasts lack myeloid and lymphoid markers (CD3 and CD19) but express CD56. These cases are classified as ALL of the natural killer cell phenotype. Blastic NK cells may show cytoplasmic CD3 and, occasionally, other T-cell markers (CD4 or CD7), and can be positive or negative for TdT. They lack evidence of T-cell receptor gene rearrangement. These cases should be distinguished from myeloid leukemia that expresses myeloid markers in addition to CD56. Expression of CD56 can also be seen in some cases that are typically lymphoblastic, with clear T-cell surface markers. Such cases should be considered precursor T-cell ALL with CD56 expression [52, 61, 71].

8.4.7 Biphenotypic and Bilineage ALL

In biphenotypic leukemia, markers specific for lymphoid as well as myeloid lineages can coexist in the same blast population. When two distinct cell populations coexist, one with lymphoid and the other with myeloid markers, the term "bilineage" applies. Biphenotypic and bilineage ALL are lumped together with other undifferentiated subtypes in the WHO classification of "acute leukemia of ambiguous lineage." Despite significant confusion over the terminology, there is agreement that cells of ALL can express CD13 or CD33 or both, especially when they are positive for Philadelphia chromosome. These cases should be called "ALL with myeloid markers" rather than "biphenotypic ALL."

Biphenotypic ALL is characterized by the expression of lymphoid markers (CD19 with TdT or CD3 with TdT) along with myeloid markers (MPO with CD13, or MPO with CD33). Several scoring systems can be used for the diagnosis of biphenotypic ALL; the Immunologic Classification of Leukemia is the most widely accepted [4, 75]. The importance of classification is to decide whether a patient should be treated for lymphoblastic leukemia or for myeloid leukemia. For practical purposes, MD Anderson Cancer Center uses a simplified approach for classifying these cases with ambiguous lineage or minimal differentiation. This approach is based on blasts being negative for MPO and NSE and positive for TdT (Fig. 8.3). If these blasts express one of the major lymphoid markers (CD10, CD19, CD3) or two of the other lymphoid markers, the case

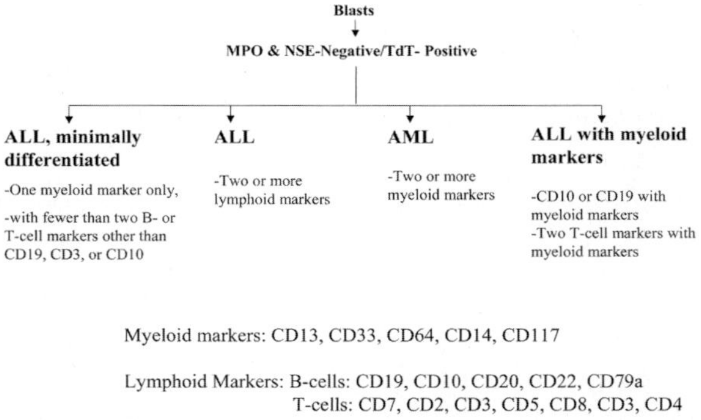

Fig. 8.3. Schematic approach for a clinically useful diagnosis of leukemia of ambiguous lineage (minimally differentiated) as used by MD Anderson Cancer Center.

is classified as lymphoblastic leukemia, irrespective of whether myeloid markers are expressed [4, 14, 31, 49, 71]. Patients who have one myeloid marker but fewer than two lymphoid markers (other than CD19, CD3, or CD10) are classified as having ALL with minimal differentiation.

8.4.8 MPO-Positive ALL

This term should be reserved for rare cases of ALL that demonstrate typical lymphoid markers without myeloid markers, except for strong positivity (20–30%) for MPO. Most of these cases show lymphoblasts with deep basophilic cytoplasm [82]. These cases should be distinguished from Burkitt cases as well as AML.

8.5 Cytogenetic and Molecular Abnormalities

Approximately 45% of ALL cases demonstrate recurrent ALL-specific cytogenetic abnormalities on conventional karyotyping studies, establishing cytogenetic study as a valuable diagnostic and prognostic tool for evaluating patients with ALL. In addition, most of these abnormalities can be detected using fluorescence in-situ hybridization (FISH), Southern blotting of genomic DNA, and reverse transcription-polymerase chain reaction (RT-PCR) of mRNA. FISH and RT-PCR are used to detect minimal residual disease and to monitor patients after therapy; real-time RT-PCR allows the quantitative monitoring of residual disease. The most common cytogenetic abnormalities are listed in Table 8.1 and discussed below.

Table 8.1. Molecular abnormalities of acute lymphoblastic leukemia (ALL)

Chromosomal abnormality	Gene	Cytogenetic lesion	% Adult ALL	% Pediatric ALL
8q24	Myc-Ig	t(8;14), t(8;22), t(2,8)	5	2
>46 chromosomes	NA	Hyperdiploidy	5	25
<46 chromosomes	NA	Hypodiploidy	5	6
12p12	*ETV6-AML1*	t(12;21)(p12;q22)	1	22
19p13.3	*E2A-PBX1*	t(1;19), t(17;19)	3	5
11q23	*MLL*	t(4;11)(q21;q23), t(9;11) (p21;q23), t(11;19) (q23;q13.3), (3;11)(q22;q23), t(x;11)(q13;q23)	8	10
9q34	*BCR-ABL*	t(9;22)(q34;q11)	25	3
14q11	T-cell antigen receptor	t(14q11)	20	15
5q35	*HOX11L2*	t(5;14)(q35;q32)	1	2.5
1p32	*TAL-1*	t(1;14)(p32;q11)	12	7
10q24	HOX11	t(10;14)(q24;q11), t(7;10)(q35;q24)	8	1
9p21	$p16^{INK4a}$, $p15^{INK4b}$	Del(9p21-22)	15	20
9q32	*TAL-2*	t(7;9)(q34;q32)	Rare	Rare
13q14	*miR15/miR16*	Del(13q14)	3	2
11q22	*ATM*	Del(11q22-23)	28*	16*
6q23	Unknown	Del(6q), t(6;12)(q23;p13)	6	5

* = As determined by loss of heterozygosity (LOH)

8.5.1 Hyperdiploidy

Hyperdiploidy, defined as the gain of additional chromosomes, is one of the most frequent cytogenetic abnormalities in ALL (25% of pediatric ALL and 5% of adult ALL). This increase in chromosomes is not random: the most commonly gained chromosomes are 4, 8, 10, and 21, followed by chromosomes 5, 6, 14, and 17. Most hyperdiploid cells contain either 47 to 50 chromosomes or 51 or more. Patients with ALL and high hyperdiploidy have longer response and survival durations after therapy, particularly those with more than 50 chromosomes. In general, hyperdiploid cells are more sensitive than nonhyperdiploid cells to chemotherapy and show more rapid induction of apoptosis [10, 13, 65].

8.5.2 Hypodiploidy

Hypodiploidy, or the presence of fewer than 46 chromosomes, is seen in 5% of ALL and this abnormality is generally considered a poor prognostic factor. However, near haploidy (23–29 chromosomes) is particularly associated with poor outcome [67].

8.5.3 Philadelphia Chromosome

The Philadelphia translocation is one of the most frequently identified chromosome abnormalities among adults with ALL (25%), while only 3% of pediatric ALL is Philadelphia chromosome positive. The presence of the Philadelphia chromosome is associated with uniformly poor outcomes [21, 26, 34].

Philadelphia chromosome results from a reciprocal translocation between the long arms of chromosomes 9 and 22 [t(9;22)(q34;q11)], which moves the *ABL* gene from 9q34 into the *BCR* (breakpoint cluster region) region of chromosome 22q11. The resulting *BCR-ABL* fusion gene encodes a tyrosine phosphokinase that is constitutively active and leads to downstream activation of several proteins, including the Crkl and AKT pathway, Ras/Raf-1 pathway, Stat 1 and 5 pathways, platelet-derived growth factor (PDGF), and the c-kit receptor tyrosine kinase [26, 34, 65]. Depending on the exact position of the translocated *ABL* gene (exon b2) within *BCR*, three different fusion products can be generated: p190 (molecular weight 190 kd, exon e1), p210 (exon b2 or b3), and p230 (exon e19). Patients with CML express mostly the p210 protein and rarely p230, whereas ALL patients mainly express p190. Some ALL patients present with p210 expression, but most of these cases represent lymphoid blast crises of CML.

8.5.4 12p12.3 Abnormalities

Translocation t(12;21)(p12;q22), which results in the ETV6 (TEL)-AML1 (CBFA2) fusion protein, is detected in 20–25% of children with B-cell precursor ALL. This is the most common cytogenetic–molecular abnormality in childhood ALL, but is relatively uncommon in adult ALL (<5%). Rare cases of prenatal t(12;21) have been documented, suggesting that the translocation may not be sufficient for overt leukemia and requires additional mutations (second hits) that occur after birth. Because the t(12;21)(p12;q22) translocation is not detected with conventional cytogenetic studies, FISH or RT-PCR should be used to identify this abnormality. Deletion in this region without translocation has also been reported. The ETV6-AML1 fusion protein in children with ALL is associated with an excellent prognosis, with longer event-free and overall survival [18, 20, 43, 65, 73].

8.5.5 11q23 Abnormalities

The *MLL* (mixed lineage leukemia) gene, located at the 11q23 locus, is involved in translocations onto other chromosomes as well as duplication. The most common *MLL* translocations in ALL are t(4;11)(q21;q23), t(9;11)(p21;q23), t(11;19)(q23;q13.3), and t(3;11)(q22;q23), which are associated with poor outcomes and a high incidence of myeloid marker expression [40, 69].

The *ATM* (ataxia telangiectasia mutated) gene, also located near chromosome 11q22-23, is frequently deleted in ALL. About 16% of pediatric ALL patients have loss of heterozygosity (LOH) at this locus. Haidar and colleagues reported that 10 of 36 (28%) adults with ALL had LOH of the *ATM* gene [35]. Only one (3%) of the 36 patients showed abnormalities involving chromosome 11q23 by conventional cytogenetic studies, indicating that most of these deletions are submicroscopic [35, 59]. The presence of this abnormality in adults is associated with better response to therapy [35].

8.5.6 8q24 Abnormalities

The c-*myc* gene is located on chromosome 8q24 and can be translocated into one of the three immunoglobulin chain loci in Burkitt leukemia: IgH on chromosome 14, Iglambda on chromosome 22, or Igkappa on chromosome 2. These translocations are detected in cytogenetic and FISH studies as t(8;14)(q24;q32), t(8;22)(q24;q11), and t(2;8)(p12;q24). Translocation of the c-*myc* gene into the T-cell receptor alpha/delta gene has been reported in T-cell ALL as translocation t(8;14)(q24;q11). All these translocations lead to quantitative increases in the expression of c-*myc* mRNA and protein, due to juxtaposition of the c-*myc* gene to the Ig or T-cell receptor gene enhancer. The c-myc protein activates the expression of genes necessary for cells to enter the S-phase and proliferate. This chromosomal abnormality is detected in approximately 80% of Burkitt ALL cases; mechanisms other than translocation are believed to be responsible for increased expression of the c-*myc* gene in the remaining cases [12, 33, 39].

8.5.7 19p13.3 Abnormalities

The E2A gene is located on chromosome 19p13.3. Translocation t(1;19)(q23;p13) forms the *E2A*-PBX1 fusion gene, leading to expression of the E2A-PBX1 fusion protein. This abnormality is seen in precursor B-cell ALL and is detected in approximately 5% of pediatric and 3% of adult ALL cases. A similar translocation t(17;19)(q22;p13) involving the E2A gene results in expression of the fusion protein E2A-HLF. The E2A-PBX1 and E2A-HLF fusion proteins are strong transcription factors that appear to activate several downstream genes [23, 32, 51, 76]; both are associated with poor outcomes.

8.5.8 5q35 Abnormalities

A recently described cryptic translocation in T-cell ALL, t(5;14)(q35;q32), moves the *HOX11L2* (HOX11like2)(RNX; TLX3) homeobox gene into close proximity of the *CTIP2* gene on chromosome 14. This translocation, which can be detected with FISH or RT-PCR, leads to overexpression of *HOX11L2*. Translocation t(5;14) appears to be restricted to T-lineage ALL and is more common in children than adults (22% vs. 13%) [6, 19].

8.5.9 1p32 Abnormalities

The *TAL-1* (*SCL; TCL-5*) gene, located on chromosome 1p32, codes for a 42-kd nuclear protein with a helix-loop-helix DNA binding motif. Found in approximately 25% of cases [3, 41, 63], *TAL-1* alterations are the most common genetic abnormalities in T-cell ALL and can be formed by translocation or deletion. The t(1;14)(p32;q11) translocation associates *TAL-1* with the T-cell receptor alpha/delta locus, whereas nonrandom, submicroscopic interstitial deletions between *SIL* and the 5′ untranslated region of the *TAL-1* gene give rise to a *SIL-TAL-1* fusion transcript. Both alterations disrupt the coding potential of *TAL-1* in a similar manner, leading to its ectopic expression in T cells.

8.5.10 10q24 Abnormalities

Translocations involving the *HOX11* homeobox gene, located on chromosome 10q24, are present in about 5% of T-cell ALL cases. Translocation t(10;14)(q24;q11) places *HOX11* under transcriptional control of the T-cell receptor alpha/delta gene, while translocation t(7;10)(q35;q24) places it under control of the T-cell receptor beta gene. Both translocations lead to transcriptional activation of *HOX11* (*TLX1; TCL3*) [30, 46, 70]. *HOX11* overexpression appears to be a favorable prognostic factor in adult T-cell ALL [30].

8.5.11 6q Abnormalities

Chromosomal bands 6q15 to 6q23 are frequently deleted in T- and B-cell ALL. Such deletions have been reported in approximately 5% of cases, but are believed to be more frequently detected if PCR analysis of LOH is used. Translocations involving this region of chromosome 6, including t(6;12)(q23;p13) (ETV-6 gene) and t(6;11)(q27;q23) (a region close to the *MLL* gene), have also been reported. There is a suggestion that this abnormality is associated with more aggressive disease [17, 38, 54, 74].

8.5.12 9q32 Abnormalities

The *TAL-2* gene encodes a helix-loop-helix protein, a transcriptional factor that activates various genes and leads to cellular proliferation [84]. The *TAL-2* gene is activated by translocation t(7;9)(q34;q32), which juxtaposes it with regulatory elements of the T-cell receptor beta gene. This abnormality is rare and best detected by cytogenetic and FISH studies, but its clinical relevance has not been established.

8.5.13 T-Cell Antigen Receptor Gene Abnormalities

The genes for T-cell receptors alpha/delta, gamma, and beta are located on chromosomes 14q11, 7q15, and 7q35, respectively; the delta receptor gene is located within the alpha gene. All of these loci are involved in chromosomal translocations that lead to activation of transcription factors or oncogenes [65]. The clinical relevance of the translocations that they are involved with is dependent on their partner gene. In most of these translocations the partner genes are deregulated and become under the influence of the promoter/enhancer of the T-cell receptors in a fashion similar to that seen in Burkitt leukemia.

8.5.14 13q14 Abnormalities

Deletion of band 13q14 is detected in ALL and many other leukemias and tumors, suggesting the presence of tumor suppressor genes in this region. Numerous genes have been investigated as targets for this deletion, including the retinoblastoma gene, but none of the potential targets investigated so far have been consistently implicated.

Micro-RNAs are short (21- or 22-nucleotide) RNAs transcribed from a family of closely related noncoding genes. Although their function is not completely understood, micro-RNAs are thought to regulate expression by binding mRNA of specific genes [15, 16, 50]. Two micro-RNA genes, *miR15* and *miR16*, were recently reported to be the target for the 13q14 deletion in chronic lymphocytic leukemia and are most likely deleted in ALL. Cytogenetic and FISH studies can detect this abnormality, but higher percentage of this abnormality has been reported when LOH is used [22].

8.5.15 9p21 Abnormalities

Abnormalities of the short arm of chromosome 9 at band p21 occur in up to 15% of patients with ALL. These patients, mainly children, tend to present with unfavorable clinical characteristics (high white blood cell and blast counts and organomegaly) and predominantly T-cell immunophenotype. Clinical outcome is characterized by high relapse rates and short overall survival. The tumor suppressor genes $p16^{INK4a}$ and $p15^{INK4b}$ are located in this region and their products are of the cyclin-dependent kinase inhibitor (CDKI) family. Deletions of $p16^{INK4a}$ and $p15^{INK4b}$ are most common in T-cell ALL, where they can be found in 60–80% of cases. Hypermethylation of the 5′-CpG promoter islands silences this gene locus [28, 60, 66].

8.5.16 Molecular Abnormalities Detected by Expression Microarrays

Expression microarrays with cDNA or oligonucleotide sequences from a few to more than 33 000 genes have been used to subclassify ALL and to stratify patients according to their risk and response to therapy. The expression microarray approach has yielded useful and interesting insights into the biology of ALL. It has proved useful as a discovery tool, and the data generated from this approach show that the number of genes required for specific diagnoses and subclassifications is small and can be adapted using standard diagnostic techniques such as real-time RT-PCR [8, 29, 48, 57, 68]. However, numerous technical issues related to the reproducibility and the practicality of this approach need to be resolved before it is accepted for clinical use.

References

1. Aboul-Nasr R, Estey EH, Kantarjian HM, Freireich EJ, Andreeff M, Johnson BJ, Albitar M (1999) Comparison of touch imprints with aspirate smears for evaluating bone marrow specimens. Am J Clin Pathol 111:753–758
2. Armitage JO, Abedi M, Albitar M, Banks PM, Chadburn A, Chang KL, Coiffier B, Cortes JE, Deitcher SR, Dunphy CH (2004) Atlas of Clinical Hematology. Lippincott Williams & Wilkins, Hagerstown, Maryland
3. Bash RO, Hall S, Timmons CF, Crist WM, Amylon M, Smith RG, Baer R (1995) Does activation of the TAL1 gene occur in a majority of patients with T-cell acute lymphoblastic leukemia? A pediatric oncology group study. Blood 86:666–676
4. Bene MC, Castoldi G, Knapp W, Ludwig WD, Matutes E, Orfao A, van't Veer MB (1995) Proposals for the immunological classification of acute leukemias. European Group for the Immunological Characterization of Leukemias (EGIL). Leukemia 9:1783–1786
5. Bennett JM, Catovsky D, Daniel MT, Flandrin G, Galton DA, Gralnick HR, Sultan C (1981) The morphological classification of acute lymphoblastic leukaemia: Concordance among observers and clinical correlations. Br J Haematol 47:553–561
6. Berger R, Dastugue N, Busson M, Van Den Akker J, Perot C, Ballerini P, Hagemeijer A, Michaux L, Charrin C, Pages MP, et al.; Groupe Francais de Cytogenetique Hematologique (GFCH) (2003) t(5;14)/HOX11L2-positive T-cell acute lymphoblastic leukemia. A collaborative study of the Groupe Francais de Cytogenetique Hematologique (GFCH). Leukemia 17:1851–1857
7. Bernasconi C, Brusamolino E, Pagnucco G, Bernasconi P, Orlandi E, Lazzarino M (1991) Burkitt's lymphoma/leukemia: A clinicopathologic study of 24 adult patients. Leukemia 5(Suppl 1):90–94
8. Bertrand FE, Spengeman JD, Shah N, LeBien TW (2003) B-cell development in the presence of the MLL/AF4 oncoprotein proceeds in the absence of HOX A7 and HOX A9 expression. Leukemia 17:2454–2459
9. Blatt J, Proujansky R, Horn M, Phebus C, Longworth D, Penchansky L (1992) Idiopathic hypereosinophilic syndrome terminating in acute lymphoblastic leukemia. Pediatr Hematol Oncol 9:151–155
10. Bloomfield CD, Lindquist LL, Arthur D, McKenna RW, LeBien TW, Nesbit ME, Peterson BA (1981) Chromosomal abnormalities in acute lymphoblastic leukemia. Cancer Res 41:4838–4843
11. Braziel RM, Arber DA, Slovak ML, Gulley ML, Spier C, Kjeldsberg C, Unger J, Miller TP, Tubbs R, Leith C, et al. (2001) The Burkitt-like lymphomas: A Southwest Oncology Group study delineating phenotypic, genotypic, and clinical features. Blood 97:3713–3720
12. Brito-Babapulle V, Crawford A, Khokhar T, Laffan M, Matutes E, Fairhead S, Catovsky D (1991) Translocations t(14;18) and t(8;14) with rearranged bcl-2 and c-myc in a case presenting as B-ALL (L3). Leukemia 5:83–87
13. Brodeur GM, Williams DL, Look AT, Bowman WP, Kalwinsky DK (1981) Near-haploid acute lymphoblastic leukemia: A unique subgroup with a poor prognosis? Blood 58:14–19
14. Brunning RD (2003) Classification of acute leukemias. Semin Diagn Pathol 20:142–153

15. Calin GA, Dumitru CD, Shimizu M, Bichi R, Zupo S, Noch E, Aldler H, Rattan S, Keating M, Rai K, et al. (2002) Frequent deletions and down-regulation of micro-RNA genes miR15 and miR16 at 13q14 in chronic lymphocytic leukemia. Proc Natl Acad Sci 99:15524–15529
16. Calin GA, Sevignani C, Dumitru CD, Hyslop T, Noch E, Yendamuri S, Shimizu M, Rattan S, Bullrich F, Negrini M, Croce CM (2004) Human microRNA genes are frequently located at fragile sites and genomic regions involved in cancers. Proc Natl Acad Sci 101:2999–3004
17. Carney LA, Kinney JS, Higgins RR, Freeman AI, Hecht BK, Woods GM (1992) X;6 translocation in a child with congenital acute lymphocytic leukemia. Cancer 69:799–803
18. Cave H, Cacheux V, Raynaud S, Brunie G, Bakkus M, Cochaux P, Preudhomme C, Lai JL, Vilmer E, Grandchamp B (1997) ETV6 is the target of chromosome 12p deletions in t(12;21) childhood acute lymphocytic leukemia. Leukemia 11:1459–1464
19. Cave H, Suciu S, Preudhomme C, Poppe B, Robert A, Uyttebroeck A, Malet M, Boutard P, Benoit Y, Mauvieux L, et al. (2004) Clinical significance of HOX11L2 expression linked to t(5;14)(q35;q32), of HOX11 expression, and of SIL-TAL fusion in childhood T-cell malignancies: Results of EORTC studies 58881 and 58951. Blood 103:442–450
20. Codrington R, O'Connor HE, Jalali GR, Carrara P, Papaioannou M, Hart SM, Hoffbrand AV, Potter M, Prentice HG, Harrison CJ, et al. (2000) Analysis of ETV6/AML1 abnormalities in acute lymphoblastic leukaemia: Incidence, alternative spliced forms and minimal residual disease value. Br J Haematol 111:1071–1079
21. Cortes JE, Kantarjian H, Freireich EJ (1996) Acute lymphocytic leukemia: A comprehensive review with emphasis on biology and therapy. Cancer Treat Res 84:291–323
22. Chung CY, Kantarjian H, Haidar M, Starostik P, Manshouri T, Gidel C, Freireich E, Keating M, Albitar M (2000) Deletions in the 13q14 locus in adult lymphoblastic leukemia: Rate of incidence and relevance. Cancer 88:1359–1364
23. Daheron L, Brizard F, Millot F, Cividin M, Lacotte L, Guilhot F, Brizard A (2003) E2A/HLF fusion gene in an acute lymphoblastic leukemia patient with disseminated intravascular coagulation and a normal karyotype. Hematol J 3:153–156
24. Evens AM, Gordon LI (2002) Burkitt's and Burkitt-like lymphoma. Curr Treat Options Oncol 3:291–305
25. Faber J, Kantarjian H, Roberts MW, Keating M, Freireich E, Albitar M (2000) Terminal deoxynucleotidyl transferase-negative acute lymphoblastic leukemia. Arch Pathol Lab Med 124:92–97
26. Faderl S, Albitar M (2000) Insights into the biologic and molecular abnormalities in adult acute lymphocytic leukemia. Hematol Oncol Clin North Am 14:1267–1288
27. Faderl S, Jeha S, Kantarjian HM (2003) The biology and therapy of adult acute lymphoblastic leukemia. Cancer 98:1337–1354
28. Faderl S, Kantarjian HM, Manshouri T, Chan CY, Pierce S, Hays KJ, Cortes J, Thomas D, Estrov Z, Albitar M (1999) The prognostic significance of p16INK4a/p14ARF and p15INK4b deletions in adult acute lymphoblastic leukemia. Clin Cancer Res 5:1855–1861
29. Ferrando AA, Look AT (2003) Gene expression profiling in T-cell acute lymphoblastic leukemia. Semin Hematol 40:274–280
30. Ferrando AA, Neuberg DS, Dodge RK, Paietta E, Larson RA, Wiernik PH, Rowe JM, Caligiuri MA, Bloomfield CD, Look AT (2004) Prognostic importance of TLX1 (HOX11) oncogene expression in adults with T-cell acute lymphoblastic leukaemia. Lancet 363 (9408):535–536
31. Fleming DR, Doukas MA, Jennings DC, Davey DD (2000) Diagnostic and clinical implications of lineage fidelity in acute leukemia patients undergoing allogeneic stem cell transplantation. Leuk Lymphoma 2000 36:309–313
32. Foa R, Vitale A, Mancini M, Cuneo A, Mecucci C, Elia L, Lombardo R, Saglio G, Torelli G, Annino L, et al. (2003) E2A-PBX1 fusion in adult acute lymphoblastic leukaemia: Biological and clinical features. Br J Haematol 120:484–487
33. Gauwerky CE, Croce CM (1993) Chromosomal translocations in leukaemia. Semin Cancer Biol 4:333–340
34. Gotoh A, Broxmeyer HE (1997) The function of BCR/ABL and related proto-oncogenes. Curr Opin Hematol 4:3–11
35. Haidar MA, Kantarjian H, Manshouri T, Chang CY, O'Brien S, Freireich E, Keating M, Albitar M (2000) ATM gene deletion in patients with adult acute lymphoblastic leukemia. Cancer 88:1057–1062
36. Harris NL, Jaffe ES, Diebold J, Flandrin G, Muller-Hermelink HK, Vardiman J, Lister TA, Bloomfield CD (2000) The World Health Organization classification of neoplasms of the hematopoietic and lymphoid tissues: Report of the Clinical Advisory Committee meeting – Airlie House, Virginia, November, 1997. Hematol J 1:53–66
37. Hay CR, Barnett D, James V, Woodcock BW, Brown MJ, Lawrence AC (1987) Granular common acute lymphoblastic leukaemia in adults: A morphological study. Eur J Haematol 39:299–305
38. Hayashi Y, Raimondi SC, Look AT, Behm FG, Kitchingman GR, Pui CH, Rivera GK, Williams DL (1990) Abnormalities of the long arm of chromosome 6 in childhood acute lymphoblastic leukemia. Blood 76:1626–1630
39. Hecht JL, Aster JC (2000) Molecular biology of Burkitt's lymphoma. J Clin Oncol 18:3707–3721
40. Hilden JM, Kersey JH (1994) The MLL (11q23) and AF-4 (4q21) genes disrupted in t(4;11) acute leukemia: Molecular and clinical studies. Leuk Lymphoma 14:189–195
41. Hsu HL, Wadman I, Tsan JT, Baer R (1994) Positive and negative transcriptional control by the TAL1 helix-loop-helix protein. Proc Natl Acad Sci 91:5947–5951
42. Invernizzi R, Rosanda C, Basso G, Conter V, di Cataldo A, Fenu S, Forni M, Frappampina V, Granchi D, Locatelli F, et al (1992) Granular acute lymphoblastic leukemia in children. "AIEOP Cooperative Group for Cytology of Acute Leukemias". Haematologica 77:30–34
43. Jalali GR, Martineau M, Ford AM, Greaves M, Stevens RF, Harrison CJ (2003) A unique variant of ETV6/AML1 fusion in a child with acute lymphoblastic leukemia. Leukemia 17:993–995
44. Kanerva J, Saarinen-Pihkala UM, Riikonen P, Makipernaa A, Mottonen M, Salmi TT (1999) Reemphasis on lymphoblast L2 morphology as a poor prognostic factor in childhood acute lymphoblastic leukemia. Med Pediatr Oncol 33:388–394
45. Kebriaei P, Anastasi J, Larson RA (2002) Acute lymphoblastic leukaemia: Diagnosis and classification. Best Pract Res Clin Haematol 15:597–621
46. Kees UR, Heerema NA, Kumar R, Watt PM, Baker DL, La MK, Uckun FM, Sather HN (2003) Expression of HOX11 in childhood T-lineage acute lymphoblastic leukaemia can occur in the absence of cytogenetic aberration at 10q24: A study from the Children's Cancer Group (CCG). Leukemia 17:887–893

47. Kita K, Shirakawa S, Kamada N (1994) Cellular characteristics of acute myeloblastic leukemia associated with t(8;21)(q22;q22). The Japanese Cooperative Group of Leukemia/Lymphoma. Leuk Lymphoma 13:229–234
48. Kohlmann A, Schoch C, Schnittger S, Dugas M, Hiddemann W, Kern W, Haferlach T (2004) Pediatric acute lymphoblastic leukemia (ALL) gene expression signatures classify an independent cohort of adult ALL patients. Leukemia 18:63–71
49. Legrand O, Perrot JY, Simonin G, Baudard M, Cadiou M, Blanc C, Ramond S, Viguie F, Marie JP, Zittoun R (1998) Adult biphenotypic acute leukaemia: An entity with poor prognosis which is related to unfavourable cytogenetics and P-glycoprotein over-expression. Br J Haematol 100:147–155
50. Liu Y, Hermanson M, Grander D, Merup M, Wu X, Heyman M, Rasool O, Juliusson G, Gahrton G, Detlofsson R, et al. (1995) 13q deletions in lymphoid malignancies. Blood 86:1911–1915
51. Look AT (1997) E2A-HLF chimeric transcription factors in pro-B cell acute lymphoblastic leukemia. Curr Top Microbiol Immunol 220:45–53
52. Macon WR, Williams ME, Greer JP, Hammer RD, Glick AD, Collins RD, Cousar JB (1996) Natural killer-like T-cell lymphomas: Aggressive lymphomas of T-large granular lymphocytes. Blood 87:1474–1483
53. Maitra A, McKenna RW, Weinberg AG, Schneider NR, Kroft SH (2001) Precursor B-cell lymphoblastic lymphoma. A study of nine cases lacking blood and bone marrow involvement and review of the literature. Am J Clin Pathol 115:868–875
54. Martineau M, Berger R, Lillington DM, Moorman AV, Secker-Walker LM (1998) The t(6;11)(q27;q23) translocation in acute leukemia: A laboratory and clinical study of 30 cases. EU Concerted Action 11q23 Workshop participants. Leukemia 12:788–791
55. Matloub YH, Brunning RD, Arthur DC, Ramsay NK (1993) Severe aplastic anemia preceding acute lymphoblastic leukemia. Cancer 71:264–268
56. Miller DR, Leikin S, Albo V, Sather H, Hammond D (1981) Prognostic importance of morphology (FAB classification) in childhood acute lymphoblastic leukaemia (ALL). Br J Haematol 48:199–206
57. Moos PJ, Raetz EA, Carlson MA, Szabo A, Smith FE, Willman C, Wei Q, Hunger SP, Carroll WL (2002) Identification of gene expression profiles that segregate patients with childhood leukemia. Clin Cancer Res 8:3118–3130
58. Mrozek K, Heerema NA, Bloomfield CD (2004) Cytogenetics in acute leukemia. Blood Rev 18:115–136
59. Oguchi K, Takagi M, Tsuchida R, Taya Y, Ito E, Isoyama K, Ishii E, Zannini L, Delia D, Mizutani S (2003) Missense mutation and defective function of ATM in a childhood acute leukemia patient with MLL gene rearrangement. Blood 101:3622–3627
60. Okuda T, Shurtleff SA, Valentine MB, Raimondi SC, Head DR, Behm F, Curcio-Brint AM, Liu Q, Pui CH, Sherr CJ, et al. (1995) Frequent deletion of p16INK4a/MTS1 and p15INK4b/MTS2 in pediatric acute lymphoblastic leukemia. Blood 85:2321–2330
61. Paietta E, Neuberg D, Richards S, Bennett JM, Han L, Racevskis J, Dewald G, Rowe JM, Wiernik PH; Eastern Cooperative Oncology Group (2001) Rare adult acute lymphocytic leukemia with CD56 expression in the ECOG experience shows unexpected phenotypic and genotypic heterogeneity. Am J Hematol 66:189–196
62. Peffault de Latour R, Legrand O, Moreau D, Perrot JY, Blanc CM, Chaoui D, Casadevall N, Marie JP (2003) Comparison of flow cytometry and enzyme cytochemistry for the detection of myeloperoxydase in acute myeloid leukaemia: Interests of a new positivity threshold. Br J Haematol 122:211–216
63. Pongers-Willemse MJ, Seriu T, Stolz F, d'Aniello E, Gameiro P, Pisa P, Gonzalez M, Bartram CR, Panzer-Grumayer ER, Biondi A, et al. (1999) Primers and protocols for standardized detection of minimal residual disease in acute lymphoblastic leukemia using immunoglobulin and T cell receptor gene rearrangements and TAL1 deletions as PCR targets: Report of the BIOMED-1 CONCERTED ACTION: Investigation of minimal residual disease in acute leukemia. Leukemia 13:110–118
64. Potter VP, Sorell M, Baglivo JA, Sather H, Miller DR (1984) Prognostic significance of vacuoles in L1 lymphoblasts in childhood acute lymphoblastic leukaemia: A report from Children's Cancer Study Group. Br J Haematol 56:215–222
65. Pui CH, Relling MV, Downing JR (2004) Acute lymphoblastic leukemia. N Engl J Med 350:1535–1548
66. Quesnel B, Preudhomme C, Fenaux P (1996) p16ink4a gene and hematological malignancies. Leuk Lymphoma 22:11–24
67. Raimondi SC, Zhou Y, Mathew S, Shurtleff SA, Sandlund JT, Rivera GK, Behm FG, Pui CH (2003) Reassessment of the prognostic significance of hypodiploidy in pediatric patients with acute lymphoblastic leukemia. Cancer 98:2715–2722
68. Ross ME, Zhou X, Song G, Shurtleff SA, Girtman K, Williams WK, Liu HC, Mahfouz R, Raimondi SC, Lenny N, et al. (2003) Classification of pediatric acute lymphoblastic leukemia by gene expression profiling. Blood 102:2951–2959
69. Rubnitz JE, Behm FG, Downing JR (1996) 11q23 rearrangements in acute leukemia. Leukemia 10:74–82
70. Salvati PD, Watt PM, Thomas WR, Kees UR (1999) Molecular characterization of a complex chromosomal translocation breakpoint t(10;14) including the HOX11 oncogene locus. Leukemia 13:975–979
71. Schumacher HR (1998) Acute leukemia: Difficult, controversial, and automated analyzers. Williams & Wilkins, Baltimore
72. Shimamoto Y, Matsuzaki M, Yamaguchi M (1992) Vacuolated Burkitt-like cells in adult T-cell leukaemia/lymphoma. Clin Lab Haematol 14:155–157
73. Slater RM, von Drunen E, Kroes WG, Weghuis DO, van den Berg E, Smit EM, van der Does-van den Berg A, van Wering E, Hahlen K, Carroll AJ, et al. (2001) t(7;12)(q36;p13) and t(7;12)(q32;p13)-translocations involving ETV6 in children 18 months of age or younger with myeloid disorders. Leukemia 15:915–920
74. Takeuchi S, Koike M, Seriu T, Bartram CR, Schrappe M, Reiter A, Park S, Taub HE, Kubonishi I, Miyoshi I, et al. (1998) Frequent loss of heterozygosity on the long arm of chromosome 6: Identification of two distinct regions of deletion in childhood acute lymphoblastic leukemia. Cancer Res 58:2618–2623
75. Thalhammer-Scherrer R, Mitterbauer G, Simonitsch I, Jaeger U, Lechner K, Schneider B, Fonatsch C, Schwarzinger I (2002) The immunophenotype of 325 adult acute leukemias: Relationship to morphologic and molecular classification and proposal for a minimal screening program highly predictive for lineage discrimination. Am J Clin Pathol 117:380–389
76. Uckun FM, Sensel MG, Sather HN, Gaynon PS, Arthur DC, Lange BJ, Steinherz PG, Kraft P, Hutchinson R, Nachman JB, et al. (1998) Clinical significance of translocation t(1;19) in childhood acute lymphoblastic leukemia in the context of contemporary therapies:

A report from the Children's Cancer Group. J Clin Oncol 16: 527–535

77. Wagner VM, Baehner RL (1977) Lack of correlation between blast cell size and length of first remission in acute lymphocytic leukemia in childhood. Med Pediatr Oncol 3:373–377
78. Walters R, Kantarjian HM, Keating MJ, Estey EH, Trujillo J, Cork A, McCredie KB, Freireich EJ (1990) The importance of cytogenetic studies in adult acute lymphocytic leukemia. Am J Med 89: 579–587
79. Weinkauff R, Estey EH, Starostik P, Hayes K, Huh YO, Hirsch-Ginsberg C, Andreeff M, Keating M, Kantarjian HM, Freireich EJ, et al. (1999) Use of peripheral blood blasts vs bone marrow blasts for diagnosis of acute leukemia. Am J Clin Pathol 111: 733–740
80. WHO (2000) In: Jaffe ES, Harris NL, Stein H, Vardiman JW (eds) World Health Organization classification of tumours. Pathology and genetics of tumours of haematopoietic and lymphoid tissues. IARC Press, Lyon, pp 111–187
81. Wibowo A, Pankowsky D, Mikhael A, Wright T, Steele PE, Schumacher H (1996) Adult acute leukemia: Hand mirror cell variant. Hematopathol Mol Hematol 10:85–98
82. Wright S, Chucrallah A, Chong YY, Kantarjian H, Keating M, Albitar M (1996) Acute lymphoblastic leukemia with myeloperoxidase activity. Am J Hematol 51:147–151
83. Wynn TT, Heerema NA, Hammond S, Ranalli M, Kahwash SB (2003) Acute lymphoblastic leukemia with hypereosinophilia: Report of a case with 5q deletion and review of the literature. Pediatr Dev Pathol 6:558–563
84. Xia Y, Brown L, Yang CY, Tsan JT, Siciliano MJ, Espinosa R III, Le Beau MM, Baer RJ (1991) TAL2, a helix-loop-helix gene activated by the (7;9)(q34;q32) translocation in human T-cell leukemia. Proc Natl Acad Sci 88:11416–11420

General Approach to the Therapy of Adult Acute Lymphoblastic Leukemia

S.H. Faderl, H.M. Kantarjian

Contents

9.1 Introduction

Remarkable progress has been made in the treatment and outcome of adult acute lymphoblastic leukemia (ALL) over the past 3 decades. This progress is the result of an accumulation of a mosaic of knowledge and experience, which have led to a more profound understanding of the biology of the disease, and at the same time the development of new drugs and treatment strategies. Advances in the understanding of the biology has highlighted significant differences between childhood and adult ALL (e.g., high frequency of Philadelphia-positive ALL and low incidence of TEL-AML1-positive disease in adults) and thus explains at least partly the divergence of outcomes that is still observed between children and adults. Moreover, ALL is increasingly recognized as a group of heterogeneous disease entities with unique responses to therapy and prognosis. The combination of further cytogenetic-molecular dissection of ALL subtypes with the emergence of new and targeted therapies will thus continue to constitute the fundament upon which further progress will hopefully occur in adult ALL.

9.2 The General Treatment Outline of ALL

Most of the initial therapeutic advances in adult ALL have arisen from successful adaptation of ALL treatment strategies in children. ALL therapy incorporates multiple drugs into regimen-specific sequences of dose and time intensity and is divided into several phases: (i) induction; (ii) a sequence of intensified consolidation; (iii) a prolonged maintenance phase; and (iv) CNS prophylaxis (Fig. 9.1). Intensive combination therapy in ALL following this pattern has resulted in complete remission (CR) rates of 80% to 90% and leukemia-free survival rates of between 30% and 40% [1–4]. Various groups in the USA and around the world are investigating modifications of these treatment blocks in an effort to improve upon the outcome. These strategies not only

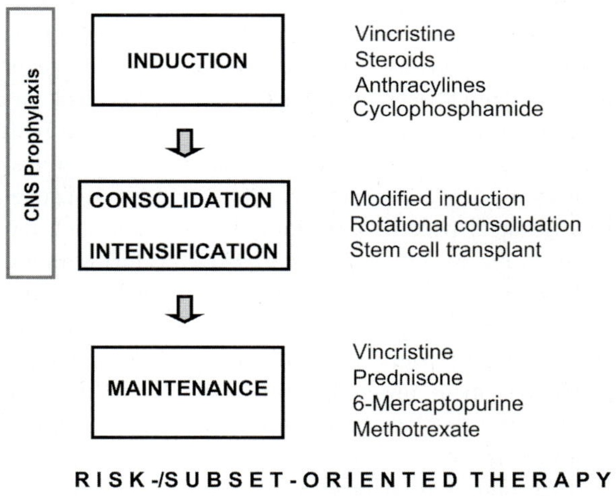

Fig. 9.1. Basic principle of ALL therapy.

include addition of known chemotherapy drugs or further intensification of chemotherapy doses, but also incorporation of new and targeted drugs (e.g., monoclonal antibodies and tyrosine kinase inhibitors), reassessment of the position of stem cell transplant as part of consolidation in first remission, use of molecular monitoring for minimal residual disease, and hence establishment of novel prognostic systems leading to more patient-specific therapy approaches based on risk profile and ALL subset (Table 9.1).

Table 9.1. New strategies in the therapy of adult ALL

Category	Question/approach
Modifications of current therapy	
Induction	Addition of other drugs to induction (cytarabine, L-asparaginase, methotrexate) Intensification of anthracycline doses Dexamethasone instead of prednisone Other induction regimens: high-dose cytarabine, mitoxantrone, liposomal daunorubicin
Consolidation	Role of high-dose anthracyclines Early use of stem cell transplant Optimal timing of consolidation (early or later during maintenance) Subtype-specific consolidation
Maintenance	Duration of therapy Intensified vs. conventional
CNS prophylaxis	Risk-adapted Intrathecal vs. craniospinal XRT
Supportive care	Use of hematopoietic growth factors (G-CSF, GM-CSF, erythropoietin) Antifungal prophylaxis Use of laminar air flow rooms
Role of stem cell transplantation	
	Consolidation in first remission vs. later after relapse Role of reduced-intensity transplants
Incorporation of novel agents	
	Monoclonal antibodies Tyrosine kinase inhibitors
Risk models	
	Molecular monitoring and role of minimal residual disease Risk-adapted and subset-specific treatment strategies
Salvage therapy	

The backbone of induction therapy consists of vincristine, steroids, and anthracyclines to which various other drugs such as L-asparaginase, cyclophosphamide, or cytarabine have been added. Dexamethasone has replaced prednisone for better antileukemia activity and achievement of higher levels in the CSF [5, 6]. Retrospective studies suggested that early dose intensification of daunorubicin would lead to superior leukemia-free survival and cure rates. Italian investigators used three cycles of daunorubicin at 30 mg/m2/day for 3 days for a total of 270 mg/m2 during induction [7]. They reported long-term disease-free survival (DFS) of 55%. Other studies have not confirmed an improvement in DFS, but noted fewer relapses after 2 years [8]. High-dose cytarabine and mitoxantrone or even single-agent high-dose idarubicin without the traditional vincristine-steroid combination as the basic therapy have been investigated, but there is little evidence of their advantage [9, 10]. Overall, it has been difficult to prove higher remission rates with these strategies. However, intensified induction may result in better quality responses and longer survival in subsets of patients. Maximum supportive care is a significant contributor to the success of induction therapy. Use of antibiotics including antifungal prophylaxis, laminar air flow rooms for older patients (≥60 years), and hematopoietic growth factors permit administration of dose-intensive therapy with relatively low induction mortality due to myelosuppression-associated complications. The Cancer and Leukemia Group B (CALGB) randomized untreated ALL patients to receive either G-CSF or placebo during intensive remission induction therapy [11]. Patients who received G-CSF experienced a shorter time to recover the neutrophil count ≥1×109/L (16 days vs. 22 days, $p<0.001$), spent fewer days in hospitals (22 days vs. 28 days, $p=0.02$), and had fewer deaths during induction (5% vs. 11%).

Consolidation strategies include repetition of a modified induction regimen, use of rotational consolidation programs frequently involving high doses of cytarabine, methotrexate, cyclophosphamide, or L-asparaginase, and stem cell transplant. There is evidence that some of these components may contribute to subset-specific improvements in outcome. For example, high-dose methotrexate may be especially effective in low-risk B-lineage ALL and T-ALL, whereas cyclophosphamide and L-asparaginase have led to improved outcome in T-lineage ALL patients [12, 13]. Early use of stem cell transplantation (SCT) remains disputed. Although recommended for patients with poor-prognosis ALL (Philadelphia-chromosome-positive, 11q23 translocations), the benefit of SCT for standard-risk patients in first CR is not established [14]. The Eastern Cooperative Oncology Group (ECOG) together with the Medical Research Council of the United Kingdom (MRC UK) is investigating early matched-related allogeneic SCT for those CR patients <50 years who have a histocompatible donor, whereas all other patients are randomized between autologous SCT and consolidation therapy followed by maintenance for 2.5 years [15]. In the standard-risk group, the 5-year EFS rates were 66% with allogeneic SCT and 45% for the randomized group ($p=0.06$) whereas the rates were 44% and 26% for high-risk patients. These data require further maturation, but may suggest that allogeneic SCT in first CR for patients <50 years may be beneficial not only for high-risk patients.

The backbone of maintenance therapy has remained fairly constant throughout the various ALL regimens and consists of vincristine, prednisone, 6-mercaptopurine, and methotrexate for the duration of 2–3 years. Although maintenance therapy is proven to be beneficial in ALL, there is so far no evidence that intensification of maintenance provides any additional benefit [16, 17]. No maintenance therapy is given to patients with Burkitt leukemia (mature B cell ALL) as these patients respond well to short-term, dose-intensive regimens and relapse after 1 year in remission is rare. Classic maintenance schedules have also not proven valuable in patients with Philadelphia chromosome-positive ALL although for the opposite reason. These patients may benefit from incorporation of tyrosine kinase inhibitors (e.g. imatinib) with or without additional chemotherapy.

Improvements have been achieved in some ALL subsets such as mature B cell ALL and T lineage ALL (including lymphoblastic lymphoma/leukemia) where the prognosis has been traditionally poor. Incorporation of high doses of cytarabine and cyclophosphamide, as well as L-asparaginase in the consolidation of T lineage ALL have increased the cure rates up to 50–60% [18]. Similar cure rates are now achieved in patients with mature B cell ALL when treated with high doses of cytarabine and methotrexate and hyperfractionated cyclophosphamide administered in short-term, dose-intensive regimens [12, 13].

9.3 New Agents

Several novel agents are being investigated in ALL (Table 9.2). The two groups of agents that have the potential to make the biggest impact currently are the tyrosine kinase inhibitors and the monoclonal antibodies (rituximab, alemtuzumab, anti-B4bR). CD20 is expressed in around 35% of ALL patients with higher expression found in Philadelphia chromosome-positive ALL and mature B-cell ALL. In addition, it was found that presence of CD20 on ALL blasts is associated with worse outcome [19]. Thus, including rituximab as part of the induction/consolidation part of therapy may improve the prognosis of ALL patients further [20]. ALL blasts also show high expression of the CD52 antigen. Unlike CD20, CD52 is also expressed on cells of T lineage and use of the anti-CD 52 monoclonal antibody alemtu-

Table 9.2. Investigational agents in ALL

Class of agent	Example
Nucleoside analogs	Clofarabine Nelarabine (Compound 506U)
Purine nucleoside phosphorylase inhibitors	BCX1777
Liposomal compounds	Liposomal vincristine Liposomal daunorubicin
Tyrosine kinase inhibitors	Imatinib, dasatinib, nilotinib Antiangiogenesis agents
Oligonucleotides	BCL-2 antisense
Monoclonal antibodies	Rituximab (anti-CD20) Alemtuzumab (anti-CD52) Anti-B4bR (anti-CD19 + ricin) Gemtuzumab (anti-CD33) Anti-CD7 + ricin
Flavones	Flavopiridol
Proteasome inhibitors	Bortezomib
Others	Pegylated asparaginase, bryostatin, arsenic trioxide

zumab may therefore provide additional benefit to patients with particularly T-cell leukemias or lymphomas. The group at M.D. Anderson has started to incorporate alemtuzumab in the hyper-CVAD induction program for patients with relapsed or refractory T-cell hematopoietic malignancies. The CALGB is testing alemtuzumab in the setting of postremission therapy for those patients whose lymphoblasts were CD52-positive at diagnosis [8]. In another randomized CALGB study, anti-B4bR (anti-CD19 monoclonal antibody conjugated to blocked ricin) during minimal residual disease showed little additional clinical evidence [21].

Imatinib is increasingly explored in Philadelphia chromosome-positive ALL. Thomas et al. pioneered imatinib-chemotherapy combinations in previously untreated patients [22]. Imatinib is added at a dose of 400 mg/day for the first 14 days of each of the eight induction/consolidation courses of the hyper-CVAD regimen which is followed by 1 year of maintenance with imatinib at 600 mg orally daily. Of 15 patients who have been treated with active disease (11 with de novo ALL and four who were primary failures following nonimatinib containing induction therapy), all achieved CR. Ten patients underwent allogeneic stem cell transplantation within a median of 3.5 months. Among 10 patients who did not undergo transplant, five remain in continuous CR for a median of 20 months. The German ALL study group (GMALL) is conducting a randomized phase II study of induction therapy with imatinib versus standard induction chemotherapy in patients >55 years with Philadelphia chromosome-positive ALL [23]. In a preliminary update, all patients treated with imatinib induction achieved CR whereas two patients assigned to chemotherapy induction failed and were crossed over to the imatinib arm. It is hoped that accumulating experience resulting from these and other regimens will establish the role of in kinase situs in Philadelphia chromosome-positive ALL and set a new standard of care for these patients.

A number of other novel agents are investigated in relapsed in refractory disease states and include new nucleoside analogs (clofarabine, nelarabine), liposomal agents (liposomal vincristine), or hypomethylating agents (decitabine).

9.4 Conclusion

ALL is a heterogeneous disease where ALL subsets are characterized by distinct clinical, biological, and thus prognostic features. In addition to developing novel therapies, adapting these therapies according to the risk profile of individual patients has become a main focus in ALL treatment in recent years [24]. Traditional risk factors such as age, white blood cell count, time to response, or cytogenetic abnormalities have shown to influence outcome. More recently, assessment of minimal residual disease has emerged as a tool to gauge individual response following achievement of a complete remission. The GMALL study group is prospectively monitoring minimal residual disease of patients during induction and early consolidation and has started to stratify patients according to residual disease levels at day 71 as low-, high-, or intermediate risk for relapse. The goal of these further refinements is clear: (i) identification of patients who should be transplanted in first CR; (ii) adjustments of intensity during consolidation; and (iii) possible modifications in the intensity and duration of maintenance therapy.

ALL therapy in adults has stepped out of the shadows from its pediatric role model. Even though battling the odds seems more cumbersome in adults, important progress has been made to combine an increasing understanding of the biology of adult ALL with the development of novel therapies and the accumulating experience of the clinical behavior of ALL during therapy. ALL therapy has become a complex endeavor and will be even more so in the future. The following articles in this section will provide a far more in-depth description of this progress and create an outlook at state-of-the art therapy in this intriguing disease.

References

1. Kantarjian HM, O'Brien S, Smith TL, et al. (2000) Results of treatment with hyper-CVAD, a dose-intensive regimen, in adult acute lymphocytic leukemia. J Clin Oncol 18:547–561
2. Larson RA, Dodge RK, Burns CP, et al. (1995) A five-drug remission induction regimen with intensive consolidation for adults with acute lymphoblastic leukemia: Cancer and Leukemia Group B Study 8811. Blood 85:2025–2037
3. Durrant IJ, Richards, SM, Prentice HG, et al. (2000) The Medical Research Council trials in adult acute lymphocytic leukemia. Hem Onc Clin North Am 14:1327–1352

4. Gökbuget N, Hoelzer D. (2002) Recent approaches in acute lymphoblastic leukemia in adults. Rev Clin Exp Hematol 6:114–141
5. Jones B, Freeman AI, Shuster JJ, et al. (1991) Lower incidence of meningeal leukemia when prednisone is replaced by dexamethasone in the treatment of acute lymphocytic leukemia. Med Pediatr Oncol 19:269–275
6. Bostrom BC, Sensel MR, Sather HN, et al. (2003) Dexamethasone versus prednisone and daily oral versus weekly intravenous mercaptopurine for patients with standard-risk acute lymphoblastic leukemia: A report from the Children's Cancer Group. Blood 101:3809–3817
7. Todeschini G, Tecchio C, Meneghini V, et al. (1998) Estimated 6-year event-free survival of 55% in 60 consecutive adult acute lymphoblastic leukemia patients treated with an intensive phase II protocol on high induction dose of daunorubicin. Leukemia 12:144–148
8. Larson RA.(2004) The US trials in adult acute lymphoblastic leukemia. Ann Hematol 83(Suppl 1):S127–128
9. Weiss M, Maslak P, Feldman E, et al. (1996) Cytarabine with high dose mitoxantrone induces rapid complete remissions in adult acute lymphoblastic leukemia (ALL) without the use of vincristine or prednisone. J Clin Oncol 14:2480–2485
10. Weiss M (2001) Induction therapyof adult acute lymphocytic leukemia without the use of vincristine or prednisone. Hem Onc Clin North Am 15:1–7
11. Larson RA, Dodge RK, Linker CA, et al. (1998) A randomized controlled trial of filgrastim during remission induction and consolidation chemotherapy for adults with acute lymphoblastic leukemia: CALGB study 9111. Blood 92:1556–1564
12. Hoelzer D. (1996) Acute lymphoblastic leukemia: Improved outcome in adult B-cell acute lymphoblastic leukemia. Blood 87:495–508
13. Thomas D, Cortes J, O'Brien S, et al. (1999) Hyper-CVAD program in Burkitt's-type adult acute lymphoblastic leukemia. J Clin Oncol 17:2461–2470
14. Thiebault A, Vernant JP, Degos L, et al. (2000) Adult acute lymphocytic leukemia study testing chemotherapy and autologous and allogeneic transplantation. A follow-up report of the French protocol LALA 87. Hem Onc Clin North Am 14:1353–1366
15. Rowe JM, Richards S, Burnett AK, et al. (2001) Favorable results of allogeneic bone marrow transplantation (BMT) for adults with Philadelphia (Ph)-chromosome-negative acute lymphoblastic leukemia (ALL) in first complete remission (CR): Results from the International ALL Trial (MRC UKALL XII/ECOG E2993). Blood 98:481a
16. Childhood ALL Cooperative Group. (1996) Duration and intensity of maintenance chemotherapy in acute lymphoblastic leukaemia: Overview of 42 trials involving 12 000 randomized children. Lancet 347:1783–1788
17. Mandelli F, Annino L, Rotoli B (1996) The GIMEMA ALL 0183 trial: Analysis of 10-year follow-up. Br J Haematol 92:665–672
18. Thomas DA, Kantarjian HM (2001) Lymphoblastic lymphoma. Hem Onc Clin North Am 15:51–95
19. Thomas DA, Cortes J, O'Brien SM, et al. (2000) Significance of CD20 positivity in de novo acute lymphocytic leukemia (ALL). Blood 96:109a
20. Thomas DA, Cortes J, Giles FJ, et al. (2001) The modified hyper-CVAD regimen in newly diagnosed adult acute lymphoblastic leukemia (ALL). Blood 98:590a
21. Szatrowski TP, Dodge RK, Reynolds C, et al. (2003) Lineage specific treatment of adult patients with acute lymphoblastic leukemia in first remission with anti-B4-blocked ricin or high-dose cytarabine: Cancer and Leukemia Group B study 9311. Cancer 97:1471–1480
22. Thomas DA, Faderl S, Cortes J, et al. (2003) Treatment of Philadelphia chromosome-positive acute lymphocytic leukemia with hyper-CVAD and imatinib mesylate. Blood [epub ahead of print]
23. Wassmann B, Gökbuget N, Scheuring UJ, et al. (2003) A randomized multicenter open label phase II study to determine the safety and efficacy of induction therapy with imatinib (Glivec, formerly STI571) in comparison with standard induction chemotherapy in elderly (>55 years) patients with Philadelphia chromosome-positive (Ph+/BCR-ABL+) acute lymphoblastic leukemia (ALL). Ann Hematol 82:716–720
24. Gökbuget N, Raff R, Brügge-Mann M, et al. (2004) Risk/MRD adapted GMALL trials in adult ALL. Ann Hematol 83(Suppl 1): S129–131

Recent Clinical Trials in Acute Lymphoblastic Leukemia by the Cancer and Leukemia Group B

Richard A. Larson, Daohai Yu, Ben L. Sanford, Wendy Stock

Contents

10.1 Introduction

The Cancer and Leukemia Group B (CALGB) has performed a series of studies evaluating different aspects of induction and postremission treatment in adults with acute lymphoblastic leukemia (ALL). In recent years, these clinical trials have been supplemented by systematic morphologic, immunophenotyping, cytogenetic and molecular genetic studies, leading to the identification of different risk groups of patients who may warrant individualized treatments. Importantly, these protocols have enrolled all adult patients older than 15 years with ALL without an upper age restriction and did not exclude Philadelphia (Ph) chromosome positive patients.

Between 1988 and 2001, the CALGB enrolled and treated 759 adults with untreated acute lymphoblastic leukemia (ALL) on one of five clinical trials using intensive multiagent therapy. The median age was 36 years (range 16 to 83 years); ≤17% were 60 years old. Of 276 centrally reviewed and evaluable cases, 28% were Ph chromosome positive; 5% had a t(4;11). Overall, complete remission (CR) was achieved in 81% of the patients [611/759, 95% confidence interval (CI), 78–83%]. The median disease-free survival (DFS) measured from time of CR was 2.0 years (95% CI, 1.6–2.3 years), and the median overall survival was 2.0 years (95% CI, 1.7–2.3 years). At 3 years, 40% (95% CI, 36–44%) remained in continuous CR, and 41% (95% CI, 37–44%) were still alive. Age was a strong determinant of patient outcomes as shown in Figs 10.1 and 10.2.

10.2 CALGB Study 8811

Intensive multiagent chemotherapy programs produce CRs in the majority of adults with ALL. CALGB study 8811 built upon observations by the CALGB and others that a more intensive remission induction program might produce more durable responses [1]. A single dose of cyclophosphamide (1200 mg/m^2) was added to a modification of the four-drug regimen (daunorubicin, vincristine, prednisone, L-asparaginase) used in earlier CALGB studies (7612 and 8011) [2, 3]. The treatment schema is shown in Table 10.1. In addition, a more intensive program of L-asparaginase administration was used during induction and the first 2 months of postremission consolidation because of reports suggesting the importance of intensive asparaginase therapy in chil-

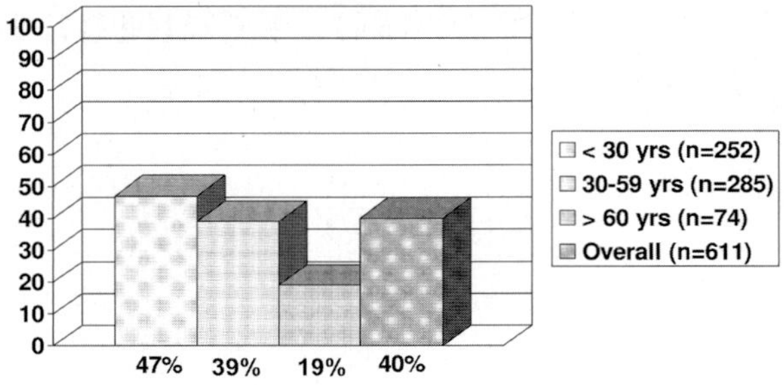

Fig. 10.1. Disease-free survival at 3 years for 611 adults who achieved a complete remission from ALL after treatment in five CALGB trials between 1988 and 2001.

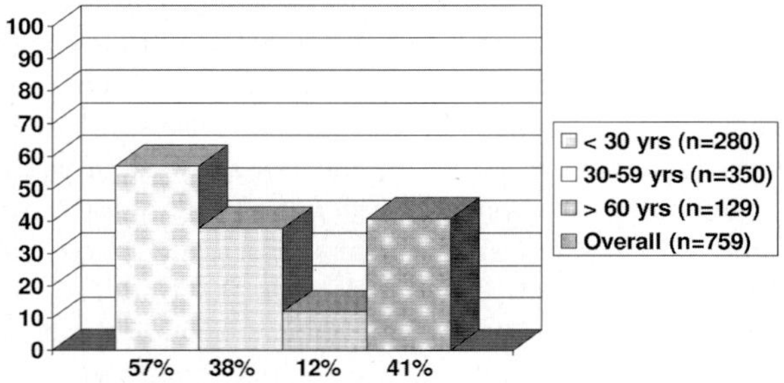

Fig. 10.2. Overall survival at 3 years for 759 adults with newly diagnosed ALL enrolled in five CALGB trials between 1988 and 2001.

dren with high-risk ALL. Other aspects of postremission therapy were patterned after that used by the adult German multicenter ALL (GMALL) study group and included a total of 2 years of scheduled chemotherapy [4].

In this trial, 85% of the 197 evaluable patients (median age, 32 years; range 16 to 80 years) achieved a CR, including 94% of patients less than 30 years old, 85% of patients aged 30–59, and 39% of patients ≥60 years old. The median duration of CR was 2.4 years (95% CI, 2.0–5.3 years) and was also age-related. Improved results were noted in patients with T-cell ALL (estimated 3-year survival, 69%) compared to B-lineage ALL (estimated 3-year survival, 38%). The most recent data indicate that 43% of patients survived >5 years (95% CI, 36–50%) and 42% (95% CI, 35–50%) were in continuous CR (CCR) for >5 years.

In contrast to earlier CALGB studies, there was no adverse impact on outcome associated with the coexpression of myeloid antigens [5]. Although the CR rate was very high, remission induction treatment was complicated by prolonged granulocytopenia requiring an average of 26 days of hospitalization. In particular, the mortality in patients >60 years of age was unacceptably high, and dose reductions of the cyclophosphamide and the daunorubicin were implemented for these patients. Similarly, the first course of consolidation therapy was also quite myelosuppressive, requiring an average of 14 days of hospitalization during this 2-month treatment.

10.3 CALGB Study 9111

The major cause of treatment-related morbidity and mortality for patients with ALL is infection due in part to bone marrow suppression by cytotoxic therapy. Therefore, the CALGB designed a double-blind, placebo-controlled clinical trial (9111) to test the effectiveness of filgrastim (granulocyte colony stimulating factor, G-CSF) in reducing the complications of treatment by potentially shortening the time to neutrophil recovery following courses of remission induction chemotherapy and postremission consolidation treatment [6].

We randomly assigned 198 adults with untreated ALL (median age, 35 years; range 16 to 79 years) to receive either placebo or G-CSF (5 μg/kg/day) subcutaneously, beginning 4 days after starting the intensive remission induction chemotherapy and continuing until the neutrophil count was ≥1000/μl for 2 days. The study assignment was unblinded when individual patients achieved a CR. Patients initially assigned to G-CSF then continued to receive G-CSF through 2 monthly courses of consolidation therapy. Patients assigned to placebo received no further study drug.

The median time to recover neutrophils ≥1000/μl during the remission induction course was 16 days (interquartile range (IQR), 15 to 18 days) for the patients assigned to receive G-CSF and 22 days (IQR, 19–29 days) for the patients assigned to placebo ($p<0.001$). Patients in the G-CSF group had significantly shorter durations of neutropenia (<1000/μl) and of thrombocytopenia (<50 000/μl) and fewer days in hospital (median, 22 days vs. 28 days, $p=0.02$) compared to patients receiving placebo. The patients assigned to receive G-CSF had a higher CR rate (87% vs. 77%) and fewer deaths during remission induction (5% vs. 11%) than did those receiving placebo. During Courses IIA and IIB of consolidation treatment, patients in the G-CSF group had significantly more rapid recovery of neutrophils ≥1000/μl than did the control group by approximately 6–9 days.

Table 10.1. CALGB chemotherapy regimen for acute lymphoblastic leukemia in adults [1, 6]

Course I: Induction (4 weeks)			
Cyclophosphamide*	IV	1200 mg/m2	Day 1
Daunorubicin*	IV	45 mg/m2	Days 1, 2, 3
Vincristine	IV	2 mg	Days 1, 8, 15, 22
Prednisone*	PO/IV	60 mg/m2/d	Days 1–21
L-Asparaginase (E. Coli)	SC/IM	6000 IU/m2	Days 5, 8, 11, 15, 18, 22
*For patients >60 years old:			
Cyclophosphamide		800 mg/m2	Day 1
Daunorubicin		30 mg/m2	Days 1, 2, 3
Prednisone		60 mg/m2/d	Days 1–7
In CALGB study 9111, patients received G-CSF 5 µg/kg subcutaneously once daily, starting on day 4 and continuing until the absolute neutrophil count was >1000/µl on two consecutive determinations >24 h apart (see text).			
Course IIA: Early intensification (4 weeks; repeat once for Course IIB)			
Intrathecal methotrexate		15 mg	Day 1
Cyclophosphamide	IV	1000 mg/m2	Day 1
6-Mercaptopurine	PO	60 mg/m2/d	Days 1–14
Cytarabine	SC	75 mg/m2/d	Days 1–4, 8–11
Vincristine	IV	2 mg	Days 15, 22
L-Asparaginase (E. Coli)	SC/IM	6000 IU/m2	Days 15, 18, 22, 25
Course III: CNS prophylaxis and interim maintenance (12 weeks)			
Cranial irradiation		2400 cGy	Days 1–12
Intrathecal methotrexate		15 mg	Days 1, 8, 15, 22, 29
6-Mercaptopurine	PO	60 mg/m2/d	Days 1–70
Methotrexate	PO	20 mg/m2	Days 36, 43, 50, 57, 64
Course IV: Late intensification (8 weeks)			
Doxorubicin	IV	30 mg/m2	Days 1, 8, 15
Vincristine	IV	2 mg	Days 1, 8, 15
Dexamethasone	PO	10 mg/m2/d	Days 1–14
Cyclophosphamide	IV	1000 mg/m2	Day 29
6-Thioguanine	PO	60 mg/m2/d	Days 29–42
Cytarabine	SC	75 mg/m2/d	Days 29–32, 36–39
Course V: Prolonged maintenance (until 24 months from diagnosis)			
Vincristine	IV	2 mg	Day 1 of every 4 weeks
Prednisone	PO	60 mg/m2/d	Days 1–5 of every 4 weeks
6-Mercaptopurine	PO	60 mg/m2/d	Days 1–28
Methotrexate	PO	20 mg/m2	Days 1, 8, 15, 22

However, the patients in the G-CSF group did not complete the planned first 3 months of chemotherapy any more rapidly than did the patients in the placebo group. Overall toxicity was not lessened by the use of G-CSF.

After a median follow-up of 4.7 years, the DFS for the patients assigned to G-CSF (median, 2.3 years) was greater compared to those assigned to placebo (median, 1.7 years), although this did not reach statistical significance. The same is true for OS in the two groups (medians, 2.4 years with G-CSF and 1.8 years with placebo). Older age (>60 years) was associated with a lower CR rate, slower neutrophil and platelet recovery, and longer hospitalization during induction, all of which were improved by G-CSF therapy. There was no adverse effect of G-CSF on the outcome of patients with myeloid antigen positive or Ph+ ALL. It was concluded that the addition of G-CSF to the CALGB induction treatment reduced the duration of hematologic toxicity and improved some measures of clinical outcomes, particularly in older patients. G-CSF was therefore added as part of the induction regimen in subsequent trials.

10.4 CALGB Study 9311

Half of all older adults with B-lineage ALL have Ph+ disease, and most of these are not able to undergo allogeneic stem cell transplantation (SCT). In addition, there is considerable room for improving the outcome for the remaining patients with B-lineage ALL. Clinical experience using the immunotoxin, anti-B4 blocked ricin (anti-B4-bR), had demonstrated reduction in tumor size in patients with B-cell lymphoproliferative disorders [7]. There was also evidence that this immunotoxin might be useful in bone marrow purging for patients with follicular lymphomas undergoing autologous bone marrow transplant. Anti-B4-bR (ImmunoGen, Inc., Cambridge, MA) is comprised of an anti-CD19 monoclonal antibody conjugated to blocked ricin, which has cytotoxic activity in lymphoid malignancies and is capable of killing malignant cells resistant to chemotherapy.

The Leukemia Committee of the CALGB therefore explored the use of anti-B4 blocked ricin in B-lineage ALL during a minimal disease state. In CALGB study 9311, two 7-day courses of the immunotoxin were given 1 week apart after completion of the first 2 months of intensive therapy given as in the 9111 protocol and prior to the central nervous system (CNS) prophylaxis phase [8]. Serial polymerase chain reaction (PCR) assays of *BCR-ABL*, immunoglobulin heavy chain (*IGH*), and T-cell receptor (*TCR*) genes were used to measure the impact of lineage-specific intensification treatment on minimal residual disease.

Eighty-two adults were enrolled; 78 were eligible. The median age was 34 years (range 17 to 81). Sixty-six patients (85%) achieved a complete remission. Forty-six patients received the anti-B4-blocked-ricin, which was generally well tolerated; 80% were able to receive both courses. The most common toxicity was asymptomatic transient elevation of liver function tests in 72%. Lymphopenia occurred in 46%. Two patients developed antibodies to the anti-B4-blocked-ricin. Molecular monitoring before and after the experimental course of intensification did not show a consistent change in the number of leukemia cells remaining, and the immediate posttreatment PCR studies did not correlate with remission duration. Although, intensification therapy with anti-B4-blocked-ricin is feasible for patients with CD19-positive ALL, there was little evidence for additional clinical benefit from the anti-B4-blocked ricin.

Six patients enrolled on study 9311 had T-cell ALL and lacked the CD19 antigen. In place of the anti-B4-bR course, these patients received one course of high-dose cytarabine (2 gm/m^2 every 12 h for 6 days) for postremission consolidation. The toxicity of this course was acceptable. Four (67%) of these patients have remained in CCR for longer than 3 years.

10.5 CALGB Study 9511

Two components of these more recent CALGB ALL trials differed from previous group trials: the more extensive use of asparaginase and the use of cyclophosphamide [9]. The addition of these agents appears to have led to improved CR rates and better DFS. CALGB 9511 was a phase II study of pegylated (PEG)-asparaginase as a replacement for E. coli asparaginase in previously untreated adult patients with ALL. The protocol otherwise used the same chemotherapy treatment schedule as delivered in CALGB studies 8811, 9111, and 9311.

ALL cells lack asparagine synthetase and are thus dependent on exogenous asparagine for survival. Rapid depletion of asparagine results in selective killing of ALL cells since normal cells are able to synthesize asparagine. Because asparaginase is not markedly myelosuppressive, it is easily added to combination chemotherapy regimens.

Three preparations of asparaginase are available. One preparation is derived from *Escherichia coli* (*E. coli*) and is commercially available for use in the USA. A second preparation is derived from Erwinia carotovora and is commercially available in Europe; it can be ordered in the USA only for patients with allergy to E. coli asparaginase. PEG-asparaginase is derived from E. coli L-asparaginase by covalently conjugating units of polyethylene glycol (PEG) to the protein. Differences between PEG-asparaginase and the other two forms of the drug include decreased immunogenicity and a longer half-life. The half-life of E. coli asparaginase is 1.2 days, Erwinia asparaginase 0.7 days, and PEG-asparaginase 5.7 days [10]. Currently, PEG-asparaginase is indicated for use in adult patients with hypersensitivity to native E. coli asparaginase at a dose of 2000 U/m^2 every 14 days.

The optimal dosing schedule of PEG-asparaginase in adults remains to be determined. Studies in children have shown that a dose of 2000 U/m^2 delivered every 2 weeks produced asparagine depletion for 14 days in more than 70% of patients despite inclusion of some patients with neutralizing antibodies [11]. We therefore chose initially to test a dose of 2000 U/m^2 (maximum, 3750 U) administered SC or IM once during each of the first three courses of therapy in newly diagnosed patients [12]. PEG-asparaginase was given on day 5 during Course I and day 15 during Courses IIA and IIB (Table 9.1). Pharmacokinetic studies of asparaginase levels were also done. Asparaginase levels provided a surrogate measure of asparagine depletion since levels >0.03 U/ml produce complete asparagine depletion. The frequency of antiasparaginase neutralizing antibodies was also measured using an enzyme-linked immunoassay (ELISA) method.

Pharmacokinetic sampling of the first 21 patients studied in this trial showed that asparaginase levels were >0.03 U/ml in all 21 patients at 7 days and in 16 of 20 patients (80%) at 14 days but in only 5 of 20 (25%) at 24 days after the initial dose of PEG-asparaginase [12, 13]. When the second dose was given on day 15 of the second chemotherapy course, 16 of 18 evaluable patients (83%) had complete asparagine depletion 7 days later, and 12 of the 18 (67%) had depletion at 14 days. A third dose was given on day 15 of the third chemotherapy course, and 14 of 16 patients (85%) had depletion at 7 days and 13 of 16 (79%) at 14 days following this final dose. Therefore, through all three doses, 67–80% of patients maintained sufficient asparaginase levels to deplete asparagine for 2 weeks. Antibodies to PEG-asparaginase developed in three patients but none before the end of the third course. No grade 3 or 4 allergic reactions or pancreatitis were observed. Hyperglycemia was reported in 38% of patients. Four patients (15%) had grade 3 phlebitis or thrombosis, and one patient had a deep vein thrombosis of the leg with embolization to the lung.

Preliminary retrospective analyses in pediatric ALL populations have suggested that the longer periods of asparagine depletion that result from the use of E. coli asparaginase are associated with better outcomes than the shorter periods of depletion that result from the use of Erwinia asparaginase. Therefore, a second cohort of patients was treated on the 9511 trial, and a second dose of PEG-asparaginase was added on day 22 of the induction course to extend the duration of asparagine depletion [13]. Pharmacokinetic analyses of this cohort of patients showed asparagine depletion in 18 of 20 patients (90%) at 14 days and 10 of 14 (71%) at 31 days. Further analyses are pending.

10.6 CALGB Study 9251

Patients with mature B-cell ALL (Burkitt-type, ALL-L3, surface immunoglobulin positive, t(8q24)) fare poorly with conventional ALL chemotherapy approaches. Early CALGB data for patients with the t(8;14) showed that none of those patients were long-term disease-free survivors. Of the eight patients with the L3 subtype enrolled on CALGB 8811, two failed to achieve CR and five relapsed after a median remission duration of only 3 months; all five developed CNS involvement.

CALGB study 9251 was derived from a series of reports, both in children and adults, which highlight a different approach to the treatment of these diseases. Repeated short courses of cyclophosphamide and high-dose methotrexate led to CR rates of 85–95% and impressive long-term DFS in a large number of patients with Burkitt-type leukemia or lymphoma. All regimens contained aggressive CNS prophylaxis and some included an initial cytoreduction using modest doses of cyclophosphamide and corticosteroids. In CALGB 9251, therapy was given over an 18-week period of time [14, 15]. We used a regimen similar to that used successfully by the German ALL study group for patients with L3 ALL [16]. The major differences between the 9251 regimen and Hoelzer's are the use of etoposide instead of teniposide and the use of cytarabine as a continuous infusion for 48 h rather than as subcutaneous injections.

We enrolled 92 adults with Burkitt leukemia or lymphoma and studied two cohorts to evaluate the efficacy of intensive chemotherapy with and without cranial radiation for CNS prophylaxis. Prophylactic cranial radiation (2400 cGy) and 12 doses of triple intrathecal chemotherapy were given to the first cohort of patients [14]. A subsequent group underwent the same chemotherapy, except intrathecal therapy was reduced to six doses and radiotherapy was given only to those at high risk [15].

The median follow-up is 6.8 years in cohort 1 and 4.1 years in cohort 2. Toxicity was significant with all patients having severe myelosuppression and most patients having grade 3 or 4 mucositis. Three occurrences of transverse myelitis, two severe neuropathies, three cases with aphasia, and one of blindness were documented in the first cohort of 52 patients. In the subsequent cohort of 40 patients, there were none of these occurrences and patients experienced less neurologic toxicity overall (61% vs. 26%, $p=0.001$). Responses were similar (74% CR overall), and the 3-year event-free survival (EFS) from diagnosis was 52% (95% confidence interval, 38–65%) for the first cohort and 45% (29–60%) for the second. The DFS rates were 66% and 67%, respectively. We concluded that intensive, short-duration chemotherapy with less intensive CNS prophylaxis controlled this sanctuary site with little neurotoxicity and may be curative for adults with Burkitt leukemia or lymphoma.

10.7 CALGB Study 19802

Aggressive combination chemotherapy for adults with ALL has resulted in CR rates of 70–90%, but overall survival (OS) remains at 30–40%. We hypothesized that early dose intensification of daunorubicin (Dnr) and cytarabine (Ara-C) may improve DFS and that aggressive high dose intravenous (IV), oral, and intrathecal (IT) methotrexate (MTX) could replace cranial radiotherapy (RT) for CNS prophylaxis. The CALGB undertook a phase II study (19802) to examine these issues [17, 18]. Treatment consisted of 6 monthly courses of intensive therapy followed by 18 months of maintenance therapy. Five drugs (cyclophosphamide [Cy], Dnr, prednisone, vincristine, l-asparaginase) were given with G-CSF support for remission induction as in study 9111. In patients <60 years old, the Dnr dose in the induction module A was increased in cohorts from 45 mg/m^2/day on days 1, 2, and 3 (used in prior CALGB ALL studies) to 60 and then to 80 mg/m^2 daily for 3 days. In patients ≥ 60 yrs old, Cy was omitted from module A, and Dnr was increased from 30 to 60 mg/m^2/day for 3 days. Cy plus high-dose Ara-C, and CNS prophylaxis with IV, oral, and IT MTX were introduced in later treatment modules for all patients. No cranial RT was given.

Between 1999 and 2001, 163 adults with untreated ALL (FAB L1 and L2) were enrolled on study. The median age was 41 years (range 16 to 82); 61% were male. The median white blood cell (WBC) count at presentation was 10 050/μl (range 500 to 348 500). A large proportion, 43% (42/97) of centrally reviewed and evaluable cases, had poor risk cytogenetics as defined in prior CALGB studies [19]. Seventy-eight percent (127/163) of patients (95% CI, 71–84%) achieved a CR, comparable to CR rates (81–85%) achieved in three prior CALGB studies with lower doses of Dnr. By age, the CR rates were 91% (43/47) for patients <30 years, 78% (65/83) for patients 30–59 years, and 58% (19/33) for patients ≥ 60 years. There were 11% induction deaths and 11% induction failures due to refractory ALL. Thirty-nine patients <60 years received Dnr at 60 mg/m^2; two of these patients (5%) died during induction and two (5%) had refractory disease. These results were similar when compared to eight (9%) induction deaths and 11 (12%) with refractory disease among the 91 patients who received Dnr at 80 mg/m^2. Thirteen high-risk patients had an allogeneic SCT in first CR and 12 more underwent transplantation after relapse.

With a median follow-up of 2.4 years for survivors, 63/163 (39%) are alive and 44/127 (35%) are in continuous CR. Relapses have occurred in 66 (52%) patients; of these, eight (5%) had isolated CNS relapses. The median DFS is 1.5 years (95% CI, 1.0–1.9) and the median OS is 1.6 years (95% CI, 1.2–2.4). Age >60 years impacted adversely on DFS. Of interest, neither poor-risk cytogenetics nor presenting WBC $>30\,000$/μl significantly affected DFS. Both older age and adverse cytogenetics were associated with shorter OS.

In conclusion, intensification of Dnr during treatment of adult ALL is feasible, and the postremission therapy piloted in CALGB 19802 was generally well tolerated and could be given in the outpatient setting. To date, intensified Dnr has not resulted in an improvement in DFS as reported by others. However, very few relapses after 2 years have been noted. CNS prophylaxis without cranial RT has been well tolerated and has not resulted in an increase in CNS relapses. Longer follow-up is needed to determine the potential benefit of intensified Dnr on late relapses. Nevertheless, further Dnr dose escalation seems unlikely to result in significant improvements in outcome. Novel agents that eradicate minimal residual disease should be introduced into clinical trials of adult ALL.

10.8 CALGB Study 19801: T-cell ALL in Relapse

There have been almost no new drugs introduced into the treatment of ALL in recent years. Nelarabine (Compound 506U78; GlaxoSmithKline) is a pro-drug of 9-D-arabinofuranosylguanine (ara-G), a deoxyguanosine analog. Previous studies have demonstrated that immature T-lymphocytes are extremely sensitive to the cytotoxic effects of deoxyguanosine [20]. The toxicity of deoxyguanosine to T-cells is related to the accumulation of deoxyguanosine triphosphate (dGTP) with subsequent inhibition of ribonucleotide reductase, inhibition of DNA synthesis, and resultant cell death. Recent information indicates that the rate of ara-GTP catabolism is similar in T-cells and B-cells, but that initial ara-G concentrations are higher in T-cells than B-cells for a given dose. Thus, T-cells have a greater intracellular exposure to ara-GTP than do B-cells.

Prior phase I studies determined a maximum tolerated dose of 40 mg/kg/day for 5 days in adult patients. The dose limiting toxicity was neurologic, consisting of seizures, obtundation and ascending paralysis. As predicted by preclinical in vitro studies, the highest response rates were observed in patients with relapsed T-cell ALL and lymphoblastic lymphoma (LBL). In order to decrease the risk of neurologic toxicities, we tested a dosing regimen of 1.5 g/m^2 given IV once per day on an alternate day schedule (days 1, 3, 5) in an intergroup study carried out by the CALGB and the Southwest Oncology Group (SWOG).

Between 1998 and 2001, a total of 40 patients were enrolled, 22 with T-ALL and 18 with LBL [21]. Patients with greater than 25% lymphoblasts within the bone marrow were considered to have ALL. The lymphoblasts had to express at least two T-cell antigens. All patients were refractory to at least one induction regimen or were in first or greater relapse after achieving a CR. Patients could not have evidence of CNS disease and had to have a calculated creatinine clearance of greater than 50 ml/min. A maximum of two induction courses was administered. Each cycle was repeated every 21 days. Those patients achieving a CR were allowed to receive an additional two courses as consolidation therapy. The median age was 34 years (range 16 to 66). There were 33 males and seven females. Of the 21 evaluable patients with ALL, there were six CRs and two partial remissions (PR) for a total response rate of 38% (95% CI, 18–62%). For the 17 evaluable patients with LBL, there were four CRs and no PRs for a total response rate of 24% (95% CI, 7–50%). The overall response rate (CR+PR) for the 38 evaluable patients was 32% (95% CI, 18–49%). One patient had a seizure and subsequent confusion, which resolved. One patient developed hallucinations but was also receiving narcotics. He was retreated without the recurrence of additional neurologic symptoms. The principal toxicity was marrow suppression. Grade 3 or 4 neutropenia and thrombocytopenia occurred in 43% and 33% of patients, respectively.

The median OS for the 40 patients was 4.6 months (95% CI, 3–10 months). The median DFS for the 10 patients achieving CR was 9.8 months (95% CI, 3–15 months). The 1-year OS is 32% (95% CI, 16–47%) and the 1-year DFS is 40% (95% CI, 10–70%). These results suggest that nelarabine is well tolerated, and has significant antitumor activity in patients with relapsed or refractory T-cell lymphoblastic leukemia/lymphoma. Studies using nelarabine in patients with newly diagnosed T-cell malignancies are warranted.

Acknowledgments

We thank the many physicians, nurses, and data managers at each of the CALGB institutions and their affiliated hospitals for their assistance with the conduct of these clinical trials. Drs. Ted P. Szatrowski, Stanley R. Frankel, Edward J. Lee, David A. Rizzieri, Daniel J. DeAngelo, and Wendy Stock have chaired the clinical studies described above. Dr. Clara D. Bloomfield chaired the central cytogenetic review study. This research was supported in part by grants from the National Cancer Institute to the Cancer and Leukemia Group B (CA31946 and CA41287), to the CALGB Statistical Center (CA33601), and to CALGB member institutions.

References

1. Larson RA, Dodge RK, Burns CP, Lee EJ, Stone RM, Schulman P, Duggan D, Davey FR, Sobol RE, Frankel SR, et al. (1995) A five-drug remission induction regimen with intensive consolidation for adults with acute lymphoblastic leukemia: Cancer and Leukemia Group B study 8811. Blood 85:2025–2037
2. Gottlieb AJ, Weinberg V, Ellison RR, Henderson ES, Terebelo H, Rafla S, Cuttner J, Silver RT, Carey RW, Levy RN, et al. (1984) Efficacy of daunorubicin in the therapy of adult acute lymphocytic leukemia: A prospective randomized trial by Cancer and Leukemia Group B. Blood 64:267–274
3. Ellison RR, Mick R, Cuttner J, Schiffer CA, Silver RT, Henderson ES, Woliver T, Royston I, Davey FR, Glicksman AS, et al. (1991) The effects of postinduction intensification treatment with cytarabine and daunorubicin in acute lymphocytic leukemia: A prospective randomized clinical trial by Cancer and Leukemia Group B. J Clin Oncol 9:2002–2015
4. Hoelzer D, Thiel E, Löffler H, Büchner T, Ganser A, Heil G. Koch P, Freund M, Diedrich H, Rühl H, et al. (1988) Prognostic factors in a multicenter study for treatment of acute lymphoblastic leukemia in adults. Blood 71:123–131
5. Sobol RE, Mick R, Royston I, Davey FR, Ellison RR, Newman R, Cuttner J, Griffin JD, Collins H, Nelson DA, et al. (1987) Clinical importance of myeloid antigen expression in adult acute lymphoblastic leukemia. N Engl J Med 316:1111–1117
6. Larson RA, Dodge RK, Linker CA, Stone RM, Powell BL, Lee EJ, Schulman P, Davey FR, Frankel SR, Bloomfield CD, et al. (1998) A randomized controlled trial of filgrastim during remission induction and consolidation chemotherapy for adults with acute lymphoblastic leukemia: CALGB study 9111. Blood 92:1556–1564
7. Grossbard ML, Freedman AS, Ritz J, Coral F, Goldmacher VS, Eliseo L, Spector N, Dear K, Lambert JM, Blättler WA, T, et al. (1992) Serotherapy of B-cell neoplasms with anti-B4-blocked ricin: A phase I trial of daily bolus infusion. Blood 79:576–585
8. Szatrowski TP, Dodge RK, Reynolds C, Westbrook CA, Frankel SR, Sklar J, Stewart C, Hurd D, Kolitz JE, Velez-Garcia E, et al. (2003) Lineage specific treatment of adult patients with acute lymphoblastic leukemia in first remission with anti-B4-blocked ricin or high-dose cytarabine: Cancer and Leukemia Group B study 9311. Cancer 97:1471–1480
9. Larson RA, Fretzin MH, Dodge RK, Schiffer CA (1998) Hypersensitivity reactions to L-asparaginase do not impact on the remission duration of adults with acute lymphoblastic leukemia. Leukemia 12:660–665
10. Asselin BL, Whitin JC, Coppola DJ, Rupp IP, Sallan SE, Cohen HJ (1993) Comparative pharmacokinetic studies of three asparaginase preparations. J Clin Onc 11:1780–1786
11. Kurtzberg J, Asselin B, Pollack B, Bernstein M, Buchanan G (1993) The Pediatric Oncology Group: PEG-L-Asparaginase (PEGasp) vs native E coli asparaginase (asp) for reinduction of relapsed acute lymphoblastic leukemia (ALL): POG #8866 Phase II trial. Proc Am Soc Clin Oncol 12:325
12. Frankel SR, Kurtzberg J, DeOleivera D, Dodge R, Peterson B, Powell BL, Larson RA, Schiffer CA (1996) Toxicity and pharmacokinetics of peg-asparaginase (peg-asp) in newly diagnosed adult acute lymphoblastic leukemia (ALL): CALGB 9511. Blood 88(Suppl 1):669a
13. Frankel SR, Kurtzberg J, DeOliveria D, Dodge R, Peterson B, Powell BL, Kolitz J, Larson RA, Schiffer CA (1997) Toxicity and pharmacokinetics of PEG-asparaginase (PEG-asn) in newly diagnosed adult acute lymphoblastic leukemia (ALL): CALGB 9511. Blood 90(Suppl 1):334a
14. Lee EJ, Petroni GR, Schiffer CA, Freter CE, Johnson JL, Barcos M, Frizzera G, Bloomfield CD, Peterson BA (2001) Brief-duration high-intensity chemotherapy for patients with small noncleaved-cell lymphoma or FAB L3 acute lymphocytic leukemia: Results of Cancer and Leukemia Group B study 9251. J Clin Oncol 19(20):4014–4022
15. Rizzieri DA Johnson JL, Niedzwiecki D, Lee EJ, Vardiman JW, Powell BL, Barcos M, Bloomfield CD, Schiffer CA, Peterson BA, et al. (2004) Intensive chemotherapy with and without cranial radiation for Burkitt leukemia and lymphoma: Final results of Cancer and Leukemia Group B study 9251. Cancer 100:1438–1448
16. Hoelzer D, Ludwig WD, Thiel E, Gabmann W, Loffler H, Fonatsch C, et al. (1996) Improved outcome in adult B-cell acute lymphoblastic leukemia. Blood 88:495–508
17. Stock W, Dodge RK, Vardiman JW, Bloomfield CD, Caligiuri MA, Frankel S, Stone RM, Larson RA (2001) Treatment of adult acute lymphoblastic leukemia: Phase II trial of dose intensification of daunorubicin and cytarabine followed by high-dose methotrexate and intrathecal methotrexate in place of cranial irradiation (CALGB 19802). Blood 98(Suppl 1):590a (#2472)
18. Stock W, Yu D, Johnson J, Bloomfield CD, Stone RM, Kolitz JE, Wetzler M, Powell B, Vardiman JW, Larson RA (2003) Intensified daunorubicin during induction and postremission therapy of adult acute lymphoblastic leukemia (ALL): Results of CALGB 19802. Blood 102:379a (#1375)
19. Wetzler M, Dodge RK, Mrozek K, Carroll AJ, Tantravahi RR, Block AMW, Pettenati MJ, Le Beau MM, Frankel SR, Stewart CC, et al. (1999) Prospective karyotype analysis in adult acute lymphoblastic leukemia: The Cancer and Leukemia Group B Experience. Blood 93:3983–3993
20. Gandhi V, Plunkett W, Rodriquez CO Jr, Nowak BJ, Du M, Ayres M, Kisor DF, Mitchell BS, Kurtzberg J, Keating MJ (1998) Compound GW506U78 in refractory hematological malignancies: Relationship between cellular pharmacokinetics and clinical response. J Clin Oncol 16:3607–3615
21. De Angelo DJ, Yu D, Johnson JL, Coutre SE, Stone RM, Stopeck AT, Gockermann JP, Mitchell BS, Appelbaum FR, Larson RA (2007) A phase II study of 2-amino-9-D-arabinosyl-6-methoxy-9H-purine (506U78) in patients with relapsed or refractory T-lineage acute lymphoblastic leukemia (ALL) or lymphoblastic lymphoma (LBL): CALGB Study 19801. Blood 109:5136–5142

Conventional Therapy in Adult Acute Lymphoblastic Leukemia: Review of the LALA Program

Xavier Thomas, Denis Fiere

Contents

11.1 Introduction

The GET-LALA (Groupe d'Etude et de Traitement de la Leucémie Aiguë Lymphoblastique de l'Adulte) group has performed a series of studies evaluating different aspects of remission induction and postremission treatment in adults with acute lymphoblastic leukemia (ALL). The LALA group was formed by interested hematologists, physicians, and statisticians in the beginning of the 1980s. The first working party was set up in 1982 with Professor Denis Fiere as chairman of the Steering Committee, and the first randomized trial involving multiple French centers was started in 1983. Since then several other trials have been opened to persons over 15 years of age. In recent years, clinical trials have been supplemented by systematic morphologic, immunophenotyping, cytogenetic, and molecular genetic studies leading to the identification of different risk groups of patients who may warrant individualized treatments. With the development of data managing and the establishment of a large network of collaborating physicians and biologists, the later trials became larger, and reporting was more reliable. The major aim of all the trials was the improvement of remission duration and survival rates of adult ALL patients, the definition of prognostic factors, and the development of risk-adapted treatment strategies. The number of participating centers in France has increased from 11 in 1982 to 47 in the LALA-94 trial that also involved 8 centers in Belgium. Since 2002 with the creation of the GRAALL (Group for Research on Adult Acute Lymphoblastic Leukemia), resulting from the fusion of the LALA and GOELAMS (Groupe Ouest-Est d'étude des Leucémies et Autres Maladies du Sang) groups, the group protocols are administered in hospitals all over France and in some Belgian centers. International collaborations were also developed with the Australasian Leukemia and Lymphoma Group (ALLG) and the Swiss Group for Clinical Cancer Research (SAKK) allowing to randomize sufficient numbers of patients to demonstrate the effects of treatments in more accurately defined risk groups. Insight into the biologic and molecular abnormalities in ALL might also provide the necessary clues that allow a clearer understanding of the crucial differences in the behavior of the different subtypes of ALL patients.

11.2 General Principles

In the 1960s, a major development in the treatment of ALL came from St. Jude Children's Research Hospital in Memphis, with Don Pinkel introducing a four-phase treatment plan for ALL, what he called "Total therapy" [1] that took into account the advantage of combination chemotherapy in overcoming initial drug resistance and inhibiting acquired resistance, as well as the superiority of some drugs for remission induction and others for its continuation. All available antileukemic agents were included in the plan. The principles that were applied resulted in the regular cure of more than 50% of children with ALL. These principles were induction therapy using vincristine and prednisone, consolidation chemotherapy, a maintenance chemotherapy using 6-mercaptopurine and methotrexate, and then radiotherapy to the central nervous system (CNS) to prevent meningeal relapse. This resulted in a tremendous increase in the survival rate of patients with ALL. This regimen also recognized the importance of early intensification chemotherapy, the need for specific CNS treatment to prevent meningeal relapse, and the idea of continuing combination chemotherapy for 2 to 3 years. With this basic therapeutic strategy, results improved regularly over time with complete remission (CR) rates above 90% with recent programs and survival approaching 70–80% [2]. Unfortunately, the success that has been achieved in children with ALL has not yet been translated into adult patients [3]. Although CR rates approach now those in children, only 30–40% of adults with ALL can expect a cure 4. Less frequent than ALL in childhood, ALL in adults has long been mishandled [4, 5]. The first cooperative studies in adults with ALL were initiated during the 1970s and the early 1980s [6–9], of which the first trial of the LALA group.

11.3 LALA-83 Trial (1983–1985)

A pilot study on 45 patients from 16 to 73 years old was initiated in 1982 to test the feasibility of an intensive and short induction phase followed by an early consolidation phase [10]. Eleven French centers participated to that pilot study. All patients received a 5-day course of induction chemotherapy with prednisone, vincristine, cytarabine, and rubidazone. An "AAA" regimen consisting of Adriamycin, cytarabine (Aracytine), and Asparaginase was used as consolidation. CR was achieved in 73% of patients and the sequence intensive induction-early consolidation was well tolerated and proved feasible. This allowed the development of a larger multicenter trial. The LALA-83 trial started at the beginning of 1983 and ran through 1985, including 225 patients from 33 French centers. The major aims of this trial were to study the usefulness of aggressive CR induction and

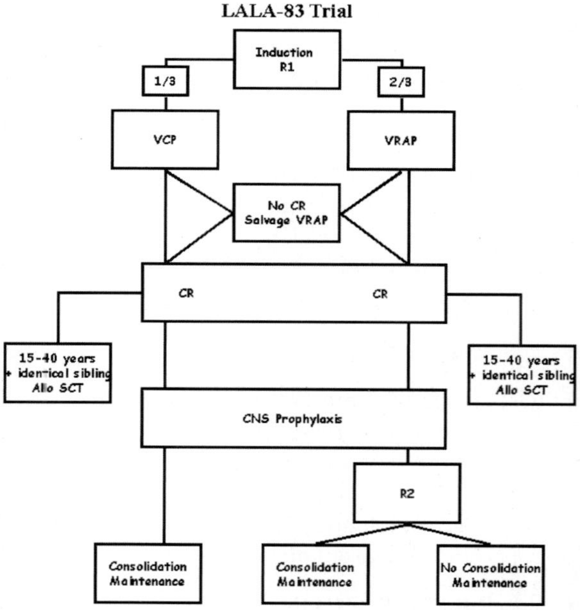

Fig. 11.1. Schema of LALA-83 trial. Induction therapy consisted of VRAP with rubidazone 450 $mg/m^2/d$ on day 1; vincristine 1.2 $mg/m^2/d$ on days 1 and 5; cytarabine 100 $mg/m^2/d$ on days 1–5; and prednisone 80 $mg/m^2/d$ on days 1–5; or VCP with vincristine 1.4 $mg/m^2/d$ on days 1, 8, 15, and 21; cyclophosphamide 400 $mg/m^2/d$ on days 1, 8, 15, and 21; and prednisone 60 $mg/m^2/d$ on days 1–15. Consolidation therapy consisted of three 1-month courses of adriamycin 40 mg/m^2 on day 1; cytarabine 60 $mg/m^2/d$ on days 3–7; and asparaginase 1000 $U/m^2/d$ on days 8–12. Maintenance chemotherapy consisted of methotrexate 15 mg/m^2/week and 6-mercaptopurine 90 $mg/m^2/d$ for 2 years. Alternating courses of reinduction consisting of either vincristine 1.4 mg/m^2 on day 1; cyclophosphamide 600 mg/m^2 on day 1; and prednisone 60 $mg/m^2/d$ on days 1–8; or adriamycin 40 mg/m^2 on day 1; and cytarabine 60 $mg/m^2/d$ on days 1–5, were performed. Abbreviations: CNS, central nervous system; R1, first randomization; R2, second randomization.

early consolidation in adult ALL, and to study the value of HLA-matched allogeneic stem cell transplantation (SCT) performed in early first CR (Fig. 11.1) [11]. One third of the patients were randomized in the VCP (vincristine, cyclophosphamide, prednisone) induction arm, while two thirds in the more aggressive VRAP (vincristine, rubidazone, cytarabine, prednisone) arm. CR rates were not statistically different with, however, a higher toxicity in the VRAP arm. Overall, the CR rate after one or two courses of induction therapy was 77.5%. Of patients evaluable for postremission therapy, 39 of 42 patients with a suitable donor were allografted in first CR, 39 patients initially treated by VCP arm received consolidation with 3 monthly courses of "AAA," followed by a 3-year maintenance therapy, 63 patients initially treated by VRAP arm were randomized to receive AAA consolidations and maintenance therapy, or only maintenance therapy. The median overall survival (OS) was 13.5 months for the entire cohort. The best results were observed after allogeneic SCT with 6-year disease-free survival (DFS) at 53% [12]. There was a significantly better survival for patients initially treated with VCP and receiving AAA consolidations followed by maintenance therapy. In the multivariate analysis, age (cut-off at 35 years) and initial white blood cell count (cut-off at 30×10^9/l) appeared as the main prognostic factors suggesting their use in a risk model further developed in subsequent trials.

11.4 LALA-85 Trial (1985–1986)

At the beginning of the 1980s, the overall probability of achieving CR exceeded 75%, and approximately 35% of patients achieving CR could be cured using chemotherapy alone [7, 13]. It was therefore appropriate to study alternative forms of treatment such as allogeneic or autologous SCT. In the LALA-83 trial, allogeneic SCT was performed in all patients aged under 40 years having an HLA-identical sibling, showing a slight advantage of SCT over optimal chemotherapy [12]. The LALA group tested, in this pilot study, the feasibility of purged autologous SCT, after an intensive induction regimen in which zorubicin was used instead of the classical daunorubicin (Fig. 11.2) [14]. The postinduction chemotherapy arm began with 3-month consolidation according to AAA regimen. The maintenance chemotherapy was similar to that of the L10 maintenance regimen, using eight drugs sequentially [4]. In patients, aged 15 to 50 years, without identical sibling donor, the chemotherapy arm was randomly compared to autologous SCT. Ex vivo purging of the stem cells was performed using mafosfamide or monoclonal antibodies plus complement. From May 1985 to December 1986, 164 patients from 33 institutions entered the trial. The overall CR rate was 83%. For the whole group, DFS was 34% and OS 42% with a median follow-up of 30 months [14]. Twenty-seven patients received autologous SCT. No difference appeared between the three arms of postremis-

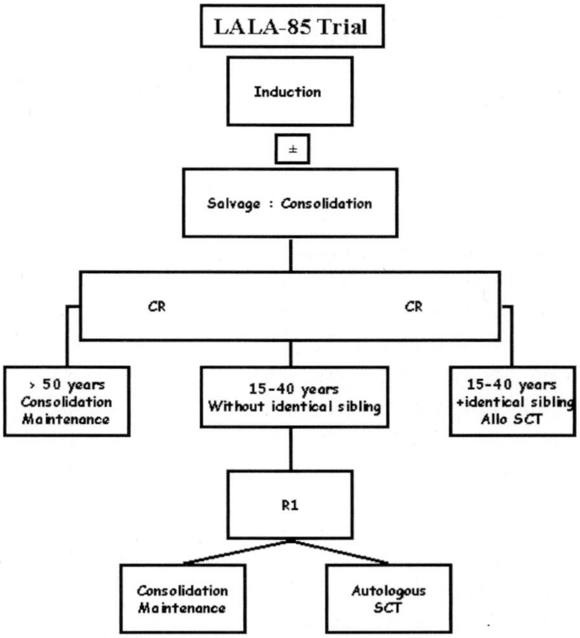

Fig. 11.2. Schema of LALA-85 trial. Induction therapy consisted of rubidazone 100 mg/m²/d on days 1–3; vincristine 1.4 mg/m²/d on days 1, 8, and 15; cyclophosphamide 400 mg/m²/d on days 1, 8, and 15; and prednisone 60 mg/m²/d on days 1–15. Consolidation therapy consisted of three 1-month courses of adriamycin 40 mg/m² on day 1; cytarabine 60 mg/m²/d on days 3–7; and asparaginase 1000 U/m²/d on days 8–12. Maintenance chemotherapy consisted of a modified L10 regimen for 4 cycles of 64 days including prednisone 60 mg/m²/d on days 1–8; adriamycin 20 mg/m² on days 15–17; vincristine 1.4 mg/m²/d on days 1 and 8; 6-mercaptopurine 60 mg/m²/d on days 25–56; methotrexate 20 mg/m²/d on days 35, 42, 49, and 56; and dactinomycin 1000 gamma/m² on day 56; alternating with 4 cycles of 64 days including prednisone 60 mg/m²/d on days 1–8; cyclophosphamide 800 mg/m² on day 15; carmustine 80 mg/m² on day 15; vincristine 1.4 mg/m²/d on days 1 and 8; 6-mercaptopurine 60 mg/m²/d on days 25–56; methotrexate 15 mg/m²/d on days 35, 42, 49 and 56; and dactinomycin 1000 gamma/m² on day 56. Abbreviations: R1, first randomization.

sion (chemotherapy, allogeneic SCT, autologous SCT) in terms of DFS or survival. However, the number of allocated patients in each arm was too small to draw any conclusions. Furthermore, 12 out of the 34 allografted patients have relapsed, of whom 10 had received T-depleted marrow.

11.5 LALA-87 Trial (1986–1991)

The previous pilot study has led the LALA group to propose a new trial (LALA-87 trial) testing the different strategies for postinduction therapy with the aim to ascertain clearly the value of transplantation and of chemotherapy in first CR [15]. The objective was therefore, first, to evaluate randomly, after consolidation chemotherapy, the benefits of autologous SCT over classical maintenance chemotherapy (L10 regimen), and second, to pursue the evaluation of allogeneic SCT in first remission. Finally, a randomized evaluation of zorubicin over daunorubicin as a part of the induction regimen was performed (Fig. 11.3). This multicentric cooperative trial was conducted between 1986 and 1991 by 43 French and Belgian institutions.

In ALL, many attempts have been made to intensify induction regimens by adding a fourth or a fifth drug [13, 16, 17], but the actual benefit of this approach remained questionable. In the LALA-87, we proposed the administration of a high-dose anthracycline added to cyclophosphamide in induction therapy. Of the 572 assessable patients, 76% achieved CR. No differences in terms of CR, DFS, or survival were observed when considering the two randomized induction regimens. The OS rate of the entire cohort was 27% at 10 years [18]. The survival rate for the 436 patients achieving CR was 30% at 10 years. All patients aged 51–60 years were treated with chemotherapy only. The 10-year survival of those patients was 18%. In the LALA-87 trial, assignment to postremission arm based on the results of HLA typing was considered as a "genetic randomization". Patients with an HLA-matched sibling donor were assigned to the allogeneic SCT arm, while those without donor were assigned to the control arm, and then secondarily randomly allocated to receive autologous SCT or chemotherapy. In the allogeneic SCT trial, based on an intent-to-treat analysis, the 10-year survival rate was 46% in the allogeneic SCT arm vs. 31% in the control arm (p = 0.04). In the autologous SCT trial, based on an intent-to-treat analysis, the 10-year survival was

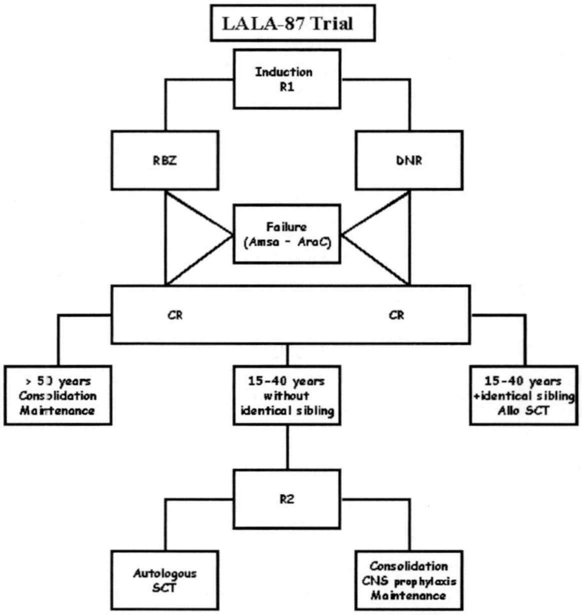

Fig. 11.3. Schema of LALA-87 trial. Induction therapy consisted of vincristine 1.5 mg/m²/d on days 1, 8, 15 and 22; cyclophosphamide 600 mg/m²/d on days 1 and 8; and prednisone 60 mg/m²/d on days 1 to 22. In addition, two anthracyclines, either rubidazone (RBZ) 100 mg/m²/d on days 1 to 3 or daunorubicin (DNR) 50 mg/m²/d on days 1 to 3, were compared (R1). In absence of CR, patients received salvage therapy including cytarabine 500 mg/m²/12 h on days 1 to 4, and amsacrine 120 mg/m²/d on days 1 to 3. Consolidation therapy consisted of three 1-month courses of either rubidazone 120 mg/m² on day 1 or daunorubicin 60 mg/m² on day 1; cytarabine 60 mg/m²/d on days 3 to 7; and asparaginase 1000 U/m²/d on days 8 to 12. Maintenance chemotherapy consisted of a modified L10 regimen for 4 cycles of 64 days including prednisone 60 mg/m²/d on days 1 to 8; daunorubicin 60 mg/m² on day 15 or rubidazone 120 mg/m² on day 15; vincristine 1.5 mg/m²/d on days 1 and 8; 6-mercaptopurine 60 mg/m²/d on days 25 to 56; methotrexate 15 mg/m²/d on days 35, 42, 49 and 56; and dactinomycin 1000 gamma/m² on day 64; alternating with 4 cycles of 64 days including prednisone 60 mg/m²/d on days 1 to 8; cyclophosphamide 800 mg/m² on day 15; carmustine 80 mg/m² on day 15; vincristine 1.5 mg/m²/d on days 1 and 8; 6-mercaptopurine 60 mg/m²/d on days 25 to 56; methotrexate 15 mg/m²/d on days 35, 42, 49 and 56; and dactinomycin 1000 gamma/m² on day 64. Abbreviations: AlloSCT, allogeneic stem cell transplantation; Amsa, amsacrine; AraC, cytarabine; Autologous SCT, autologous stem cell transplantation; CNS, central nervous system; DNR, daunorubicin; RBZ, rubidazone; R1, first randomization; R2, second randomization.

34% in the autologous SCT arm vs. 29% in the chemotherapy arm (p = NS). Overall results were in the range of those published by most larger cooperative groups. The LALA-87 confirmed the efficacy of allogeneic SCT [19–21]. In the second trial comparing autologous SCT and chemotherapy, there was only a trend for better results in the autologous SCT arm.

11.6 LALA-91 Pilot Study (1991–1993)

Between 1991 and 1993, 57 patients were included in a pilot multicenter trial in which we used sequential administration of prednisone from day 1 to day 7, and day 15 to day 21, in combination with a conventional chemotherapy combining vincristine, daunorubicin, and cyclophosphamide, with the aim of decreasing the risk of complications in relation with steroid administration [22]. A high rate of CR (89%) was observed without severe toxicity. Severe infectious complications occurred in only 14% of cases. Sequential use of prednisone seemed at least as effective as continuous administration at the expense of a few adverse side effects and was therefore included in the further trials (LALAG-92 and LALA-94).

11.7 LALA-94 Trial (1994–2002)

The prognosis of adult patients with ALL, treated with modern chemotherapeutic regimens, is dependent on a number of variables. These features have been utilized to identify patients with low and high risk of relapse. Treatment tailored to individual risk groups has resulted in dramatic improvements in outcome for pediatric patients with ALL, and risk-adapted strategies based on biological and clinical features were also applied to adults with ALL to improve survival. The major prognostic factors in adults are age, cytogenetics, immunologic subtype, white blood cell count, and time to achieve CR [23]. Risk-adapted strategy is based on a dose efficacy scheme and the optimal treatment strategy is related to a perfect knowledge of prognostic factors. However, prognostic factors are regimen-dependent and could therefore change according to the period of study.

Based on the LALA-87 trial results [15], aggressive induction plus more potent intensification programs with chemotherapy plus SCT have been proposed to improve treatment results. We introduced in the LALA-94 trial a risk-adapted postremission strategy according to initial features and to initial response to therapy, and we re-evaluated transplantation for high-risk ALL [24]. Between 1994 and 2002, a total of 1000 untreated ALL patients (excluding mature B-cell ALL) from 68 French, Belgian, Swiss, and Australian centers entered the LALA-94. All patients received a standard 4-drug/4-week induction course. After one course of induction chemotherapy, patients were systematically stratified, by initial clinical and biological characteristics (based on cytogenetic analysis and molecular examination) and by their response to initial therapy, in different risk groups. Postinduction intensity was designed according to the risk level (Fig. 11.4). Standard-risk ALL comprised all T-cell lineage ALL patients achieving CR after one course of chemotherapy and B-cell lineage ALL patients defined by the absence of CNS-positive ALL, the absence of Philadelphia chromosome, t(4;11), t(1;19), or other abnormalities involving 11q23 rearrangements, a white blood cell count $<30\times10^9$/l, an immunophenotype characterized by $CD10^+/CD19^+$, or $CD20^+/CD19^+$ and the absence of myeloid markers, and achievement of CR after one course of chemotherapy. Standard-risk ALL followed a chemotherapy program for 2 years with a randomization on day 35 between either an intensive consolidation chemotherapy, combining mitoxantrone and intermediate-dose cytarabine (HAM), followed by maintenance therapy or only maintenance chemotherapy. Philadelphia chromosome-positive ALL and CNS-positive ALL were individualized. On the basis of intention-to-treat principle, these patients achieving CR, after an induction course followed by HAM intensive consolidation, were distributed in one of the following groups: matched related allogeneic SCT if they had a sibling donor, or autologous SCT if they did not meet criteria for the first group. High-risk ALL was defined as nonstandard-risk ALL without Philadelphia chromosome or CNS involvement. In this group, all patients with a HLA sibling were scheduled for allogeneic SCT. Patients without a sibling donor were randomly assigned between the chemotherapy program and autologous SCT.

Report on 922 eligible patients showed a CR rate of 84%. Median OS was 23 months and median DFS was 17.5 months with 3-year DFS at 37%. In standard-risk ALL, the 3-year DFS rate was 41%, with no difference between arms of postremission randomization. In high-risk ALL and ALL with CNS involvement, the 3-year DFS rates were 38% and 44%, respectively. In high-risk ALL, autologous SCT and chemotherapy resulted in not significantly different outcome. Patients with an HLA-matched sibling had improved DFS [24].

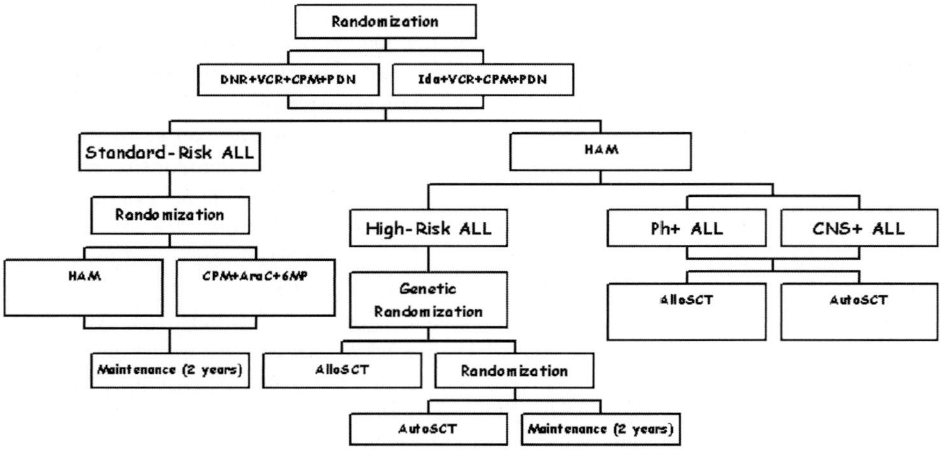

Fig. 11.4. Schema of LALA-94 trial. The induction course was administered over a 4-week period and consisted of either idarubicin 9 mg/m^2/d on days 1, 2, 3, and 8, or daunorubicin 30 mg/m^2/d on days 1–3, and 15 and 16; vincristine 2mg/d on days 1, 8, 15, and 16; cyclophosphamide 750 mg/m^2/d on days 1 and 8; and prednisone 60 mg/m^2/d on days 1–7, and 15–21. Postinduction chemotherapy varied according to risk-groups. It could consist of either cytarabine 1 g/m^2/12h on days 1–4, and mitoxantrone 10 mg/m^2/d on days 3–5; or cyclophosphamide 1 g/m^2/d on days 1, 15, and 29; cytarabine 75 mg/m^2/d on days 3–6, 10–13, and 17–20; and 6-mercaptopurine 60 mg/m^2/d on days 1–28. Maintenance chemotherapy was a program for 2 years with alternating courses of methotrexate 1.5 g/m^2 on day 1, and L-asparaginase 1000 U/m^2 on day 2 (9 courses); vincristine 0.4 mg/d on days 1–4, doxorubicin 12 mg/m^2/d on days 1–4, and dexamethasone 40 mg/d on days 1–4 (2 courses); and cyclophosphamide 1 g/m2 on day 1, and cytarabine 500 mg/m^2 on day 1 (8 courses). Methotrexate 15 mg/m^2/week and 6-mercaptopurine 60 mg/m^2/d were administered between maintenance courses from day 220 to month 30. Abbreviations: AlloSCT, allogeneic stem cell transplantation; AutoSCT, autologous stem cell transplantation; AraC, cytarabine; CNS+, central nervous system-positive; CPM, cyclophosphamide; DNR, daunorubicin; HAM, high-dose cytarabine plus mitoxantrone; Ida, idarubicin; PDN, prednisone; Ph+, Philadelphia-positive; VCR, vincristine; 6MP, 6-mercaptopurine.

Philadelphia-positive and/or BCR-ABL-positive ALL confirmed a poor outcome with a 3-year OS rate of 28%. Median DFS values for autografted patients and for allografted patients were 6.5 and 15.5 months with 3-year DFS rates at 15% and 34%, respectively ($p=0.001$) [25]. After each course, minimal residual disease (MRD) was tested by specific reverse transcriptase-polymerase chain reaction (RT-PCR) with a median sensitivity of 10^{-5}.

Better results in terms of CR may be obtained by using more intensive chemotherapy and better supportive care to reduce early deaths [26]. In the LALA-94 trial, encouraging results in terms of remission proportion could be explained by reduced toxicity with fewer infections related to lower doses corticosteroids [22] and the use of hematologic growth factors in some centers [27], and efficacy of HAM salvage therapy [26, 28–30]. In Philadelphia-positive ALL, HAM-associated salvage rate was higher in patients with M-BCR than in those with m-BCR ALL (55% vs. 30%, $p=0.05$). BCR-ABL status after HAM was predictive of remission duration and survival [25].

11.8 Results of Stem Cell Transplantation in LALA Study Group

11.8.1 Allogeneic Stem Cell Transplantation

The optimal consolidation therapy for adults with ALL in first complete remission remains unclear. Trials evaluating allogeneic stem cell transplantation have uniformly shown higher treatment-related mortality and decreased disease relapse, resulting in centers favoring a conservative approach and recommending transplantation only for patients <30 years old with very high-risk ALL, such as Philadelphia-positive ALL [20, 31]. In the LALA-87 trial, allogeneic SCT was compared to chemotherapy or autologous SCT in first CR [18, 32]. Based on an intent-to-treat analysis, the survival rate

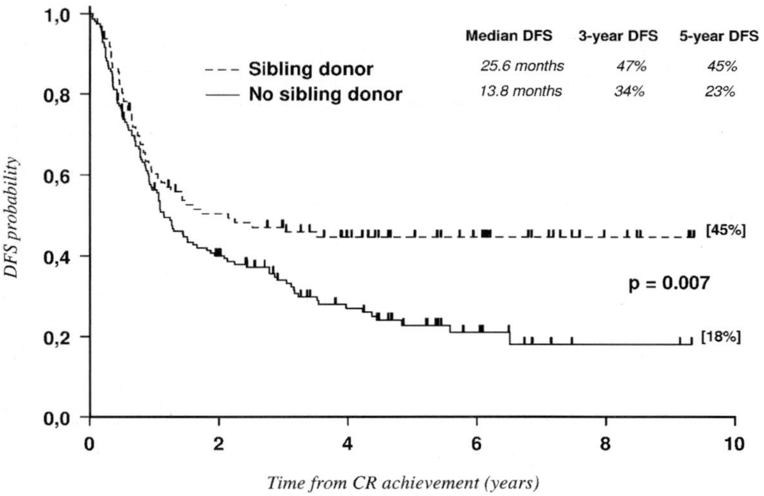

Fig. 11.5. DFS according to genetic randomization in the LALA-94 trial.

was 46% with allogeneic SCT vs. 31% with chemotherapy or autologous SCT (p = 0.04). In the high-risk group (including Philadelphia-positive ALL), survival rates at 10 years were 44% in the allogeneic SCT group vs. only 11% in the control arm (p = 0.009). In the standard-risk group, the corresponding numbers were 49% and 39%, respectively. These results supported the value of allogeneic SCT in first CR in patients with high-risk ALL [18].

Actually, non-Philadelphia-positive high-risk ALL represents the majority of ALL cases. In the LALA-94 trial, allogeneic SCT did better than the other postremission therapeutic strategies in terms of DFS in Philadelphia-negative high-risk patients using the results of the HLA typing as a random allocation (5-year DFS: 45% vs. 23%; p = 0.007) (Fig. 11.5) [24]. Furthermore, allogeneic SCT appeared definitively of benefit to Philadelphia chromosome-positive ALL [25], t(4;11) ALL, and t(1;19) ALL [33]. These results, together with recent data showing no difference in related compared with unrelated transplant in first CR [34], suggest the feasibility of using matched unrelated donor SCT in future clinical trials for those patients in absence of a sibling donor.

Our results confirmed those of the Medical Research Council UKALL XII/Eastern Cooperative Oncology Group E2993 trial, in which data suggested that allogeneic SCT was beneficial in first CR, regardless of the risk group, challenging the current approach of restricting allogeneic SCT to high-risk ALL patients in first CR only [35].

11.8.2 Autologous Stem Cell Transplantation

In the LALA-87 trial, based on an intent-to-treat analysis, survival at 10 years was 34% in the autologous SCT arm vs. 29% in the chemotherapy arm (p = NS). Sixty-six percent of patients actually received transplantation. After stratification according to standard-risk and high-risk criteria, the difference was still not significant. In high-risk ALL (including Philadelphia-positive ALL), the OS rate at 10 years was 10% for the autologous SCT arm vs. 16% for the chemotherapy arm. In standard-risk ALL, the 10-year OS rate was 49% in the autologous SCT arm and 40% in the chemotherapy arm [18]. In the LALA-94 trial, autologous SCT and chemotherapy resulted in high-risk ALL in comparable median DFS (15.2 vs. 11 months) with 3-year DFS of 39% and 24%, respectively (p = NS). However, there were some flaws in all studies: the number of patients in each arm was small, and some patients allocated to the transplantation group actually did not undergo transplantation.

In a retrospective study including adult patients randomized in the three successive trials—LALA-85, LALA-87, and LALA-94—autologous SCT did not show superiority over chemotherapy in high-risk ALL patients, although a different pattern of relapse was observed after autologous SCT with fewer late relapses [36]. The use of autologous SCT in first remission was, however, not advocated.

11.9 Prognostic Factors

The majority of adults with ALL now achieve CR. Unfortunately, despite these achievements, the majority of these patients still relapse. One way of approaching this challenge is to examine options for postremission therapy based on the prognostic factors. Different classifications have been proposed [13, 16, 37], identifying roughly three risk groups: a standard-risk group that contains patients with B- or T-lineage ALL who have no adverse cytogenetics [absence of t(9;22)/BCR-ABL, t(4;11)/MLL-AF4, or t(1;19)/E2A-PBX1], are under age 30, present with white blood cell counts of less than 30×10^9/l, and achieve CR in less than 4 to 6 weeks; a poor-risk group that contains patients with adverse cytogenetics, present with WBC counts of more than 100×10^9/l, or who achieve late CR, and patients aged more than 60 years; and an intermediate-risk group that contains patients with prognostic characteristics of neither the standard-risk nor the poor-risk group. These prognostic factors were also considered in the LALA trials, in which other factors were identified. In the LALA-87 trial, T-cell lineage ALL had a more favorable outcome than B-cell lineage ALL [38]. T-ALL patients had a significantly more favorable outcome than favorable outcome than B-cell lineage ALL patients only in the chemotherapy arm. A useful measure in risk assessment could be the rate of clearance of leukemic cells from the blood or bone marrow during the early phase of therapy. Slow clearance of the cells has proved to be an indicator of poor prognosis, requiring intensification therapy [39].

Improved understanding of the molecular pathogenesis of ALL, as well as the development of innovative molecular monitoring techniques, is beginning to provide both new prognostic information and insights into future therapeutic strategies. The identification of new molecular markers of disease may also increase our ability to tailor treatment for specific risk groups in ALL. Both T cell receptor (TCR) and genotypic stratification have been shown to contribute to risk-adapted management of adult T-cell lineage ALL [40]. Detection of MRD is also beginning to provide important prognostic information that may affect postremission strategies. This was applied in the GRAALL-03 trial, in which treatment decisions were based on the detection and quantification of leukemia cells at different times during postremission treatment [41]. Ultimately, the goal of risk-stratification was to provide the rationale for successful subset-specific therapeutic strategies to improve outcome for all adults with ALL.

11.10 Treatment of Elderly Patients

A number of clinical and laboratory characteristics influence the response to treatment and thus the survival of patients with ALL. Among them, age is one of the most important prognostic variables [7]. Only few reports have been published on ALL in the elderly, but all confirmed the poor prognosis in elderly patients with ALL with survival rates of less than 10% at 5 years [42]. This may be related to the biology of leukemia in the elderly [7, 43] and/or could be related to an increase in the number of early deaths during induction [44, 45]. Toxicity is probably not mainly hematologic since regeneration after chemotherapy is not significantly delayed, but mainly extrahematologic. This may lead to incomplete application of a proposed treatment schedule, which additionally worsens the outcome. Another major reason for the poor outcome in elderly ALL patients is a higher prevalence of disease refractory to standard chemotherapy programs related to the higher incidence of adverse risk factors, particularly the increasing frequency of Philadelphia chromosome-positive ALL with age.

The LALA group has developed special schedules for elderly patients with ALL since 1992. The LALA group initiated a study (LALAG-92) aimed at improving the prognosis of ALL in older patients [46]. Induction therapy was derived from the young adult protocol LALA-87 [15] with chemotherapy administered at lower dose and tailored according to the response assessed on day 15. In addition, the feasibility of maintenance with interferon (IFN) combined with chemotherapy was assessed (Fig. 11.6). The introduction of IFN in the treatment of ALL was supported by anecdotal reports suggesting that IFN may prove effective in some relapsing ALL [47, 48]. Moreover, in patients receiving IFN after bone marrow transplantation, the risk for subsequent relapse was reduced [49], and a hemizygous or homozygous deletion of the IFN gene has been reported in 30% of ALL patients, which led to the hypothesis that a functional or

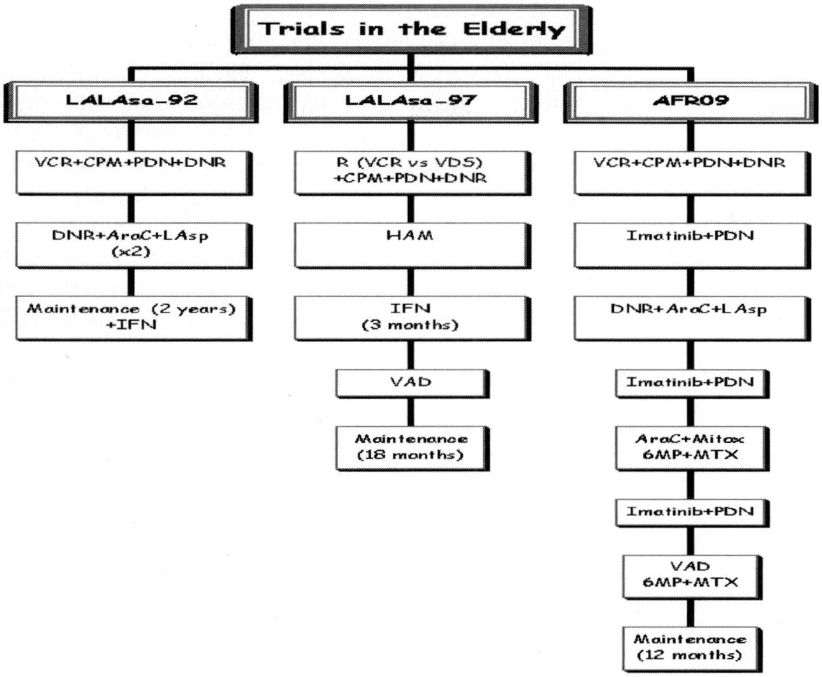

Fig. 11.6. LALA trials in the elderly. Abbreviations: AraC, cytarabine; CPM, cyclophosphamide; DNR, daunorubicin; IFN, interferon-α; HAM, intermediate-dose cytarabine + mitoxantrone; Imatinib, imatinib mesylate; Lasp, L-asparaginase; Mitox, mitoxantrone; MTX, mitoxantrone; PDN, prednisone; R, randomization; VAD, vincristine + adriamycin + dexamethasone; VCR, vincristine; VDS, vindesine; 6MP, 6-mercaptopurine.

quantitative defect of endogenous IFN may be involved in the pathogenesis of ALL [50]. From 1992 to 1995, 40 patients from 11 French and Belgian centers were included in the LALAG-92 study [46]. Compared with younger adults treated according to the LALA-87 protocol, elderly patients did not present with more adverse prognostic features, except for a lower incidence of T-cell ALL. After completion of induction therapy, 85% achieved a CR, while treatment-related mortality during induction was 7.5%. Median OS and DFS were 14.3 months and 14 months, respectively, which, although inferior to results obtained in younger adults, compared favorably with available data in the elderly. Treatment with IFN proved feasible in most patients, but had to be discontinued in 32% of cases because of toxicity.

In 1997, The LALA group initiated a study (LALAG-97) derived from the 1992 study, with as main purposes to better understand the value of IFN and to assess the toxicity and the impact on OS of an intensified induction and of a double consolidation (Fig. 11.6). At inclusion, patients were randomly allocated to therapy with vincristine or with vindesine during induction and the dose of daunorubicin was increased. The consolidation phase was intensified. A 3-month course of IFN was started after the first consolidation phase. A second consolidation phase and maintenance were given after IFN therapy. From 1997 to 1999, 58 patients were included in this study [51]. A CR was obtained in 58% of patients. OS and DFS were also inferior to those observed in the previous trial [46]. The pattern of relapses over time suggested that the 3-month IFN treatment phase with no additional chemotherapy might have contributed to the comparatively poor outcome of this cohort.

Despite the poor prognosis in this type of leukemia, improvements have been observed over time. The development of supportive care and the introduction of growth factors could have been responsible for notable improvements in outcome related to complete applications of proposed treatment schedules. This was also probably due to an improvement of specific therapy against leukemia. "Personalized" treatments, administered until 1987, have been progressively given up, and

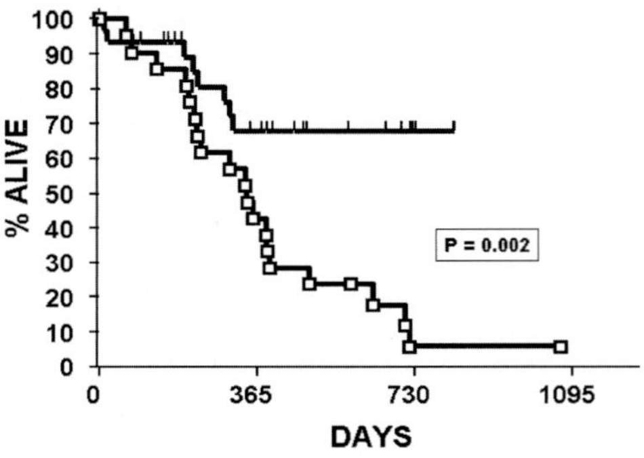

Fig. 11.7. Comparison of Philadelphia-positive ALL patients treated in the elderly with imatinib mesylate and chemotherapy (AFR09) with those treated according to our previous protocol (LALAG-97).

replaced, in all patients with WHO performance status <3, by therapeutic schedules either similar to those administered to adults under 60 years of age, or specifically design for elderly patients. However, "age-adapted" therapies did not show any advantage in terms of DFS. Higher toxicity of "young adult-like" therapy was contrabalanced by a higher relapse rate after "age-adapted" therapy probably related to lighter maintenance therapy [52].

Prognosis of Philadelphia-positive elderly ALL could be transformed by the introduction of imatinib mesylate [53] and could become even better than that of the other subtypes of ALL in the elderly. This prompted the GRAALL to treat apart Philadelphia-positive and Philadelphia-negative ALL and to implement a treatment protocol alternating chemotherapy and imatinib in previously untreated elderly patients with Philadelphia-positive ALL (AFR09 trial) (Fig. 11.6). Our first results showed very encouraging data with a projected 1-year event-free survival (EFS) at 57% for patients treated with imatinib and a 1-year OS at 71% (Fig. 11.7) [54].

11.11 GRAALL Trials (2003–Present)

Despite improvements in outcome of adult patients with ALL, several questions were still open. Is the current stratification using standard-risk and high-risk ALL absolutely adequate in adults? Although risk models have been proposed, the prevailing view was that the vast majority of affected adults should be considered having a high risk of recurrence and that all adult ALL patients should be treated with intensive protocols. Encouraging results of T-cell lineage ALL after allografting in a recent retrospective study [55], together with the poor outcomes observed in the LALA-94 trial with chemotherapy alone [24] and the identification of T-cell lineage subtypes associated with a poor outcome [39], suggested further studies examining allografts compared with more intensive chemotherapy regimens.

The use of more intensive chemotherapy regimens was supported by a retrospective study comparing the characteristics and outcome of 100 adolescents treated in the French adult LALA-94 trial and 77 adolescents treated during the same period in the French pediatric FRALLE (French Acute Lymphoblastic Leukemia)-93 trial [56]. In this study, the comparison pointed out that adolescents treated in the pediatric protocol had a significantly better outcome in terms of CR achievement and EFS. Such a more favorable evolution was not explained by a difference in patients characteristics, and was already remarkable after the induction course, suggesting the major role of drugs and global treating attitude disparities between pediatric and adults departments. These results incited not only treatment of adolescents using pediatric protocols but also the design of new trials inspired by pediatric protocols to treat young adults over 20 years. Disparity was particularly observed in patients with B-cell lineage ALL, but was also present in patients with T-cell ALL. Differences in induction courses, which could underlie this gain in CR rates, were essentially the continuous administration of higher doses of prednisone and the use of L-asparaginase in the FRALLE-93 protocol. Higher doses of major drugs in the treatment of ALL were used in the pediatric protocol within a shorter period of time. The 3-time daily administration schedule of steroids has early been demonstrated superior to more spaced administration in children ALL [57]. Moreover, a recent study of the Dana-Farber Cancer Institute demonstrated improved response to increased steroids dose in pediatric patients [58]. Children aged 9–18 years have been shown to benefit from higher doses of L-asparaginase despite an increased related toxicity, and repeated doses of L-asparaginase during early treatment significantly improved outcome in pediatric patients with T-ALL [59]. Moreover, the pediatric delayed intensifications appeared to contribute to an improve outcome. This strategy, initially proposed by the Berlin-Frankfurt-Munster study group [60], has been demonstrated in children older than 10 years [61], with increased benefit of an

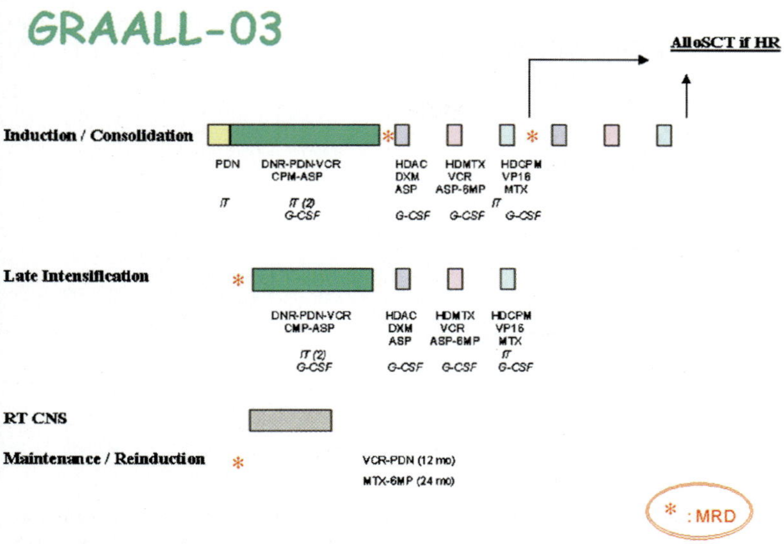

Fig. 11.8. Overall outline of GRAALL-03 protocol. Abbreviations: AlloSCT, allogeneic stem cell transplantation; ASP, L-asparaginase; CPM, cyclophosphamide; DNR, daunorubicin; DXM, dexamethasone; G-CSF, granulocyte colony-stimulating factor; HDAC, high-dose cytarabine; HDCPM, high-dose cyclophosphamide; HDMTX, high-dose methotrexate; HR, high-risk; IT, intrathecal; MRD, minimal residual disease; MTX, methotrexate; PDN, prednisone; RT CNS, central nervous system irradiation; VCR, vincristine; VP16, etoposide; 6MP, 6-mercaptopurine.

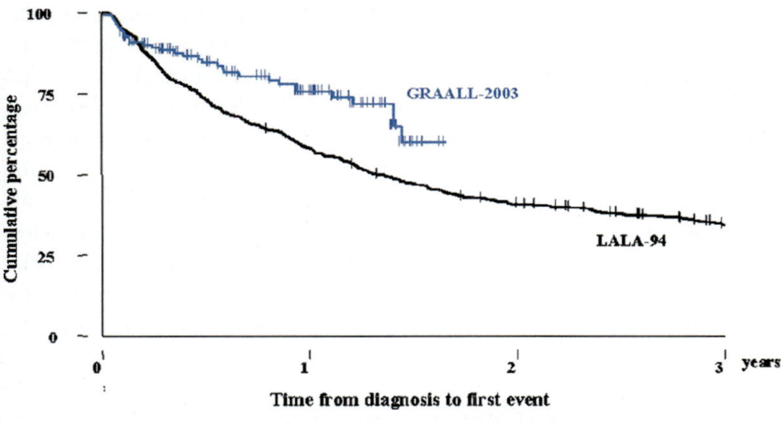

Fig. 11.9. Philadelphia-negative ALL: Comparison of GRAALL-03 and LALA-94 trials in terms of EFS.

augmented therapy including double delayed intensifications in slow early responder patients [62].

Based on these results and those from the LALA-94 study, a prospective Phase 2 study (GRAALL-03) was initiated in 2003 (Fig. 11.8). The major goals of this trial were to increase the indications of allogeneic SCT in both Philadelphia chromosome-negative B-lineage ALL and T-lineage ALL depending on initial prognostic factors; to evaluate the initial response to a prephase of corticosteroids; to evaluate the response to initial chemotherapy evaluated on day 8 and day 28; and to define a therapeutic strategy adapted to the evaluation of MRD. A total of 144 patients were included between 2003 and 2005. CR was achieved in 91% of patients after one or two chemotherapy courses. Estimated 18-month EFS and OS were 65% and 74% respectively (Fig. 11.9) [41].

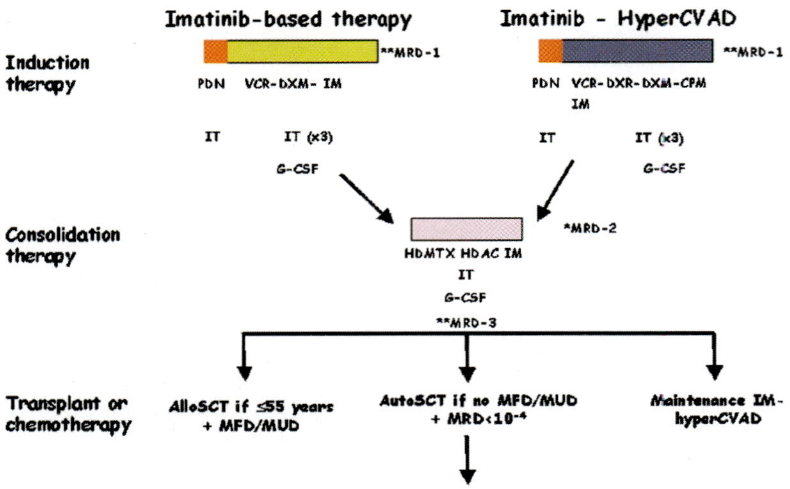

Fig. 11.10. Overall outline of GRAAPH-05 protocol. Abbreviations: AlloSCT, allogeneic stem cell transplantation; AutoSCT, autologous stem cell transplantation; MRD, minimal residual disease (* decisional, ** not decisional); CPM, cyclophosphamide; DXM, dxamethasone; DXR, doxorubicin; G-CSF, granulocyte colony-stimulating factor; HDAC, high-dose cytarabine; HDMTX, high-dose methotrexate; HyperCVAD, regimen of hyperfractionated cyclophosphamide, vincristine, doxorubicin, and dexamethasone; IM, imatinib mesylate; IT, intrathecal; MFD, matched familial donor; MUD, matched unrelated donor; PDN, prednisone; VCR, vincristine.

Early response to initial therapy (response to corticosteroid prephase and response to chemotherapy at day 8) was not correlated to baseline high-risk factors and should be considered in further adult ALL studies. The evaluation of morphological early response correlated closely with postinduction MDR measurement. The hyperfractionated cyclophosphamide (HyperC) reinforcement in patients with a poor early response appeared to be a promising approach to improve their outcome and will be randomly tested in the further GRAALL-05 study.

In the LALA-94 trial, negative BCR-ABL MRD and allogeneic donor availability were two independent good-risk factors for survival in Philadelphia-positive ALL patients reaching hematologic CR after standard induction followed by intensive HAM consolidation [25]. In a phase 1/2 study initiated in 2003, we combined increasing dosages of imatinib mesylate with HAM with an attempt to increase the fraction of patients achieving molecular remission, and to evaluate the safety of the combination regimen and the feasibility of autologous peripheral blood stem cell collection after HAM [63]. The recommended dosage of imatinib was 600 mg per day for further combinations of imatinib and intensive chemotherapy. After HAM, peripheral blood stem cell collection was feasible under imatinib administration. Failure to improve the molecular remission rate as compared to our historical control could be explained by the relatively short exposure to imatinib and/or by the absence of in vivo synergism between imatinib and cytarabine or mitoxantrone. More benefit might be anticipated by incorporating imatinib early in the treatment. This is currently tested in the GRAAPH-05 (Fig. 11.10) comparing an induction therapy "based" on imatinib to an induction therapy combining the regimen of hyperfractionated cyclophosphamide, vincristine, doxorubicin, and dexamethasone (HyperCVAD) chemotherapy with imatinib as conceived by the M.D. Anderson Cancer Center [64, 65].

References

1. George P, Hernandez K, Hustu O, Borella L, Holton C, Pinkel D (1968) A study of "total therapy" of acute lymphocytic leukemia in children. J Pediatr 72:399–408
2. Pui CH (2000) Acute lymphoblastic leukemia in children. Curr Opin Oncol 12:3–12
3. Gee TS, Haghbin M, Dowling MD, Cunningham I, Middleman MP, Clarkson BD (1976) Acute lymphoblastic leukemia in adults and children. Differences in response with similar therapeutic regimens. Cancer 37:1256–1264
4. Clarkson B, Ellis S, Little C, Gee T, Arlin Z, Mertelsmann R, Andreeff M, Kempin S, Koziner B, Chaganti R, et al. (1985) Acute lymphoblastic leukemia in adults. Semin Oncol 12:160–169

5. Jacobs AD, Gale RP (1984) Recent advances in the biology and treatment of acute lymphoblastic leukemia in adults. N Engl J Med 311:1219–1231
6. Baccarani M, Corbelli G, Amadori S, Drenthe-Schronk A, Willemze R, Meloni G, Cardozo PL, Haanen C, Mandelli F, Tura S (1982) Adolescent and adult acute lymphoblastic leukemia: Prognostic features and outcome of therapy: A study of 293 patients. Blood 60:677–684
7. Hoelzer D, Thiel E, Löffler H, Bodenstein H, Plaumann L, Büchner T, Urbanitz D, Koch P, Heimpel H, Engelhardt R, et al. (1984) Intensified therapy in acute lymphoblastic and acute undifferentiated leukemia in adults. Blood 64:38–47
8. Lister TA, Whitehouse JMA, Beard MEJ, Brearley RL, Wrigley PF, Oliver RT, Freeman JE, Woodruff RK, Malpas JS, Paxton AM, Crowther D (1978) Combination chemotherapy for acute lymphoblastic leukaemia in adults. Br Med J 1:199–203
9. Schauer P, Arlin ZA, Mertelsmann R, Cirrincione C, Friedman A, Gee TS, Dowling M, Kempin S, Straus DJ, Koziner B, et al. (1983) Treatment of acute lymphoblastic leukemia in adults: Results of the L-10 and L-10M protocols. J Clin Oncol 462–470
10. Fiere D, Marty M, Solal-Celigny P, Harousseau JL, Gorin NC, Desablens B, Brière J, David B, Bordessoule D, Hayat M, et al. (1989) Induction massive et consolidation précoce des leucémies aigus lymphoïdes de l'adulte. Etude pilote de faisabilité et évolution lointaine. Presse Méd (Paris) 18:221–223
11. Fiere D, Extra JM, David B, Witz F, Vernand JP, Gastaut JA, Dauriac C, Pris J, Marty M (1987) Treatment of 218 adult acute lymphoblastic leukemias. Semin Oncol 14:64–66
12. Vernant JP, Marit G, Maraninchi D, Guyotat D, Kuentz M, Cordonnier C, Reiffers J (1988) Allogeneic bone marrow transplantation in adults with acute lymphoblastic leukemia in first complete remission. J Clin Oncol 6:227–231
13. Gaynor J, Chapman D, Little C, McKenzie S, Miller W, Andreeff M, Arlin Z, Berman E, Kempin S, Gee T, et al. (1988) A cause specific hazard rate analysis of prognostic factors among 199 adults with acute lymphoblastic leukemia. The Memorial Hospital experience since 1969. J Clin Oncol 6:1014–1030
14. Fiere D, Broustet A, Leblond V, Maraninchi D, Castaigne S, Flesch M, Varet B, Vernant JP, Milpied N, Troussard X, et al. (1990) Comparison of chemotherapy and autologous and allogeneic transplantation as postinduction regimen in adult acute lymphoblastic leukemia: A preliminary multicentric study. Hamatol Bluttransfus 33:409–412
15. Fiere D, Lepage E, Sebban C, Boucheix C, Gisselbrecht C, Vernant JP, Varet B, Broustet A, Cahn JY, Rigal-Huguet F, et al. for the French Group on Therapy for Adult Acute Lymphoblastic Leukemia (1993) Adult acute lymphoblastic leukemia: A multicentric randomized trial testing bone marrow transplantation as postremission therapy. J Clin Oncol 11:1990–2001
16. Hoelzer D, Thiel E, Löffler H, Büchner T, Ganser A, Heil G, Koch P, Freund M, Diedrich H, Rühl H, et al. (1988) Prognostic factors in a multicenter study for treatment of acute lymphoblastic leukemia in adults. Blood 71:123–131
17. Linker CA, Levitt LJ, O'Donnell M, Forman SJ, Ries CA (1991) Treatment of adult acute lymphoblastic leukemia with intensive cyclical chemotherapy: A follow-up report. Blood 78:2814–2822
18. Thiebaut A, Vernant JP, Degos L, Rigal Huguet F, Reiffers J, Sebban C, Lepage E, Thomas X, Fiere D (2000) Adult acute lymphocytic leukemia study testing chemotherapy and autologous and allogeneic transplantation. A follow-up report of the French protocol LALA 87. Hematol Oncol Clin North Am 14:1353–1365
19. Horowitz MM, Messerer D, Hoelzer D, Gale RP, Neiss A, Atkinson K, Barrett AJ, Büchner T, Freund M, Heil G, et al. (1991) Chemotherapy compared with bone marrow transplantation for adults with acute lymphoblastic leukemia in first remission. Ann Intern Med 115:13–18
20. Oh H, Gale RP, Zhang MJ, Passweg JR, Ino T, Murakami H, Ohno R, Rowlings PA, Sobocinski KA, Tanimoto M, et al. (1998) Chemotherapy vs. HLA-identical sibling bone marrow transplants for adults with acute lymphoblastic leukemia in first remission. Bone Marrow Transplant 22:253–257
21. Gale RP, Park RE, Dubois RW, Herzig GP, Hocking WG, Horowitz MM, Keating A, Kempin S, Linker CA, Schiffer CA, et al. (1998) Delphi-panel analysis of appropriateness of high-dose therapy and bone marrow transplants in adults with acute lymphoblastic leukemia in first remission. Leuk Res 22:973–981
22. Thomas X, Danala C, Bach QK, Dufour P, Christian B, Corront B, Bosly A, Bastion Y, Gratecos N, Leblay R, et al. (1995) Sequential induction chemotherapy with vincristine, daunorubicin, cyclophosphamide and prednisone in adult acute lymphoblastic leukemia. Ann Hematol 70:65–69
23. Hoelzer D (1994) Treatment of acute lymphoblastic leukemia. Semin Hematol 31:1–15
24. Thomas X, Boiron JM, Huguet F, Dombret H, Bradstock K, Vey N, Kovacsovics T, Delannoy A, Fegueux N, Fenaux P, et al. (2004) Outcome of treatment in adults with acute lymphoblastic leukemia: Analysis of the LALA-94 trial. J Clin Oncol 22:4075–4086
25. Dombret H, Gabert J, Boiron JM, Rigal-Huguet F, Blaise D, Thomas X, Delannoy A, Buzyn A, Bilhou-Nabera C, Cayuela JM, et al. for the Groupe d'Etude et de Traitement de la Leucémie Aiguë Lymphoblastique de l'Adulte (GET-LALA Group) (2002) Outcome of treatment in adults with Philadelphia chromosome-positive acute lymphoblastic leukemia – Results of the prospective multicenter LALA-94 trial. Blood 100:2357–2366
26. Weiss M, Maslak P, Felman E, Berman E, Bertino J, Gee T, Megherian L, Seiter K, Scheinberg D, Golde D (1996) Cytarabine with high dose mitoxantrone induces rapid complete remission in adult acute lymphoblastic leukemia without the use of vincristine or prednisone. J Clin Oncol 14:2480–2485
27. Thomas X, Boiron JM, Huguet F, Reman O, Sutton L, Turlure P, Garban F, Gardin C, Espinouse D, Boulat O, et al. for the Groupe d'Etude et de Traitement de la Leucémie Aiguë Lymphoblastique de l'Adulte (GET-LALA Group) (2004) Efficacy of granulocyte and granulocyte-macrophage colony-stimulating factors in the induction treatment of adult acute lymphoblastic leukemia: A multicenter randomized study. Hematol J 5:384–394
28. Rohatiner AZ, Bassan R, Battista R, Barnett MJ, Gregory W, Lim J, Amess J, Oza A, Barbui T, Horton M (1990) High dose cytosine arabinoside in the initial treatment of adults with acute lymphoblastic leukaemia. Br J Cancer 62:454–458
29. Cassileth PA, Andersen JW, Bennett JM, Hoagland HC, Mazza JJ, O'Connell MC, Paietta E, Wiernik P (1992) Adult acute lymphocytic leukemia: The Eastern Cooperative Oncology Group experience. Leukemia 6(Suppl 2):178–181
30. Hoelzer D, Thiel E, Ludwig WD, Löffler H, Büchner T, Freund M, Heil G, Hiddemann W, Maschemeyer G, Volkers B (1992) The German

multicentre trials for treatment of acute lymphoblastic leukemia in adults. Leukemia 6(Suppl 2):175–177

31. Zhang MJ, Hoelzer D, Horowitz MM, Gale RP, Messerer D, Klein JP, Löffler H, Sobocinski KA, Thiel E, Weisdorf DJ (1995) Long-term follow-up of adults with acute lymphoblastic leukemia in first remission treated with chemotherapy or bone marrow transplantation. Ann Intern Med 123:428–431
32. Sebban C, Lepage E, Vernant JP, Gluckman E, Attal M, Reiffers J, Sutton L, Racadot E, Michallet M, Maraninchi D, et al. for the French Group of Therapy of Adult Acute Lymphoblastic Leukemia (1994) Allogeneic bone marrow transplantation in adult acute lymphoblastic leukemia in first complete remission: A comparative study. J Clin Oncol 12:2580–2587
33. Charrin C, Thomas X, Ffrench M, Le QH, Andrieux J, Mozziconacci MJ, La JL, Bilhou-Nabera C, Michaux L, Bernheim A, et al. (2004) A report of the LALA-94 and LALA-SA groups on hypodiploidy with 30 to 39 chromosomes and near-triploidy: 2 possible expressions of a sole entity conferring poor prognosis in adult acute lymphoblastic leukemia (ALL). Blood 104:2444–2451
34. Kiehl MG, Kraut L, Schwerdtfeger R, Hertenstein B, Remberger M, Kroeger N, Stelljes M, Bornhaeuser M, Martin H, Scheid C, et al. (2004) Outcome of allogeneic hematopoietic stem-cell transplantation in adult patients with acute lymphoblastic leukemia: No difference in related compared with unrelated transplant in first complete remission. J Clin Oncol 22:2816–2825
35. Rowe JM, Richards S, Burnett AK, Wiernik PH, Harrison G, Lazarus HM, Franklin IM, Prentice GH, Durrant JI, Tallman MS, et al. (2001) Favorable results of allogeneic bone marrow transplantation (BMT) for adults with Philadelphia (Ph)-chromosome-negative acute lymphoblastic leukemia (ALL) in first complete remission (CR): Results from the International ALL trial (MRC UKALL XII/ECOG E2993). Blood 98:481a
36. Dhedin N, Thomas X, Huguet F, Lhéritier V, Boiron JM, Micléa JM, Vey N, Kuentz M, Charrin C, Boucheix C, et al. for the LALA Group (2002) No superiority of autologous stem cell transplantation over chemotherapy alone in adult Ph-negative ALL in first complete remission: A long follow-up report combining results of LALA 85, 87 and 94 trials. Blood 100(Suppl 1):217a
37. Kantarjian HM, Walters RS, Keating MJ, Smith TL, O'Brien S, Estey EH, Huh YO, Spinolo J, Dicke K, Barlogie B, et al. (1990) Results of the vincristine, doxorubicin, and dexamethasone regimen in adults with standard and high-risk acute lymphocytic leukemia. J Clin Oncol 8:994–1004
38. Boucheix C, David B, Sebban C, Racadot E, Bene MC, Bernard A, Campos L, Jouault H, Sigaux F, Lepage E, et al. for the French Group on Therapy for Adult Acute Lymphoblastic Leukemia (1994) Immunophenotype of adult acute lymphoblastic leukemia, clinical parameters and outcome: An analysis of a prospective trial including 562 tested patients (LALA-87). Blood 84:1603–1612
39. Sebban C, Browman GP, Lepage E, Fiere D (1995) Prognostic value of early response to chemotherapy assessed by the day 15 bone marrow aspiration in adult acute lymphoblastic leukemia: A prospective analysis of 437 cases and its application for designing induction chemotherapy trials. Leuk Res 19:861–868
40. Asnafi V, Buzyn A, Thomas X, Huguet F, Vey N, Boiron JM, Reman O, Cayuela JM, Lhéritier V, Vernant JP, et al. (2005) Impact of TCR status and genotype on outcome in adult T-cell acute lymphoblastic leukemia: A LALA-94 study. Blood 105:3072–3078
41. Huguet F, Pigneux A, Delabesse E, Thomas X, Beldjord K, Escoffre-Barbe M, Harousseau JL, Reman O, Garban F, Buzyn A, et al. for the Group for Reseach on Adult Acute Lymphoblastic Leukemia (GRAALL) (2005) Blood 106(Suppl 1):(abstr 874)
42. Ellison RR, Mick R, Cuttner J, Schiffer CA, Silver RT, Henderson ES, Woliver T, Royston I, Davey FR, Glicksman AS, et al. (1991) The effect of postinduction intensification treatment with cytarabine and daunorubicin in adult acute lymphoblastic leukemia: A prospective randomized clinical trial by Cancer and Leukemia Group B. J Clin Oncol 9:2002–2015
43. Taylor PRA, Reid MM, Bown N, Hamilton PJ, Proctor SJ (1992) Acute lymphoblastic leukemia in patients aged 60 years and over: A population-based study of incidence and outcome. Blood 80:1813–1817
44. Kantarjian HM, O'Brien S, Smith T, Estey EH, Beran M, Preti A, Pierce S, Keating MJ (1994) Acute lymphocytic leukaemia in the elderly: Characteristics and outcome with the vincristine-adriamycin-dexamethasone (VAD) regimen. Br J Haematol 88:94–100
45. Delannoy A, Ferrant A, Bosly A, Chatelain C, Doyen C, Martiat P, Michaux JL, Sokal G (1990) Acute lymphoblastic leukemia in the elderly. Eur J Haematol 45:90–93
46. Delannoy A, Sebban C, Cony-Makhoul P, Cazin B, Cordonnier C, Bouabdallah R, Cahn JY, Dreyfus F, Sadoun A, Vernant JP, et al. (1997) Age-adapted induction treatment of acute lymphoblastic leukemia in the elderly and assessment of maintenance with interferon combined with chemotherapy. A multicentric prospective study in forty patients. Leukemia 11:1429–1434
47. Einheim S, Ost A, Grimfors G, Grander D, Bjorkholm M (1990) Prolonged remission induced by interferon in a patient with refractory T-cell ALL. Lancet i:794–795
48. Ochs J, Brecher ML, Mahoney D, Vega R, Pollock BH, Buchanan GR, Whitehead VM, Ravindranath Y, Freedman AI (1991) Recombinant interferon alfa given before and in combination with standard chemotherapy in children with acute lymphoblastic leukemia in first marrow relapse: A Pediatric Oncology group pilot study. J Clin Oncol 9:777–782
49. Meyers JD, Flournoy N, Sanders JE, McGuffin RW, Newton BA, Fisher LD, Lum LG, Appelbaum FR, Doney K, Sullivan KM, et al. (1987) Prophylactic use of human leukocyte interferon after allogeneic marrow transplantation. Ann Intern Med 107:809–816
50. Diaz MO, Rubin CM, Harden A, Ziemin S, Larson RA, Le Beau MM, Rowley JD (1990) Deletions of interferon genes in acute lymphoblastic leukemia. New Engl J Med 322:77–82
51. Delannoy A, Cazin B, Thomas X, Bouabdallah R, Boiron JM, Huguet F, Straetmans N, Zerazhi H, Vernant JP, Dombret H, et al. (2002) Treatment of acute lymphocytic leukemia in the elderly: An evaluation of vindesine during induction and of interferon alpha given as a single agent after comlete remission. Leuk Lymphoma 43:75–81
52. Thomas X, Olteanu N, Charrin C, Lhéritier V, Magaud JP, Fiere D (2001) Acute lymphoblastic leukemia in the elderly: The Edouard Herriot Hospital experience. Am J Hematol 67:73–83
53. Ottmann OG, Druker BT, Sawyers CL, Goldman JM, Reiffers J, Silver RT, Tura S, Fischer T, Deininger MW, Schiffer CA, et al. (2002) A phase 2 study of imatinib in patients with relapsed or refractory Philadelphia chromosome-positive acute lymphoid leukemias. Blood 100:1965–1971

54. Delannoy A, Lhéritier V, Thomas X, Castaigne S, Rigal-Huguet F, Raffoux E, Garban F, Legrand O, Witz F, Dubruille V, et al. (2005) Treatment of Philadelphia-positive acute lymphocytic leukemia (Ph+ ALL) in the elderly with imatinib mesylate (STI571) and chemotherapy. Blood 106(Suppl 1):(abstr 146)
55. Thomas X, Danala C, Le QH, Sebban C, Troncy J, Charrin C, Lhéritier V, Michallet M, Magaud JP, Fiere D (2001) Long-term follow-up of patients with newly diagnosed adult acute lymphoblastic leukemia: A single institution experience of 378 consecutive patients over a 21-year period. Leukemia 15:1811–1822
56. Boissel N, Auclerc MF, Lhéritier V, Perel Y, Thomas X, Leblanc T, Rousselot P, Cayuela JM, Gabert J, Fegueux N, et al. (2003) Should adolescents with acute lymphoblastic leukemia be treated as old children or young adults? Comparison of the French FRALLE-93 and LALA-94 trials. J Clin Oncol 21:774–780
57. Leikin SL, Brubaker C, Hartmann JR, Murphy ML, Wolff JA, Perrin E (1968) Varying prednisone dosage in remission induction of previously untreated childhood leukemia. Cancer 21:346–351
58. Schwartz CL, Thompson EB, Gelber RD, Young ML, Chilton D, Cohen HJ, Sallan SE (2001) Improved response with higher corticosteroid dose in children with acute lymphoblastic leukemia. J Clin Oncol 19:1040–1046
59. Amylon MD, Shuster J, Pullen J, Berard C, Link MP, Wharam M, Katz J, Yu A, Laver J, Ravindranath Y, et al. (1999) Intensive high-dose asparaginase consolidation improves survival for pediatric patients with T cell acute lymphoblastic leukemia and advanced stage lymphoblastic lymphoma: A Pediatric Oncology Group study. Leukemia 13:335–342
60. Riehm H, Gadner H, Henze G, Kornhuber B, Lampert F, Niethammer D, Reiter A, Schelong G (1990) Results and significance of six randomized trials in four consecutive ALL-BFM studies. Hamatol Bluttransfus 33:439–450
61. Tubergen DG, Gilchrist GS, O'Brien RT, Coccia PF, Sather HN, Waskerwitz MJ, Hammond GD (1993) Improved outcome with delayed intensification for children with acute lymphoblastic leukemia and intermediate presenting features: A Childrens Cancer Group phase III trial. J Clin Oncol 11:527–537
62. Nachman JB, Sather HN, Sensel mg, Trigg ME, Cherlow JM, Lukens JM, Wolff L, Uckun FM, Gaynon PS (1998) Augmented post-induction therapy for children with high-risk acute lymphoblastic leukemia and a slow response to initial therapy. N Engl J Med 338:1663–1671
63. Dombret H, Witz F, de Botton S, Cayuela JM, Delabesse E, Preudhomme C, Huguet-Rigal F, Vekhoff A, Dauriac C, Hayette S, et al. for the Group for Research on Adult Acute Lymphoblastic Leukemia (GRAALL) (2004) Imatinib combined with intensive HAM chemotherapy as consolidation of Philadelphia chromosome-positive acute lymphoblastic leukemia (Ph1-ALL). Preliminary results of the AFR03 phase I/II study. Blood 104(Suppl 1):749a
64. Kantarjian HM, O'Brien S, Smith TL, Cortes J, Giles FJ, Beran M, Pierce S, Huh Y, Andreeff M, Koller C, et al. (2000) Results of treatment with Hyper-CVAD, a dose-intensive regimen, in adult acute lymphocytic leukemia. J Clin Oncol 18:547–561
65. Thomas DA, Faderl S, Cortes J, O'Brien S, Giles FJ, Kornblau SM, Garcia-Manero G, Keating MJ, Andreeff M, Jeha S, et al. (2004) Treatment of Philadelphia chromosome-positive acute lymphocytic leukemia with hyper-CVAD and imatinib mesylate. Blood 103:4396–4407

ALL Therapy: Review of the MD Anderson Program

S. Faderl, D.A. Thomas, Hagop M. Kantarjian

Contents

12.1 Introduction

Prognosis of adult ALL has improved over the last few decades. Following the lead from the pediatric experience, dose-intense multiagent regimens now achieve remission rates exceeding 80% with 5-year survival probabilities of around 40%. In addition, ALL is more and more recognized as a heterogeneous group of diseases. Definition of subgroups based on cytogenetic-molecular markers has important practical implications including better delineation of prognostic groups, design of risk-adapted therapies, and eventually integration of novel agents into existing therapies that target pathways relevant for ALL pathophysiology. The hyper-CVAD program is one example of a regimen that has been successfully patterned after a previous pediatric regimen and that has developed along advances based on better understanding of ALL biology and availability of new drugs with activity in ALL. This article summarizes the rationale for the development of hyper-CVAD, experience with this regimen in adult ALL, and recent modifications and subtype-specific approaches.

12.2 The Hyper-CVAD Regimen in Adult ALL

12.2.1 Development and Treatment Outline

To address the problem of poor prognosis in children with mature B-cell ALL (Burkitt's leukemia/lymphoma), Murphy, et al. developed a short-term dose-intense chemotherapy regimen that consisted of a combination of fractionated cyclophosphamide, followed by vincristine and adriamycin in combination with CNS prophylaxis of intrathecal methotrexate and cytarabine [1]. Following hematologic recovery, patients would receive a second cycle, this time with a noncross-resistant combination of high-dose intravenous methotrexate and cytarabine. This sequence was repeated four times for a total of eight courses. The rationale of the combination was based on the cell cycle characteristics of the rapidly proliferating mature B ALL cells. Given a generation time of the ALL cells of about 25 h and a plasma half-life of cyclophosphamide of around 6 h, fractionation of cyclophosphamide every 12 h would indicate that the leukemic blasts are exposed to the active metabolite at least twice during their doubling time and thus exert a more powerful effect than would be possible with once daily dosing [2, 3]. Of 29 children treated, 27 (93%) achieved complete remission (CR) with an estimated 2-year disease-free survival of 81%. Although highly effective, significant myelosuppression-associated morbidity, as well as renal and neurotoxic complications occurred. Use of hematopoietic growth factor support and additional supportive care measures ameliorated some of these problems and made the regimen adaptable to adult ALL patients.

The Hyper-CVAD regimen follows the principles common to other contemporary adult ALL programs: (1) dose-intense systemic chemotherapy to induce remission quickly followed by an intensified consolidation; (2) prolonged maintenance therapy; (3) effective CNS prophylaxis; and (4) accompanying supportive care measures including hematopoietic growth factors and prophylactic antibiotics [4]. Dose and schedule of hyper-CVAD are summarized in Table 12.1. CNS prophylaxis consists of intrathecal (IT) therapy with alternating methotrexate and cytarabine, the number of IT injections depending on the risk of CNS relapse. Mature B-cell ALL, serum lactate dehydrogenase (LDH) levels, and a high proportion of bone marrow cells in a proliferative state (>14% of cells in S+G2M phase of the cell cycle) have been associated with a higher risk of CNS disease in adults. Those patients with low-risk of CNS disease receive four intrathecal treatments (two IT injections per treatment cycle), those with intermediate risk eight, and those with high-risk disease 16 intrathecal treatments including all patients with mature B-cell ALL.

Maintenance consists of daily 6-mercaptopurine, weekly methotrexate, and monthly pulses of vincristine and prednisone, given over 2–3 years (POMP). Extension of maintenance beyond 3 years has not shown additional benefits, whereas omission of maintenance therapy has been associated with shorter DFS rates [5, 6]. No maintenance therapy is given in mature B-cell ALL; these patients respond well to short-term dose-intense regimens, and relapses beyond the first year in remission are rare. Patients with most other immunophenotypes continue to receive standard POMP maintenance. Differences of current programs for patients with Philadelphia chromosome-positive ALL are outlined in more detail below.

Accompanying supportive care measures include antibiotic prophylaxis and hematopoietic growth factor support. Granulocyte colony-stimulating factor (G-CSF) is administered at 10 mcg/kg/day starting 24 h following completion of chemotherapy and is continued until neutrophil recovery to at least 1×10^9/L. Antibiotic prophylaxis during induction and intensified consolidation consists of a combination of fluoroquinolones, antifungals, and antivirals, and is changed to trimethoprim-sulfamethoxazole and an antiviral drug (e.g., valacyclovir, famciclovir, acyclovir) during maintenance.

Outcome of hyper-CVAD has been reported on 204 adults with newly diagnosed ALL [7]. Median age was 39.5 years and about one third of patients were at least 50 years old. Mature B-cell ALL was diagnosed in 9% and T-cell ALL in 17%. Philadelphia chromosome (Ph)-positive ALL occurred in 16% of patients. CNS disease was demonstrated at the time of diagnosis in 7%. Of 204 patients, 185 (91%) achieved CR. Seven patients (3%) had resistant disease and 12 patients (6%) died during induction. The median time to CR was 21 days with 81% of patients achieving CR following the first course. The estimated median survival was 35 months with a 5-year estimated survival rate of 39%. Younger age was associated with a better outcome: 54% estimated 5-year survival for patients younger than 30 years and 25% for those older than 60 years. Other factors that correlated with poor outcome included Ph-positive disease, thrombocytopenia, hepatomegaly, hyperbilirubinemia, and hypoalbuminemia. Compared with the earlier and less intense VAD (vincristine, adriamycin, dexamethasone) program, CR rate (91% vs. 75%, $p>0.01$) and survival ($p>0.01$) have been superior with hyper-CVAD. Hyper-CVAD has thus been established as an active induction regimen in adult ALL demonstrating superior outcome to previous regimens used at MDACC [8].

12.2.2 Modifications of Hyper-CVAD

A number of issues emerged related to Hyper-CVAD, which were addressed in subsequent modifications of the regimen. These issues included the still higher induction mortality in patients over age 60 years (17% vs. 3% in younger patients), reports that suggested longer disease-free survival with early anthracycline intensification [9], expression of CD20 and impact on outcome, differing CNS relapse rates between low and high risk patients, and occurrence of late relapses following completion of therapy.

To respond to the higher induction mortality in older patients, patients over age 60 are offered to undergo the induction course in a laminar airflow room in which they will remain for the duration of the induction (which is typically about 21 days). CNS prophylaxis re-

Table 12.1. Outline of the hyper-CVAD regimen

Therapy stage	Dose and schedule
Induction and intensified consolidation	Hyper-CVAD (courses 1, 3, 5, and 7) – Cyclosphosphamide 300 mg/m^2 i.v. over 3 h q 12 h for 6 doses on days 1–3 – Mesna 600 mg/m^2 as a continuous i.v. continuous infusion over 24 h daily on days 1–3 (starting with cyclophosphamide and finishing 6 h after the last dose) – Doxorubicin 50 mg/m^2 i.v. continuous infusion over 24 h on day 4 – Vincristine 2 mg i.v. days 4 and 11 – Dexamethasone 40 mg/day days 1–4, and 11–14 Methotrexate (MTX) and high-dose cytarabine (courses 2, 4, 6, and 8) – MTX 200 mg/m^2 i.v. over 2 h followed by 800 mg/m^2 i.v. over 22 h on day 1 – Citrovorum factor rescue 15 mg q 6 h for 8 doses (starting 24 h after completion of MTX) – Cytarabine 3 g/m^2 i.v. over 2 h q 12 h for 4 doses on days 2 and 3 – Methylprednisolone 50 mg i.v. twice daily on days 1–3
CNS prophylaxis	IT MTX 12 mg on day 2 and cytarabine 100 mg on day 7 of each course Low- risk patients: 4 IT (courses 1–2) Standard and unknown-risk patients: 8 IT (courses 1–4) High-risk patients: 16 IT (courses 1–8)
Maintenance therapy	POMP – 6-mercaptopurine 50 mg orally three times per day – MTX 20 mg/m^2 orally weekly – Prednisone 200 mg orally days 1–5 q month – Vincristine 2 mg i.v. q month
Supportive care	– Antibiotic prophylaxis (e.g., levaquin, fluconazole, valacylovir) – Hematopoietic growth factor support during induction and consolidation – Use of laminar air flow rooms (patients ≥60 years of age)

mains a mainstay of the hyper-CVAD regimen. As among 35 patients with "unknown CNS risk" who received eight IT injections none experienced a CNS relapse, and as among 51 patients with low-risk for CNS relapse, the CNS relapse rate was 6%, the number of IT therapies was changed to six for low-risk disease, and eight for all other risk categories except mature B ALL where patients still receive 16 IT treatments. Because of late relapses, maintenance was extended to 3 years. In addition, two intensification courses of hyper-CVAD followed by methotrexate and L-asparaginase, each, at months 6 and 18 of maintenance were added. Thomas, et al. demonstrated that expression of CD20 has been associated with a worse prognosis with both conventional [e.g., vincristine, adriamycin, dexamethasone (VAD)], or intensive ALL therapy (hyper-CVAD) [10]. Of 324 patients with de novo ALL (mature B ALL excluded) and of whom complete flow cytometry data were available, 120 cases (37%) were CD20-positive (defined as >20% expression by flow cytometry). Although remission rates were comparable, 3-year remission duration (28% vs. 58% with hyper-CVAD; $p = 0.02$) and 3-year survival (27% vs. 52%; $p < 0.001$) were significantly worse in the CD20-positive group compared with those patients whose blasts were CD20-negative. Consequently, anti-CD20 therapy (rituximab) was added to those patients whose blasts expressed CD20. The modifications are summarized in Table 12.2. Approaches to specific ALL subsets (Ph-positive and mature B ALL) are detailed below.

Table 12.2. Modifications of hyper-CVAD

Rationale	Modification
Worse prognosis of CD20-positive ALL than CD20-negative disease	Addition of rituximab to hyper-CVAD in CD20-positive patients
Anthracycline intensification reported to be associated with better DFS	Anthracycline intensification following induction course
Ph-positive ALL continues to have poor prognosis	Addition of imatinib to hyper-CVAD and change of maintenance based on continuous exposure to imatinib
Late relapses following completion of therapy	Extension of maintenance from 2 to 3 years with 2 additional courses of hyper-CVAD plus MTX/L-asparaginase on months 6 and 18 of maintenance
CNS prophylaxis	Number of IT injections was changed from 4 for low-risk and 8 for standard-risk patients to 6 IT injections for both groups. High-risk patients receive 8 injections and patients with mature B ALL a total of 16
Improvement of supportive care	Routine use of antibiotic prophylaxis and hematopoietic growth factors. In addition, laminar airflow rooms for patients ≥60 years

In a recent update, 77 patients with newly diagnosed or primary refractory (after one course only) ALL were treated with the modified regimen [11]. Patients with mature B ALL were excluded. Their median age was 40 years with >20% aged ≥60 years. Overall response rate was 98%. Mortality remained higher in patients ≥60 years (6/18) compared to younger patients (2/59). With a median follow up of 17 months, the 2-year DFS rate was 50% overall, and 73% vs. 40% for CD20-positive and CD20-negative ALL, respectively. Although anthracycline intensification did not appear to improve outcome, addition of rituximab in CD20-positive patients may have a favorable impact on prognosis. Longer follow up and more patients are needed to validate this observation.

12.3 Subset-Specific Approaches

Based on cytogenetic-molecular markers and immunophenotypic features, specific approaches are pursued in ALL subsets such as Ph-positive disease and mature B ALL. A summary of a subtype-specific treatment algorithm is presented in Fig. 12.1.

12.3.1 Ph-Positive ALL

Ph-positive ALL remains a distinct poor-prognosis group in ALL [12]. Although remission rates following a standard hyper-CVAD induction are comparable to Ph-negative patients, remissions are brief with median CR durations of 16 months [13]. Imatinib mesylate, a highly active BCR-ABL tyrosine kinase inhibitor, has shown encouraging results in Ph-positive ALL where the response rate was 20% when given as single agent in patients with relapsed and refractory disease [14]. Over the last few years, several combination programs of imatinib with dose-intensive chemotherapy to increase response rates and improve durability of responses in Ph-positive ALL have been investigated [15–19]. Thomas, et al. were the first to combine imatinib with hyper-CVAD [18, 19]. In a recent update, 25 of 26 patients (96%) with active disease at study entry achieved CR at a median time to response of 21 days [19]. Thirteen of the patients were able to proceed with allogeneic stem cell transplant within a median of 3 months from start of therapy. Molecular responses as assessed by RT-PCR for BCR-ABL occurred in 9 of 19 patients. Two-year DFS was 87% with the hyper-CVAD imatinib combination compared with 28% with hyper-CVAD alone. The input of next generation tyrosine kinases (dasatinib, nilotinib) is currently evaluated.

12.3.2 Mature B ALL (Burkitt Leukemia)

Response of mature B-cell ALL to conventional ALL therapy used to be poor, with long-term disease-free survival rates hardly exceeding 10% [20, 21]. Use of dif-

		Pre B				
		CD20 -	CD20 +	Mature B	Ph +	T
Induction/ Consolidation	HCVAD + MTX/AC x 8	✓	✓	✓	✓	✓
	Rituximab		✓	✓[1]	✓[1]	
	Tyrosine kinase inhibitor[3]				✓	
	Mediastinal XRT					✓[2]
Maintenance	POMP x 36 months	✓	✓		(✓)	✓
	Intensification	✓	✓		(✓)	✓
	Imatinib				✓	
CNS	CNS N° of IT inj.					
	Low risk	6	6	16	6	6
	High risk	8	8	16	8	8
MRD	Residual disease				PCR	

Fig. 12.1. Subtype-specific approach to ALL therapy. MTX, methotrexate; AC, cytarabine; POMP, vincristine, prednisone, 6-mercaptopurine, methotrexate; IT inj., intrathecal injections; MRD, minimal residual disease; PCR, polymerase chain reaction. *1* Rituximab is added if CD-positive. *2* mediastinal irradiation is performed if bulky mediastinal mass/adenopathy existed at diagnosis. *3* Imatinib, dasatinib, nilotinib

ferent noncross-resistant agents in tandem and in dose- and schedule-intense regimens such as Hyper-CVAD formed the basis of many contemporary programs with significant improvement in outcome [1, 22, 23]. Complete remissions were attained in >80% of patients; 2-year DFS rates increased to 60–80%. Relapses are rare after the first year in remission. Intensive early prophylactic intrathecal therapy (with or without cranial irradiation), in addition to intensive systemic methotrexate and ara-C, significantly reduced the CNS relapse rate.

In the modified hyper-CVAD program by Thomas, et al., induction courses were administered in the laminar airflow room for patients over age 60 years and rituximab was added for high expression of CD20, which is virtually ubiquitous in mature B ALL [24]. Thirty-one human immunodeficiency virus (HIV)-negative patients with either mature B ALL or Burkitt lymphoma were treated. Median age was 46 years (range 17 to 77 years). A total of eight courses were planned with two IT treatments accompanying each course for a total of 16 IT treatments. Of 23 evaluable patients, the CR rate was 91%. All nine patients over age 60 achieved a complete remission. No induction deaths occurred. Among 17 patients who were followed for at least 1 year, no one relapsed. Compared to a historical control population of 48 patients with mature B ALL who were treated with hyper-CVAD without addition of rituximab, response rates (regardless of age) and 2-year survival rates were superior with the modified hyper-CVAD approach.

Treatment of patients with mature B ALL associated with the acquired immunodeficiency syndrome (AIDS) or HIV remains challenging. Cortes, et al. reported the hyper-CVAD experience in 13 patients [25]. Median age was 43 years (range 32 to 55 years). Nine of the patients received concomitant highly active antiretroviral therapy (HAART). Nine patients were diagnosed with HIV at diagnosis, whereas the remaining four patients had a history of known HIV infection for a median of 37 months prior to the diagnosis of the leukemia/lymphoma. Median absolute CD4 count was 77 cells/μL (range 9 to 544 cell/ L) with only one patient maintaining CD4 counts >200 cells/μL. CR rate was 92%. Median time of survival was 12 months and 48% of patients were still alive at 2 years. Therapy with HAART is an essential component of therapy for mature B ALL. Of seven patients who received HAART from the start of therapy, six were still alive and in CR after a median of 29 months, whereas none of the four patients who didn't receive HAART survived. Toxicities were comparable to that of non-HIV patients with mature B ALL.

12.4 Summary

The developments of dose-intensive, multiagent therapy programs, which were patterned after experience in childhood ALL have created the current standard of approach in adult ALL. Further improvement will depend on dissecting the biologic heterogeneity of ALL further, identifying targets for therapy, and developing novel agents in clinical trials. The goal of these developments remains subtype-specific and risk-adapted therapy, which will eventually improve long-term outcome for adults with ALL.

References

1. Murphy SB, Bowman WP, Abromowitch M, et al. (1986) Results of treatment of advanced-stage Burkitt's lymphoma and B cell (sIg+) acute lymphoblastic leukemia with high-dose fractionated cyclophosphamide and coordinated high-dose methotrexate and cytarabine. J Clin Oncol 4:1732–1739
2. Bagley CM Jr, Bostick FW, DeVita VT Jr (1973) Clinical pharmacology of cyclphosphamide. Cancer Res 33:226–233
3. Iversen OH, Iversen U, Ziegler JL, et al. (1974) Cell kinetics in Burkitt lymphoma. Eur J Cancer 10:155–163
4. Garcia-Manero G, Kantarjian HM (2000) The hyper-CVAD regimen in adult acute lymphocytic leukemia. Hematol Oncol Clin North Am 6:1381–1396
5. Childhood ALL Collaborative Group (1996) Duration and intensity of maintenance chemotherapy in acute lymphoblastic leukaemia: Overview of 42 trials involving 12 000 randomized children. Lancet 347:1783–1788
6. Dekker AW, van't Veer MB, Sizoo W, et al. (1997) Intensive postremission chemotherapy without maintenance therapy in adults with acute lymphoblastic leukemia. Dutch Hemato-Oncology Research Group. J Clin Oncol 15:476–482
7. Kantarjian HM, O'Brien S, Smith TL, et al. (2000) Results of treatment with hyper-CVAD, a dose-intensive regimen, in adult acute lymphocytic leukemia. J Clin Oncol 18:547–561
8. Kantarjian HM, O'Brien S, Smith T, et al. (1994) Acute lymphocytic leukaemia in the elderly: Characteristics and outcome with the vincristine-adriamycin-dexamethasone (VAD) regimen. Br J Haematol 88:94–100
9. Todeschini G, Tecchio C, Meneghini V, et al. (1998) Estimated 6-year event-free survival of 55% in 60 consecutive adult acute lymphoblastic leukemia patients treated with an intensive phase II protocol based on high induction dose of daunorubicin. Leukemia 12:144–149
10. Thomas DA, Cortes J, O'Brien S, et al. (2000) Significance of CD20 positivity in de novo acute lymphocytic leukemia (ALL). Blood 96:109a
11. Thomas DA, Cortes J, Giles F, et al. (2003) Update of the modified hyper-CVAD regimen in newly diagnosed adult acute lymphocytic leukemia (ALL). Blood 102:880a
12. Dombret H, Gabert J, Boiron J-M, et al. (2002) Outcome of treatment in adults with Philadelphia chromosome-positive acute lymphoblastic leukemia – Results of the prospective multicenter LALA-94 trial. Blood 100:2357–2366
13. Faderl S, Kantarjian HM, Thomas DA, et al. (2000) Outcome of Philadelphia chromosome-positive adult acute lymphoblastic leukemia. Leuk Lymphoma 36:263–273
14. Druker BJ, Sawyers CL, Kantarjian H, et al. (2001) Activity of a specific inhibitor of the BCR-ABL tyrosine kinase in the blast crisis of chronic myeloid leukemia and acute lymphoblastic leukemia with the Philadelphia chromosome. N Engl J Med 344:1038–1042
15. Ottmann OG, Druker BJ, Sawyers CL, et al. (2002) A phase 2 study of imatinib in patients with relapsed or refractory Philadelphia chromosome-positive acute lymphoid leukemias. Blood 100:1965–1971
16. Ottmann OG, Wassmann B, Pfeifer H, et al. (2004) Imatinib given concurrently with induction chemotherapy is superior to imatinib subsequent to induction and consolidation in newly diagnosed Philadelphia-positive acute lymphoblastic leukemia (Ph+ALL). Blood 104:197a
17. Towatari M, Yanada M, Usui N, et al. (2004) Combination of intensive chemotherapy and imatinib can rapidly induce high-quality complete remission for a majority of patients with newly diagnosed BCR-ABL-positive acute lymphoblastic leukemia. Blood 104:3507–3512
18. Thomas DA, Faderl S, Cortes J, et al. (2004) Treatment of Philadelphia chromosome-positive acute lymphocytic leukemia with hyper-CVAD and imatinib mesylate. Blood 103:4396–4407
19. Thomas DA, Faderl S, Cortes J, et al. (2004) Update of the Hyper-CVAD and imatinib mesylate regimen in Philadelphia (Ph) positive acute lymphocytic leukemia (ALL). Blood 104:748a
20. Gill PS, Meyer PR, Pavlova Z, et al. (1986) B cell acute lymphoblastic leukemia in adults. Clinical, morphological, and immunologic findings. J Clin Oncol 4:737–743
21. Fenaux P, Bourhuis JH, Ribrag V (2001) Burkitt's acute lymphocytic leukemia (L3 ALL) in adults. Hematol Oncol Clin North Am 15:37–50
22. Patte C, Philip T, Rodary C, et al. (1986) Improved survival rate in children with stage III and stage IV B cell non-Hodgkin's lymphoma and leukemia using multi-agent chemotherapy: Results of a study of 114 children from the French Pediatric Oncology Society. J Clin Oncol 4:1219–1226
23. Reiter A, Schrappe M, Ludwig W-D, et al. (1992) Favorable outcome of B-cell acute lymphoblastic leukemia in childhood: A report of three consecutive studies of the BFM group. Blood 80:2471–2478
24. Thomas DA, Cortes J, Faderl S, et al. (2005) Hyper-CVAD and rituximab therapy in HIV-negative Burkitt (BL) or Burkitt-like (BLL) leukemia/lymphoma and mature B-cell acute lymphocytic leukemia (B-ALL). J Clin Oncol 23(16S):567s
25. Cortes J, Thomas D, Rios A, et al. (2002) Hyperfractionated cyclophosphamide, vincristine, doxorubicin, and dexamethasone and highly active antiretroviral therapy for patients with acquired immunodeficiency syndrome-related Burkitt lymphoma/leukemia. Cancer 94:1492–1499

Treatment of Adult ALL According to Protocols of the German Multicenter Study Group for Adult ALL (GMALL)

Nicola Gökbuget, Renate Arnold, Angelika Böhme, Rainer Fietkau, Matthias Freund, Arnold Ganser, Michael Kneba, Thomas Lipp, Wolf-Dieter Ludwig, Georg Maschmeyer, Dorle Messerer, Harald Rieder, Eckhard Thiel, and Dieter Hoelzer for the German Multicenter Study Group for Adult ALL (GMALL)

Contents

13.1 Introduction

Since 1978 more than 4500 adult ALL patients have been treated according to the protocols of the German Multicenter Study Group for Adult Acute Lymphoblastic Leukemia (GMALL). GMALL protocols are administered in hospitals all over Germany and the number of participating centers in Germany increased from 25 in 1981 to 120 in the most recent trial. Up to now seven consecutive trials for adult de novo ALL have been conducted. The major aim of all trials was the improvement of remission duration and survival of adult ALL patients, detailed diagnostic characterization, the development of prognostic models and the evaluation of risk-adapted, individualized and targeted treatment strategies. The time-periods and further aims of these studies are briefly summarized in Table 13.1.

Several accompanying trials of the GMALL have been initiated in parallel, such as treatment protocols for:

- Elderly patients with ALL and B-ALL
- Ph+ ALL
- B-ALL, Burkitt's Lymphoma, and other high-grade lymphoma
- T-lymphoblastic lymphoma
- Relapsed ALL

These strategies can only partly be described in the following sections.

Table 13.1. Studies of the German Multicenter Study Group for Adult ALL

Studies	Period	Aims	Patients (~)
01/81	1978–1983	Application of a modified pediatric treatment protocol in adult ALL Central diagnosis review (morphology/cytochemistry, immunophenotyping)	384
02/84	1983–1987	Stratification to standard and high-risk patients Intensified consolidation therapy for high-risk patients B-NHL81 protocol for mature B-ALL	569
03/87	1987–1989	High-dose cytarabine/mitoxantrone as consolidation therapy in high-risk patients B-NHL84 protocol for mature B-ALL	350
04/89	1989–1993	Extended central diagnosis review (cytogenetics, molecular genetics) Randomized evaluation of high-dose consolidation therapy in high-risk patients Allogeneic stem cell transplantation in all high-risk patients in CR1	580
05/93	1993–1999	Risk-adapted, intensified consolidation therapy with 3 risk groups Randomized evaluation of conventional vs. intensified maintenance therapy Pilot study for evaluation of minimal residual disease B-NHL90 protocol for mature B-ALL and B-NHL	1200
06/99	1999–2003	Pilot study for GMALL 07/03	830
07/03	2003–ongoing	Shortened and intensified induction therapy Evaluation of a combined risk stratification according to conventional risk factors and MRD Risk-adapted postremission therapy Stem cell transplantation (allogeneic sibling, unrelated, and autologous) in high-risk and very-high-risk patients	680

13.2 Therapy for Younger (15–65 Years) Patients with B-Precursor and T-Lineage ALL

13.2.1 GMALL Trials 01/81–07/03

In the earlier trials (01/81–05/93), an 8-week induction therapy with two phases was scheduled with several minor modifications [1]. All patients received reinduction therapy, and maintenance therapy with methotrexate (M) and 6-mercaptopurine (MP) was scheduled for a total treatment duration of approximately 2 1/2 years. The overall treatment outline of GMALL studies 01/81–07/03 is given in Fig. 13.1.

The results of earlier trials (01/81–04/89) have been summarized previously [1–4]. Major findings referred to identification of new prognostic factors, development of subgroup-specific and risk-adapted regimens, intensified consolidation and maintenance, and extended indications for stem cell transplantation (SCT). In study 03/87 it was shown that postponed (standard risk = SR patients) or omitted (high risk = HR patients) CNS irradiation was associated with inferior overall outcome and a higher rate of CNS relapse [1]. Complete remission (CR) rates, remission duration, and survival improved stepwise with significant differences between subgroups.

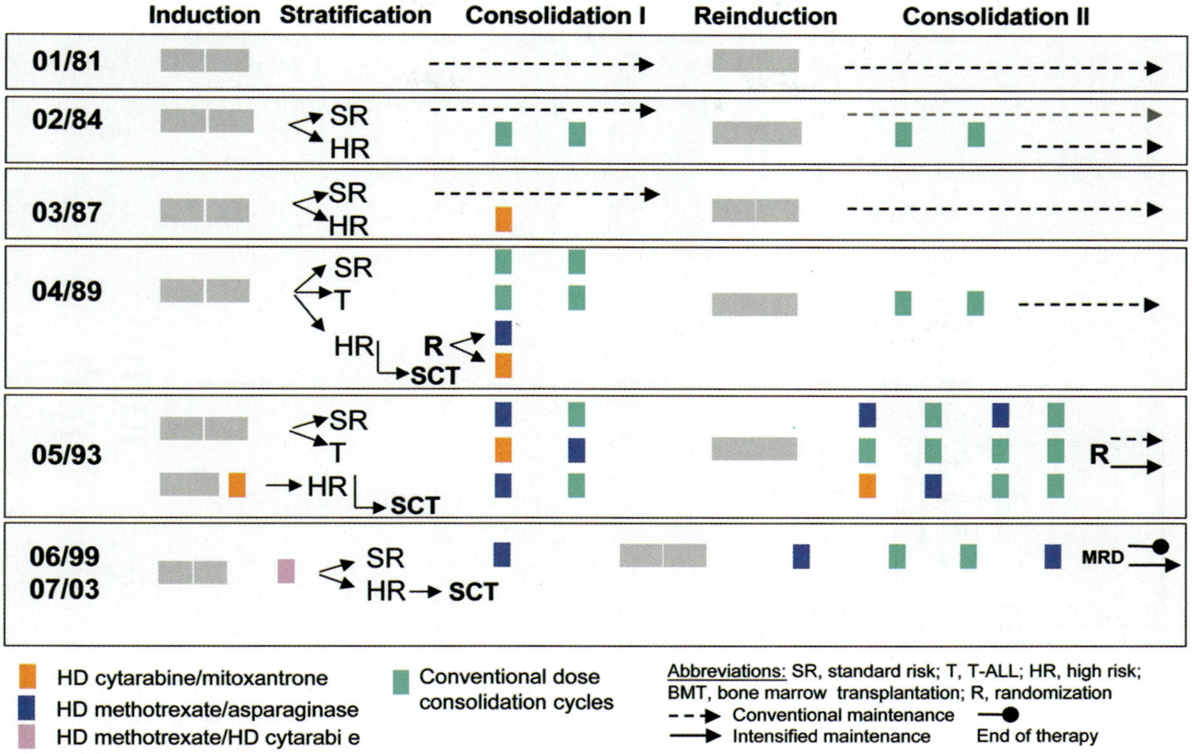

Fig. 13.1. Overview on treatment approaches in seven consecutive GMALL studies. SR, standard risk; T, T-ALL; HR, high risk; BMT, bone marrow transplantation; R, randomization.

13.2.2 Study 05/93

Based on improved knowledge of clinical and biological features as prognostic factors (PF) and specific effectiveness of distinct treatment elements in subtypes of ALL, a subgroup-specific consolidation therapy was initiated in study 05/93. The trial had four treatment arms: (1) SR B-precursor ALL (patients without adverse PF); (2) HR B-precursor ALL (at least one PF); (3) T-ALL; and (4) older patients above 50 years (Elderly) (PFs of the trial are listed in Fig. 13.4). The general principle was to intensify treatment with high-dose methotrexate (HDM) in SR B-lineage ALL, with cyclophosphamide (CP) and cytarabine (AC) in T-ALL, and with HDM and HDAC followed by SCT in HR B-lineage ALL. Furthermore, there was a randomized comparison of intensified versus conventional maintenance therapy in SR and T-ALL.

Twelve hundred patients with a median age of 35 (15–65) years were included. The CR rate was 83% with a range of 70% in older patients to 87% in SR B-lineage ALL (Table 13.2). In T-ALL, immunologic subtypes had a substantial impact on outcome, with a rate of continuous complete remission (CCR) of 63% for thymic, 28% for mature, and 25% for early T-ALL, and ruled out the prognostic impact of WBC and time to CR.

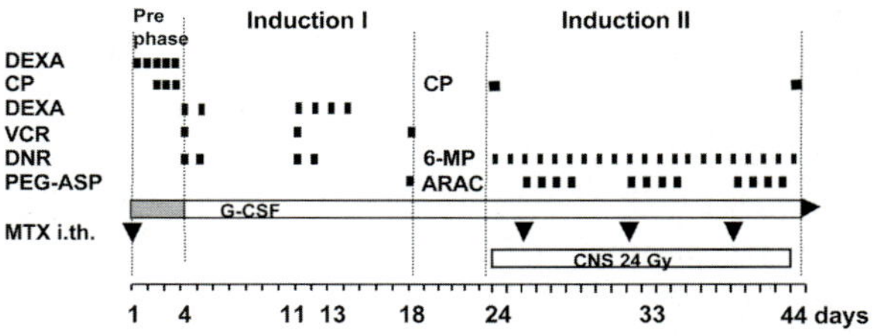

Fig. 13.2. Induction therapy in GMALL Study 07/03. DEXA, dexamethasone; CP, cyclophosphamide; VCR, vincristine; DNR, daunorubicine; PEG-ASP, PEG-L-asparaginase; MTX, methotrexate; i.th., intrathecal; CNS 24 Gy, CNS irradiation; 6-MP, mercaptopurine; ARAC, cytarabine.

Table 13.2. Results of the GMALL Trial 05/93 [5]

	SR	HR	Elderly	T-ALL
Evaluable	291	352	216	304
CR	87%	85%	70%	86%
Early death <56 days	3%	3%	17%	5%
Continuous CR at 5 years (CCR)	47%	27%	16%	51%

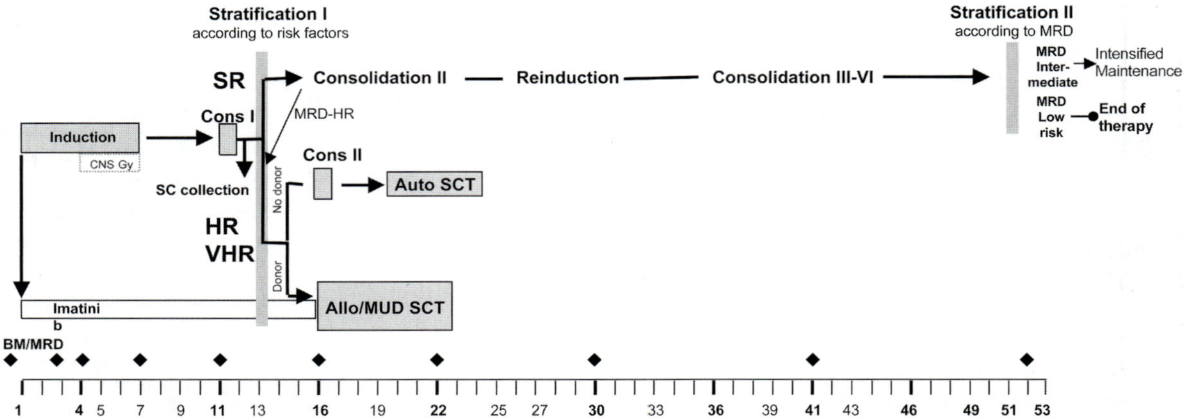

Fig. 13.3. Overall outline of GMALL Trial 07/03. BM, bone marrow evaluation; MRD, evaluation for minimal residual disease; CNS Gy, 24 Gy CNS irradiation; SC, stem cell; SR, standard risk; HR, high risk; VHR, very high risk; SCT, stem cell transplantation; auto, autologous; allo, allogeneic; MUD, matched unrelated.

In SR, high CR and CCR rates were obtained, but relapses occurred continuously up to 6 years. In HR, intensified induction/consolidation did not improve overall CR and CCR with the exception of pro-B-ALL with a reasonable CCR of 41%, whereas CCR was only 19% in other HR patients (WBC late CR as only PF). In Ph+ ALL, CCR improved slightly to 21% at 3 years (9% in study 04/89). This may be due to extended indications for SCT [5]. Based on the results in the ER group (>50 years) the GMALL study group decided to initiate a trial with dose-reduced chemotherapy for older patients (>55–65 years according to biological age).

13.2.3 Study 06/99 and 07/03

The GMALL study 06/99 was initiated as a pilot trial. One major aim was to develop a new, shortened, and intensified induction regimen based on the following new principles compared to previous GMALL trials: (1) Dexamethasone (DEXA) instead of prednisone to improve antileukemic activity and prophylaxis of CNS relapse; (2) prephase with CP; (3) G-CSF parallel to chemotherapy; (4) intensified daunorubicin with two 2-day cycles (DNR) vs. 4 weekly applications; and (5) one dose PEG-L-ASP instead of 14 days conventional ASP. Induction I was followed by GMALL induction phase II as previously reported (Fig. 13.2) and a uniform consolidation I. Thereafter treatment was risk adapted. Patients with HR features and with very HR ALL (Ph+) were transferred to SCT in first CR including allogeneic sibling, matched-unrelated, and autologous SCT. Patients with SR ALL received six consolidation cycles and a reinduction therapy. Maintenance therapy was stratified according to the course of minimal residual disease (MRD) (see below). Figure 13.3 gives an overview on the study design.

Overall, 843 patients with a median age of 36 years were included. The CR rate was 83%, with 12% failure/PR and 7% early death (ED). The CR rate improved after

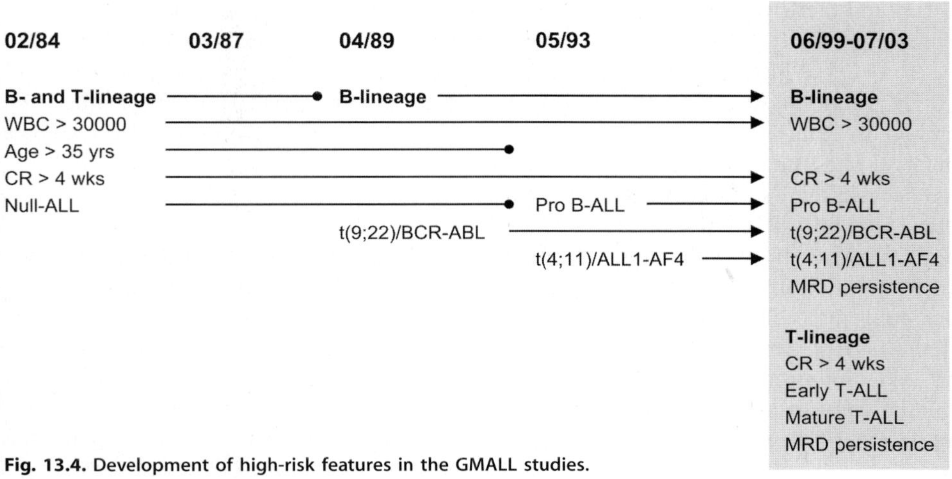

Fig. 13.4. Development of high-risk features in the GMALL studies.

modifications of the DEXA regimen. With lower doses of DEXA, the rate of ED and severe infections decreased significantly. The earlier application of G-CSF during phase I of induction contributed to a significant decrease of grade III/IV granulocytopenias and probably also mucositis [6]. The optimized regimen for induction (Fig. 13.2) was used in the ongoing study 07/03. Interim results confirmed the high antileukemic activity with CR rates of 89% and the feasibility with 4% ED. Beside the optimized induction, the use of Imatinib in Ph+ ALL parallel to induction (see below) contributed to the improvement. Further progress is attempted by additional use of rituximab in CD20-positive patients. The aim of this trial is to improve overall survival (OS) to above 50%, and according to interim results this goal seems to be achievable.

13.2.4 Results of Stem Cell Transplantation

The general principle was to administer allogeneic SCT in CR1 only for HR patients (definition Fig. 13.4) starting with study 04/89. Patients with Ph+ ALL were also eligible for matched, unrelated BMT (starting with study 05/93). Starting with study 06/99 sibling and unrelated SCT were used on an equal footing.

In GMALL study 05/93 survival after SCT in CR1 in HR patients was 34% for sibling (n = 68) and 51% for unrelated donors (n = 31). The most favorable results for sibling SCT were obtained in pro-BALL (59%). In Ph+ ALL, unrelated SCT improved survival (50%) compared to sibling SCT (25%) [7]. Equal survival rates for matched related (45%) or unrelated (42%) SCT in 1st CR were also reported from an overview analysis of nine German SCT centers [8].

In the GMALL study 06/99, also high-risk T-lineage ALL patients were candidates for SCT in CR1. The OS after sibling SCT (n = 50) was 53% and after unrelated SCT (n = 71) 44%. Results of SCT differed significantly between the subgroups ranging from 74% in ProB and 64% in HR-T-ALL to 44% in Ph+ALL and 18% in HR-B-lineage ALL. Thus it could be demonstrated that pro B-ALL and HR T-ALL profit substantially from allogeneic SCT. The results for Ph+ALL were promising and underlined the value of MUD SCT. HR-B-lineage ALL did poorly with chemotherapy alone as well as with SCT [9].

13.3 Therapy of Ph/BCR-ABL-Positive (Ph+) ALL

Treatment of this formerly most unfavorable subtype was revolutionized by the invention of imatinib as the first therapy targeted to the increased tyrosine-kinase (TK) activity induced by the bcr-abl rearrangement. An early phase II trial in relapsed/refractory Ph+ ALL demonstrated a CR rate of 29% [10]. Resistance and relapse developed rapidly in the majority of patients, although a proportion of patients could be transferred to allogeneic SCT [11]. It could be demonstrated furthermore that treatment response was significantly correlated to the quantitative course of BCR-ABL levels in bone marrow and blood [12] and thereby MRD evaluation provided an excellent method for response evaluation.

In younger patients (<55 years), the GMALL group therefore integrated imatinib in front-line therapy of Ph+ ALL – first in the interval after induction therapy. With this schedule, no molecular remissions could be achieved. In the next step imatinib was administered parallel to chemotherapy in phase II of induction. With this schedule, the CR rate increased to 96% and half of the patients achieved molecular remissions [13]. More than 70% of the patients were transferred to SCT, and OS of Ph+ ALL improved significantly. Neither toxicity of chemotherapy nor mortality after SCT increased. Therefore, in the most recent trial imatinib is given parallel to phase I of induction to increase the number of molecular remissions and the risk of resistance.

The application of imatinib after SCT proved to be very promising due to synergisms with graft-versus-leukemia effects. These effects, however, depend on molecular response. The majority of patients, who obtained a molecular remission with SCT and imatinib, achieved a long-term survival, whereas most of the patients who did not respond to imatinib relapsed eventually [14]. In an ongoing trial, the GMALL evaluates now whether prophylactic use of imatinib after SCT is superior to the application in patients with positive MRD status.

In older patients (>55 years), a GMALL pilot trial for elderly ALL showed a very poor response rate in Ph+ ALL (19%) [15]. Therefore, the GMALL group started a randomized trial for elderly Ph+ ALL comparing induction chemotherapy with imatinib only (600 mg) with a dose-reduced chemotherapy induction. After induction all patients received imatinib together with consolidation chemotherapy. The CR rate was 93% for the imatinib induction compared to 54% with chemotherapy. However, LFS and survival were similar in both arms due to a high rate of relapse [16], and only one third of the patients achieved a molecular CR.

Most probably pre-existing or developing resistance to imatinib is a major problem. With gene expression analysis it was demonstrated that resistance to imatinib is associated with a set of 56 differentially expressed genes [17]. A high proportion of patients develop resistance mutations in the TK domain at relapse (90%) and in a considerable proportion these mutations are already present at diagnosis (40%) [18]. These results may help to predict response to imatinib and other TK inhibitors. Also a less genotoxic chemotherapy in combination with imatinib or other TK-inhibitors will be evaluated in the next GMALL studies for Ph+ ALL.

13.4 Studies for Mature B-ALL and High-Grade B-Cell Non-Hodgkin's Lymphomas

Major advances in the treatment of mature B-ALL were achieved by innovative childhood B-ALL studies with short, intensive cycles including high doses of fractionated CP and HDM in combination with conventional drugs. The GMALL study group developed such a regimen in two consecutive trials as described previously. Both protocols were based on six short, intensive and alternating cycles at 21-day intervals (ABABAB) with differences in the dose of HDM (0.5 g/m^2 in study B-NHL83 and 1.5 g/m^2 in study B-NHL86) [19]. A significant improvement with a CR rate of 63% and 74%, respectively, was obtained and the CCR rate increased from 53% in study B-NHL83 to 71% in study B-NHL86 [19].

13.4.1 B-NHL90 Protocol

In the protocol B-NHL90 the dose level for M was doubled to 3 g/m^2 (patients <50 years). The protocol was also opened for patients with Burkitt's lymphoma and other high-grade B-cell NHL. Overall 270 patients were included. The CR-rate was 83% in Burkitt NHL (n=118), 75% in B-ALL (n=89), 70% in B-lymphoblastic lymphoma (n=10), 76% in large cell anaplastic NHL (n=21), and 66% in diffuse large cell B-NHL (n=32) with survival rates of 70, 38, 64, 80, and 61%, respectively. Despite substantial hematoxicity and mucositis, the ED rate of overall 4% (mostly B-ALL: 11%) and death in CR of 3% were low. Higher age had no impact on CCR in Burkitt's NHL. It was concluded that dose intensification for HDM did not lead to a further improvement of outcome in B-ALL. On the other hand, results in Burkitt's NHL were very promising with less toxicity than in B-ALL [20].

13.4.2 B-ALL/NHL 2002 Protocol

More than 80% of patients with mature B-ALL show a CD20-positive phenotype. Therefore, in the subsequent trial two major changes of the protocol were implemented: (1) introduction of rituximab before each of the six chemotherapy cycles followed by two consolidation doses of rituximab, and (2) implementation of a HDAC- and HDM-based cycle C in younger patients (<55 years) changing the schedule to ABCABC. The dose of M was reduced to 1.5 g/m^2. Older patients received a dose-reduced version of the schedule without cycle C.

According to an interim analysis in 53 patients who had completed the first two cycles, CR was achieved after only two cycles (AB) in 10/11 B-ALL patients (91%). In 26 Burkitt's NHL patients, the response rate (15 CR/10 PR) after two cycles was 96%. Fifty out of 53 patients were alive after a median follow-up of 137 days. Rituximab was administered without excess toxicity. The survival rate was improved significantly to approximately 90% in younger patients with B-ALL, in BuNHL, and other B-NHL. In older patients with B-ALL, mortality is not negligible, and more frequent relapses are observed [21]. It was also demonstrated that the protocol is applicable in HIV-positive patients with B-ALL or Burkitt's lymphoma [22]. In the future, the reduction of toxicity, namely mucositis, and further improvement of outcome in older patients with mature B-ALL will be the focus of the study group.

13.5 Prognostic Factors

Central diagnostic review in all patients including morphology/cytochemistry, immunophenotyping, cytogenetics, molecular genetics, and eventually MRD made a major contribution to the identification of prognostic factors in the GMALL studies.

13.5.1 Immunophenotyping

The refined classification according to surface and intracytoplasmatic markers of ALL blasts by flow cytometry contributed to a better characterization of ALL subtypes, their specific clinical and biologic features, and revealed their prognostic relevance [4, 23–25]. In the GMALL, immunophenotype contributes substantially to the prognostic model and also to treatment stratification, e.g., application of rituximab in all CD20-positive patients. In an early paper, prethymic phenotype (cyCD3+, CD2−, sCD3−) was identified as a poor prognostic feature [26] and the unfavorable outcome of mature T-ALL was detected later [5, 27]. Therefore, early and mature T-ALL is now considered a high-risk subgroup and patients are candidates for SCT in first CR. The prognostic relevance of phenotype rules out all other prognostic factors including WBC >100 000/µl.

Similar observations have been made for early B-lineage ALL (also referred to as pro B-ALL, CD10-negative ALL). This subtype was associated with an inferior prognosis in GMALL studies [4]. In study 04/89, an improved outcome was observed for early B-lineage ALL patients treated according to the high-risk protocol with either HDAC consolidation or allogeneic SCT [28]. More recently it was demonstrated that CD10-negative pre-B-ALL has a similarly unfavorable outcome as pro-B-ALL [29].

13.5.2 Cytogenetic and Molecular Analysis

t(9;22) or the corresponding BCR-ABL fusion transcript is the most frequent aberration in adult ALL. In the GMALL trials, initial detection and follow-up for MRD are performed by central laboratories [30], and prospective analysis of MRD has a major impact on treatment decisions. Recently, the presence of a fusion gene NUP214-ABL1 also conferring increased TK activity was also detected in 4% of the T-ALL patients. This may represent a target for therapy with TK-inhibitors [31]. Quantitative analysis of MRD is also established for t(4;11) and the corresponding fusion gene ALL1-AF4 [32].

More recently, the GMALL group has focussed on the application of gene expression analysis in T-ALL. For the GMALL studies, the most important question is whether new adverse prognostic factors can be identified within the favorable subgroup of thymic T-ALL in order to select additional patients who could benefit from SCT in first CR. It was demonstrated that overexpression of the HOX11 oncogene confers a favorable prognosis but is mostly confined to thymic T-ALL. Within thymic T-ALL it did not show prognostic relevance. HOX11L2 overexpression is a rare feature that is observed in 10% of T-ALL cases and identifies within thymic T-ALL patients with poor prognosis [33]. Furthermore, it was demonstrated that high expression of the ETS transcription factor ERG, which has an incidence of 50% within T-ALL, is associated with an inferior survival in T-ALL. The prognostic relevance was confirmed in a multivariate analysis together with immunophenotype (early/mature), presence of HOX11L2 and absence of HOX11. Most importantly, within thymic T-ALL high ERG and HOX11L2 were confirmed as adverse prognostic factors [34]. The overexpression of ERG was then correlated to the overexpression of the BAALC gene, which is present in 25% of adult T-ALL cases. The latter is also correlated with inferior prognosis. The prognostic significance of BAALC increased if combined with ERG. Patients with low BAALC/low ERG had a favorable prognosis compared to an unfavorable prognosis in patients with high BAALC/high ERG [35].

13.5.3 MRD Analysis

The GMALL central laboratory for MRD analysis has demonstrated in a large patient cohort that persistence of MRD above 10^{-4} until week 16 (after consolidation 1), which is observed in 25% of the patients, confers a very poor prognosis with a relapse rate above 90%. On the other hand, there is a small proportion of patients (10%) who decline rapidly below 10^{-4} at day 11 and day 24 (after induction 1). These patients have an excellent prognosis. In the remaining patients the relapse rate was nearly 50% [36].

Thanks to the frequent MRD analyses during first year of therapy, it was possible to identify molecular relapses in patients who had already achieved a molecular remission. If the MRD level increased during the second year to more than 10^{-4}, 89% of the patients relapsed. As a result of this study molecular relapse is treated in the GMALL trials similarly to cytologic relapse and identifies patients for salvage therapy and SCT [37].

Based on these findings, the ongoing GMALL trial 07/2003 comprises a risk stratification based on MRD analysis in patients with SR according to conventional factors. Patients with high level of MRD after consolidation I ($>10^{-4}$) were allocated to a MRD-HR group and to SCT in first CR. Patients with low level of MRD after induction and consolidation I were defined as MRD low risk and received no maintenance therapy. The remaining patients (MRD intermediate risk) with inconclusive course of MRD or technical problems were scheduled for intensified maintenance (Table 13.3).

According to an interim analysis of MRD risk stratification at month 12 in 98 SR patients, the risk groups according to MRD were distributed as follows: MRD-LR 36%, MRD-HR 9%, and MRD-IMR 55%. The major reasons for allocation to MRD-IMR were lack of a second marker (58%), insufficient sensitivity (51%), and inconclusive course of MRD (28%). Most patients in the MRD-IMR group had, however, combinations of several reasons. Further treatment after MRD risk stratification was evaluable in 88 patients. In nearly all MRD-LR patients therapy was stopped. The relapse risk (RR) in this cohort was so far 20–30%. In MRD-HR less than half of the patients could receive SCT. In several cases the relapses occurred shortly after the end of the first year of therapy and before the MRD results were available.

Table 13.3. MRD-based stratification in GMALL study 07/03

MRD risk group	Day 71[a]		Week 16 until week 52[b]
MRD low risk (MRD-LR)	$<10^{-4}$	and	Always $<10^{-4}$ Negative in week 52
MRD high risk (MRD-HR)	$>10^{-4}$	and	$>10^{-4}$
MRD intermediate risk (MRD-IMR)	MRD evaluation not possible Technical prerequisites not fulfilled[c] Inconclusive course of MRD		
Molecular relapse	Increase of MRD above 10^{-4} later than week 16 after previous negative status		

[a] after induction, before first consolidation

[b] during consolidation

[c] Technical prerequisites: At least 2 clone-specific markers, minimum sensitivity of 10^{-4} material from decisive time-points available

Only patients with immediate SCT remained relapse free in the MRD-HR group. In MRD-IMR half of the patients received intensified maintenance. In this group the RR was overall also around 20–30% with lowest RR for intensified maintenance and highest RR for premature stop of therapy. Unexpectedly the MRD-IMR group was large (>50%) partly due to strict quality standards for MRD evaluation as mandatory for a prospective study. Further characterization of this subgroup also by other means e.g. gene profiling is attempted. Overall the interim results demonstrate that the treatment recommendations for the MRD risk groups are reasonable although the relapse rate was higher than expected. Nevertheless the major question is still whether the intermediate risk group can be reduced and whether any type of treatment de-escalation is justified in adult ALL [38].

13.5.4 Development of Risk Models in the GMALL Studies

The risk model for adult ALL first described for study 01/81 [2] was continuously developed in subsequent trials (Fig. 13.4). It is important to note that in the meantime prognostic factors are different for B-precursor and T-ALL and individualized factors such as course of MRD are added. Furthermore, although increasing age is one of the most significant adverse prognostic features, it is not included in the risk stratification. The aim of risk stratification is to identify patients who could benefit from SCT and since outcome of SCT also decreases with age, it is not an adequate feature for this purpose.

13.6 Future Risk Stratification and Treatment Concepts for Adult ALL

Risk and subtype adjusted treatment strategies led in the GMALL studies to considerable improvement of outcome in mature B-ALL, T-ALL and Ph-positive ALL but to a lesser extent in B-precursor ALL. Future concepts will integrate a variety of additional factors thereby resulting in a more complex, flexible and patient specific treatment approach [39]. These approaches include:

- Subgroup adjusted treatment e.g. for mature B-ALL and Burkitt's NHL
- Age adapted treatment e.g. specific protocols for elderly fit, elderly frail and adolescent patients.
- Individualized treatment e.g. according to MRD, drug resistance or TK domain mutations
- Risk adapted indications for SCT
- Targeted therapies e.g. with kinase inhibitors in Ph+ ALL, monoclonal antibodies and other new drugs e.g. subtype specific therapy in T-ALL
- Evaluation of new cytostatic drugs

Beside these sophisticated approaches a better adherence to protocols, support of patients to improve their compliance and documentation of compliance would be warranted. Treatment should be done at experienced centers and closer cooperation between internal medicine and pediatrics including cooperative studies is attempted.

References

1. Gökbuget N, Hoelzer D, Arnold R, et al. (2000) Treatment of adult ALL according to the protocols of the German Multicenter Study Group for Adult ALL (GMALL). Hemat/Oncol Clin North Am 14:1307–1325
2. Hoelzer D, Thiel E, Löffler H, et al. (1984) Intensified therapy in acute lymphoblastic and acute undifferentiated leukemia in adults. Blood 64:38–47
3. Hoelzer D, Thiel E, Ludwig WD, et al. (1993) Follow-up of the first two successive German multicentre trials for adult ALL (01/81 and 02/84). German Adult ALL Study Group. Leukemia 7(Suppl 2):S130–S134
4. Hoelzer D, Thiel E, Löffler H, et al. (1988) Prognostic factors in a multicenter study for treatment of acute lymphoblastic leukemia in adults. Blood 71:123–131
5. Gökbuget N, Arnold R, Buechner TH, et al. (2001) Intensification of induction and consolidation improves only subgroups of adult ALL: Analysis of 1200 patients in GMALL study 05/93. Blood 98:802a(abstr)
6. Gökbuget N, Baur K-H, Beck J, et al. (2005) Dexamethasone dose and schedule significantly influences remission rate and toxicity of induction therapy in adult acute lymphoblastic leukemia (ALL): Results of the GMALL pilot trial 06/99 [abstract]. Blood 106:1832
7. Arnold R, Bunjes D, Ehninger G, et al. (2002) Allogeneic stem cell transplantation from HLA-identical sibling donor in high risk ALL patients is less effective than transplantation from unrelated donors. Blood 100:77a (abstr 279)
8. Kiehl MG, Kraut L, Schwerdtfeger R, et al. (2004) Outcome of allogeneic hematopoietic stem-cell transplantation in adult patients with acute lymphoblastic leukemia: No difference in related compared with unrelated transplant in first complete remission. J Clin Oncol 22:2816–2825

9. Arnold R, Beelen D, Bunjes D, et al. (2003) Phenotype predicts outcome after allogeneic stem cell transplantation in adult high risk ALL patients. Blood 102:(abstr #1719)
10. Ottmann OG, Druker BJ, Sawyers CL, et al. (2002) A phase II study of imatinib mesylate (Glivec) in patients with relapsed or refractory Philadelphia chromosome-positive acute lymphoid leukemias. Blood 100:1965–1971
11. Wassmann B, Pfeifer H, Scheuring U, et al. (2002) Therapy with imatinib mesylate (Glivec) preceding allogeneic stem cell transplantation (SCT) in relapsed or refractory Philadelphia-positive acute lymphoblastic leukemia (Ph+ALL). Leukemia 16:2358–2365
12. Scheuring UJ, Pfeifer H, Wassmann B, et al. (2003) Early minimal residual disease (MRD) analysis during treatment of Philadelphia chromosome/Bcr-Abl-positive acute lymphoblastic leukemia with the Abl-tyrosine kinase inhibitor imatinib (STI571). Blood 101:85–90
13. Wassmann B, Pfeifer H, Gökbuget N, et al. (2006) Alternating versus concurrent schedules of Imatinib and chemotherapy as frontline therapy for Philadelphia-positive acute lymphoblastic leukemia (Ph+ALL). Blood 108:1469–1477
14. Wassmann B, Pfeifer H, Stadler M, et al. (2005) Early molecular response to posttransplantation imatinib determines outcome in MRD+ Philadelphia-positive acute lymphoblastic leukemia (Ph+ ALL). Blood 106:458–463
15. Gökbuget N, de Wit M, Gerhardt A, et al. (2000) Results of a shortened, dose reduced treatment protocol in elderly patients with acute lymphoblastic leukemia (ALL). Blood 96:3104a(abstr)
16. Ottmann OG, Wassmann B, Pfeifer H, et al. (2007) Imatinib compared with chemotherapy as front-line treatment of elderly patients with Philadelphia chromosome-positive acute lymphoblastic leukemia (Ph+ALL). Cancer 109:2068–2076
17. Hofmann WK, de Vos S, Elashoff D, et al. (2002) Relation between resistance of Philadelphia-chromosome-positive acute lymphoblastic leukaemia to the tyrosine kinase inhibitor STI571 and gene-expression profiles: A gene-expression study. Lancet 359: 481–486
18. Pfeifer H, Wassmann B, Pavlova A, et al. (2007) Kinase domain mutations of BCR-ABL frequently precede imatinib-based therapy and give rise to relapse in patients with de novo Philadelphia-positive acute lymphoblastic leukemia (Ph+ ALL). Blood 110:727–734
19. Hoelzer D, Ludwig W-D, Thiel E, et al. (1996) Improved outcome in adult B-cell acute lymphoblastic leukemia. Blood 87:495–508
20. Hoelzer D, Arnold R, Diedrich H, et al. (2002) Successful treatment of Burkitt's NHL and other high-grade NHL according to a protocol for mature B-ALL. Blood 100:159a(abstr 595)
21. Hoelzer D, Baur K-H, Giagounidis A, et al. (2003) Short intensive chemotherapy with rituximab seems successful in Burkitt NHL, mature B-ALL and other high-grade B-NHL. Blood 102:(abstr 236)
22. Hoffmann C, Wolf E, Wyen C, et al. (2006) AIDS-associated Burkitt or Burkitt-like lymphoma: Short intensive polychemotherapy is feasible and effective. Leuk Lymphoma 47:1872–1880
23. Thiel E, Hoelzer D, Dörken B, et al. (1987) Clinical relevance of blast cell phenotype as determined with monoclonal antibodies in acute lymphoblastic leukemia of adults. Haematol Blood Transf 30:95–103
24. Bene MC, Castoldi G, Knapp W, et al. (1995) Proposal for the immunological classification of acute leukemias. Leukemia 9:1783–1786
25. Ludwig WD, Raghavachar A, Thiel E (1994) Immunophenotypic classification of acute lymphoblastic leukemia. Bailliere's Clin Haematol 7(2):235
26. Thiel E, Kranz BR, Raghavachar A, et al. (1989) Prethymic phenotype and genotype of pre-T(CD+/ER–)-cell leukemia and its clinical significance within adult acute lymphoblastic leukemia. Blood 73:1247–1258
27. Hoelzer D, Arnold R, Freund M, et al. (1999) Characteristics, outcome and risk factors in adult T-lineage acute lymphoblastic leukemia (ALL). Blood 94:2926a
28. Ludwig WD (1996) Immunophenotypic features of childhood and adult acute lymphoblastic leukemia (ALL): experience of the German Multicentre Trials ALL-BFM and GMALL. Leuk Lymphoma 13:71
29. Gleissner B, Gökbuget N, Rieder H, et al. (2005) CD10-negative pre-B acute lymphoblastic leukemia (ALL): A distinct high-risk subgroup of adult ALL associated with a high frequency of MLL aberrations. Results of the German Multicenter Trials for Adult ALL (GMALL). Blood 106:4054–4056
30. Gleissner B, Gökbuget N, Bartram CR, et al. (2002) Leading prognostic relevance of the BCR-ABL translocation in adult acute B-lineage lymphoblastic leukemia: A prospective study of the German Multicenter Trial Group and confirmed polymerase chain reaction analysis. Blood 99:1536–1543
31. Burmeister T, Gökbuget N, Reinhardt R, et al. (2006) NUP214-ABL1 in adult T-ALL: The GMALL study group experience. Blood 108:3556–3559
32. Burmeister T, Marschalek R, Schneider B, et al. (2006) Monitoring minimal residual disease by quantification of genomic chromosomal breakpoint sequences in acute leukemias with MLL aberrations. Leukemia 20:451–457
33. Baak U, Burmeister T, Gökbuget N, et al. (2004) Prognostic impact of the expression of the TLX1 (HOX11) and TLX3 (HOX11L2) oncogenes in adult ALL: Experience of the German Multicenter Acute Lymphoblastic Leukemia (GMALL) Therapy Study Group. Session Type: Poster Session 229-I. Blood 104:#1075
34. Baldus CD, Burmeister T, Martus P, et al. (2006) High expression of the ETS transcription factor ERG predicts adverse outcome in acute T-lymphoblastic leukemia in adults. J Clin Oncol 24:4714–4720
35. Baldus CD, Martus P, Burmeister T, et al. (2007) Low ERG and BAALC expression identifies a new subgroup of adult acute T-lymphoblastic leukemia with a highly favorable outcome. J Clin Oncol (accepted)
36. Bruggemann M, Raff T, Flohr T, et al. (2006) Clinical significance of minimal residual disease quantification in adult patients with standard-risk acute lymphoblastic leukemia. Blood 107:1116–1123
37. Raff T, Gökbuget N, Luschen S, et al. (2007) Molecular relapse in adult standard-risk ALL patients detected by prospective MRD monitoring during and after maintenance treatment: Data from the GMALL 06/99 and 07/03 trials. Blood 109:910–915
38. Gökbuget N, Raff R, Brugge-Mann M, et al. (2004) Risk/MRD adapted GMALL trials in adult ALL. Ann Hematol 83(Suppl 1): S129–S131
39. Gökbuget N, Hoelzer D (2006) Treatment of adult acute lymphoblastic leukemia. Hematology Am Soc Hematol Educ Program 1:133–141

Philadelphia Chromosome-Positive Acute Lymphoblastic Leukemia

Olga Sala-Torra, Jerald P. Radich

Contents

14.1 Introduction

The Philadelphia chromosome (Ph) is the shortened chromosome 22 resulting from the reciprocal translocation between 5′ part of the BCR gene from chromosome 22 combines with the 3′ part of the ABL gene, resulting in an chimeric BCR-ABL tyrosine kinase that is constitutively activated and oncogenic. The Ph is the genetic hallmark of chronic myeloid leukemia (CML), and it is also the most frequent cytogenetic abnormality in adult acute lymphoblastic leukemia (Ph+ ALL), where it is present in roughly 25% of cases. The Ph occurs less often in pediatric ALL, with a prevalence of <5%. In both age groups the Ph chromosome describes a subgroup of ALL with a poor prognosis. Thus, patients with Ph+ ALL are usually offered a hematopoietic stem cell transplant if a suitable donor is available. The tyrosine kinase inhibitor, imatinib mesylate, has been found to block the activity of the BCR-ABL tyrosine kinase and has made an impact in the short-term management of Ph+ ALL. Unfortunately the effect of Imatinib monotherapy tends to be short-lived in Ph+ ALL, and it is by no means curative. Therefore, recent approaches are investigating combinations of Imatinib with either other small molecular inhibitors, chemotherapy, and transplant regimens. Although the numbers of patients reported are still small, the results suggest that these combinations using Imatinib with other therapies may improve clinical outcomes for this highly recalcitrant malignancy.

14.2 Molecular Biology of the Ph Chromosome

The most common breakpoints of the BCR and ABL sequences yield two fusion BCR-ABL genes in Ph+ ALL (Fig. 14.1) [1–4]. These two different BCR-ABL variants result from the different breakpoint locations in the BCR gene, while the breakpoint in ABL occurs reliably 5′ to ABL exon 2, except in rare circumstances. The typical 210 kD BCR-ABL fusion protein, found in CML and Ph+ ALL, involves a break in the major breakpoint clus-

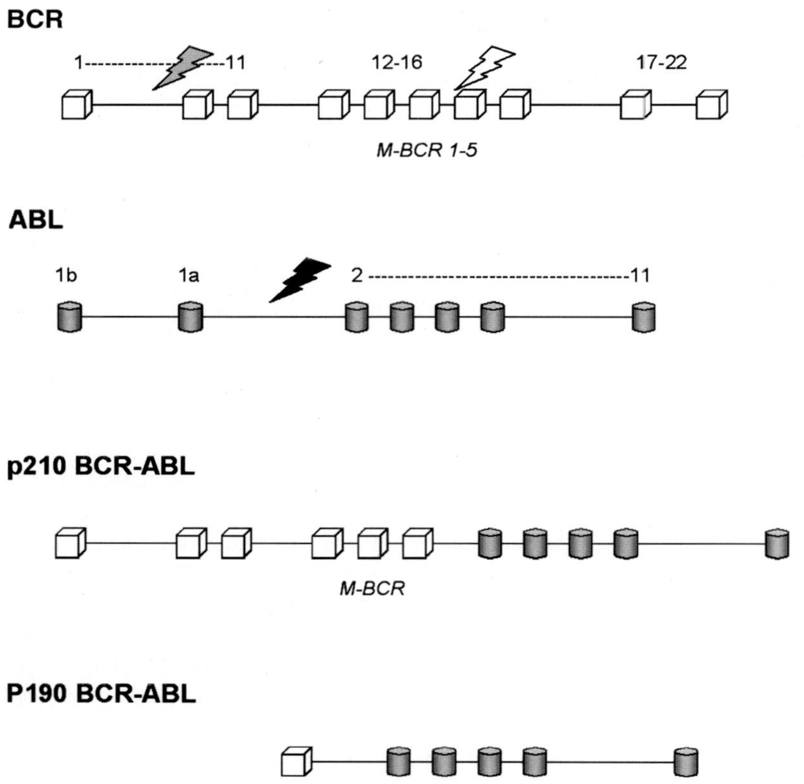

Fig. 14.1. A schematic of the BCR-ABL breakpoint. The p210 BCR-ABL variant (found in both CML and ALL) stems from a breakpoint in the M-BCR region of the BCR gene (*bold*) combining with the downstream domains of ABL exposed after a break between exons 1 and 2. The p190 BCR-ABL (found in ALL) occurs when the BCR break occurs more upstream. *Boxes* and *cylinders* are exons, and the *lines* connecting them are introns.

ter region (M-*bcr*), linking the (5′ upstream domains of the BCR gene to the tyrosine kinase domains of ABL. The alternative BCR-ABL oncoprotein found in Ph+ ALL involves a more proximal break in the BCR gene at the minor breakpoint cluster region (m-bcr). This chimeric mRNA yields a 190 kD BCR-ABL fusion protein, which is often referred to as p190 Ph variant (note that some investigators refer to this fusion protein as "p185").

While conventional cytogenetic evaluation cannot discriminate between the p210 and p190 BCR-ABL forms, molecular biology methods make the determination of the type of BCR-ABL breakpoint straightforward. Polymerase chain reaction- (PCR) based assays accomplish this task [3, 5, 6] by using different oligonucleotide primers specific to the BCR sequences involved in either the p190 or p210 breakpoints. PCR methods also have revealed rare alternative breakpoints utilizing BCR exon 2 (e2) coupled to ABL exon 2 [7], or the use of ABL exon 3 rather than exon 2 [8]. The biological significance of these rare BCR-ABL variants is unknown.

The frequency of BCR-ABL subtypes varies with the lineage of Ph+ leukemia. Thus, CML is almost always associated with p210 BCR-ABL. In pediatric Ph+ ALL, nearly 90% of cases are p190 BCR-ABL, yet in adult ALL approximately 25–50% of cases harbor the p210 BCR-ABL fusion variant. Indeed, the ratio of p210/p190 BCR-ABL may increase by decade of patient age [9]. Also, low and variable amounts of p190 BCR-ABL transcripts can be detected in patients with p210 BCR-ABL [10–12] by RT-PCR assays. This dual transcript expression suggests an mRNA splicing preference resulting in a vast predominance of the p210 BCR-ABL transcript. The mechanisms controlling such splicing processes, and the potential effect on disease activity, are unknown.

14.2.1 Lineage Restriction of the Ph Chromosome

The fact that the same p210 BCR-ABL translocation can be found in both CML and ALL, begs the question whether or not CML lymphoid blast crisis (CML-LBC) and Ph+ ALL are the same, or different, diseases. Since CML is thought to arise in a multipotent "stem cell," the Ph might be expected to be found both in lymphoid blasts and myeloid cells in CML-LBC, whereas ALL arises in a lymphoid restricted progenitor, the Ph might be expected to be found in lymphoid blasts, but not myeloid cells in true Ph+ ALL. Unfortunately, studies of lineage involvement in Ph+ ALL patients have not yielded such a straightforward answer. There are cases described of both p190 and p210 Ph+ ALL lymphoid lineage restricted disease [13–21], in addition to cases showing multilineage [13–17, 20–22]. In addition, cases with convincingly documented CML-LBC have been shown, predictably, to have multilineage involvement [15, 19]. There is a suggestion that Ph+ ALL with involvement of the myeloid lineage has a better outcome than lymphoid-restricted disease [14, 15, 17]. Thus, under the Ph+ ALL term a somewhat heterogeneous group of diseases seem to be included: (1) a lymphoid lineage restricted ALL that can be either p190 or p210, the majority of p190 cases would be included in this group; (2) a "stem cell" ALL with the Ph (either p190 or p210) present in both lymphoid and myeloid lineages, bearing BCR-ABL; and (3) occasionally misclassified CML-LBC, a "stem cell" leukemia with the p210 BCR-ABL variant.

More recent reports argue that the leukemic stem cell (LSC) in p190 ALL originates in the hematopoietic stem cell compartment. This p190 bearing cell has the ability to renew itself, although it appears to be a lymphoid-restricted precursor that does not express B-lineage markers [23, 24]. Moreover, Castor et al. [21] found that in the mouse model system, CD34+CD38-CD19- cells from p210 Ph+ ALL leukemia would not reconstitute NOD-SCID mice with leukemia, while CD19+ precursors could. Thus, while the Ph may arise in progenitors in different stages of differentiation yielding different lineage involvement, the leukemic stem cell with the ability to self perpetuate seems to be lymphoid committed in Ph+ ALL.

14.2.2 The Molecular and Cell Biology of the Ph Chromosome

The abnormal activation of ABL, a result of the chimeric BCR-ABL, has a central role in the transformation of Ph+ leukemic cells. Aberrant expression of the BCR-ABL tyrosine kinase increases proliferation, inhibits apoptosis, and alters cell-adhesion properties. Several animal models have been used in transplantation or transgenic approaches to demonstrate that BCR-ABL activity is sufficient to cause leukemogenesis. Such effects can be demonstrated using either the p210 or p190 BCR-ABL construct. However, the introduction of the p190 or p210 BCR-ABL gene appears to yield somewhat different types of leukemia. Transgenic 190 BCR-ABL mice develop a virulent leukemia that is restricted to the pre-B lymphocytes. These mice typically die of disease early, with 50% mortality by 10 weeks [25, 26]. In contrast, p210 BCR-ABL mice develop B, T, and myeloid leukemias, and have a more chronic disease, with the 50% mortality occurring at approximately 30 weeks [27]. A bone marrow transduction model has been used to place a p210 BCR-ABL retroviral construct in mice [28]. These animals typically developed clonal myeloproliferative disease followed by the onset of acute lymphoma/leukemia similar to blast crisis. The data suggest that p190 BCR-ABL drives a more virulent, lymphoid-biased disease process, whereas p210 BCR-ABL tends to target a disease more resembling CML.

The wild-type ABL protein, a nonreceptor tyrosine kinase, has low enzymatic activity and is predominantly localized to the cytoplasm, with a lower level of presence in the nucleus. BCR-ABL, both p210 and p190, are cytoplasmic in leukemic cell lines reflecting the normal BCR location [29]. It is unclear which of the genetic pathways inappropriately activated by BCR-ABL are necessary for malignant transformation, and whether additional genetic "hits" are required (or if the oncogenic process is different between CML and Ph+ ALL). Thus, pathways involved in cell proliferation, namely the RAS-MAPK, JAK-STAT, and PI3K pathways, are aberrantly activated by BCR-ABL. The anomalous activation of the *RAS* signaling cascade is achieved when BCR-ABL complexes directly with the adaptor protein Grb2, which, when coupled to the *RAS* guanine nucleotide releasing protein SOS, interacts with and activates *RAS* [30]. Stat5 appears to phosphorylated in BCR-ABL cells, though neither Stat5a nor Stat5b appear to be indispensable for the transformation process induced by BCR-ABL, at least in murine models, as lethally irradiated mice deficient for STAT5 a/b and infected with p210 or p190 leukemia develop myeloid and B-cell tumors [31]. The p190 form of BCR-ABL phosphorylates phospholipase gamma, and phosphatidylinositol 3′ kinase [32], that in turn likely activate proliferative pathways. In addition, there is evidence that BCR-ABL acts to inhibit apoptotic pathways [33]. Moreover in CML, BCR-ABL appears to influence adhesion to bone marrow stromal elements, thus releasing immature cells into the periphery, as well as divorcing the cell from adherence-mediated cell cycle control [34, 35]. It is not known whether this occurs in Ph+ ALL.

An interesting observation is the fact that the Src kinases (Lyn, Hck and Fgr), while essential for the induction of B-ALL by BCR-ABL in mouse models, are not required for the induction of CML, and the inhibition of Src kinases independent of the inhibition of BCR-ABL (by CP76030) inhibits the lymphoid transformation [36]. This again reinforces that the leukemogenesis of p190 and p210 ALL and CML may be subtlety but fundamentally different.

14.2.3 The Biology of p190 Versus p210 BCR-ABL

Several differences among the p190 and p210 fusion genes have been described in different biological models. The first characteristic that differentiates both transcripts is the in vitro kinase activity. The kinase activity of the chimeric BCR-ABL protein is higher in p190 BCR-ABL than in the p210 variant (and p210 activity is greater than the rare p230 BCR-ABL variant, caused by a more downstream BCR break) [37, 38]. Li et al. uncovered significant additional differences among the three different BCR-ABL chimeric proteins [38]. The three BCR-ABL types transformed in vitro murine myeloid and lymphoid IL-3 dependent cells, but the transformation of lymphoid cells (BA/F3) with p190 resulted in the highest proliferative rate. Furthermore, in a bone marrow transduction/transplantation system with marrow enriched for myeloid precursor cells (with donors treated with 5-FU), mice transplanted with precursors transduced with any of the three fusion genes developed a CML-like disease. On the other hand, when using untreated-donors, a greater percentage of mice transplanted with p190-transfected marrow developed B-ALL, and they developed it faster than mice transplanted with p210- or p230-transfected marrow. The activation of STAT6, induced by p190 but not by p210, may be involved in the preferred lymphoid transformation by p190 BCR-ABL [39].

In addition, there are some clinical data that suggest that patients with the p190 BCR-ABL do worse than those with p210 after conventional chemotherapy [40]. Different prognostic value of the persistence of minimal residual disease after transplant for the two breakpoints, with p190 BCR-ABL having a worse prognosis [10, 41] also favors that the different transcripts determine somewhat different diseases.

14.3 Treatment of Ph+ ALL

Despite modern chemotherapy regimens having improved the outcome of pediatric and adult ALL in the last decades, the improved results in the aggregate have not translated into an improvement in Ph+ ALL, where treatment with chemotherapy alone still affords dismal survival statistics [42, 43]. Newer strategies incorporating Imatinib appear promising for short-term benefits, but their impact in long-term survival remains to be seen.

14.3.1 Pediatric Ph+ ALL

Childhood ALL is a paradigm of a malignancy curable with chemotherapy alone. However, despite cure rates exceeding 80% with current treatment protocols [44], children with Ph+ ALL (Table 14.1) have an extremely poor prognosis when compared to those with Ph-negative ALL [45–49]. Although most (80–100%) Ph+ ALL patients will obtain an initial complete remission (CR) [42, 45–48, 50–55], their event-free survival (EFS) and overall survival (OS) range from 28–50% and 40–50% at 5 years. More recent studies incorporate related or unrelated allogeneic hematopoietic stem cell transplantations (HSCT) for first CR Ph+ ALL patients, preferring to treat these patients with ablative regimens sooner rather than later [42, 45–48, 54, 56, 57].

Despite the overall poor prognosis in Ph+ ALL, several studies have defined prognostic subgroups among pediatric patients with Ph+ ALL. In a meta-analysis of ten different trials, Arico et al. [42] found that age and initial WBC, included in the Rome/NCI criteria

Table 14.1. Outcomes after chemotherapy in pediatric Ph+ ALL

Ref.	Author	Years	N (%)	CR	EFS/DFS^{years}	HSCT
[49]	Crist, et al.	1981–1989	52 (2%)	78%	–	7 CR1
[53]	Ribeiro, et al.	1984–1994	18 (5%)	72%	20%^{4y}	4 CR1
[51]	Schrappe, et al.	1986–1995	61 (1%)	75%	38%^{4y}	24 CR1
[54]	Forestier, et al.	1986–1997	17 (1.3%)	–	41%^{4y}	6 CR1
[50]	Uckun, et al.	1988–1995	30 (2%)	97%	20%^{4y}	10 CR1
[55]	Hann, et al.	1990–1997	25 (2%)	–	27%^{5y}	--
[48]	Silverman, et al.	1991–1995	6 (1.6%)	100%	50%^{5y}	6 CR1
[46]	Pui, et al.	1994–1998	7 (2.9%)	85.7%	28.6%^{5y}	4 CR1
[42]	Arico, et al.	1986–1996	326 (?)	82%	28%^{5y}	79 CR1
[47]	Arico, et al.	1995–1999	30 (15.2%)	86.6%	46% ^{4y*}	–
[45]	Roy, et al.	1997–2002	42 (2.3%)	86%	52%^{3y}	28 CR1

(%) refers to the % of ALL patients who were Ph positive in the study. Estimates of median survival were made by analysis of the published survival curves, or when possible, directly from the text. HSCT: Indicates number of patients who underwent a transplant in first CR. (–): not reported. * EFS in this study were calculated on 26 patients who achieved CR.

for childhood ALL classification [58, 59], could discriminate Ph+ ALL patients into better (age <10 years, WBC at diagnosis <50 000/μl), intermediate, and worse (WBC at diagnosis >100 000/μl) prognosis groups that demonstrated 5-year DFS rates of 49%, 30%, and 20%, respectively. While secondary cytogenetic abnormalities are relatively common (~60%) in pediatric Ph+ ALL, it is not clear that they have a detrimental influence on outcome [60].

The prognostic value of in vivo steroid response during induction chemotherapy in pediatric ALL patients was initially reported in the ALL-BFM 83 study [61]. "Good" and "poor" responders to an initial 7-day course of prednisone ("good" defined as <1000 peripheral blasts/μl vs. >1000 blasts/μl in poor responders at day 8) had significant differences in their EFS (76% vs. 43%, respectively). Schrappe et al. [51] studied prednisone response in the subgroup of childhood ALL presenting with Ph chromosome. While all good steroid-responsive patients achieved CR after induction, only 30% of poor prednisone-responsive patients obtained a CR, and the probability of EFS after 4 years was more favorable for the good responder group (52% vs. 10%, respectively). In a Cox regression model, poor prednisone response was the only independent risk factor for survival (WBC, age, nonresponse to induction therapy, and coexpression of myeloid markers were not independently associated with outcome). Notably, the prevalence of poor responders among Ph+ ALL children was three times higher than in unselected pediatric ALL patients (32% vs. 10%).

The marrow blast response to induction chemotherapy without steroid use has been used to differentiate two different outcome groups in the ALL 97 trial [45]. The reduction of bone marrow blasts to less than 25% within the first 2 weeks on induction therapy discriminated the good response group (OS 74%, compared to 40% in patients without such a reduction in marrow blast percentage). In addition, a recent publication stratified risk by in vitro drug sensitivity testing and found that patients with resistance to multiple drugs had worse EFS compared to those whose blasts were sensitive in vitro [62].

14.3.2 Adult Ph+ ALL

(Table 14.2). The implementation of more intensive chemotherapy regimens for the treatment of adult ALL, designed after pediatric trials, has resulted in notable improvement of outcomes. These treatment protocols have raised the CR rates for Ph+ ALL to 70–90% [43, 63–67]. Unfortunately, despite these promising CR rates, remissions are short, median overall survivals are measured in months, and treatment options after relapse have little impact in long-term survival [68].

Table 14.2. Outcomes after chemotherapy for adult Ph+ ALL

Ref.	Author	Years	N (%)	CR	EFS/DFS^{year}	HSCT
[69]	Preti, et al.	1980–1993	41 (12%)	56%	–	6 CR1
[64]	Faderl, et al.	1980–1997	67 (13%)	@55%/90%	10%^{3y}	–
[66]	Thomas, et al.	1984–1996	43	64%	–	11 CR1
[65]	Secker-Walker, et al.	1985–1992	40 (11%)	83%	13%^{3y}	11 CR1
[67]	Westbrook, et al.	1987–1990	17 (30%)	71%	–	–
[63]	Annino, et al.	1988–1996	47 (6%)	83%	–	14 CR1
[43]	Gleissner, et al.	1992–1999	175 (37%)	69%	#6%/13%^{3y}	57 CR1
[*84]	Lee, et al.	2000–2003	29	86%	78.1%^{3y}	25 CR1
[*80]	Thomas, et al.	2001–2003	32	96%	87%^{2y}	10 CR1
[*82]	Lee, et al.	2001–2004	20	90%	–	15 CR1
[*83]	Towatari, et al.	2002–2003	24	96%	68%^{1y}	15 CR1

(%) refers to the % of ALL patients who were Ph-positive in the study. HSCT: Indicates number of patients who underwent a transplant in first CR. (-): not reported. (*): Chemotherapy included Imatinib. (@): CR rate for patients treated with Pre-hyper-CVAD chemotherapy (55%)/CR rate for patients treated with hyper-CVAD chemotherapy (90%). (#): 3 years DFS for patients who did not undergo transplant (6%) / patients who underwent transplant (13%).

The prevalence of Ph+ ALL increases with age, and is usually linked with a higher WBC, two factors considered to be associated with worse prognosis in and of themselves [43, 65, 69]. Efforts to classify adult Ph+ ALL into prognostic subgroups in adults have been attempted, as in the pediatric trials, but the studies lack the statistical power of their younger counterparts. Between 65–70% of Ph+ ALL patients present with secondary karyotype aberrations [66, 70–73]. Supernumerary Philadelphia chromosome, monosomy 7, trisomy 8, and del 9p21 have been associated with an inferior prognosis. The GIMEMA 0288 study [63] evaluated the value of prednisone response before induction in a very similar way to the previously mentioned pediatric studies. In adult ALL in general, prednisone response was an independent factor for CR, OS, and DFS. Among 36 patients with Ph+ ALL, 72% were good prednisone responders, and 83% achieved CR. Seven of 36 patients in this study had a initial low WBC and a good prednisone response, and enjoyed a prolonged CR without HSCT. The trial LALA-94 evaluated the value of early response to chemotherapy to predict outcome in adult Ph+ ALL and found that the lack of response to chemotherapy by day 8 predicted a lower likelihood of CR and worse survival [74, 75].

14.3.3 Imatinib-based Therapy of Ph+ ALL

Since the discovery of Imatinib, new options in the treatment of Ph+ leukemia have been embraced. This small molecule, 2-phenylamino pyrimidine, binds competitively to the ATP binding site in the Abl kinase domain and inhibits the phosphorylation of its substrates. Phase I and II [76–78] clinical trials showed Imatinib alone has an effective cytoreduction activity in 60% of patients with relapsed or refractory Ph+ ALL, with 20% of patients achieving complete hematologic responses (that is, normalization of the peripheral blood WBC). However, the relatively short responses achieved with Imatinib as a single agent in these studies (median estimated times to progression and OS were 2.2 and 4.9 months, respectively), have enticed investigators to incorporate this drug in different stages of the treatment of Ph+ ALL in combination with other therapies. Moreover, there is concern with regard to a possible high risk of CNS disease in patients treated with Imatinib alone [79–81] that may reflect the low penetration of the blood/brain barrier by the drug.

Multiple protocols incorporating Imatinib in the chemotherapy-based treatment of Ph+ ALL have been published. A recent study of 20 Ph+ ALL cases combined Imatinib to the hyper-CVAD induction regime (consisting of eight courses of hyper-CVAD alternating with consolidation with high dose methotrexate and Ara-C) and followed by maintenance with Imatinib [80]. Remarkably, CR was achieved in 100% of patients (93% after the first treatment course, compared to the historical rate of 66% with hyper-CVAD alone), including five patients with primary refractory disease. More encouraging, of the 10 patients treated on protocol who were not eligible for subsequent HSCT, five remained in continuous CR with a median follow-up of 20 months, while only two relapsed. The OS and DFS results with the Imatinib/hyper-CVAD regimen appeared superior to the historical results obtained with hyper-CVAD alone [64]. Similarly, Imatinib has been administered in conjunction with Linker-type chemotherapy, yielding CR rates >90% [82, 83].

Imatinib has also been used as a single agent during the interim period between induction chemotherapy and consolidation, and then later between consolidation and HSCT. This strategy achieved a reduction BCR-ABL mRNA of 0.77 and 0.34 logs after each cycle of therapy, and was accompanied by a lower relapse rate (compared to historical controls) in patients during consolidation (4.3 vs. 40.7%); a higher rate of patients proceeded to transplant in first CR (86.2 vs. 51.5%). The DFS after transplant for patients successfully getting to transplant at 3 years was 78% [84, 85].

Imatinib has been used as a treatment for minimal residual disease (MRD) after transplantation in order to abort relapse. In a prospective multicenter trial, 52% of patients became BCR-ABL negative after 1.5 months of treatment with Imatinib. Patients who became PCR negativity early after the initiation of Imatinib had a significantly higher DFS and OS at 1 year than patients who did not become BCR-ABL negative (91% and 100% vs. 23% and 13%, respectively) [86].

The effectiveness of Imatinib alone is limited by the relatively frequent development of resistance [87]. Compared to patients treated for chronic phase CML, the rate of response to Imatinib in Ph+ ALL is not only substantially lower but also much shorter. Progression on Imatinib has been associated with the presence of point mutations (either in the ATP binding domain or the activation loop of Abl) that interferes with Imatinib binding to Abl, or amplification of BCR-ABL [88]. The short time span from response to relapse in Ph+ ALL suggests the pre-existence of a mutated clone that expands under the selective pressure of Imatinib. Indeed, the presence of Abl point mutations affecting the ATP-binding pocket have been described in Imatinib naïve patients [89, 90].

New strategies are being developed to overcome resistance to Imatinib. First of all, as described above, Imatinib is being incorporated in poly-chemotherapy regimens. Secondly, new Abl inhibitors are being developed and tested in clinical trials: AMN 107 has been found to inhibit the proliferation of Imatinib-resistant BCR-ABL expressing cells [91], and BMS-354825 [92], a small molecule that inhibits kinases of the Src family as well as Abl, is able to overcome most of the clinically relevant described mutations. This last compound may be of special interest in Ph+ ALL as Src kinases are involved in the transformation of BCR-ABL induced B-ALL in the murine model. Remarkably, the mutation T315I maintains its resistance to both new Abl inhibitors. Other approaches to overcome resistance include the delivery of Imatinib at a much higher dose to specific cell types therefore overcoming resistance and avoiding nonspecific toxicity. For example, high-dose cell-specific Imatinib distribution may be achieved by engineering Imatinib encapsulated in liposomes that carry antibodies specific for CD19 [93].

14.4 Hematopoietic Stem Cell Transplantation

Given the short remission duration of Ph+ ALL after chemotherapy, allogeneic HSCT is considered the treatment of choice in the setting of a suitable patient and donor (Table 14.3). Results of HSCT are difficult to evaluate and compare given the heterogeneity of transplant regimens, patient cohorts, and merciful rarity of the disease. But it is clear that allogeneic HSCT can achieve a cure in a significant proportion of patients [94]. Reports of autologous HSCT are few [42, 74, 95, 96]. The data suggests that incidence of relapse is higher following autologous transplant when compared to allogeneic HSCT recipients [74]. The factors that are associated most strongly with successful outcome after HSCT are stage of disease (first remission being the most favorable), and the occurrence of graft-versus-host disease [41, 96–101]. In a review of 121 patients from three different French adult and pediatric protocols, Esperou et al. [97] found the disease status at the time of transplant was the only independent factor predictor for survival (estimated OS 4 years for patients undergoing HSCT in first CR 42%, compared to 5% for patients transplanted in more advanced disease stages), consistent with previous reports [101, 102]. The type of donor (HLA matched-related or matched-unrelated) does not

Table 14.3. Outcomes after hematopoietic stem cell transplant

Ref.	Author	Years	N	EFS^{years}	Comments
[94]	Barrett, et al.	1978–1990	67	31%^{2y}	Similar results for CR1 and >CR1
[101]	Snyder, et al.	1984–1997	23	64%^{3y}	All patients studied in CR1
[95]	Dunlop, et al.	1986–1995	19	@26%/22%^{3y}	EFS: 2/9 autologous, 2/11 MRD (12 CR1, 3 CR, 5 RLPS)
[42]	Arico, et al.	1986–1996	38	*65%^{5y}	EFS with autologous transplant: 6/25
[100]	Sierra, et al.	1988–1995	18	49%^{2y}	All matched unrelated donors
[96]	Kroger, et al.	1990–1997	14	38%^{3y}	13 MRD, 6 URD, 5 autologous. DFS for allogeneic transplants in 1st CR 46% at 3y.
[97]	Esperou, et al.	1992–2000	121	–	2 yr OS: 50% for CR1 and 17% for >CR1
[75]	Thomas, et al.	1994–2002	140	**24%^{5y}	75 allogeneic, 65 autologous. 3 year DFS 15% for autografted patients and 34% for allografted

MRD: matched related donor. URD: unrelated donor. (@): 26% 3y DFS for autologous bone marrow transplantation; 22% 3y DFS for allogeneic bone marrow transplantation. (-) Not reported. (*) Estimated EFS in patients treated with HLA-Matched related donor. (**) Reported on 198 patients diagnose with Ph+ ALL and treated on protocol LALA-94.

appear to have a significant effect on outcome, as the higher risks of relapse in the related setting is offset by problems with GVHD in the unrelated setting [41].

14.5 The Detection of Minimal Residual Disease

As noted above, disease burden at the time of transplant has a strong impact on survival. This effect is also evident when looking at more subtle levels of disease that can be detected by sensitive methods of MRD detection (especially RT-PCR assays for BCR-ABL). Thus, the detection of MRD after induction and consolidation therapy is fairly common in Ph+ ALL, and is associated with an increase risk of relapse [103–105]. By using quantitative RT-PCR for BCR-ABL, Pane et al. [104] found that patients who achieved >3 log reduction after consolidation had a significantly better DFS and OS. Moreover, analysis of the MRD during the phase II Imatinib studies showed that the kinetics in the reduction in the number BCR-ABL predicted the group of "good responders" with a longer time to progression [106]. Furthermore, high levels of MRD at diagnosis, and an increase in the level of MRD ≥2 logs predicted patients at a high risk of relapse [107].

MRD after HSCT also predicts relapse. Unlike the chemotherapy setting, a significant percentage of patients who undergo allogeneic HSCT become BCR-ABL negative after transplant. The detection of MRD by RT-PCR correlates strongly with subsequent relapse, usually within 3 months; the risk seems to be higher for patients with the p190 BCR-ABL transcript compared to the p210 variant [10, 41, 98, 103, 105, 108, 109]. Moreover, the MRD status prior to transplant has been shown to be significantly predictive of EFS [41, 74, 110].

14.6 Conclusion

Despite advances in conventional chemotherapy and targeted therapy, Ph+ ALL continues to be a very poor prognostic variable in adult and pediatric ALL. A better understanding of the molecular biology of BCR-ABL may lead to advances in more active targeted therapies, but for now, the only curative modality remains stem cell transplantation. As advances in this modality increase, the likelihood of potential cures with transplantation combined with novel targeted therapy likely looms at the best strategy for curative therapy.

References

1. Rubin CM, Carrino JJ, Dickler MN, Leibowitz D, Smith SD, Westbrook CA (1988) Heterogeneity of genomic fusion of BCR and ABL in Philadelphia chromosome-positive acute lymphoblastic leukemia. Proc Natl Acad Sci 85(8):2795–2799

2. Kurzrock R, Shtalrid M, Gutterman JU, Koller CA, Walters R, Trujillo JM, et al. (1987) Molecular analysis of chromosome 22 breakpoints in adult Philadelphia-positive acute lymphoblastic leukaemia. Br J Haematol 67(1):55–59
3. Hooberman AL, Carrino JJ, Leibowitz D, Rowley JD, Le Beau MM, Arlin ZA, et al. (1989) Unexpected heterogeneity of BCR-ABL fusion mRNA detected by polymerase chain reaction in Philadelphia chromosome-positive acute lymphoblastic leukemia. Proc Natl Acad Sci 86(11):4259–4263
4. Hermans A, Heisterkamp N, von Linden M, van Baal S, Meijer D, van der Plas D, et al. (1987) Unique fusion of bcr and c-abl genes in Philadelphia chromosome positive acute lymphoblastic leukemia. Cell 51(1):33–40
5. Gehly GB, Bryant EM, Lee AM, Kidd PG, Thomas ED (1991) Chimeric BCR-abl messenger RNA as a marker for minimal residual disease in patients transplanted for Philadelphia chromosome-positive acute lymphoblastic leukemia. Blood 78(2):458–465
6. Maurer J, Kinzel H, Nentwig T, Thiel E (1990) Molecular diagnosis of the Philadelphia chromosome in chronic myelogenous and acute lymphoblastic leukemias by PCR. Dis Markers 8(4):211–218
7. Okamoto K, Karasawa M, Sakai H, Ogura H, Morita K, Naruse T (1997) A novel acute lymphoid leukaemia type BCR/ABL transcript in chronic myelogenous leukaemia. Br J Haematol 96(3):611–613
8. Inukai T, Sugita K, Suzuki T, Ijima K, Goi K, Tezuka T, et al. (1993) A novel 203 kD aberrant BCR-ABL product in a girl with Philadelphia chromosome positive acute lymphoblastic leukaemia. Br J Haematol 85(4):823–825
9. Secker-Walker LM, Craig JM, Hawkins JM, Hoffbrand AV (1991) Philadelphia positive acute lymphoblastic leukemia in adults: Age distribution, BCR breakpoint and prognostic significance. Leukemia 5(3):196–199
10. Radich J, Gehly G, Lee A, Avery R, Bryant E, Edmands S, et al. (1997) Detection of bcr-abl transcripts in Philadelphia chromosome-positive acute lymphoblastic leukemia after marrow transplantation. Blood 89(7):2602–2609
11. Saglio G, Pane F, Gottardi E, Frigeri F, Buonaiuto MR, Guerrasio A, et al. (1996) Consistent amounts of acute leukemia-associated P190BCR/ABL transcripts are expressed by chronic myelogenous leukemia patients at diagnosis. Blood 87(3):1075–1080
12. Lichty BD, Keating A, Callum J, Yee K, Croxford R, Corpus G, et al. (1998) Expression of p210 and p190 BCR-ABL due to alternative splicing in chronic myelogenous leukaemia. Br J Haematol 103(3):711–715
13. Secker-Walker LM, Cooke HM, Browett PJ, Shippey CA, Norton JD, Coustan-Smith E, et al. (1988) Variable Philadelphia breakpoints and potential lineage restriction of bcr rearrangement in acute lymphoblastic leukemia. Blood 72(2):784–791
14. Haferlach T, Winkemann M, Ramm-Petersen L, Meeder M, Schoch R, Weber-Matthiesen K, et al. (1997) New insights into the biology of Philadelphia-chromosome-positive acute lymphoblastic leukaemia using a combination of May-Grunwald-Giemsa staining and fluorescence in situ hybridization techniques at the single cell level. Br J Haematol 99(2):452–459
15. Anastasi J, Feng J, Dickstein JI, Le Beau MM, Rubin CM, Larson RA, et al. (1996) Lineage involvement by BCR/ABL in Ph+ lymphoblastic leukemias: Chronic myelogenous leukemia presenting in lymphoid blast vs Ph+ acute lymphoblastic leukemia. Leukemia 10(5):795–802
16. Estrov Z, Talpaz M, Kantarjian HM, Zipf TF, McClain KL, Kurzrock R (1993) Heterogeneity in lineage derivation of Philadelphia-positive acute lymphoblastic leukemia expressing p190BCR-ABL or p210BCR-ABL: Determination by analysis of individual colonies with the polymerase chain reaction. Cancer Res 53(14):3289–3293
17. Secker-Walker LM, Craig JM (1993) Prognostic implications of breakpoint and lineage heterogeneity in Philadelphia-positive acute lymphoblastic leukemia: A review. Leukemia 7(2):147–151
18. Craig JM, Hawkins JM, Yamada T, Ganeshaguru K, Mehta AB, Secker-Walker LM (1990) First intron and M-bcr breakpoints are restricted to the lymphoid lineage in Philadelphia positive acute lymphoblastic leukemia. Leukemia 4(10):678–681
19. Pajor L, Vass JA, Kereskai L, Kajtar P, Szomor A, Egyed M, et al. (2000) The existence of lymphoid lineage restricted Philadelphia chromosome-positive acute lymphoblastic leukemia with heterogeneous bcr-abl rearrangement. Leukemia 14(6):1122–1126
20. Kasprzyk A, Harrison CJ, Secker-Walker LM (1999) Investigation of clonal involvement of myeloid cells in Philadelphia-positive and high hyperdiploid acute lymphoblastic leukemia. Leukemia 13(12):2000–2006
21. Castor A, Nilsson L, Astrand-Grundstrom I, Buitenhuis M, Ramirez C, Anderson K, et al. (2005) Distinct patterns of hematopoietic stem cell involvement in acute lymphoblastic leukemia. Nat Med 11(6):630–637
22. Schenk TM, Keyhani A, Bottcher S, Kliche KO, Goodacre A, Guo JQ, et al. (1998) Multilineage involvement of Philadelphia chromosome positive acute lymphoblastic leukemia. Leukemia 12(5): 666–674
23. Cobaleda C, Gutierrez-Cianca N, Perez-Losada J, Flores T, Garcia-Sanz R, Gonzalez M, et al. (2000) A primitive hematopoietic cell is the target for the leukemic transformation in human philadelphia-positive acute lymphoblastic leukemia. Blood 95(3): 1007–1013
24. Hotfilder M, Rottgers S, Rosemann A, Schrauder A, Schrappe M, Pieters R, et al. (2005) Leukemic stem cells in childhood high-risk ALL/t(9;22) and t(4;11) are present in primitive lymphoid-restricted CD34+CD19- cells. Cancer Res 65(4):1442–1449
25. Voncken JW, Morris C, Pattengale P, Dennert G, Kikly C, Groffen J, et al. (1992) Clonal development and karyotype evolution during leukemogenesis of BCR/ABL transgenic mice. Blood 79(4):1029–1036
26. Heisterkamp N, Jenster G, ten Hoeve J, Zovich D, Pattengale PK, Groffen J (1990) Acute leukaemia in bcr/abl transgenic mice. Nature 344(6263):251–253
27. Voncken JW, Kaartinen V, Pattengale PK, Germeraad WT, Groffen J, Heisterkamp N (1995) BCR/ABL P210 and P190 cause distinct leukemia in transgenic mice. Blood 86(12):4603–4611
28. Pear WS, Miller JP, Xu L, Pui JC, Soffer B, Quackenbush RC, et al. (1998) Efficient and rapid induction of a chronic myelogenous leukemia-like myeloproliferative disease in mice receiving P210 bcr/abl-transduced bone marrow. Blood 92(10):3780–3792
29. Wetzler M, Talpaz M, Van Etten RA, Hirsh-Ginsberg C, Beran M, Kurzrock R (1993) Subcellular localization of Bcr, Abl, and Bcr-Abl proteins in normal and leukemic cells and correlation of expression with myeloid differentiation. J Clin Invest 92(4):1925–1939

30. Puil L, Liu J, Gish G, Mbamalu G, Bowtell D, Pelicci PG, et al. (1994) Bcr-Abl oncoproteins bind directly to activators of the Ras signalling pathway. EMBO J 13(4):764–773
31. Sexl V, Piekorz R, Moriggl R, Rohrer J, Brown MP, Bunting KD, et al. (2000) Stat5a/b contribute to interleukin 7-induced B-cell precursor expansion, but abl- and bcr/abl-induced transformation are independent of stat5. Blood 96(6):2277–2283
32. Gotoh A, Miyazawa K, Ohyashiki K, Toyama K (1994) Potential molecules implicated in downstream signaling pathways of p185BCR-ABL in Ph+ ALL involve GTPase-activating protein, phospholipase C-gamma 1, and phosphatidylinositol 3′-kinase. Leukemia 8(1):115–120
33. Amarante-Mendes GP, Naekyung Kim C, Liu L, Huang Y, Perkins CL, Green DR, et al. (1998) Bcr-Abl exerts its antiapoptotic effect against diverse apoptotic stimuli through blockage of mitochondrial release of cytochrome C and activation of caspase-3. Blood 91(5):1700–1705
34. Lewis JM, Baskaran R, Taagepera S, Schwartz MA, Wang JY (1996) Integrin regulation of c-Abl tyrosine kinase activity and cytoplasmic-nuclear transport. Proc Natl Acad Sci 93(26): 15174–15179
35. Verfaillie CM, Hurley R, Zhao RC, Prosper F, Delforge M, Bhatia R (1997) Pathophysiology of CML: Do defects in integrin function contribute to the premature circulation and massive expansion of the BCR/ABL positive clone? J Lab Clin Med 129(6):584–591
36. Hu Y, Liu Y, Pelletier S, Buchdunger E, Warmuth M, Fabbro D, et al. (2004) Requirement of Src kinases Lyn, Hck and Fgr for BCR-ABL1-induced B-lymphoblastic leukemia but not chronic myeloid leukemia. Nat Genet 36(5):453–461
37. Lugo TG, Pendergast AM, Muller AJ, Witte ON (1990) Tyrosine kinase activity and transformation potency of bcr-abl oncogene products. Science 247(4946):1079–1082
38. Li S, Ilaria RL, Jr., Million RP, Daley GQ, Van Etten RA (1999) The P190, P210, and P230forms of the BCR/ABL oncogene induce a similar chronic myeloid leukemia-like syndrome in mice but have different lymphoid leukemogenic activity. J Exp Med 189(9):1399–1412
39. Ilaria RL, Jr, Van Etten RA (1996) P210 and P190(BCR/ABL) induce the tyrosine phosphorylation and DNA binding activity of multiple specific STAT family members. J Biol Chem 271(49):31704–31710
40. Radich JP, Kopecky KJ, Boldt DH, Head D, Slovak ML, Babu R, et al. (1994) Detection of BCR-ABL fusion genes in adult acute lymphoblastic leukemia by the polymerase chain reaction. Leukemia 8(10):1688–1695
41. Stirewalt DL, Guthrie KA, Beppu L, Bryant EM, Doney K, Gooley T, et al. (2003) Predictors of relapse and overall survival in Philadelphia chromosome-positive acute lymphoblastic leukemia after transplantation. Biol Blood Marrow Transplant 9(3):206–212
42. Arico M, Valsecchi MG, Camitta B, Schrappe M, Chessells J, Baruchel A, et al. (2000) Outcome of treatment in children with Philadelphia chromosome-positive acute lymphoblastic leukemia. N Engl J Med 342(14):998–1006
43. Gleissner B, Gokbuget N, Bartram CR, Janssen B, Rieder H, Janssen JW, et al. (2002) Leading prognostic relevance of the BCR-ABL translocation in adult acute B-lineage lymphoblastic leukemia: A prospective study of the German Multicenter Trial Group and confirmed polymerase chain reaction analysis. Blood 99(5): 1536–1543
44. Pui CH, Relling MV, Downing JR (2004) Acute lymphoblastic leukemia. N Engl J Med 350(15):1535–1548
45. Roy A, Bradburn M, Moorman AV, Burrett J, Love S, Kinsey SE, et al. (2005) Early response to induction is predictive of survival in childhood Philadelphia chromosome positive acute lymphoblastic leukaemia: Results of the Medical Research Council ALL 97 trial. Br J Haematol 129(1):35–44
46. Pui CH, Sandlund JT, Pei D, Campana D, Rivera GK, Ribeiro RC, et al. (2004) Improved outcome for children with acute lymphoblastic leukemia: Results of Total Therapy Study XIIIB at St Jude Children's Research Hospital. Blood 104(9):2690–2696
47. Arico M, Valsecchi MG, Conter V, Rizzari C, Pession A, Messina C, et al. (2002) Improved outcome in high-risk childhood acute lymphoblastic leukemia defined by prednisone-poor response treated with double Berlin-Frankfurt-Muenster protocol II. Blood 100(2):420–426
48. Silverman LB, Gelber RD, Dalton VK, Asselin BL, Barr RD, Clavell LA, et al. (2001) Improved outcome for children with acute lymphoblastic leukemia: Results of Dana-Farber Consortium Protocol 91-01. Blood 97(5):1211–1218
49. Crist W, Carroll A, Shuster J, Jackson J, Head D, Borowitz M, et al. (1990) Philadelphia chromosome positive childhood acute lymphoblastic leukemia: Clinical and cytogenetic characteristics and treatment outcome. A Pediatric Oncology Group study. Blood 76(3):489–494
50. Uckun FM, Nachman JB, Sather HN, Sensel MG, Kraft P, Steinherz PG, et al. (1998) Clinical significance of Philadelphia chromosome positive pediatric acute lymphoblastic leukemia in the context of contemporary intensive therapies: A report from the Children's Cancer Group. Cancer 83(9):2030–2039
51. Schrappe M, Arico M, Harbott J, Biondi A, Zimmermann M, Conter V, et al. (1998) Philadelphia chromosome-positive (Ph+) childhood acute lymphoblastic leukemia: Good initial steroid response allows early prediction of a favorable treatment outcome. Blood 92(8):2730–2741
52. Schlieben S, Borkhardt A, Reinisch I, Ritterbach J, Janssen JW, Ratei R, et al. (1996) Incidence and clinical outcome of children with BCR/ABL-positive acute lymphoblastic leukemia (ALL). A prospective RT-PCR study based on 673 patients enrolled in the German pediatric multicenter therapy trials ALL-BFM-90 and CoALL-05-92. Leukemia 10(6):957–963
53. Ribeiro RC, Broniscer A, Rivera GK, Hancock ML, Raimondi SC, Sandlund JT, et al. (1997) Philadelphia chromosome-positive acute lymphoblastic leukemia in children: Durable responses to chemotherapy associated with low initial white blood cell counts. Leukemia 11(9):1493–1496
54. Forestier E, Johansson B, Gustafsson G, Borgstrom G, Kerndrup G, Johannsson J, et al. (2000) Prognostic impact of karyotypic findings in childhood acute lymphoblastic leukaemia: A Nordic series comparing two treatment periods. For the Nordic Society of Paediatric Haematology and Oncology (NOPHO) Leukaemia Cytogenetic Study Group. Br J Haematol 110(1):147–153
55. Hann I, Vora A, Harrison G, Harrison C, Eden O, Hill F, et al. (2001) Determinants of outcome after intensified therapy of childhood lymphoblastic leukaemia: Results from Medical Research Council United Kingdom acute lymphoblastic leukaemia XI protocol. Br J Haematol 113(1):103–114

56. Mori T, Manabe A, Tsuchida M, Hanada R, Yabe H, Ohara A, et al. (2001) Allogeneic bone marrow transplantation in first remission rescues children with Philadelphia chromosome-positive acute lymphoblastic leukemia: Tokyo Children's Cancer Study Group (TCCSG) studies L89-12 and L92-13. Med Pediatr Oncol 37(5):426–431
57. Sharathkumar A, Saunders EF, Dror Y, Grant R, Greenberg M, Weitzman S, et al. (2004) Allogeneic bone marrow transplantation vs. chemotherapy for children with Philadelphia chromosome-positive acute lymphoblastic leukemia. Bone Marrow Transplant 33(1):39–45
58. Mastrangelo R, Poplack D, Bleyer A, Riccardi R, Sather H, D'Angio G (1986) Report and recommendations of the Rome workshop concerning poor-prognosis acute lymphoblastic leukemia in children: Biologic bases for staging, stratification, and treatment. Med Pediatr Oncol 14(3):191–194
59. Smith M, Arthur D, Camitta B, Carroll AJ, Crist W, Gaynon P, et al. (1996) Uniform approach to risk classification and treatment assignment for children with acute lymphoblastic leukemia. J Clin Oncol 14(1):18–24
60. Heerema NA, Harbott J, Galimberti S, Camitta BM, Gaynon PS, Janka-Schaub G, et al. (2004) Secondary cytogenetic aberrations in childhood Philadelphia chromosome positive acute lymphoblastic leukemia are nonrandom and may be associated with outcome. Leukemia 18(4):693–702
61. Riehm H, Reiter A, Schrappe M, Berthold F, Dopfer R, Gerein V, et al. (1987) [Corticosteroid-dependent reduction of leukocyte count in blood as a prognostic factor in acute lymphoblastic leukemia in childhood (therapy study ALL-BFM 83)]. Klin Padiatr 199(3):151–160
62. Hongo T, Okada S, Inoue N, Yamada S, Yajima S, Watanabe C, et al. (2002) Two groups of Philadelphia chromosome-positive childhood acute lymphoblastic leukemia classified by pretreatment multidrug sensitivity or resistance in in vitro testing. Int J Hematol 76(3):251–259
63. Annino L, Vegna ML, Camera A, Specchia G, Visani G, Fioritoni G, et al. (2002) Treatment of adult acute lymphoblastic leukemia (ALL): Long-term follow-up of the GIMEMA ALL 0288 randomized study. Blood 99(3):863–871
64. Faderl S, Kantarjian HM, Thomas DA, Cortes J, Giles F, Pierce S, et al. (2000) Outcome of Philadelphia chromosome-positive adult acute lymphoblastic leukemia. Leuk Lymphoma 36(3-4):263–273
65. Secker-Walker LM, Prentice HG, Durrant J, Richards S, Hall E, Harrison G (1997) Cytogenetics adds independent prognostic information in adults with acute lymphoblastic leukaemia on MRC trial UKALL XA. MRC Adult Leukaemia Working Party. Br J Haematol 96(3):601–610
66. Thomas X, Thiebaut A, Olteanu N, Danaila C, Charrin C, Archimbaud E, et al. (1998) Philadelphia chromosome positive adult acute lymphoblastic leukemia: Characteristics, prognostic factors and treatment outcome. Hematol Cell Ther 40(3):119–128
67. Westbrook CA, Hooberman AL, Spino C, Dodge RK, Larson RA, Davey F, et al. (1992) Clinical significance of the BCR-ABL fusion gene in adult acute lymphoblastic leukemia: A Cancer and Leukemia Group B Study (8762). Blood 80(12):2983–2990
68. Camera A, Annino L, Chiurazzi F, Fazi P, Cascavilla N, Fabbiano F, et al. (2004) GIMEMA ALL – Rescue 97: A salvage strategy for primary refractory or relapsed adult acute lymphoblastic leukemia. Haematologica 89(2):145–153
69. Preti HA, O'Brien S, Giralt S, Beran M, Pierce S, Kantarjian HM (1994) Philadelphia-chromosome-positive adult acute lymphocytic leukemia: Characteristics, treatment results, and prognosis in 41 patients. Am J Med 97(1):60–65
70. Wetzler M, Dodge RK, Mrozek K, Stewart CC, Carroll AJ, Tantravahi R, et al. (2004) Additional cytogenetic abnormalities in adults with Philadelphia chromosome-positive acute lymphoblastic leukaemia: A study of the Cancer and Leukaemia Group B. Br J Haematol 124(3):275–288
71. Rieder H, Ludwig WD, Gassmann W, Maurer J, Janssen JW, Gokbuget N, et al. (1996) Prognostic significance of additional chromosome abnormalities in adult patients with Philadelphia chromosome positive acute lymphoblastic leukaemia. Br J Haematol 95(4):678–691
72. Primo D, Tabernero MD, Perez JJ, Rasillo A, Sayagues JM, Espinosa AB, et al. (2005) Genetic heterogeneity of BCR/ABL+ adult B-cell precursor acute lymphoblastic leukemia: Impact on the clinical, biological and immunophenotypical disease characteristics. Leukemia 19(5):713–720
73. Ko BS, Tang JL, Lee FY, Liu MC, Tsai W, Chen YC, et al. (2002) Additional chromosomal abnormalities and variability of BCR breakpoints in Philadelphia chromosome/BCR-ABL-positive acute lymphoblastic leukemia in Taiwan. Am J Hematol 71(4): 291–299
74. Dombret H, Gabert J, Boiron JM, Rigal-Huguet F, Blaise D, Thomas X, et al. (2002) Outcome of treatment in adults with Philadelphia chromosome-positive acute lymphoblastic leukemia–results of the prospective multicenter LALA-94 trial. Blood 100(7):2357–2366
75. Thomas X, Boiron JM, Huguet F, Dombret H, Bradstock K, Vey N, et al. (2004) Outcome of treatment in adults with acute lymphoblastic leukemia: Analysis of the LALA-94 trial. J Clin Oncol 22(20):4075–4086
76. Druker BJ, Sawyers CL, Kantarjian H, Resta DJ, Reese SF, Ford JM, et al. (2001) Activity of a specific inhibitor of the BCR-ABL tyrosine kinase in the blast crisis of chronic myeloid leukemia and acute lymphoblastic leukemia with the Philadelphia chromosome. N Engl J Med 344(14):1038–1042
77. Champagne MA, Capdeville R, Krailo M, Qu W, Peng B, Rosamilia M, et al. (2004) Imatinib mesylate (STI571) for treatment of children with Philadelphia chromosome-positive leukemia: Results from a Children's Oncology Group phase 1 study. Blood 104(9):2655–2660
78. Ottmann OG, Druker BJ, Sawyers CL, Goldman JM, Reiffers J, Silver RT, et al. (2002) A phase 2 study of imatinib in patients with relapsed or refractory Philadelphia chromosome-positive acute lymphoid leukemias. Blood 100(6):1965–1971
79. Takayama N, Sato N, O'Brien SG, Ikeda Y, Okamoto S (2002) Imatinib mesylate has limited activity against the central nervous system involvement of Philadelphia chromosome-positive acute lymphoblastic leukaemia due to poor penetration into cerebrospinal fluid. Br J Haematol 119(1):106–108
80. Thomas DA, Faderl S, Cortes J, O'Brien S, Giles FJ, Kornblau SM, et al. (2004) Treatment of Philadelphia chromosome-positive acute lymphocytic leukemia with hyper-CVAD and imatinib mesylate. Blood 103(12):4396–4407

81. Leis JF, Stepan DE, Curtin PT, Ford JM, Peng B, Schubach S, et al. (2004) Central nervous system failure in patients with chronic myelogenous leukemia lymphoid blast crisis and Philadelphia chromosome positive acute lymphoblastic leukemia treated with imatinib (STI-571). Leuk Lymphoma 45(4):695–698
82. Lee KH, Lee JH, Choi SJ, Seol M, Lee YS, Kim WK, et al. (2005) Clinical effect of imatinib added to intensive combination chemotherapy for newly diagnosed Philadelphia chromosome-positive acute lymphoblastic leukemia. Leukemia 19(9):1509–1516
83. Towatari M, Yanada M, Usui N, Takeuchi J, Sugiura I, Takeuchi M, et al. (2004) Combination of intensive chemotherapy and imatinib can rapidly induce high-quality complete remission for a majority of patients with newly diagnosed BCR-ABL-positive acute lymphoblastic leukemia. Blood 104(12):3507–3512
84. Lee S, Kim YJ, Min CK, Kim HJ, Eom KS, Kim DW, et al. (2005) The effect of first-line imatinib interim therapy on the outcome of allogeneic stem cell transplantation in adults with newly diagnosed Philadelphia chromosome-positive acute lymphoblastic leukemia. Blood 105(9):3449–3457
85. Lee S, Kim DW, Kim YJ, Chung NG, Kim YL, Hwang JY, et al. (2003) Minimal residual disease-based role of imatinib as a first-line interim therapy prior to allogeneic stem cell transplantation in Philadelphia chromosome-positive acute lymphoblastic leukemia. Blood 102(8):3068–3070
86. Wassmann B, Pfeifer H, Stadler M, Bornhauser M, Bug G, Scheuring UJ, et al. (2005) Early molecular response to posttransplantation imatinib determines outcome in MRD+ Philadelphia-positive acute lymphoblastic leukemia (Ph+ ALL). Blood 106(2): 458–463
87. von Bubnoff N, Peschel C, Duyster J (2003) Resistance of Philadelphia-chromosome positive leukemia towards the kinase inhibitor imatinib (STI571, Glivec): A targeted oncoprotein strikes back. Leukemia 17(5):829–838
88. Gorre ME, Mohammed M, Ellwood K, Hsu N, Paquette R, Rao PN, et al. (2001) Clinical resistance to STI-571 cancer therapy caused by BCR-ABL gene mutation or amplification. Science 293(5531): 876–880
89. Hato T, Yamanouchi J, Tamura T, Hojo N, Niiya Y, Kohno M, et al. (2004) Existence of leukemic clones resistant to both imatinib mesylate and rituximab before drug therapies in a patient with Philadelphia chromosome-positive acute lymphocytic leukemia. Int J Hematol 80(1):62–66
90. Hofmann WK, Komor M, Wassmann B, Jones LC, Gschaidmeier H, Hoelzer D, et al. (2003) Presence of the BCR-ABL mutation Glu255Lys prior to STI571 (imatinib) treatment in patients with Ph+ acute lymphoblastic leukemia. Blood 102(2):659–661
91. Weisberg E, Manley PW, Breitenstein W, Bruggen J, Cowan-Jacob SW, Ray A, et al. (2005) Characterization of AMN107, a selective inhibitor of native and mutant Bcr-Abl. Cancer Cell 7(2):129–141
92. Shah NP, Tran C, Lee FY, Chen P, Norris D, Sawyers CL (2004) Overriding imatinib resistance with a novel ABL kinase inhibitor. Science 305(5682):399–401
93. Harata M, Soda Y, Tani K, Ooi J, Takizawa T, Chen M, et al. (2004) CD19-targeting liposomes containing imatinib efficiently kill Philadelphia chromosome-positive acute lymphoblastic leukemia cells. Blood 104(5):1442–1449
94. Barrett AJ HM, Ash RC, Atkinson K, Gale RP, Goldman JM, Henslee-Downey PJ, Herzig RH, Speck B, Zwaan FE, et al. (1992) Bone marrow transplantation for Philadelphia chromosome-positive acute lymphoblastic leukemia. Blood 79(30):67–70
95. Dunlop LC PR, Singhal S, Treleaven JG, Swansbury GJ, Meller S, Pinkerton CR, Horton C, Mehta J (1996) Bone marrow transplantation for Philadelphia chromosome-positive acute lymphoblastic leukemia. Bone Marrow Transplant 17(36):5–9
96. Kroger N, Kruger W, Wacker-Backhaus G, Hegewisch-Becker S, Stockschlader M, Fuchs N, et al. (1998) Intensified conditioning regimen in bone marrow transplantation for Philadelphia chromosome-positive acute lymphoblastic leukemia. Bone Marrow Transplant 22(11):1029–1033
97. Esperou H, Boiron JM, Cayuela JM, Blanchet O, Kuentz M, Jouet JP, et al. (2003) A potential graft-versus-leukemia effect after allogeneic hematopoietic stem cell transplantation for patients with Philadelphia chromosome-positive acute lymphoblastic leukemia: Results from the French Bone Marrow Transplantation Society. Bone Marrow Transplant 31(10):909–918
98. Lee S, Kim DW, Cho B, Kim YJ, Kim YL, Hwang JY, et al. (2003) Risk factors for adults with Philadelphia-chromosome-positive acute lymphoblastic leukaemia in remission treated with allogeneic bone marrow transplantation: The potential of real-time quantitative reverse-transcription polymerase chain reaction. Br J Haematol 120(1):145–153
99. Matsue K, Tabayashi T, Yamada K, Takeuchi M (2002) Eradication of residual bcr-abl-positive clones by inducing graft-versus-host disease after allogeneic stem cell transplantation in patients with Philadelphia chromosome-positive acute lymphoblastic leukemia. Bone Marrow Transplant 29(1):63–66
100. Sierra J, Radich J, Hansen JA, Martin PJ, Petersdorf EW, Bjerke J, et al. (1997) Marrow transplants from unrelated donors for treatment of Philadelphia chromosome-positive acute lymphoblastic leukemia. Blood 90(4):1410–1414
101. Snyder DS, Nademanee AP, O'Donnell MR, Parker PM, Stein AS, Margolin K, et al. (1999) Long-term follow-up of 23 patients with Philadelphia chromosome-positive acute lymphoblastic leukemia treated with allogeneic bone marrow transplant in first complete remission. Leukemia 13(12):2053–2058
102. Chao NJ, Blume KG, Forman SJ, Snyder DS (1995) Long-term follow-up of allogeneic bone marrow recipients for Philadelphia chromosome-positive acute lymphoblastic leukemia. Blood 85(11):3353–3354
103. Preudhomme C, Henic N, Cazin B, Lai JL, Bertheas MF, Vanrumbeke M, et al. (1997) Good correlation between RT-PCR analysis and relapse in Philadelphia (Ph1)-positive acute lymphoblastic leukemia (ALL). Leukemia 11(2):294–298
104. Pane F, Cimino G, Izzo B, Camera A, Vitale A, Quintarelli C, et al. (2005) Significant reduction of the hybrid BCR/ABL transcripts after induction and consolidation therapy is a powerful predictor of treatment response in adult Philadelphia-positive acute lymphoblastic leukemia. Leukemia 19(4):628–635
105. Mitterbauer G, Nemeth P, Wacha S, Cross NC, Schwarzinger I, Jaeger U, et al. (1999) Quantification of minimal residual disease in patients with BCR-ABL-positive acute lymphoblastic leukaemia using quantitative competitive polymerase chain reaction. Br J Haematol 106(3):634–643
106. Scheuring UJ, Pfeifer H, Wassmann B, Bruck P, Atta J, Petershofen EK, et al. (2003) Early minimal residual disease (MRD) analysis during treatment of Philadelphia chromosome/Bcr-Abl-positive

acute lymphoblastic leukemia with the Abl-tyrosine kinase inhibitor imatinib (STI571). Blood 101(1):85–90

107. Scheuring UJ, Pfeifer H, Wassmann B, Bruck P, Gehrke B, Petershofen EK, et al. (2003) Serial minimal residual disease (MRD) analysis as a predictor of response duration in Philadelphia-positive acute lymphoblastic leukemia (Ph+ALL) during imatinib treatment. Leukemia 17(9):1700–1706
108. Miyamura K, Tanimoto M, Morishima Y, Horibe K, Yamamoto K, Akatsuka M, et al. (1992) Detection of Philadelphia chromosome-positive acute lymphoblastic leukemia by polymerase chain reaction: Possible eradication of minimal residual disease by marrow transplantation. Blood 79(5):1366–1370
109. Kohler S, Galili N, Sklar JL, Donlon TA, Blume KG, Cleary ML (1990) Expression of bcr-abl fusion transcripts following bone marrow transplantation for Philadelphia chromosome-positive leukemia. Leukemia 4(8):541–547
110. Knechtli CJ, Goulden NJ, Hancock JP, Grandage VL, Harris EL, Garland RJ, et al. (1998) Minimal residual disease status before allogeneic bone marrow transplantation is an important determinant of successful outcome for children and adolescents with acute lymphoblastic leukemia. Blood 92(11):4072–4079

Burkitt's Acute Lymphoblastic Leukemia (L_3ALL) in Adults

Vincent Ribrag, Philippe Casassus, Pierre Fenaux

Contents

15.1 Introduction

Accounting for 1–3% of all cases of acute lymphoblastic leukemias (ALL), Burkitt cell ALL (L_3ALL) is characterized by the morphology of blast cells, the presence of monoclonal surface immunoglobulins (sIg), and by chromosomal translocations, usually t(8;14) (q24;q32) and less commonly its variants t(2;8) (p12;q24) or t(8;22) (q24;q11) [1–4]. These translocations lead to rearrangements of the protooncogene c-myc, located at band 8q24 [5]. Recently, the World Health Organization (WHO) classification of lymphoid diseases recognized the Burkitt lymphoma and the L_3ALL as a single entity; a mature B-cell neoplasm with an oncogenic c-myc overexpression [6].

L_3ALL predominates in children and adolescents, and is less common in adults [7]. Its prognosis, both in children and adults, had long been regarded as uniformly poor, because of frequent central nervous system (CNS) involvement and early relapses. Over the last 15 years, however, survival has improved in children, with the use of aggressive protocols combining intensive induction and consolidation chemotherapy and early CNS disease treatment. The impact of these new approaches on the outcome of adult ALL_3 has also been subsequently demonstrated.

15.2 Clinical and Hematological Characteristics of L_3ALL in Adults and Outcome with "Conventional" ALL Treatment

15.2.1 Clinical and Hematological Characteristics of L_3ALL

No clearcut separation can be made between Burkitt's lymphoma (BL) with marrow involvement and L_3ALL. Diagnosis of L_3ALL rather than BL therefore somewhat varies between authors, but is generally considered when bone marrow blasts are greater than 25%, in the absence of massive extramedullary tumor mass, especially in the abdomen, and when the presentation consists mainly of signs of marrow failure. Marrow infiltration, in L_3ALL, is in fact generally massive, with greater than 50% blasts. The disease largely predominates in males (by about 3 to 1), and median age ranges between 25 and 35 years, but about one quarter of the patients are older than 50. Hepatosplenomegaly and moderately enlarged lymph nodes are seen in 50–60% of the cases. The frequency of CNS involvement at diagnosis has been reported to vary greatly, from 12% to greater than 70%. This variation may have different causes. One of them could be taking into account clinical findings like mental neuropathy. Mental neuropathy is indeed a frequent clinical finding in BL and L_3ALL, rarely seen in other lymphomas or acute leukemias. It appears to result from infiltration of inferior dental nerves, and therefore can reasonably be considered as a sign of CNS disease, even when isolated [8]. We observed it in 60% of our L_3ALL cases, and only one half of those patients had other signs of CNS involvement. CNS disease, in L_3ALL, is also often diagnosed in the presence of other cranial nerve palsies, not always associated to the presence of blasts in the CSF. Other organs are involved in about 30% of the L_3ALL cases, including mediastinal tumors, and stomach, abdomen, skeleton and epidural masses, leading to paraplegia, which can be a presenting sign of the disease.

Thrombocytopenia is present in most patients, but anemia is less frequent; leukocytosis is found in two thirds of the cases but exceeds 50×10^9/l in only 10–20% of the patients. Circulating blasts are often associated to myelocytes and metamyelocytes, a rather unusual finding in most other types of acute leukemias.

A high correlation is found, in ALL, between L_3 morphology and the presence of surface immunoglobulins, (sIg) although cases of morphologically L_1 or L_2 ALL with sIg, and cases of morphologically L_3ALL without sIg have been reported, both in children and adults [9–12]. In the study of Hoelzer, et al., six of the 68 patients included had discrepancies between morphological and immunological diagnosis: Five were positive for sIg but had L_1 or L_2 morphology; one had L_3 morphology but no sIg. Patients with sIg and L_1 or L_2 morphology had a very poor outcome, and probably constitute (both in adults and children) a subtype of ALL different from L_3ALL, that requires other therapeutic approaches. In the same report, three additional patients with L_3 morphology were found to have a different immunophenotype (c-ALL in two cases and preB-ALL in one case). Kantarjian et al. also reported L_3 morphology in only 11 of their 18 cases of mature B cell ALL.

t(8;14) is the most frequent translocation observed in blasts cells, t(2;8) and t(8;22) being only occasionally seen. In recent series, 38–68% of L_3ALL had typical t(8;14) or t(2;8) and t(8;22) abnormality detected [9, 13–15]. Comparative genomic hybridization (CGH) analysis also showed that L_3ALL had higher number of cytogenetic changes, including a high level of genetic amplification than BLs [16]. Additional chromosomal abnormalities are found in 30–40% of the patients when karyotype is assessed by conventional cytogenetic analysis, and do not appear to carry prognostic value [17].

15.2.2 Outcome of Adult L_3ALL Treated with Conventional ALL Regimens

A relatively large number of small series of L_3ALL (with 3–10 patients) treated with conventional ALL regimens have been reported, and their results have been uniformly poor [17–26]. Conventional ALL treatments, usually combining vincristine (VCR) an anthracycline (ANTHR), prednisone (PR), L asparaginase (L-ASP) and 5–6 intrathecal injections of MTX (the latter being mainly given during consolidation therapy) yielded CR rates of only 30–50%, with most patients subsequently relapsing, especially in the CNS. In addition to rapid progression in many patients, failure to achieve CR was often due to early death associated with acute tumor lysis syndrome. We also observed, in some cases treated with conventional protocols, eradication of marrow blasts but concomitant rapid progression of CNS disease, leading to early death [18]. Median survival, in those series, did not exceed a few months and almost no patients were cured.

Due to similar poor results in disseminated BL and L_3ALL in children, several pediatric groups, especially the St. Jude's group, the BFM German group and the French SFOP attempted new strategies which dramatically improved prognosis in children.

15.3 Improved Strategies in the Treatment of Disseminated BL and L_3ALL in Children

Experience accumulated over the years by pediatric groups had indeed shown that "classical" ALL regimens, or "lymphoma regimens" combining relatively moderate doses of cyclophosphamide (CPM), ANTHR, VCR, and PR plus "conventional" CNS prophylaxis, that could cure localized BL, were not sufficient to eradicate systemic and CNS disease in disseminated BL and L_3ALL [27–30] (HD MTX, 3 g/m^2). Several groups then showed that considerable improvement in the outcome of disseminated BL and L_3ALL in children could be obtained. The St. Jude's group, French SFOP, and German BFM group introduced treatment protocols that included, in particular, fractionated high doses of CPM (or ifosfamide), intermediate or high dose (HD) methotrexate and Ara C, and VM26 or VP16 in addition to doxorubicin and VCR (Tables 15.1, 15.2). Very early CNS treatment, with repeated intrathecal therapy and CNS irradiation (which could often be replaced by courses of HD-MTX at 3 g/m^2) was added to reduce the incidence of CNS disease.

Those groups also showed that, in order to reduce the risk of potentially lethal tumor lysis syndrome, treatment had to start by a small dose ("prephase," generally combining CPM, VCR, and PR), high-dose chemotherapy being usually started 1 week later. The combination of urate oxidase with induction therapy can also reduce the risk of severe renal injury during early phase of induction therapy [31]. With these intensified protocols, and introduction of a treatment prephase, the prognosis of stage III and stage IV BL had greatly improved, 70–75% of the patients achieving cure. This large pediatric experience also showed that virtually no relapse occurred after 1 year of diagnosis.

However, patients with CNS involvement and L_3ALL still had poor outcome using such protocols and had many relapses involving in particular the CNS, and finally cure rates of only 20–30%. This led to start approaches using further intensification of CNS treatment with HDMTX (at 5 g/m^2 in BFM trials and 8 g/m^2 in SFOP trials), a greater number of triple intrathecal injections (with AraC, MTX, hydrocortisone), consolidation with VP16 and HD Ara C, and cranial irradiation [28, 32, 33]. With those protocols, about 75% of BL with CNS involvement and L_3ALL could be cured in the experience of the French SFOP and the German BFM group. Those results were recently confirmed by a UK group, using a SFOP protocol [34].

15.4 Current Treatment of Newly Diagnosed L_3ALL in Adults

The approaches that showed improved results in children were rapidly proposed to adults. In particular, the SFOP and BFM protocols were applied to adults, with no or minor modifications (Tables 15.1, 15.2). Groups involved in the treatment of adult ALL also used the bases of those protocols to adapt their treatment of L_3ALL. Results of the published experience with such treatments are shown in Table 15.3.

Application of those reinforced protocols to adult L_3 ALL rapidly led to improved results. For example, all the seven adult L_3ALL patients treated by our group from 1981 to 1984 with conventional (or with slightly reinforced CNS prophylaxis) ALL protocols died within 1 year of diagnosis [18]. By contrast, six of the nine subsequent adult L_3ALL cases, treated by SFOP 86 protocol, were cured of their disease. Favorable results of SFOP programs, especially SFOP 86 protocol in adult L_3ALL, were more recently confirmed by Soussain et al. in 24 patients [35]. Nineteen of them achieved CR, and 14 of them were alive in prolonged first CR. Importantly, eight of the 18 patients who achieved CR in that series were allografted (six cases) or autografted (two cases) in first CR. Three of them died from toxicity, two relapsed and only three were cured of their disease. By comparison, all the 11 patients consolidated with chemotherapy alone remained disease free. This transplantation series may have had especially poor results, notably when compared with a previous French series of allogeneic BMT performed in first CR in adult BL with initial CNS and/or marrow involvement, where seven of nine patients had favorable outcome [36]. Still, results of Soussain, et al. and the recent EBMT series [37] suggest that intensification with an allo or autograft is not justified in L_3ALL in first CR.

Pees et al. [38] and Todeschini et al. [39] also applied childhood BL and L_3ALL trials to adults (BFM-NHL and POG protocols, respectively) with favorable results, although on smaller numbers of cases. POG 86 trial consists of six courses alternating a cycle A and a cycle B, which are largely similar to BFM-NHL trials, but include, like SFOP 86 trial, HDAraC. Magrath et al. [33] also found that adults with disseminated BL treated with a childhood BL protocol that included the same drugs at similar doses as BFM and SFOP trials achieved as favorable results as with children.

Table 15.1. Principles of SFOP Protocols 84 and 86

Prephase: COP			
	VCR	1 mg/m^2	
	CPM	300 mg/m^2	
	MTX (CIT)		
	PRED	60 mg/m^2 (in 2 fractions)	
COPADM 1			
	VCR	2 mg/m^2 (max. 2 mg)	d_1
	CPM	500 mg/m^2/d (in 2 fractions)	d_2 to d_4
	ADR	60 mg/m^2	d_2
	HDM	3 g/m^2	d_1
	MTX (IT)		d_1 and d_6
	PRED	60 mg/m^2 (in 2 fractions)	d_1 to d_6
COPADM 2: idem but			
	VCR		d_1 and d_6
	CPM	1 g/m^2/d	d_2 to d_4
CYM 2 courses			
	HD MTX	3 g/m^2	d_1
	MTX (IT)		d_2
	Ara-C cont. inf.	100 mg/m^2/d	d_2 to d_6
	Ara-C (IT)		d_6
	Sequence 1		
	– VCR	2 mg/m^2 (max. 2 mg)	d_1
	– CPM	500 mg/m^2	d_1 and d_2
	– ADR	60 mg/m^2	d_2
	– HD MTX	3 g/m^2	d_1
	– MTX + (IT)		d_2
	– PRED	60 mg/m^2 (in 2 fractions)	d_1 to d_6
	Sequence 2 (SFOP 86 only)		
	– ARA C	100 mg/m^2/d	d_1 to d_5
	– VP 16	150 mg/m^2/d	d_1 to d_5

In SFOP 84 trial, treatment is stopped after the first sequence 1. In SFOP protocol 86, CYM courses were replaced by 2 CYVE courses: Ara C 3 g/m^2/d d_2 to d_5 and VP16: 200 mg/m^2/d d_2 to d_5 and cranial irradiation. Patients received four maintenance courses alternating sequence 1 and 2. Subsequent trials (SFOP 89 and SFOP 95) followed the same approach with relatively minor changes, intermediate risk patients receiving an LMB 84 type protocol, and high risk patients (including L_3ALL) receiving an LMB 86 type protocol.

The German adult ALL group experience of intensified treatment of L_3ALL currently remains the largest published in this disorder. Hoelzer et al. [9], who had observed no cure in nine L_3ALL patients treated with a conventional ALL trial, subsequently decided to start a specific L_3 trial (B-NHL83) which, like the SFOP and BFM trials, included a prephase, followed by repeated cycles with intermediate dose MTX, fractionated CPM and VCR (Table 15.4). The CR rate was 63%, and 47% of the patients who had achieved CR relapsed. Relapses

Table 15.2. Principles of BFM 90 trial

Prephase	Prednisone (orally/IV)	30 mg/m^2	d_1 to d_5
	Cyclophosphamide (IV 1 h)	200 mg/m^2	d_1 to d_5
	Methotrexate IT	12 mg	d_1
	Cytarabine IT	30 mg	d_1
	Prednisolone IT	10 mg	d_1
Course A	Dexamethasone (orally/IV)	10 mg/m^2	d_1 to d_5
	Ifosfamide (IV 1 h)	800 mg/m^2	d_1 to d_5
	Methotrexate IV 24 h	5 g/m^2	d_1
	Methotrexate IT	6 mg	d_4 and d_6
	Cytarabine IT	15 mg	d_1 and d_6
	Prednisolone IT	5 mg	d_1 and d_6
	Vincristine IV	1.5 mg/m^2	d_1
	Cytarabine IV 1 h	150 mg/m^2	d_4 and d_5
	Etoposide IV 1 h	100 mg/m^2	d_4 and d_5
Course B	Dexamethasone	10 mg/m^2	d_1 to d_5
	Cyclophosphamide (IV 1 h)	200 mg/m^2	d_1 to d_5
	Methotrexate IV 24 h	5 g/m^2	d_1
	Methotrexate IT	6 mg	d_1 and d_6
	Cytarabine IT	15 mg	d_1 and d_6
	Prednisolone IT	5 mg	d_1 and d_6
	Vincristine IV	1.5 mg/m^2	d_1
	Doxorubicin IV 1 h	25 mg/m^2	d_4 and d_5

Patients with L_3ALL receive six courses alternating A and B (ABABAB).

involved the CNS in 57% cases, and the marrow in 43% of the cases. Forty nine per cent of the patients were eventually considered to be cured of their disease. Subsequently, this group used another trial, with higher doses of MTX, of VM26 and Ara C (B-NHL 86). With this trial, the CR rate slightly increased to 74%, and the relapse rate dropped to 23%. Furthermore, only 17% of the relapses involved the CNS. Long-term survival, however, was similar (51%) in the B-NHL 86 trial, due in part to older age of patients and death from allogeneic BMT in two cases. In studies B-NHL 83 and B-NHL 86, five patients were allografted, four in first CR and one in PR, and one was autografted in first CR. Three allografted patients died, two from toxicity and the patient who had achieved PR from progressive disease. Those results, like results of the French group, confirmed that allogeneic BMT seems to have no or limited place in the first line treatment of L_3ALL.

The CALGB chose to adapt the German adult ALL protocol where etoposide replaced teniposide. Patients with an L_3ALL or a Burkitt lymphoma with a CNS involvement were included in two successive phase II trials [13, 14]. For L_3ALL, 18 out of the 24 patients reached CR (75%). Seven of them relapsed. Overall survival for L_3ALL was 45% with a median follow-up of 5 years. Most of the relapsing occurred during the first year. Only two patients experienced relapse more than 1 year after the start of therapy. CNS prophylaxis was modified between these two successive trials. The initial trial planned 12 doses of triple intrathecal chemotherapy combined with early radiotherapy (given halfway through therapy). A high neurological toxicity was ob-

Table 15.3. Previous experience of treatment of adult L_3ALL with specific intensive protocols

Author (year of publication)	Protocol	No. of patients	Median age	CNS in-volvement	WBC $>50\times10^9$/l	CR rate	Early death rate	LFS	Survival
Fenaux (1989)	SFOP86	9	38	100%	11%	8/9	1/9	2/8 relapses	6/9 long survivors
Soussain (1995)	SFOP84 SFOP86	24	NK	33%	NK	9/24	2/24	14/19 leukemia free	14/24 long survivors
Hoelzer (1996)	B-NHL83	24	33	8%	17%	63%	8%	50% at 4 years	49% at 4 years
	B-NHL86	35	36	17%	20%	74%	9%	71% at 4 years	51% at 4 years
Pees (1992)	BFM-NHL	5	35	2/5	NK	3/5	1/5	no relapse	3/5 long survivors
Todeschini (1997)	POG	6	35	1/6	NK	6/6	0	no relapse	6/6 long survivors
Kantarjian (1999)	HyperCVAD	11	NK	NK	NK	8/11	NK		33% 5 year survival
Lee (2001)	Modified BFM	24	NK	NK	NK	8/11	NK		33% 5 year survival
Cabanillas (1) (2003)	R-HyperCVAD	20	52	17%	NK	89%	0	12/14 non-HIV at 12 months	NK
Hoelzer (2) (2003)	R-GMALL	11	NK	NK	NK	91%	1/11	NK	NK

NK: not known. 1-including Burkitt and Burkitt-like lymphomas (with 6/20 HIV patients). Including Rituximab and HyperCVAD2-including 82 patients with 11 mature B-ALL. Rituximab was added to German GMALL regimen.

Table 15.4. Protocols of the German ALL group

B-NHL 83			
Prephase			
– CP	200 mg/m^2	i.v. (1 h)/d	d_1–d_5
– PRED	3×20 mg/m^2	p.o./d	d_1–d_5
Block A			
– MTX	12 mg	i.th.	
– MTX	500 mg/m^2	i.v. (24 h)	d_1
– CP	200 mg/m^2	i.v./d	d_1–d_5
– VM26	165 mg/m^2	i.v.	d_5
– ARAC	300 mg/m^2	i.v.	d_5
– PRED	60 mg/m^2	p.o.	d_1–d_5
Block B			
– MTX	12 mg	i.th.	
– MTX	500 mg/m^2	i.v.	d_1
– CP	200 mg/m^2	i.v./d	d_1–d_5
– ADR	50 mg/m^2	i.v.	d_5
– PRED	60 mg/m^2	p.o./d	d_1–d_5
B-NHL 86			
Prephase			
– CP	200 mg/m^2		
– PRED	3×20 mg/m^2		
Block A			
– MTX, ARAC, DEXA		i.th.	
– VCR	2 mg	i.v.	d_1
– MTX	1500 mg/m^2	i.v.	d_1
– IFO	800 mg/m^2	i.v./d	d_1–d_5
– VM26	100 mg/m^2	i.v./d	d_4 and d_5
– ARAC	150 mg/m^2	i.v./12 h	d_4 and d_5
– DEXA	10 mg/m^2	p.o./d	d_1–d_5
Block B			
– MTX, ARAC, DEXA		i.th.	
– VCR	2 mg	i.v.	d_1
– MTX	1500 mg/m^2	i.v.	d_1
– CP	200 mg/m^2	i.v./d	d_1–d_5
– ADR	25 mg/m^2	i.v. (15 m)/d	d_4 and d_5
– DEXA	10 mg/m^2	p.o./d	d_1–d_5

In B-NHL 83 and 86, patients received six cycles alternating block A and B (ABABAB). In the protocol B-NHL 93, cranial irradiation was omitted, and MTX escalated to 3 g/m^2.

served with this protocol, which was then modified [14]. The second group of patients received only six intrathecal chemotherapy injections and radiotherapy was given later in the course of the protocol (after chemotherapy). Neurological toxicity was significantly reduced with this less-intensive CNS prophylaxis. CNS relapses and overall treatment efficacy were not modified [13, 14].

Kantarjian et al. [41] reported results of a protocol alternating eight cycles of hyper-CVAD (with fractionated CPM and high dose VAD) and HD MTX (3 g/m^2) combined to HD AraC (3 g/m^2) and overall 16 intrathecal injections in 11 cases of L_3ALL. Eight achieved CR, but the 5-year survival rate was only 33%. Causes of failure were not detailed. When all mature B cell ALL cases were considered, only 29% of the cases could be cured.

The combination of Rituximab and "Burkitt-tailored" chemotherapy has recently been tested in Burkitt and Burkitt-like leukemia and lymphoma [42, 43]. Preliminary results in HIV-positive and HIV-negative patients showed a high response rate in patients with Burkitt leukemia/lymphoma. Patients with ALL have not been evaluated separately and it remains to be seen whether the favorable response rate observed with these new combinations will translate into improved survival.

Finally, like in children, almost all relapses in adult disseminated BL and L_3ALL occur within 1 year of diagnosis, and prolonged maintenance treatment therefore is also unnecessary in those patients.

15.5 Prognostic Factors in Adult L_3ALL

The considerable improvement that has been observed in the outcome of L_3ALL in adults makes delineation of the patient population still at high risk of failure with those regimens particularly important. In the two published series with sufficiently large numbers of L_3ALL patients treated "optimally," patients with poor performance status at diagnosis [35] and older patients [9] had somewhat lower CR rates. Patients with CNS involvement or other extramedullary disease had poorer outcome in the study of Hoelzer et al. [9]. In the French SFOP 84 trial, CNS involvement was also a poor prognostic factor. However, it was no more a prognostic factor in the SFOP 86 trial, which incorporated higher dose MTX (8 g/m^2), high-dose Ara C 3 g/m^2, and cranial irradiation at 24 Gy [28].

Hoelzer, et al. [9] also found high WBC counts ($>50\times10^9$/l) and hemoglobin <8 g/dl to be associated with a higher risk of relapse whereas LDH levels had borderline significance. No other biological prognostic with prognostic importance clearly exists in L_3ALL. We found in particular that p53 mutations had no prognostic value in BL or L_3ALL, contrary to most other hematological malignancies [44].

Recently, additional cytogenetic abnormalities to the classical c-myc rearrangement were found to be associated with a poor outcome [45–46]. The prognostic value of additional cytogenetic abnormalities needs to be validated on more adult cases but represent new biological prognostic factors of special interest. Abnormalities in 1q and 7q detected by CGH analysis could be associated with a poor outcome in patients with Burkitt lymphoma or L_3ALL [16].

15.6 Treatment of Resistant and Relapsing Disease

Experience in the treatment of childhood BL has suggested that salvage chemotherapy, followed by intensification with autologous SCT could salvage about 40% of relapsing patients and patients who achieved only PR with first-line therapy. Drugs used for salvage chemotherapy included in particular HD MTX and high-dose AraC, and/or etoposide and cisplatin.

This relatively high incidence of durable salvage, however, was mostly reported in selected series of patients that often had received less than optimal first-line therapy, and who were able to reach autologous SCT. It was less clear if similar efficacy could be observed in unselected patients who had only partial response or relapsed after first-line treatment using recent intensive multiagent protocols. For example, Philip et al. [47] reported the outcome of 27 patients with BL who had relapsed after the SFOP 84 trial (14% of the patients who had achieved CR). Three of them had early death; 15 of the remaining 24 patients had at least partial response to salvage regimens (VP16 and HD AraC, VP16 and cisplatin or MIME) and could be autografted. Four of them had prolonged survival, whereas none of the patients who could not be autografted survived. Thus, only four of the 27 patients who relapsed could be durably salvaged.

In the case of adult L_3ALL initially treated with conventional ALL protocols, reports suggest that virtually none of the patients who relapsed could be durably salvaged [17–19]. Those patients generally had failure, only PR, or had rapid relapse after salvage treatment, and rarely achieved sufficient tumor reduction to envisage subsequent intensification by allogeneic or autologous SCT.

Outcome of adult L_3ALL patients who had PR or relapsed after first-line, more optimal intensive protocols (SFOP, BFM or German ALL trials) also appeared dismal. In the French experience [35], four of the six adult L_3ALL patients refractory or who relapsed after first line treatment were refractory to salvage treatment. The remaining two patients, who had sufficient tumor response with salvage chemotherapy, could be intensified by allo (one case) or auto (one case) SCT. However, they also rapidly died from relapse. Only two patients in the report of Soussain et al. [35] on adult BL and L_3ALL could be salvaged after a relapse, but they initially had stage I and stage II_E BL. Outcome of relapses was not detailed in Hoelzer's et al. study [9], but none of the patients who relapsed appeared to have obtained subsequent disease cure.

The EBMT recently assessed the benefit of allogeneic bone marrow transplant when compared to high-dose therapy and autologous stem cell reinjection in lymphomas including Burkitt lymphomas [45]. No benefit was observed with allogeneic bone marrow transplant when compared to autologous bone marrow transplant in this series including 71 patients who received an allograft compared to 416 patients who received an autograft. Most of the patients were intensified when their disease remained chemosensitive, but results with allogeneic or autologous bone marrow transplant were disappointing. Allogeneic bone marrow transplant gave similar results to autologous bone marrow transplant, with a median survival of 4.7 months from the date of transplant and a progression-free survival of 2.5 months [37].

15.7 L_3ALL in Adults Positive for the Human Immunodeficiency Virus (HIV)

Although the number of HIV-associated NHL is now decreasing with improvement of treatment of HIV infection in industrialized countries, this virus has led to a major increase in BL cases. For example, the National Cancer Institute of Italy recently reported, during an 8-year period, 131 cases of HIV-associated NHL, of which 46 (35%) were BL. During the same time, only 29 of the 1004 (2.8%) negative NHL diagnosed at the same institution were BL [48]. Large studies have shown that, in HIV-positive patients, BL tended to develop at a stage when immune functions are still relatively preserved, whereas other types of HIV-associated NHL (including large cell NHL, immunoblastic NHL, and Burkitt-like NHL), tend to develop at a stage of profound immunodeficiency. EBV infection is also found less often in HIV-associated BL than in HIV-associated immunoblastic NHL [49].

Bone marrow involvement is reported in 20–60% of HIV-associated BL. However, it is unclear from most published series how many of those patients fulfilled criteria for L_3ALL [49]. Only occasional cases clearly described as HIV-associated L_3ALL have been reported [17–19].

The outcome of HIV-associated NHL is generally poorer than that of NHL occurring in HIV-negative patients, due both to greater aggressiveness of the disease and to the underlying poor general condition and immune deficiency. In HIV-associated BL, CR rates of 20–45%, and median survival of 3–6 months have generally been reported with chemotherapy [19, 50–51]. Details regarding patients with bone marrow involvement were not available in those reports, however. In the report of the Italian NCI [48], treatment results in HIV-positive adult BL, regardless of disease stage, were less favorable than in HIV-negative BL: CR rate of 40% vs. 65% ($p = 0.03$). The difference was due to a higher incidence of deaths from opportunistic infections in HIV-associated BL, but also to the fact that HIV-positive cases were generally treated less intensively. Survival was also poorer in HIV-positive BL (median 7 months) as compared to HIV-negative BL (median not reached). DFS at 4 years was, however, identical in the two groups (74 vs. 73%). The French BL study group also reported 18 cases of BL, among 103 cases of HIV-positive NHL [52]. Only two of the 18 patients met criteria for AIDS before the diagnosis of NHL. Bone marrow involvement was reported in seven of them, but the degree of marrow infiltration was not known. Those seven patients received high-dose CHOP plus CNS prophylaxis. Only two of them achieved CR, and they both had prolonged response.

Treatment results in the rare cases of precisely described L_3ALL in HIV-positive patients were uniformly poor [17–19]. The possible impact of highly active antiretroviral therapy (HAART) in combinations with intensive Burkitt protocols has recently been investigated in HIV-positive Burkitt lymphomas and leukemias [53, 54]. The combination of HAART and intensive chemotherapy was feasible and resulted in long-term survivors in both series, which suggests that HAART should be combined with chemotherapy in L_3ALL patients. However those patients had generally received "classical" ALL protocols, and it is difficult to determine if underlying HIV infection worsened prognosis.

The impact of intensive protocols now applied to non-HIV related cases of disseminated BL and L_3ALL on the prognosis of HIV-related cases is also difficult to determine. Such protocols should probably be applied whenever possible, i.e., in patients without advanced AIDS symptoms and without very low CD_4 counts.

15.8 Conclusion

L_3ALL is a rare type of adult ALL, probably difficult to distinguish from disseminated BL involving the bone marrow. This tumor is highly proliferative, and tends to involve the CNS at diagnosis or rapidly during the disease course. It shows rapid chemosensitivity, initially leading to the risk of severe acute tumor lysis syndrome. Principles of its treatment, by comparison to the other types of ALL, include (i) a low-dose chemotherapy "prephase" to prevent acute tumor lysis syndrome; (ii) multiagent chemotherapy using high-dose cyclophosphamide, an anthracycline, high-dose MTX, high-dose Ara C and probably VP16. A short and intensive treatment (6–8 months) without maintenance, is indicated; (iii) early, intensive CNS treatment, with multiple triple intrathecal injections, high-dose MTX and high-dose Ara C, and possibly cranial irradiation. Autologous or allogeneic stem cell transplantation do not appear to be useful in first CR.

Using such approaches, recent results suggest that about two thirds of L_3ALL in adults can be cured, i.e., more than in any other type of adult ALL.

References

1. Bennett JM, Catovsky D, Daniel MT, et al. (1976) Proposals for the classification of the acute leukaemias. French-American-British (FAB) co-operative group. Br J Haematol 33(4):451
2. Bloomfield CD, Goldman AI, Alimena G, et al. (1986) Chromosomal abnormalities identify high-risk and low-risk patients with acute lymphoblastic leukemia. Blood 67(2):415
3. Flandrin G, Brouet JC, Daniel MT, Preudhomme JL (1975) Acute leukemia with Burkitt's tumor cells: A study of six cases with special reference to lymphocyte surface markers. Blood 45:183
4. Berger R, Bernheim A (1982) Cytogenetic studies on Burkitt's lymphoma-leukemia. Cancer Genet Cytogenet 7(3):231
5. Dalla-Favera R, Gregni M, Erikson J, et al. (1982) Human C-myc oncogene is located on the region of chromosome 8 that is translocated in Burkitt's lymphoma cells. Proc Natl Acad Sci 79:7824
6. Jaffe ES, Harris NL, Stein H, Vardiman JW (2001) World Health Organization Classification of Tumours. Pathology and genetics. Tumours of hematopoietic and lymphoid tissues. IARC Press, Lyon, pp 181–184
7. Vassal G, Leverger G, Schaison G, Castaigne S (1986) Leucémies aiguës lymphoblastiques á cellules de Burkitt. Aspects cliniques, thérapeutiques et évolutifs. Nouv Rev Fr Hematol 28(3):141
8. Massey EW, Moore J, Schold SC, Jr (1981) Mental neuropathy from systemic cancer. Neurology 31(10):1277
9. Hoelzer D, Ludwig WD, Thiel E, et al. (1996) Improved outcome in adult B-cell acute lymphoblastic leukemia. Blood 87(2):495
10. Navid F, Mosijczuk AD, Head DR, et al. (1999) Acute lymphoblastic leukemia with the (8;14)(q24;q32) translocation and FAB L3 morphology associated with a B-precursor immunophenotype: The Pediatric Oncology Group experience. Leukemia 13(1):135
11. Hammami A, Chan WC, Michels SD, Nassar VH (1991) Mature B-cell acute leukemia: A clinical, morphological, immunological, and cytogenetic study of nine cases. Hematol Pathol 5(3):109
12. Sullivan MP, Pullen DJ, Crist WM, et al. (1990) Clinical and biological heterogeneity of childhood B cell acute lymphocytic leukemia: Implications for clinical trials. Leukemia 4(1):6
13. Lee EJ, Petroni GR, Schiffer CA, Freter CE, Johnson JL, Barcos M, Frizzera G, Bloomfield CD, Peterson BA (2001) Brief-duration high-intensity chemotherapy for patients with small non-cleaved-cell lymphoma or FAB L3 acute lymphocytic leukemia: Results of cancer and leukemia group B study 9251. J Clin Oncol 19:4014–4022
14. Rizzieri DA, Johnson JL, Niedzwiecki D, Lee EJ, Vardiman JW, Powell BL, Barcos M, Bloomfield CD, Schiffer CA, Peterson BA, et al. (2004) Intensive chemotherapy with and without cranial radiation for Burkitt leukemia and lymphoma: Final results of Cancer and Leukemia Group B Study 9251.Cancer 100(7): 1438–1448
15. Thomas DA, Cortes J, O'Brien S, Pierce S, Faderl S, Albitar M, Hagemeister FB, Cabanillas FF, Murphy S, Keating MJ, et al. (1999) Hyper-CVAD program in Burkitt's-type adult acute lymphoblastic leukemia. J Clin Oncol. 17:2461–2470
16 Garcia JL, Hernandez JM, Gutierrez NC, Flores T, Gonzalez D, Calasanz MJ, Martinez-Climent JA, Piris MA, Lopez-Capitan C, Gonzalez MB, et al. (2003) Abnormalities on 1q and 7q are associated with poor outcome in sporadic Burkitt's lymphoma. A cytogenetic and comparative genomic hybridization study. Leukemia 17: 2016–2024
17. Bernasconi C, Brusamolino E, Pagnucco G, Bernasconi P, Orlandi E, Lazzarino M (1991) Burkitt's lymphoma/leukemia: A clinicopathologic study on 24 adult patients. Leukemia 5(Suppl 1):90
18. Fenaux P, Lai JL, Miaux O, Zandecki M, Jouet JP, Bauters F (1989) Burkitt cell acute leukaemia (L3 ALL) in adults: A report of 18 cases [see comments]. Br J Haematol 71(3):371

19. Gill PS, Meyer PR, Pavlova Z, Levine AM (1986) B cell acute lymphocytic leukemia in adults. Clinical, morphologic, and immunologic findings. J Clin Oncol 4(5):737
20. Baccarani M, Corbelli G, Amadori S, et al. (1982) Adolescent and adult acute lymphoblastic leukemia: Prognostic features and outcome of therapy. A study of 293 patients. Blood 60(3):677
21. Lazzarino M, Morra E, Alessandrino EP, et al. (1982) Adult acute lymphoblastic leukemia. Response to therapy according to presenting features in 62 patients. Eur J Cancer Clin Oncol 18(9):813
22. van der Reijden HJ, van Wering ER, van de Rijn JM, et al. (1983) Immunological typing of acute lymphoblastic leukaemia. Scand J Haematol 30(4):356
23. Lerede T, Bassan R, Rossi A, et al. (1996) Therapeutic impact of adult-type acute lymphoblastic leukemia regimens in B-cell/L3 acute leukemia and advanced-stage Burkitt's lymphoma. Haematologica 81(5):442
24. Clarkson B, Ellis S, Little C, et al. (1985) Acute lymphoblastic leukemia in adults. Semin Oncol 12(2):160
25. Walters R, Kantarjian H, Keating M, et al. (1986) Effective, low-morbidity, outpatient induction therapy for adult acute lymphocytic leukemia (ALL). Proc Am Soc Clin Oncol 4:737
26. Barnett MJ, Greaves MF, Amess JA, et al. (1986) Treatment of acute lymphoblastic leukaemia in adults. Br J Haematol 64(3): 455
27. Patte C, Philip T, Rodary C, et al. (1986) Improved survival rate in children with stage III and IV B cell non-Hodgkin's lymphoma and leukemia using multi-agent chemotherapy: Results of a study of 114 children from the French Pediatric Oncology Society. J Clin Oncol 4(8):1219
28. Patte C, Michon J, Frappaz D, et al. (1994) Therapy of Burkitt and other B-cell acute lymphoblastic leukaemia and lymphoma: Experience with the LMB protocols of the SFOP (French Paediatric Oncology Society) in children and adults. Baillieres Clin Haematol 7(2):339
29. Murphy SB, Bowman WP, Abromowitch M, et al. (1986) Results of treatment of advanced-stage Burkitt's lymphoma and B cell (SIg+) acute lymphoblastic leukemia with high-dose fractionated cyclophosphamide and coordinated high-dose methotrexate and cytarabine. J Clin Oncol 4(12):1732
30. Rosanda C, Cantu-Rajnoldi A, Invernizzi R, et al. (1992) B-cell acute lymphoblastic leukemia (B-ALL): A report of 17 pediatric cases. Haematologica 77(2):151
31. Patte C, Sakiroglu C, Ansoborlo S, Baruchel A, Plouvier E, Pacquement H, Babin-Boilletot A; Societe Francaise d'Oncologie Pediatrique (2002) Urate-oxidase in the prevention and treatment of metabolic complications inpatients with B-cell lymphoma and leukemia, treated in the Societe Francaise d'Oncologie Pediatrique LMB89 protocol. Ann Oncol 13:789–795
32. Reiter A, Schrappe M, Tiemann M, et al. (1999) Improved treatment results in childhood B-cell neoplasms with tailored intensification of therapy: A report of the Berlin-Frankfurt-Munster Group Trial NHL-BFM 90. Blood 94(10):3294
33. Patte C, Auperin A, Michon J, et al. (2001) The société française d'oncologie pédiatrique LMB89 protocol: Highly effective multiagent chemotherapy tailored to the tumor burden and initial response in 561 unselected children with B-cell lymphomas and L3 leukemia. Blood 97:3370–3379
34. Mead GM, Sydes MR, Walewski J, Grigg A, Hatton CS, Pescosta N, Guarnaccia C, Lewis MS, McKendrick J, Stenning SP, et al.; UKLG LY06 collaborators (2002) An international evaluation of CODOX-M and CODOX-M alternating with IVAC in adult Burkitt's lymphoma: Results of United Kingdom Lymphoma Group LY06 study. Ann Oncol 13:1264–1274
35. Soussain C, Patte C, Ostronoff M, et al. (1995) Small noncleaved cell lymphoma and leukemia in adults. A retrospective study of 65 adults treated with the LMB pediatric protocols. Blood 85(3):664
36. Troussard X, Leblond V, Kuentz M, et al. (1990) Allogeneic bone marrow transplantation in adults with Burkitt's lymphoma or acute lymphoblastic leukemia in first complete remission. J Clin Oncol 8(5):809
37. Peniket AJ, Ruiz de Elvira MC, Taghipour G, Cordonnier C, Gluckman E, de Witte T, Santini G, Blaise D, Greinix H, Ferrant A,et al.; European Bone Marrow Transplantation (EBMT) Lymphoma Registry (2003) An EBMT registry matched study of allogeneic stem cell transplants for lymphoma: Allogeneic transplantation is associated with a lower relapse rate but a higher procedure-related mortality rate than autologous transplantation. Bone Marrow Trans 31:667–678
38. Pees HW, Radtke H, Schwamborn J, Graf N (1992) The BFM-protocol for HIV-negative Burkitt's lymphomas and L3 ALL in adult patients: A high chance for cure. Ann Hematol 65(5):201
39. Todeschini G, Tecchio C, Degani D, et al. (1997) Eighty-one percent event-free survival in advanced Burkitt's lymphoma/leukemia: No differences in outcome between pediatric and adult patients treated with the same intensive pediatric protocol. Ann Oncol 8(Suppl 1):77
40. Magrath I, Adde M, Shad A, et al. (1996) Adults and children with small non-cleaved-cell lymphoma have a similar excellent outcome when treated with the same chemotherapy regimen. J Clin Oncol 14(3):925
41. Kantarjian HM, O'Brien S, Smith TL, et al. (2000) Results of treatment with hyper-CVAD, a dose-intensive regimen, in adult acute lymphocytic leukemia. J Clin Oncol 18(3):547
42. Hoelzer D, Baur K-H, Giagounidis A, et al. (2003) Short intensive chemotherapy with Rituximab seems successful in Burkitt NHL, mature B-ALL and other high-grade B-NHL. Blood 102:70 a, (abstr 236)
43. Cabanillas ME, Thomas DA, Cortes J, et al. (2002) Outcome with hyper-CVAD and Rituximab in Burkitt (BL) and Burkitt-like (BLL) leukemia/lymphoma. Proc Am Soc Clin Oncol 22:574, (abstr 2309)
44. Preudhomme C, Dervite I, Wattel E, et al. (1995) Clinical significance of p53 mutations in newly diagnosed Burkitt's lymphoma and acute lymphoblastic leukemia: A report of 48 cases. J Clin Oncol 13(4):812
45. Harbott J, Harder S, Haas OA, et al. (2003) Secondary chromosomal aberrations in childhood Burkitt's leukemia/lymphoma-analysis of 182 complete caryotypes of patients treated according to the German-Austrian-Swiss BFM-NHL trials. Blood 102:11, 887a
46. Poirel HA, Heerema N, Swansbury J, et al. (2003) Prognostic value of recurrent chromosomal alterations in pediatric B-cell non-Hodgkin's lymphoma: Report of 238 cases from the International FAB/LMB96 study. Blood 102:11, 391a
47. Philip T, Hartmann O, Pinkerton R, et al. (1993) Curability of relapsed childhood B-cell non-Hodgkin's lymphoma after intensive first line therapy: A report from the Societe Francaise d'Oncologie Pediatrique. Blood 81(8):2003

48. Spina M, Tirelli U, Zagonel V, et al. (1998) Burkitt's lymphoma in adults with and without human immunodeficiency virus infection: A single-institution clinicopathologic study of 75 patients. Cancer 82(4):766
49. Levine AM (1992) Acquired immunodeficiency syndrome-related lymphoma [see comments]. Blood 80(1):8
50. Knowles DM, Chamulak GA, Subar M, et al. (1988) Lymphoid neoplasia associated with the acquired immunodeficiency syndrome (AIDS). The New York University Medical Center experience with 105 patients (1981–1986). Ann Intern Med 108(5):744
51. Odajnyk C, Subar M, Dugan M, et al. (1986) Clinical features and correlates with immunopathology and molecularbiology of a large group of patients with AIDS associated small non-cleaved lymphoma (SNCL). Blood 68:131a
52. Davi F, Delecluse HJ, Guiet P, et al. (1998) Burkitt-like lymphomas in AIDS patients: Characterization within a series of 103 human immunodeficiency virus-associated non-Hodgkin's lymphomas. Burkitt's Lymphoma Study Group. J Clin Oncol 16(12):3788
53. Cortes J, Thomas D, Rios A, Koller C, O'Brien S, Jeha S, Faderl S, Kantarjian H (2002) Hyperfractionated cyclophosphamide, vincristine, doxorubicin, and dexamethasone and highly active antiretroviral therapy for patients with acquired immunodeficiency syndrome-related Burkitt lymphoma/leukemia. Cancer 94:1492–1499
54. Wang ES, Straus DJ, Teruya-Feldstein J, Qin J, Portlock C, Moskowitz C, Goy A, Hedrick E, Zelenetz AD, Noy A (2003) Intensive chemotherapy with cyclophosphamide, doxorubicin, high-dose methotrexate/ifosfamide, etoposide, and high-dose cytarabine (CODOX-M/IVAC) for human immunodeficiency virus-associated Burkitt lymphoma.Cancer 98:1196–1205

Treatment of Lymphoblastic Lymphoma in Adults

Nicola Gökbuget, Dieter Hoelzer

Contents

16.1 Introduction

Lymphoblastic lymphoma (LBL) is a rare entity of non-Hodgkin's lymphoma (NHL) with an incidence of less than 2% (1.7% for T- and less than 1% for B-lymphoblastic lymphoma) within all NHL [1]. In the USA, the population-based incidence was 0.2/100 000 in males and 0.1/100 000 in females between 1978 and 1995. The age distribution is bimodal with higher rates in individuals younger than 20 and in those older than 50 years [2]. LBL represents a distinctive lymphoma entity with cytological and histological features similar to those of acute lymphoblastic leukemia (ALL). LBL and ALL are generally separated by an arbitrary cut-point of 25% bone marrow (BM) infiltration. Patients with BM infiltration below 25% are considered as LBL. In the new WHO classification of lymphatic neoplasia both are summarized as B- or T-precursor lymphoblastic leukemia/lymphoma [3].

Despite the generally accepted viewpoint that ALL and LBL represent different manifestations of the same disease, a recent gene expression analysis showed that a clear segregation of T-ALL and T-LBL based on differentially expressed genes is possible. Thus the study demonstrated an overexpression of the MLL-1 gene in T-LBL and of CD47 in T-ALL. Furthermore, adhesion molecules and extracellular matrix proteins were upregulated in T-LBL. Some of the latter differences may be due to mechanisms in stroma cells. However, there is also evidence that important growth regulatory pathways may be different in T-ALL and T-LBL, which may partly explain the different clinical presentation of both diseases [4].

16.2 Immunophenotype

Most published studies in adults summarize patients with LBL of B- and T-cell origin. Approximately 80% of LBL carry T-markers which is different from ALL with >70% B-markers [5, 6] (Table 16.1). The reported disease features of LBL are therefore dominated by the T-cell subtype.

T-LBL can be separated in subtypes according to differentiation markers similarly to T-ALL. The thymic subtype (CD1 positive) is found most frequently. In a childhood ALL series the incidences for early, thymic, and mature T-ALL were 18, 71, and 10%, respectively [7]. For adult LBL the incidence of immunologic subtypes has not been reported so far. Whereas in T-ALL the immunophenotype is an important prognostic marker with inferior outcome for early and mature T-ALL and superior outcome for thymic T-ALL [8], it's impact on outcome is unknown in T-LBL.

16.3 Clinical Features

LBL generally has a male preponderance (61–75%). The majority of patients show advanced disease with stage III-IV in 58–95%. B symptoms (16–48%) and elevated LDH (48–84%) were present in a considerable proportion of patients. The incidence of initial CNS involvement is similar to ALL (0–10%) (Table 16.1).

T-LBL patients showed, compared to B-LBL younger age [9], a higher rate of mediastinal [10] or BM [9, 10] involvement and stage IV disease [9] whereas extranodal involvement was more frequent in B-LBL [10].

In the so far largest study on T-LBL in adults, 89% of the patients showed a mediastinal involvement often (40%) associated with pleural effusion. Seventy percent of the patients had lymph node or organ involvement (11%) and most of them (72%) had advanced stage III/IV disease with LDH values increased above two times the normal in 33% of the patients [11].

In contrast to T-ALL, peripheral blood values – particularly hemoglobin and platelet counts – were generally near to normal in this patient cohort indicating a potentially better BM reserve and tolerability of chemotherapy [11].

16.4 Therapeutic Approaches

Therapeutic approaches for adult LBL included in the past conventional protocols for NHL, intensive combination chemotherapy protocols designed for high grade NHL, and protocols for the treatment ALL, with or without prophylactic cranial irradiation (as in most ALL protocols) and with or without prophylactic or therapeutic mediastinal irradiation. Furthermore, stem cell transplantation (SCT) – particularly autologous SCT – was included to a different extent in treatment strategies. These different treatment approaches in conjunction with differences in patient characteristics – particularly median age and the proportion of patients with stage III/IV disease – may explain the considerable variations in outcome. The cumulative results of different approaches are summarized in Table 16.2.

16.4.1 Chemotherapy Regimens Designed for NHL

Earlier reports on conventional NHL protocols such as CHOP-based regimens yielded relatively low complete remission (CR) rates (53–71%) and rates for disease-free survival (DFS) (23–53%) [14, 16, 19–21] (Table 16.2).

Improved results for adult patients with LBL were later reported for a *modified CHOP regimen* with additional application of asparaginase, CNS prophylaxis, and maintenance therapy. With this regimen, known as "Stanford/NCOG," CR rates of 79–100% and DFS rates of 23–56% were achieved [22–25]. Thus there was growing evidence that intensified and prolonged chemotherapy together with CNS prophylaxis is beneficial in LBL.

With more *intensive NHL regimens*, designed for childhood NHL such as the LSA2-L2 or LNH-84 regimen, the CR rates were higher (73–84%) but not the DFS rates (35–44%) [14, 26]. Two studies which both included SCT yielded a more favorable DFS of 75% [27] or overall survival of 85% in T-LBL [28].

16.4.2 Chemotherapy Regimens Designed for ALL

The largest experience on treatment of adult LBL is available from ALL-type regimens (Table 16.3). In earlier studies at the Memorial Sloan Kettering Cancer

Table 16.1. Clinical characteristics of lymphoblastic lymphoma

	Bernasconi, et al. [12]	Santini, et al. [13]	Morel, et al. [14]	Zinzani, et al. [15]	Bouabdallah, et al. [16]	Sweetenham, et al. [17]	Hoelzer, et al. [11]	Thomas, et al. [18]
Year	1990	1991	1992	1996	1998	1997	2002	2004
N	31	40	54	53	62	95	45	33
Age	25 (15–64)	22 (15–51)	34 (15–76)	37 (15–78)	35 (14–70)	25 (>14)	25 (15–61)	28 (17–59)
Male gender	61%	62%	65%	74%	75%	69%	73%	82%
B-symptoms	16%	n.r.	48%	23%	n.r.	34%	27%	30%
Stage III/IV	68%	95%	58%	66%	73%	70%	73%	70%
Med. involvement	61%	85%	61%	57%	63%	n.r.	91%	70%
CNS involvement	10%	8%	2%	4%	6%	n.r.	0%	9%
Subtype T-cell	n.r.	77%	85%	62%	n.r.	68%	100%	79%
Subtype B-cell	n.r.	17%	2%	38%	n.r.	32%	0%	18%
LDH increased	n.r.	n.r.	62%	60%	79%	48%	84%	24%

Table 16.2. Cumulative* treatment results in adult patients with lymphoblastic lymphoma

Author	N Studies	N patients	Age (median)	CR	DFs
Conventional NHL	5	114	28–45	58% (53–71%)	36% (23–53%)
Modified NHL	5	112	14–22	92% (79–100%)	49% (23–56%)
High grade NHL	4	64	25–34	67% (57–84%)	51% (35–75%)
ALL Protocols	9	282	22–37	80% (55–100%)	56% (45–67%)

* according to [29]

Table 16.3. Results of ALL-type regimens in adult patients with lymphoblastic lymphoma

Author	Year	N pts	Age (median)	Induction	CNS prophylaxis	CR rate	DFS
Slater, et al. [30]	1986	20	22	MSKCC L10/17	i.th.	80%	45%
Bernasconi, et al. [12]	1990	18 13	25	V,P,D,C + c/m V,P,AD,C + c/m	i.th, CRT i.th.	78% 77%	45% (both)
Morel, et al. [14]	1992	22	34	FRALLE	i.th. +/– CRT	91%	52%
Daenen, et al. [33]	1995	18 (T)	22	V,P,AD + c/m +/– SCT	i.th.	100%	66%
Engelhard, et al. [9]	1996	35 18 (T) 8 (B)	26	V,P,D,A,AC,TG,C + c/m	i.th., CRT	66% 72% 50%	67%
Zinzani, et al. 15	1996	53	37	L17-L20 +/– SCT	i.th.	55%	56%
Bouabdallah, et al. [16]	1998	38	30	ALL protocols +/– SCT	i.th., +/– CRT	89%	45%
Hoelzer, et al. [11]	2002	45	25	GMALL 04/89 GMALL 05/93	i.th., CRT	93%	62%
Thomas, et al. [18]	2004	33	28	fC,V,AD,DX, HDM, HDAC repeated	i.th.	91%	70%
Song, et al. [34]	2007	34	26	ALL-type induction + auto SCT	i.th. +/– TBI	n.r.	72%

c/m, consolidation/maintenance; SCT, stem cell transplantation; i.th., intrathecal; CRT, cranial irradiation; V, vincristine; P, prednisone; D, daunorubicin; C, cyclophosphamide; AD, adriamycin; A, asparaginase; AC, cytarabine; TG, thioguanine; fC, fractionated cyclophosphamide; DX, dexamethasone; HDM, high dose methotrexate; HDAC, high dose cytarabine; (T), T-LBL; (B), B-LBL

Center, CR rates of 80% and DFS of 45% could be achieved with different ALL-type regimens (L2, L10, L17) [30]. Similar or even better results with CR rates between 55 and 100% and DFS rates between 45 and 67% were reported later for ALL-type regimens [9, 11, 12, 14–16, 31, 32].

16.4.2.1 MDACC

The MD Anderson Cancer Center (MDACC) reported the results of 33 patients treated according to the Hyper-CVAD regimen. The schedule is based on alternating cycles with fractionated cyclophosphamide (CYCLO) combined with other drugs and cycles with HD-ARAC and methotrexate (HD-MTX). The majority of patients received consolidative mediastinal irradiation after eight cycles. The cohort included mainly T-LBL (80%) with 70% stage III-IV disease.

The CR rate was 91% with 9% partial responses. The progression-free survival at 3 years was 66% and the survival 70% with 62% and 67% for the T-cell subtype, respectively. The major relapse localization was the mediastinum (50% of the relapses). Ten percent of the CR patients developed CNS involvement at relapse. Except CNS involvement at diagnosis, no prognostic factors could be identified [18].

16.4.2.2 GMALL

The largest cohort of T-LBL was reported by the German Multicenter Study Group for Adult ALL (GMALL). Forty-five patients were treated with standard 8-drug induction including prophylactic CNS irradiation and mediastinal irradiation followed by consolidation and reinduction therapy. In the majority of patients, treatment ended after reinduction at about 30 weeks.

The CR rate was 93%. Thirty-six percent of the patients relapsed. No late relapses after the first year from diagnosis were observed. The majority of relapses (47%) involved the mediastinum, although six out of seven patients had received mediastinal irradiation with 24 Gy. The survival was 51% at 7 years, 65% for CR patients, and the DFS was 62%. Advanced stage, age, LDH and other parameters had no prognostic impact [11].

16.4.3 Summary

These studies provide strong evidence that intensive chemotherapy in T-LBL may lead to favourable outcome without SCT in first CR even in patients with advanced disease and that particularly late relapses may be avoided to a large extent. Additional evidence for the high effectivity of ALL-type chemotherapy in T-LBL comes from a report on 105 children with T-LBL. The event-free survival of 90% was superior to previous studies in childhood T-LBL [7].

16.5 CNS Prophylaxis

Initial CNS involvement is observed in approximately 7% of LBL patients, which is similar to the incidence in ALL [11, 12, 14, 18, 19, 30, 35]. As in ALL, a high rate of CNS relapse (32–50%) was observed in earlier studies where patients did not receive specific CNS-directed prophylaxis [19, 35]. The inclusion of i.th. therapy leads to a substantial reduction of the CNS relapse rate [19] which ranged from 0% to 36% in studies with CNS prophylaxis based on i.th. therapy only [12, 19, 23, 30, 35] and from 3% to 21% in studies with i.th. therapy and CNS irradiation [12, 23, 26, 35].

Several historical comparisons underline the potential role of prophylactic CNS irradiation [23, 36]. In the GMALL study, 91% of the study patients received CNS irradiation and all of them had intensive i.th. therapy. This approach proved to be effective since only one of 42 CR patients experienced a CNS relapse [11]. CNS irradiation is not part of the Hyper-CVAD regimen, which, however, included i.th. therapy and systemic high-dose therapy. CNS involvement at relapse was seen in three of 30 CR patients [18].

Overall published results underline the importance of effective CNS prophylaxis in LBL and there is some evidence that CNS irradiation is a successful approach. It may be reasoned, however, whether CNS irradiation could be omitted in patients with stage I-II disease in order to avoid toxicity and treatment delays during induction therapy.

16.6 Mediastinal Tumors

One major specific issue in T-LBL is the role of mediastinal tumors (MedTu) as a cause for initial treatment failure and as relapse localization. Most patients show large MedTu at diagnosis, which in some patients even leads to emergency situations with acute respiratory distress and/or acute vena cava superior syndrome.

After induction, residual MedTu are sometimes difficult to assess and hamper the confirmation of CR. The mediastinum is also the most frequent site of recurrence. Several questions arise from this issue, such as prognostic impact of residual tumors, useful diagnostic procedures, and additional directed treatment of MedTu, which may either be prophylactic or therapeutic.

16.6.1 Prognostic Impact of Residual Mediastinal Tumors

The rapid achievement of CR had a prognostic impact in childhood LBL. Three out of 64 T-LBL patients with complete response at day 33 of induction showed local progress (5%) compared to three out of 35 (9%) with only partial remission [7]. In this study, however, the overall incidence of local progression was very low. One pediatric study demonstrated an inferior survival in patients without normalization of chest radiography after induction [37]. Also in adult T-LBL an inferior outcome was observed in patients with incomplete response to induction therapy, which was mainly due to residual MedTu [11]. On the other hand, in patients treated with a HD-MTX based regimen none of three patients with residual mass after induction relapsed [28].

16.6.2 Diagnostic Procedures

Not surprisingly, in T-LBL patients with large MedTu often residual structures are detectable after induction therapy by X-ray or computed tomography (CT). Additional diagnostic procedures aim to answer the question whether this is necrotic or scar tissue or whether vital tumor cells are present. When resection or biopsy was performed in 10 pediatric T-LBL patients with residual tumor after induction therapy, necrotic tissue was found in all cases [7]. Imaging techniques such as positron emission tomography (PET) are probably not helpful very early after induction therapy due to the ongoing effects of the chemotherapy. They are, however, important for staging at later time-points. Recently it was reported that persistently positive PET results were highly predictive for residual or recurrent disease in NHL [38]. In the GMALL studies PET diagnostics are performed in patients with residual mediastinal structures after induction and first consolidation.

Altogether there is some evidence that residual MedTu after induction therapy are associated with increased relapse risk. In addition to the intensification of systemic chemotherapy, the most frequently discussed approach for prevention of mediastinal recurrence and treatment of residual tumors is mediastinal irradiation (MedRad) with two principally different strategies: irradiation of all patients with MedTu or irradiation in patients with residual tumor only.

16.6.3 Mediastinal Irradiation

Mott et al. reported a significant advantage in terms of DFS for pediatric T-LBL patients with low-dose irradiation (15 Gy) (66%) compared to 18% for those without in an early study with probably suboptimal chemotherapy [39]. Other strategies in childhood T-LBL included MedRad in case of emergency only [7, 40, 41]. In the latter study the local recurrence rate (7%) was very low although no MedRad was administered. This may be due to a more rigorous early application of cyclophosphamide and ARAC and HD MTX, specifically designed as "extra compartment protocol" during consolidation [7]. This is underlined by the results of an HDMTX-based NHL protocol in adult T-LBL where only three of 14 relapses occurred in the mediastinum [28].

In the GMALL series of adult T-LBL, the mediastinal relapse rate was higher (47% of all relapses), despite an induction therapy similar to the pediatric approach and prophylactic MedRad with 24 Gy in 85% of the patients early during or after induction chemotherapy. Consolidation with HD-MTX was, however, less intensive. Mediastinal relapses occurred in patients with complete resolution of MedTu as well as in those with residual tumors after induction therapy [11].

In the cohort of the MDACC, the majority (74%) of patients had received MedRad with 30–39 Gy after eight cycles of chemotherapy. Three patients progressed before this time-point and one out of three patients without MedRad due to other reasons experienced mediastinal relapse. The mediastinal relapse rate was 12% in those who had received MedRad [18].

Altogether these findings underline that effective treatment of MedTu is an important specific issue in the treatment of adult T-LBL. In pediatric LBL low mediastinal recurrence rates are achieved by intensive chemotherapy, which may, however, not be feasible in adult patients. Therefore MedRad still has a role in adult LBL. Since an irradiation dose of 24 Gy may not be sufficient in the new GMALL protocol for T-LBL, patients receive prophylactic MedRad at a dose of 36 Gy similar to the dose included in NHL protocols for local irradiation. Irradiation is delivered after induction therapy without parallel chemotherapy in order to reduce hematotoxicity. On the other hand, MedRad leads to delays of systemic chemotherapy and since hematopoietic tissue is involved, toxicity of subsequent chemotherapy cycles may be increased. Due to this dilemma the optimal strategy remains to be defined.

16.7 Prognostic Factors

One important issue in adult LBL is the identification of prognostic factors in order to define indications for SCT in first CR. A variety of risk factors for relapse have been described in single studies such as higher age (>30–40 years) [12, 14, 15, 30, 42], increased LDH (either above normal or above 2× normal) [11, 12, 14, 15, 21, 23], CNS [12, 18, 23, 30], bone marrow [12, 23, 24, 42, 43] or extranodal involvement [21], stage IV disease [12, 15, 23, 42, 43], presence of B-symptoms [14], or decreased hemoglobin [14]. The majority of them are indicators for advanced disease or large tumor mass. Partial or late response was also associated with a poorer outcome [11, 14, 30].

Both recent larger trials with intensive chemotherapy hardly identified prognostic factors in adult LBL. In the GMALL series on T-LBL, the only significant prognostic factor for survival was elevated LDH. No single risk factor for relapse risk could be identified. Particularly the stage of disease and age did not have a prognostic impact [11]. In the MDACC series only CNS involvement at diagnosis was significantly associated with poorer outcome [18]. Similarly no prognostic factors were identified in the largest series in childhood T-LBL. Neither age, stage, LDH, nor immunophenotype appeared to have an impact on DFS [7]. The decreased relevance of single prognostic factors may therefore be a consequence of more effective chemotherapy in adult as well as in childhood LBL.

A convincing prognostic model has not yet been defined for adult LBL. New prognostic factors are required to define indications for SCT in CR1. The better characterization of biologic markers, e.g., immunophenotype of T-LBL, may contribute to this aim. Rational assessment of individual treatment response and relapse risk may be based on evaluation of minimal residual disease from bone marrow or peripheral blood. Furthermore, analysis of gene expression profiles, as recently published for T-ALL [44] and T-LBL [4], may help to identify new prognostic markers in T-LBL.

16.8 Results of Stem Cell Transplantation in LBL

SCT was included to a different extent in published studies and sometimes restricted to high risk LBL patients (Table 16.4).

16.8.1 Autologous SCT

The majority of studies evaluated the role of autologous (auto) SCT with a weighted mean for DFS of 61 (31–77)% [13–16, 45–47, 49, 50]. One prospective study was based on treatment with two sequential high-dose induction courses (without HDAC or HDMTX) followed by BEAM and autologous SCT. Thirteen patients with LBL were included and the CR rate was 73%. At 5 years the survival was 46% and the DFS 40%, which is inferior to chemotherapy studies. Surprisingly, results with this regimen were significantly better in Burkitt's lymphoma [52].

This favorable result for auto SCT in de novo and advanced disease may be at least partly due to selection mechanism, e.g., part of the patients reaching auto SCT after intensive front-line therapy may have been already cured by chemotherapy and the few patients reaching auto SCT after relapse of LBL may represent those few with chemosensitive disease at relapse.

16.8.2 Allogeneic SCT

Less experience exists with allogeneic (allo) SCT in LBL [16, 45, 50] with a mean DFS of 74 (59–91%) in a few small series (Table 16.4). In a survey of the European Bone Marrow Transplantation Registry (EBMTR), the survival of 222 LBL patients with allo SCT in first remission or advanced disease was 38% with a considerable rate of transplant related mortality (TRM) (31%). In this

Table 16.4. Results of SCT in lymphoblastic lymphoma

Author	Year	N	DFS
Auto CR1			
Milpied, et al. [45]	1989	13	68% [a]
Baro, et al. [46]	1992	14	77%
Morel, et al. [14]	1992	5	60% [b]
Bouabdallah, et al. [16]	1998	16	62% [b]
Verdonck, et al. [47]	1992	9	67% [b]
Santini, et al. [13]	1991	21	66%
Sweetenham, et al. [48]	1994	105	63% [c]
Jost, et al. [42]	1995	17	31% [d]
Zinzani, et al. [15]	1996	10	70% [b]
Conde, et al. [49]	1999	58	76%
Sweetenham, et al. [50]	2001	31	55%
Song, et al. [34]	2007	25	69%
Total		241	61 (31–77)%
Auto > CR1			
Baro, et al. [46]	1992	8	50%
Morel, et al. [14]	1992	7	43% [b]
Conde, et al. [49]	1999	11	36%
Total		15	47 (43–50)%
Allo CR1			
Milpied, et al. [45]	1989	12	68% [a]
Bouabdallah, et al. [16]	1998	11	91% [b]
Sweetenham, et al. [50]	2001	7	59%
Total		30	74 (59–91)%
Allo > CR1			
Morel, et al. [14]	1992	7	14% [b]
Van Besien, et al. [51]	1996	25	17%
Total		32	16 (14–17)%

According to [11]

[a] for allo and auto together; no difference observed

[b] percentage, not probability

[c] overall survival

[d] including Burkitt's lymphoma

study the lower relapse rate after allo SCT was outweighed by higher mortality [53].

16.8.3 Auto Versus Allo SCT

In several reports, results of auto and allo SCT were compared. Milpied, et al. reported a series of 25 patients with stage III-IV LBL. The LFS was 68% with no difference between allo and auto SCT [45]. Another group reported results of allo SCT in LBL which was performed in younger patients with advanced disease. Ten out of 12 patients mainly transplanted in CR1 survived disease free. LFS after allo SCT was superior (78%) to auto SCT (50%) in this study [16].

Results of SCT (auto N = 128; allo N = 76) in 204 LBL patients at different stages of disease are available from an analysis performed by the International Bone Marrow Transplantation Registry (IBMTR) and the Autologous Blood and Marrow Transplantation Registry (ABMTR). Not surprisingly, there was a higher TRM after allo (18%) compared to auto (3%) SCT. On the other hand, the authors observed a lower relapse rate of 34% for allo compared to 56% for auto SCT after longer observation time. Altogether there was no difference of survival at 5 years with 44% for auto and 39% for allo SCT. Prognostic factors for DFS were donor source, BM involvement, and disease stage [54]. As these are registry data, the options for interpretation are limited. The overall result is not superior to chemotherapy, but includes patients with advanced disease. The risk profile of the patients and the effects of previous therapy, which may be particularly important for auto SCT, are not analyzed. However, there seems to be a graft-versus-lymphoma effect in LBL. Since TRM may be lowered in more recent trials, allo SCT could be an option for high-risk T-LBL. In patients after relapse allo SCT should probably be preferred to auto SCT in patients with an available donor.

16.8.4 Auto SCT Versus Chemotherapy

In the largest prospective trial with randomized comparison of auto SCT and conventional consolidation/maintenance, however, only 65 of 98 eligible patients were actually randomized. The DFS for conventional chemotherapy was 24% compared to 55% for auto SCT. No difference was detected for survival (45 vs. 56%).

In this study, however, the overall CR rate of 56% and the DFS for chemotherapy were suboptimal [50].

It is a well-known fact that results of chemotherapy and SCT cannot be easily compared since retrospectively analyzed SCT patients generally represent a selected patient cohort excluding patients not achieving CR, with early relapse or poor general condition. Particularly patients with LBL generally achieve remission rapidly and if they relapse, they do it early. Thus it can be assumed that these patients are not represented in the transplantation cohort and that a significant number of the transplanted patients are already cured by previous chemotherapy.

A recent study tried to circumvent these issues by an intent-to-treat analysis. In 34 T-LBL patients, SCT was planned upfront after an NHL/ALL-type induction regimen. SCT was actually realized in 29 patients (24 auto, 4 allo), which is a high proportion. The overall survival was 72% for all patients and 79% for those who actually proceeded to SCT. For auto SCT the DFS is 69% [34]. This is the first study showing convincingly that auto SCT may yield similar results as chemotherapy in an intent-to-treat analysis.

16.8.5 Summary

Auto or allo SCT may confer an advantage in survival for high-risk LBL. However, in recent studies survival after chemotherapy is similar to the reported results of allo or auto SCT; furthermore, no convincing risk model for LBL is available at present and therefore clear indications for SCT in first CR are missing. Particularly for allo SCT results are still scarce and treatment-related morbidity and mortality is high; it should therefore probably be restricted to relapse patients.

16.9 Outcome of Salvage Therapy

The outcome of patients with relapsed LBL was poor in most studies. The disease generally shows a rapid progression and response rates after salvage chemotherapy are low. Results of auto SCT are also inferior beyond first CR (Table 16.4). In a report from the EBMTR, the DFS for auto SCT in CR2 or in resistant disease was 31 and 15%, respectively, compared to 63% in CR1 [48]. Also in another large cohort, the DFS after auto SCT in CR1 was 76% compared to 38% for CR2 [49]. From single studies DFS rates between 14 and 50% have been reported for auto SCT in CR2 [14, 46, 55]. For allo SCT beyond first CR the DFS was low (16%), which seems to be a realistic result.

The major problem is to achieve a stable second remission. Several new treatment options may be evaluated. Salvage treatment should aim to refer the patients to an allo SCT as soon as possible. In patients without a compatible donor auto SCT in second remission is an option if stem cells are available or may be performed as interim therapy before allo SCT. Therefore storage of peripheral stem cells during front-line treatment appears to be reasonable since particularly in patients without a sibling donor, the search for an unrelated donor may be too time-consuming.

16.10 Summary and Future Prospects

For the development of future treatment strategies in adult LBL various questions remain open since no randomized studies are available. The use of ALL-type regimens appears to be justified although a prospective comparison with intensive NHL regimens is desirable. In this rare disease this aim could, however, only be achieved with large cooperative studies.

The requirement for intensive prophylaxis of CNS relapse in T-LBL is evident. It remains, however, open whether this aim can be achieved by intensive intrathecal therapy and systemic high dose chemotherapy, whether CNS irradiation is required or whether it may be restricted to patients with stage III/IV disease.

The major problem of local disease control is the effective treatment of mediastinal tumors. This may be achieved by increased dose for mediastinal irradiation, although this approach may compromise further chemotherapy due to bone marrow suppression.

At the same time intensification of systemic treatment can be attempted since treatment-related mortality is generally low in LBL. The value of cytostatic drugs with particular effectivity in T-ALL should be analyzed. From adult T-ALL it is known that CYCLO and ARAC contributed to an improvement of overall results [29]. In childhood T-ALL intensive use of asparaginase [56] and MTX [57] contributed to better outcome. In T-LBL superior results were attributed to intensive treatment including cyclophosphamide, MTX, and dexamethasone during early phase of treatment. As a result no relapses occurred later than 1 year compared to other studies with relapses up to 5 years [7]. Also pretreatment with CYCLO pulses may play a role in T-LBL. In T-ALL the introduction of pretreatment with fractionated CYCLO in one study lead to a reduction of failure rate from 5/39 without CYCLO pretreatment to 0/8 with pretreatment [58]. The efficacy of fractionated CYCLO is also underlined by the successful hyper-CVAD regimen [18].

New cytostatic drugs such as 2-CDA, forodesine Hydrochloride, and nelarabine with specific activity on T-cells or immunotherapy with T-cell specific antibodies such as anti-CD3 and anti-CD52 (Campath) deserve evaluation in relapsed and refractory patients. For nelarabine it was shown recently that it is equally effective in relapsed T-ALL and T-LBL with response rates of 42 and 38%, respectively [59]. This drug is of interest not only for salvage therapy but also for integration in front-line therapy of T-LBL

SCT may have a role in the treatment of high-risk patients with T-LBL although it is still not clear how high-risk patients have to be defined in the context of contemporary intensive ALL-type regimens. Particularly before auto SCT, intensive chemotherapy aiming to a high CR rate and effective tumor reduction seems to be necessary. New prognostic factors are required to define indications for SCT in first remission. The better characterization of biologic markers, e.g., immunophenotype of T-LBL, may contribute to this aim. Methods for MRD evaluation from bone marrow or even peripheral blood have to be established. Microarray analyses may contribute to characterization of disease biology and identification of new prognostic markers. It was already demonstrated that the majority of T-LBL patients show individual T-cell receptor rearrangements similarly to T-ALL. Thus, in the future, indications for SCT may be based at least partly on the evaluation of MRD.

References

1. The Non-Hodgkin's Lymphoma Classification Project (1997) A clinical evaluation of the International Lymphoma Study Group classification of non-Hodgkin's lymphoma. Blood 89:3909–3918
2. Groves FD, Linet MS, Travis LB, Devesa SS (2000) Cancer surveillance series: Non-Hodgkin's lymphoma incidence by histologic subtype in the United States from 1978 through 1995. J Natl Cancer Inst 92:1240–1251
3. Harris NL, Jaffe ES, Diebold J, et al. (2000) The World Health Organization classification of neoplastic diseases of the haematopoietic and lymphoid tissues: Report of the Clinical Advisory Committee Meeting, Airlie House, Virginia, November 1997. Histopathology 36:69–86
4. Raetz EA, Perkins SL, Bhojwani D, et al. (2006) Gene expression profiling reveals intrinsic differences between T-cell acute lymphoblastic leukemia and T-cell lymphoblastic lymphoma. Pediatr Blood Cancer 47:130–140
5. Foon KA, Herzog P, Billing RJ, Terasaki PI, Feig SA (1981) Immunologic classification of childhood acute lymphocytic leukemia. Cancer 47:280–284
6. Jaffe ES, Berard CW (1978) Lymphoblastic lymphoma, a term rekindled with new precision. Ann Intern Med 89:415–417
7. Reiter A, Schrappe M, Ludwig WD, et al. (2000) Intensive ALL-type therapy without local radiotherapy provides a 90% event-free survival for children with T-cell lymphoblastic lymphoma: A BFM group report. Blood 95:416–421
8. Gökbuget N, Hoelzer D (2006) Treatment of adult acute lymphoblastic leukemia. Hematology Am Soc Hematol Educ Program, pp 133–141
9. Engelhard M, Brittinger G, Gerhartz HH, Kuse R, Steinke B (1996) Lymphoblastic lymphoma: Results of a prospective treatment trial (BMFT study). Br J Haematol 93:1391a
10. Soslow RA, Baergen RN, Warnke RA (1999) B-lineage lymphoblastic lymphoma is a clinicopathologic entity distinct from other histologically similar aggressive lymphomas with blastic morphology. Cancer 85:2648–2654
11. Hoelzer D, Gökbuget N, Digel W, et al. (2002) Outcome of adult patients with T-lymphoblastic lymphoma treated according to protocols for acute lymphoblastic leukemia. Blood 99:4379–4385
12. Bernasconi C, Brusamolino E, Lazzarino M, et al. (1990) Lymphoblastic lymphoma in adult patients: Clinicopathological features and response to intensive multiagent chemotherapy analogous to that used in acute lymphoblastic leukemia. Ann Oncol 1:141–146
13. Santini G, Congiu AM, Coser P, et al. (1991) Autologous bone marrow transplantation for adult advanced stage lymphoblastic lymphoma in first CR. A study of the NHLCSG. Leukemia 5(Suppl)1: 42–45
14. Morel P, Lepage E, Brice P, et al. (1992) Prognosis and treatment of lymphoblastic lymphoma in adults: A report on 80 patients. J Clin Oncol 10:1078–1085
15. Zinzani PL, Bendandi M, Visani G, et al. (1996) Adult lymphoblastic lymphoma: Clinical features and prognostic factors in 53 patients. Leuk Lymphoma 23:577–582
16. Bouabdallah R, Xerri L, Bardou VJ, et al. (1998) Role of induction chemotherapy and bone marrow transplantation in adult lymphoblastic lymphoma: A report on 62 patients from a single center. Ann Oncol 9:619–625
17. Sweetenham JW, Pearce R, Taghipour G, et al. (1997) Adult Burkitt's and Burkitt-like non-Hodgkin's lymphoma – Outcome for patients treated with high-dose therapy and autologous stem-cell transplantation in first remission or at relapse: Results from the European Group for Blood and Marrow Transplantation. J Clin Oncol 14:2465–2472
18. Thomas DA, O'Brien S, Cortes J, et al. (2004) Outcome with the hyper-CVAD regimens in lymphoblastic lymphoma. Blood 104:1624–1630

19. Voakes JB, Jones SE, McKelvey EM (1981) The chemotherapy of lymphoblastic lymphoma. Blood 57:186–188
20. Liang R, Todd D, Chan TK, et al. (1991) Intensive chemotherapy for adult lymphoblastic lymphomas. Cancer Chemother Pharmacol 29:80–82
21. Kaiser U, Uebelacker I, Havemann K (1999) Non-Hodgkin's lymphoma protocols in the treatment of patients with Burkitt's lymphoma and lymphoblastic lymphoma: A report on 58 patients. Leuk Lymphoma 36:101–108
22. Coleman CN, Cohen JR, Burke JS, Rosenberg SA (1981) Lymphoblastic lymphoma in adults: Results of a pilot protocol. Blood 57:679–684
23. Coleman CN, Picozzi VJ Jr, Cox RS, et al. (1986) Treatment of lymphoblastic lymphoma in adults. J Clin Oncol 4:1628–1637
24. Colgan JP, Andersen J, Habermann TM, et al. (1994) Long-term follow-up of a CHOP-based regimen with maintenance therapy and central nervous system prophylaxis in lymphoblastic non-Hodgkin's lymphoma. Leuk Lymphoma 15:291–296
25. Chen YC, Ho CL, Kao WY, et al. (2001) Adult lymphoblastic lymphoma in Taiwan: An analysis of treatment results of 26 patients. Ann Hematol 80:647–652
26. Levine AM, Forman SJ, Meyer PR, et al. (1983) Successful therapy of convoluted T-lymphoblastic lymphoma in the adult. Blood 61:92–98
27. Santini G, Congiu A, D'Amico T, et al. (1989) Lymphoblastic lymphoma (LBL) and acute lymphoblastic leukaemia (ALL) in adults: Relationships and therapeutic perspectives. Bone Marrow Transplant 4(Suppl)1:106–107
28. Jabbour E, Koscielny S, Sebban C, et al. (2006) High survival rate with the LMT-89 regimen in lymphoblastic lymphoma (LL), but not in T-cell acute lymphoblastic leukemia (T-ALL). Leukemia 20:814–819
29. Hoelzer D, Gökbuget N (2002) Treatment of lymphoblastic lymphoma in adults. Best Pract Res Clin Haematol 15:713–728
30. Slater DE, Mertelsmann R, Koziner B, et al. (1986) Lymphoblastic lymphoma in adults. J Clin Oncol 4:57–67
31. Daenen S, van Imhoff GW, Haaxma-Reiche H, et al. (1995) Acute lymphoblastic leukemia: Single center experience with modified chemotherapy. Blood 86(S1):754 a
32. Thomas DA, Cortes J, O'Brien S, et al. (1999) Hyper-CVAD program in Burkitt's-type adult acute lymphoblastic leukemia. J Clin Oncol 17:2461–2470
33. Daenen S, van Imhoff GW, Haaxma-Reiche H, et al. (1995) Outcome of a hybrid chemotherapy regimen with mediastinal irradiation in leukemic T-lymphoblastic lymphoma. Blood 86:754 a
34. Song K, Barnett M, Gascoyne R, et al. (2007) Primary therapy for adults with T-cell lymphoblastic lymphoma with hematopoietic stem-cell transplantation results in favorable outcomes. Ann Oncol 18:535–540
35. Salloum E, Henry-Amar M, Caillou B, et al. (1988) Lymphoblastic lymphoma in adults: A clinicopathological study of 34 cases treated at the Institut Gustave-Roussy. Eur J Cancer Clin Oncol 24:1609–1616
36. Yeh KH, Cheng AL, Su IJ, et al. (1997) Prognostic significance of immunophenotypes in adult lymphoblastic lymphomas. Anticancer Res 17:2269–2272
37. Shepherd SF, A'Hern RP, Pinkerton CR (1995) Childhood T-cell lymphoblastic lymphoma – Does early resolution of mediastinal mass predict for final outcome? The United Kingdom Children's Cancer Study Group (UKCCSG). Br J Cancer 72:752–756
38. Spaepen K, Stroobants S, Dupont P, et al. (2001) Prognostic value of positron emission tomography (PET) with fluorine-18 fluorodeoxyglucose ([18F]FDG) after first-line chemotherapy in non-Hodgkin's lymphoma: Is [18F]FDG-PET a valid alternative to conventional diagnostic methods? J Clin Oncol 19:414–419
39. Mott MG, Eden OB, Palmer MK (1984) Adjuvant low dose radiation in childhood non-Hodgkin's lymphoma (report from the United Kingdom Childrens' Cancer Study Group–UKCCSG). Br J Cancer 50:463–469
40. Camitta BM, Lauer SJ, Casper JT, et al. (1985) Effectiveness of a six-drug regimen (APO) without local irradiation for treatment of mediastinal lymphoblastic lymphoma in children. Cancer 56: 738–741
41. Weinstein HJ, Cassady JR, Levey R (1983) Long-term results of the APO protocol (vincristine, doxorubicin [adriamycin], and prednisone) for treatment of mediastinal lymphoblastic lymphoma. J Clin Oncol 1:537–541
42. Jost LM, Jacky E, Dommann-Scherrer C, et al. (1995) Short-term weekly chemotherapy followed by high-dose therapy with autologous bone marrow transplantation for lymphoblastic and Burkitt's lymphomas in adult patients. Ann Oncol 6:445–451
43. Mazza P, Bertini M, Macchi S, et al. (1986) Lymphoblastic lymphoma in adolescents and adults. Clinical, pathological and prognostic evaluation. Eur J Cancer Clin Oncol 22:1503–1510
44. Ferrando AA, Neuberg DS, Staunton J, et al. (2002) Gene expression signatures define novel oncogenic pathways in T cell acute lymphoblastic leukemia. Cancer Cell 1:75–87
45. Milpied N, Ifrah N, Kuentz M, et al. (1989) Bone marrow transplantation for adult poor prognosis lymphoblastic lymphoma in first complete remission. Br J Haematol 73:82–87
46. Baro J, Richard C, Sierra J, et al. (1992) Autologous bone marrow transplantation in 22 adult patients with lymphoblastic lymphoma responsive to conventional dose chemotherapy. Bone Marrow Transplant 10:33–38
47. Verdonck LF, Dekker AW, de Gast GC, Lokhorst HM, Nieuwenhuis HK (1992) Autologous bone marrow transplantation for adult poor-risk lymphoblastic lymphoma in first remission. J Clin Oncol 10:644–646
48. Sweetenham JW, Liberti G, Pearce R, et al. (1994) High-dose therapy and autologous bone marrow transplantation for adult patients with lymphoblastic lymphoma: Results of the European Group for Bone Marrow Transplantation. J Clin Oncol 12:1358–1365
49. Conde E, Zuazu J, Lopez-Guillermo A, et al. (1999) Autologous stem cell transplantation (ASCT) for lymphoblastic lymphoma (LBL). Blood 94:2130 a
50. Sweetenham JW, Santini G, Qian W, et al. (2001) High-dose therapy and autologous stem-cell transplantation versus conventional-dose consolidation/maintenance therapy as postremission therapy for adult patients with lymphoblastic lymphoma: Results of a randomized trial of the European Group for Blood and Marrow Transplantation and the United Kingdom Lymphoma Group. J Clin Oncol 19:2927–2936
51. van Besien KW, Mehra RC, Giralt SA, et al. (1996) Allogeneic bone marrow transplantation for poor-prognosis lymphoma: Response, toxicity and survival depend on disease histology. Am J Med 100:299–307

52. van Imhoff GW, van der HB, MacKenzie MA, et al. (2005) Short intensive sequential therapy followed by autologous stem cell transplantation in adult Burkitt, Burkitt-like and lymphoblastic lymphoma. Leukemia 19:945–952
53. Peniket AJ, Ruiz de Elvira MC, Taghipour G, et al. (1997) Allogeneic transplantation for lymphoma produces a lower relapse rate than autologous transplantation but survival is worse because of higher treatment related mortality – A report of 764 cases from the EBMT lymphoma registry. Blood 90:1121a
54. Levine JE, Harris RE, Loberiza FR Jr, et al. (2003) A comparison of allogeneic and autologous bone marrow transplantation for lymphoblastic lymphoma. Blood 101:2476–2482
55. van Besien K, Przepiorka D, Mehra R, et al. (1996) Impact of preexisting CNS involvement on the outcome of bone marrow transplantation in adult hematologic malignancies. J Clin Oncol 14: 3036–3042
56. Amylon MD, Shuster J, Pullen J, et al. (1999) Intensive high-dose asparaginase consolidation improves survival for pediatric patients with T cell acute lymphoblastic leukemia and advanced stage lymphoblastic lymphoma: A Pediatric Oncology Group study. Leukemia 13:335–342
57. Schrappe M, Reiter A, Ludwig WD, et al. (2000) Improved outcome in childhood acute lymphoblastic leukemia despite reduced use of anthracyclines and cranial radiotherapy: Results of trial ALL-BFM 90. German-Austrian-Swiss ALL-BFM Study Group. Blood 95:3310–3322
58. Bassan R, Pogliani E, Lerede T, et al. (1999) Fractionated cyclophosphamide added to the IVAP regimen (idarubicin-vincristine-L-asparaginase-prednisone) could lower the risk of primary refractory disease in T-lineage but not B-lineage acute lymphoblastic leukemia: First results from a phase II clinical study. Haematologica 84:1088–1093
59. Deangelo DJ, Yu D, Johnson JL, et al. (2007) Nelarabine induces complete remissions in adults with relapsed or refractory T-lineage acute lymphoblastic leukemia or lymphoblastic lymphoma: Cancer and leukemia group B study 19801. Blood Mar 7 [Epub ahead of print]

The Role of Allogeneic Stem Cell Transplantation in the Therapy of Adult Acute Lymphoblastic Leukemia (ALL)

Partow Kebriaei, Richard Champlin

Contents

17.1 Introduction

Adult patients with acute lymphoblastic leukemia (ALL) can now achieve complete remission (CR) rates of 80–90% [1–3]. However, only 25–50% of these patients achieve long-term, disease-free survival. Current research efforts are focused on innovative postremission strategies with the goal of improving disease-free (DFS) and overall survival (OS). The identification of different prognostic groups based on the biology of the malignant clone and prognostic factors allows for risk-adapted therapy. Multiple randomized trials have demonstrated that hematopoietic stem cell transplantation (SCT) improves the outcome of patients with high-risk ALL. In this chapter, we will define the different disease risk groups, the clinical outcomes of major transplant trials for ALL, and the therapeutic factors that affect outcome after SCT.

17.2 Prognostic Factors in Adult ALL

Several biologic features and specific clinical characteristics have been consistently noted to influence the outcome of adult ALL and impact on risk-stratification (Table 17.1). Older age, a high white blood cell count (WBC) at presentation, and failure to achieve a clinical remission within the first 4 weeks of treatment are generally accepted adverse clinical features. The detection of spe-

Table 17.1. Adverse prognostic features in Adult ALL

Age greater than 60 years*
WBC count greater than 30000/μL
Cytogenetics: t(9;22)(q34;q11), trisomy 8, t(4;11)(q21;q23), monosomy 7, a hypodiploid karyotype, t(1;19)(q23;p13)
Delayed time to complete remission, greater than 4 weeks

* Established in US series; German series use age 30, 35, or 50 years as cut-off.

cific recurring cytogenetic abnormalities has emerged as the most important prognostic factor for risk stratification of adults with ALL [4]. Clonal chromosomal aberrations can be detected in cells from 62% to 85% of adult ALL patients, and numerous studies have shown their significance as predictors of outcome [5, 6]. In one review of this literature, six abnormalities were associated with unfavorable outcome, defined as having a 0.25 or less probability of continuous CR at 5 years. These included, in decreasing frequency, t(9;22)(q34;q11), trisomy 8, t(4;11)(q21;q23), monosomy 7, a hypodiploid karyotype, and t(1;19)(q23;p13) [7, 8].

In addition to the adverse prognostic factors listed in Fig. 17.1, the detection of minimal residual disease (MRD) using qualitative or semiquantitative polymerase chain reaction (PCR) or flow cytometric techniques also provides important prognostic information [9]. MRD levels have been investigated both before and after transplantation, and this topic is addressed in a separate chapter of this book. In brief, persistent MRD positivity postinduction appears to be associated with an increased risk of relapse [10]. Brisco, et al. studied 27 adults with B-lineage ALL for MRD in first complete remission (CR1). Relapse occurred in eight of nine patients with a high level of disease detected using semiquantitative PCR (levels $>10^{-3}$), compared to six of 13 patients with lower MRD levels (levels $<10^{-3}$) [11].

MRD positivity after transplant has been most extensively studied in Philadelphia chromosome (Ph)-positive ALL. In 28 patients evaluated, Radich, et al. found that the relative risk (RR) for relapse was significantly higher for patients with a detectable *BCR/ABL* transcript following transplantation than for those without detectable *BCR/ABL* (RR = 5.7, p = 0.025) [12]. The prognostic significance of the PCR assay remained after controlling for other prognostic variables. The risk of relapse was greater for patients with a p190 fusion transcript than for those with p210 *BCR/ABL*. The median time from detection of a positive PCR result to relapse was 94 days. Other investigators have found similar results [13–16]. Generally, patients who are persistently *BCR/ABL* negative following transplantation are unlikely to relapse. Conversely, patients who are *BCR/ABL*+ following transplantation are at high risk for subsequent relapse.

17.3 Results with Allogeneic Transplantation for High-Risk ALL

17.3.1 First Complete Remission

Review of a number of small, phase II trials in high-risk adult ALL who have undergone ASCT in CR1 suggests a higher DFS when compared with historic controls based on conventional chemotherapy [17–23]. High-risk in these studies was defined as patients having at least one or more of the following: age greater than 30 years, WBC greater than 30×10^9/L at presentation, extramedullary disease, unfavorable cytogenetic abnormalities, and requiring more than 4 weeks to achieve CR. As shown in Table 17.2, DFS ranges broadly from 21% to 71%, with a 3- to 8-year follow-up. The large difference in the outcome of these phase II studies is influenced by multiple variables, including differences in patient selection, type of graft vs. host disease (GVHD) prophylaxis, and different supportive care regimens. The choice of preparative regimen may have played a smaller role since all received a total body irradiation (TBI)-based conditioning regimen.

Two large, prospective controlled trials have directly compared transplant with chemotherapy in patients in CR1. The French Leucemie Aigue Lymphoblastique de l'Adulte LALA 87 protocol was a cooperative study that examined the role of chemotherapy and SCT for adult ALL patients. This was a prospective, randomized study, initiated in November 1986 and completed in July 1991, which enrolled 634 newly diagnosed patients. After exclusions, 572 patients were analyzed with 10-year follow-up results. The median age of patients entered in this trial was 33 years. Patients received induction chemotherapy with cyclophosphamide, vincristine, prednisone, and one of two anthracyclines. Central nervous system prophylaxis was administered. Complete remission was achieved in 436 (76%) patients. After CR was achieved, patients older than 50 years received postremission chemotherapy. Patients between 15 and

Table 17.2. Allogeneic transplantation for ALL in CR1

Study	No. pts	Med. age (yrs)	Preparative regimen	GVHD prophylaxis	II-IV GVHD3	3-yrs DFS%
Wingard, 1990 [23]	18	24 (5–36)	CY/TBI	CSA +/– MP	8	42
Blaise, 1990 [17]	25	22 (4–36)	CY/fTBI, ML/fTBI CY/ML/fTBI	MR	7	71
Chao, 1991 [18]	53	28 (1–45)	Ara-C/CY/TBI CY/TBI VP-16/TBI	CSA +/– MP MTX +/– MP	6	61
Doney, 1991 [20]	41	22 (18–50)	CY/fTBI or Single dose TBI	MR	7	21 (5 yrs)
Sutton, 1993 [21] (retrospective review)	184	25 (15–44)	CY/TBI (majority)	MR	15 deaths	49.5 (6 yrs)
Vey, 1994 [22]	29	24 (16–41)	CY/TBI	CSA/MTX	7	62 (8 yrs)
DeWitte, 1994 [19]	22	15–51	CY/TBI	CSA	NR	58

CY, cyclophosphamide; TBI, total body irradiation; fTBI, fractionated TBI; VP-16, etoposide; MR, multiple regimens; NR, not reported; CSA, cyclosporine; MTX, methotrexate; MP, methylprednisolone.

40 years of age were assigned to allogeneic SCT if they had an HLA-matched sibling donor. Patients between ages 40 and 50, and those under the age of 40 without a matched sibling donor, were further randomized to consolidation chemotherapy or autologous SCT using bone marrow purged with antibodies or mafosfamide. Consolidation chemotherapy consisted of three monthly courses of daunorubicin or zorubicin, Ara-C, and asparaginase followed by long-term maintenance therapy. The transplant preparative regimen consisted of TBI and cyclophosphamide. The study separately evaluated high- and standard-risk subsets. High-risk was defined as having one or more of the following factors: presence of the Ph chromosome, null ALL, age >35 years, WBC count $>30\times10^9$/L, time to CR >4 weeks. The remaining patients were considered standard risk.

This study showed that survival at 10 years was significantly greater for the allogeneic SCT group compared to consolidation chemotherapy (46% SCT vs. 31% chemotherapy, $p=0.04$). Furthermore, when these groups were stratified into high and standard risk, there was a highly significant benefit for allogeneic SCT in the high-risk subset, but no statistically significant benefit seen for the standard risk subset (high risk: 44% SCT, 11% chemotherapy, $p=0.009$; standard risk: 49% SCT, 43% chemotherapy, $p=0.6$) [24, 25]. There was no statistically significant difference in outcome between patients who received autologous SCT versus consolidation chemotherapy (34% SCT, 29% chemotherapy, $p=0.6$), with no difference detected in either the high- or standard-risk subset.

The United Kingdom Medical Research Council's (MRC) UKALL XII/Eastern Cooperative Oncology Group (ECOG) E2993 is also conducting a prospective trial to define the role of allogeneic SCT, autologous SCT, and conventional dose chemotherapy in adult patients with ALL in CR1. Initiated in 1993, over 1200 patients have been enrolled to date. All patients received two phases of induction therapy, and continued to allogeneic SCT if they achieved CR and had a histocompatible donor. The remaining patients were randomized to standard consolidation/maintenance therapy for 2.5 years vs. a single autologous SCT. The conditioning regimen for both allogeneic and autologous transplants was fractionated TBI (1320 cGy) and VP-16 (60 mg/kg). Based on the data presented in an abstract in 2001 [26], 239 patients received an allogeneic SCT (170 Ph–) and 291 patients received chemotherapy or autologous SCT. The overall event-free survival (EFS) for the allogeneic SCT group was 54 vs. 34% ($p=0.04$) for the chemotherapy or autologous BMT group. Excluding the t(9;22) karyotype, when patients were stratified into high or standard risk, the difference in EFS becomes more dramatic in the high-risk subset (allogeneic BMT 44% vs. chemotherapy/autologous BMT 26%, p=0.06).

In conclusion, both of these large prospective controlled studies determined that allogeneic SCT improved the outcome for adults with high-risk ALL in CR1.

17.3.2 Beyond CR1

There are no data suggesting that durable remissions can be achieved with standard chemotherapy for adults with ALL who fail to achieve an initial complete remission or have recurrent disease. Second complete remissions can often be achieved, but are typically of shorter duration than the initial response. Patients who undergo an allogeneic SCT in CR2 have achieved long-term, leukemia-free survival (LFS) rates between 14% to 43%, as illustrated in Table 17.3 [20, 23, 27–30]. Therefore, if patients are in remission, allogeneic SCT results in greater LFS when compared to chemotherapy. The primary cause of failure is relapse (>50%).

Table 17.3. Allogeneic transplantation for ALL in CR2

Study	No. patients	LFS (%)	Risk of relapse
IBMTR, 1989 [27]	208 (high risk)	22 (4 yrs)	56
	97 (standard risk)	36 (4 yrs)	49
Barrett, 1989 [28]	391	26 (5 yrs)	52
Wingard, 1990 [23]	36	43 (5 yrs)	26
Doney, 1991 [20]	48	15 (5 yrs)	64
Greinix, 1998 [29]	27	14 (3 yrs)	78
Michallet, 2000 [30]	47	30 +/- 8% (5 yrs)	44+/- 12%

17.3.3 Primary Refractory ALL

With current induction regimens, only 5–10% of adults with newly diagnosed ALL fail to achieve remission. These patients often have poor prognostic factors at presentation, and additional attempts at induction chemotherapy are usually of limited benefit. Several studies suggest that patients with an HLA-identical sibling benefit by receiving allogeneic transplantation without undergoing a second attempt at induction therapy [31–33]. In the largest of these studies, 38 patients with ALL failing to achieve remission received HLA-identical sibling transplants. Approximately 35% of these patients with refractory disease became long-term, disease-free survivors. In a retrospective review of patients with primary refractory and relapsed ALL, the records of 314 adults were reviewed for disease outcome at MD Anderson Cancer Center between 1980 and 1997. Allogeneic SCT was performed in 29 patients (13 in salvage and 16 in CR2). The rates for durable CR posttransplant were comparable between the two groups; 5/13 (38%) in the salvage group and 5/16 (31%) in the remission group. Although patient numbers are small and a variety of transplant conditioning regimens were used, these results corroborate the findings of earlier studies, and suggest that allogeneic transplant should be considered for these patients with an otherwise dismal chance of long-term survival [34, 35].

17.4 Philadelphia Chromosome-Positive ALL

Philadelphia chromosome-positive (Ph+) acute lymphoblastic leukemia is well established to have a very poor prognosis. The recent incorporation of imatinib mesylate into combination chemotherapy has been a major development. Imatinib is a highly effective, targeted therapy directed against the *BCR/ABL* tyrosine kinase that is overexpressed as a result of the t(9;22)(q34;q11) in chronic myeloid leukemia and Ph+ ALL [34]. The rapid initial response to therapy and minimal side effects make imatinib an ideal drug for incorporation into clinical trials for treatment of newly diagnosed Ph+ ALL. In a study by Thomas et al., 20 patients with newly diagnosed Ph+ ALL received concurrent hyper-CVAD (cyclophosphamide, vincristine, Adriamycin, dexamethasone) and imatinib at the 400 mg dose. All patients achieved CR. Ten patients received allogeneic SCT in first CR within a median of 3.5 months, with nine remaining alive in CR with a median follow-up of 12 months. Among ten patients ineligible for SCT, one relapsed after 12 months, two died in CR from comorbid conditions at 15 and 16 months, and five remained in continuous CR for a median of 20 months [36]. Although this is an early study with very short follow-up, these results are very encouraging for a subset of patients with a traditionally very poor prognosis.

Data from the MRC UKALL XII/ECOG E2993 study described earlier revealed similar poor results for Ph+ patients treated with chemotherapy only. In this ongoing, prospective, randomized study, 167 Ph+ patients were treated on the MRC UKALL XII/ECOG E2993 protocol between 1993 and 2000. Seventy-two patients received a matched-related or unrelated donor transplant in CR1, while seven received an autologous transplant and 88 received chemotherapy due to lack of donors. As expected, the 5-year EFS and OS were significantly higher for the allogeneic transplant group, 36% and 42%, respectively, compared to 17% and 19% for the nonallogeneic transplant groups [37]. These results suggest that the presence of the Ph chromosome is most detrimental to maintaining long-term remission, and underscore the need for long-term follow-up of ongoing studies with imatinib. Until long-term results are obtained, all Ph+ patients should still receive an allogeneic SCT in CR1 if a donor is available.

Disease outcome from a series of single-center retrospective studies are listed in Table 17.4 [19, 38–40]. It is difficult to draw conclusions from these small series that vary considerably with respect to type of patient (CR1 or beyond), type of preparative regimen, GVHD prophylaxis, and supportive care. The reported DFS rate varies widely between 20% to 80%, and it is difficult to determine if a particular preparative regimen is superior. Generally, data from most series suggest that Ph+ patients fare best when transplanted in CR1. Follow-up from the prospective MRC UKALL XII/ECOG E2993 study is eagerly anticipated.

It is hoped that the incorporation of imatinib into the transplant conditioning regimen or early posttransplant will further improve results. The Cancer and Leukemia Group B (CALGB), in combination with the Southwest Oncology Group (SWOG) are enrolling patients in a Phase II trial of sequential chemotherapy, imatinib, and allogeneic or autologous SCT for adults with newly diagnosed Ph+ ALL. The primary objectives of this study will be to determine the ability of imatinib to produce a complete molecular response (achieve *BCR/ABL-* status by RT-PCR) following sequential chemotherapy, imatinib therapy, and transplantation, and to determine the ability of imatinib to improve DFS and OS in this high-risk group of patients. The safety and efficacy of concurrent imatinib administration with high dose chemotherapy is being investigated in blast phase CML patients currently enrolled in clinical trials at MD Anderson Cancer Center, and results may be applicable to Ph+ ALL patients.

The feasibility of alternative donor transplants has also been investigated in Ph+ ALL patients in efforts to provide allogeneic transplantation to patients who lack a matched sibling. At the Fred Hutchinson Cancer Research Center, matched unrelated donor (MUD) transplantation was investigated in 18 patients with Ph+ ALL between 1988 and 1995. The study included children and adults, with the median age being 25 years. Seven patients were in CR1, one in CR2, three in first relapse, and seven with advanced disease. The preparative regimen involved TBI and cyclophosphamide. Six patients who were transplanted in CR1, one in CR1, and two while in second remission remained leukemia-free at a median follow-up of 17 months. The probability of LFS at 2 years was 49%, similar to rates reported for matched-sibling-SCT [41]. However, it must be emphasized that this was a highly selected population of relatively young patients. Too few adults with Ph+ ALL have received cord blood or haploidentical donor transplants to comment on results.

Table 17.4. Allogeneic transplantation for Ph+ ALL

Study	No. pts	Med. age (years)	Prep. regimen	3-year DFS%
Stockschlader, 1995 [39]	10	31	VP-16/CY/TBI	46
Dunlop, 1996 [40]	11	27	TBI-based	21.8
Snyder, 1999 [38]	23	30	VP-16/fTBI	65 (SCT before 1992)
				81 (SCT after 1992)

CY, cyclophosphamide; TBI, total body irradiation; fTBI, fractionated TBI; VP-16, etoposide.

Donor lymphocyte infusion (DLI) has also been investigated in patients with Ph+ ALL. DLI is most effective as treatment for Ph+ chronic phase CML, but has little benefit for patients with either myeloid or lymphoid blast crisis. Although peptides derived from bcr-abl may be immunogenic, the immunologic target of DLI is unknown and minor histocompatibility antigens and overexpressed myeloid lineage related proteins might be involved.

DLI has had very limited efficacy in Ph+ ALL [42, 43]. It is not known whether this disparity in efficacy stems from differences in the immunogenicity of the p190 *BCR/ABL* (most Ph+ ALL) vs. the p210 *BCR/ABL* (most CML), differences in growth kinetics of Ph+ ALL relapse (high tumor burden) vs. those in CML (lower tumor burden), or other disease specific factors. Interestingly, in a study of 11 patients, including one with Ph+ ALL, second allogeneic PBSC transplants from the original donor were administered for treatment of relapse. All patients achieved CR, but responses were not durable. The patient with Ph+ ALL achieved a complete clinical and molecular response, but died at 12 weeks due to CNS relapse. This was the only site of disease at time of death [44].

17.5 Factors Influencing Transplant Outcome

17.5.1 Preparative Regimens

17.5.1.1 Radiation-based

Several different preparative regimens for allogeneic SCT have been described in attempts to decrease transplant related mortality (TRM) and improve DFS. The most widely used regimen is the combination of total body irradiation (TBI) and cyclophosphamide developed by Thomas and colleagues. TBI can be administered as single dose, or fractionated over 3–5 days. A comparative analysis of fractionated-dose vs. single-dose TBI in adult ALL patients showed a significantly higher TRM in the single-dose group ($p = 0.017$), but an increase in the relapse rate of the fractionated-dose group; consequently, there were no differences in the overall LFS between the two groups [21]. The Minnesota Group compared TBI/cyclophosphamide with TBI/Ara-C in a study including both adults and children, and found no outcome difference in regards to toxicity or outcome [45]. The City of Hope group studied fractionated TBI with etoposide followed by SCT in patients with advanced leukemia. A Phase I/II trial indicated that etoposide at 60 mg/kg is the maximum tolerated dose when combined with TBI. In that study, 36 ALL patients were treated; 20 had relapsed disease. The DFS was 57%, with a 32% relapse rate suggesting that the regimen has significant activity in advanced ALL [46].

Novel methods to allow selective delivery of radiation to sites of leukemia without increasing systemic toxicity are currently under investigation. One method with great potential is the incorporation of radiolabeled monoclonal antibodies (MoAb) into the conditioning regimen. A Phase I transplant trial using ^{131}I-labeled anti-CD45 antibody combined with cyclophosphamide at 120 mg/kg and 12-Gy TBI was recently published [47]. All patients had advanced hematologic malignancies. The dose limiting toxicity was grade III/IV mucositis. Nine patients with ALL (five with relapsed/refractory ALL; four in CR2 or CR3) received allogeneic (six patients) or autologous (3 patients) transplants using this preparative regimen; three patients were disease-free 19, 54, and 66 months posttransplant. A more recent study evaluated the feasibility of using ^{188}rhenium (^{188}Re)-labeled anti-CD66 in combination with standard high-dose chemotherapy/TBI (12 Gy) in 50 advanced leukemia patients, including 11 with ALL, undergoing allogeneic or autologous SCT. All patients achieved primary engraftment. After a median follow-up of 11 months, 28/50 (56%) patients were in CR, nine (5%) patients relapsed, and 13 (7%) died from treatment-related causes [48]. The ultimate benefits of this approach with respect to safety and improvements in survival will be defined by Phase II studies for patients with ALL. Much more clinical data has been gathered for nonradiolabeled MoAbs as discussed below.

17.5.1.2 Nonradiation-based

Nonradiation-containing regimens, most commonly busulfan and cyclophosphamide, have been investigated in hopes of decreasing radiation-related complications. Fractionated TBI/etoposide was compared with busulfan/cyclophosphamide in a prospective, randomized study conducted by the Southwest Oncology Group (SWOG 8612). One hundred twenty-two patients with leukemia beyond CR1 received either FTBI/etoposide or busulfan/cyclophosphamide in preparation for SCT. One hundred fourteen (93%) proceeded to SCT. All patients received cyclosporine and prednisone for posttransplant immunosuppression. There was no significant difference with respect to toxicity, incidence of acute GVHD, OS, or DFS between the two groups. The leading cause for treatment failure was leukemic relapse (39%) [56]. Furthermore, retrospective analysis of registry data from the International Bone Marrow Transplant Registry (IBMTR) shows similar rates for LFS and relapse when busulfan/cyclophosphamide is compared to TBI/cyclophosphamide [49].

The addition of monoclonal antibodies to the transplant conditioning regimen is another method of developing potentially more effective, and less toxic, regimens. Antibody therapy is generally considered to be an option when the target antigen is expressed on at least 30% of the targeted cells [50]. ALL blasts express a variety of B- or T-cell differentiation antigens, such as CD19, CD20, CD22, CD33, and CD52, which can serve as targets for directed therapy [50]. The greatest clinical data has been gathered for rituximab, a chimeric MoAb directed against CD20, which has demonstrated efficacy in patients with non-Hodgkin's lymphoma. At the MD Anderson Cancer Center, rituximab has been incorporated in both the upfront induction regimen for ALL patients who present with CD20 positive disease, as well as in the transplant conditioning regimen for these patients. Preliminary results for rituximab combined with hyper-CVAD for induction therapy have been favorable (Thomas, abstract). The transplant protocol utilizing rituximab, cyclophosphamide, and TBI is still in the process of patient accrual, but no excess adverse results have been noted thus far (Khouri, personal communication).

CD19 is expressed in a large portion of B-lineage ALL patients, and several antibodies have been developed against the CD19 antigen. Since this antigen readily modulates internally, studies have generally involved anti-CD19 MoAb-based immunotoxins. Preliminary results from small phase I studies suggest that they are feasible as an adjunct to chemotherapy, but that efficacy for MoAbs as monotherapy is limited, especially in the setting of overt relapse or rapidly progressive disease [51, 52].

Campath-1H, a humanized MoAb developed against the CD52 antigen, is particularly interesting since it targets a subset of ALL for disease eradication, as well as a novel method of T-cell depletion to prevent GVHD in the allogeneic transplant setting. The clinical efficacy has been limited in the nontransplant setting [53, 54], but the agent may be potentially more useful with allogeneic SCT. Campath-1H either as an intravenous treatment or for ex vivo purging of the allogeneic cells, is effective to reduce the incidence and severity of graft-vs.-host disease following allogeneic SCT. Novitzky et al. evaluated 13 patients with ALL (eight in CR1) and 37 patients with AML (33 in CR1), who had undergone HLA-identical sibling transplants. The conditioning regimen consisted of TBI/cyclophosphamide. Bone marrow or PBSC were exposed to CAMPATH-1H ex-vivo. Patients received no posttransplant immunosuppression. All but one patient engrafted, and only 22% of all patients developed grade I or II GVHD; there was no severe GVHD. There is concern that the immunosuppressive effect of Campath-1H may inhibit the immune graft-vs.-malignancy effect and 54% (7/13) of the ALL patients in this study relapsed [55]. A study is ongoing at MD Anderson combining Campath-1H with cyclophosphamide and TBI to provide both disease eradication and in vivo T-cell purging in a transplant protocol for CD52+ lymphoid malignancies at MD Anderson Cancer Center. The trial is currently in the process of accruing patients, and preliminary results are promising (Khouri, personal communication). Large, randomized studies will be required to determine whether inclusion of Campath-1H will improve the overall outcome for patients undergoing transplantation for ALL.

17.5.1.3 Nonmyeloablative SCT (NMSCT)

Numerous studies have now demonstrated successful donor stem cell engraftment with NMSCT for hematologic and solid organ malignancies. These regimens use reduced doses of chemotherapy +/− low dose TBI as immune suppression to prevent graft rejection and allow development of an immune graft-vs.-malignancy (GVM) effect. GVM appears to be operative against ALL; the major evidence being a reduced rate of relapse in patients who have GVHD. However, ALL appears less effected by GVM than the other major forms of leukemia and the role of NMSCT requires further evaluation. The major benefit of NMSCT is a lower risk of drug toxicity and treatment-related morbidity and mortality, which is most relevant to older or debilitated patients unable to tolerate ablative preparative regimens. This option would be particularly attractive for patients with Ph+ ALL where the majority of patients are older than 50 years.

Martino et al. reported on the largest published cohort of adult ALL patients receiving NMSCT [56]. He analyzed the results of 27 patients with high-risk ALL that were included in four prospective studies. Similar to other reduced-intensity transplant series, these were older patients with advanced disease. The median age was 50 years; 23 (85%) patients were beyond CR1, 44% were chemorefractory, and 41% were Ph+. Donors were mismatched related donors or volunteer unrelated donors in 12 cases (44%). The incidence of grades II-IV acute GVHD was 48%, and 13 of 18 evaluable patients (72%) developed chronic GVHD. With a median follow-up of 809 days, the incidence of TRM was 23%, the probability of OS was 31%, and the incidence of disease progression was 49% at 2 years. The incidence of disease progression in patients with and without GVHD, 35% and 47%, respectively, approached statistical significance ($p=0.05$). The incidence of disease relapse was 33% in patients transplanted in CR compared to 60% in those with overt disease.

These observations for NMSCT must be validated in well-defined prospective trials. NMSCT, as an immunotherapeutic approach, is probably most appropriate in patients with low-bulk disease. In this study, and others, a higher relapse rate was observed for patients transplanted with overt disease [57]. Thus, NMSCT does not appear indicated for patients with overt relapsed or resistant ALL. The initial studies appear most promising for older patients transplanted in remission, and the reported OS and TRM rates were quite favorable considering the advanced disease state of the patients and the number of unrelated transplants included in this series. Thus, it is reasonable to enroll older patients (age >50 years) and those with a high risk of TRM onto prospective studies of NMSCT. Younger allogeneic transplant candidates without major comorbidities, should still receive high dose therapy with ablative preparative regimens, as established effective treatment for ALL.

17.5.2 Source of Stem Cells

17.5.2.1 Bone Marrow vs. Peripheral Blood Stem Cells

Bensinger et al. published a prospective, randomized trial comparing bone marrow (BM) to peripheral blood as the source of stem cells. Between March 1996 and July 1999, 172 patients, including 22 with ALL, with a median age of 42 years, were randomly assigned to receive BM or filgrastim-mobilized peripheral blood stem cells (PBSC) from HLA-identical relatives for hematopoietic rescue after dose-intensive chemotherapy. After randomization, patients were stratified according to age and stage of cancer, with roughly equal numbers in the two groups. It was concluded from this study that allogeneic PBSC result in faster engraftment without an increased risk of GVHD (median day to neutrophil recovery defined as $>500/mm^3$, 16 vs. 21, p-value <0.001; median day to platelet recovery defined as $>20\,000/mm^3$, 13 vs. 19, p-value <0.001). It was also observed that patients who received PBSC had a lower incidence of relapse at 2 years, and higher OS and DFS [55]. While similar subsequent series have confirmed that PBSC result in faster engraftment, a large retrospective analysis from the IBMTR and EBMT showed that the incidence of chronic GVHD was significantly higher with the use of PBSC (65 vs. 53%, $p=0.02$). In addition, the risk of relapse was not significantly different between these two groups [58]. Thus, a large, multicenter, prospective study was developed to help define the role of PBSC in allogeneic SCT. In this collaborative effort by the BMT-CTN, adult leukemia patients requiring MUD transplantation will be randomized to BM or PBSC donors. Results of this trial are eagerly anticipated.

17.5.2.2 Umbilical Cord Blood (UCB)

Recently, UCB transplantation (UCBT) is beginning to emerge as a viable alternative hematopoietic stem cell source for patients who lack an HLA-matched donor. UCBT is less likely to produce severe GVHD compared to bone marrow transplantation, and thus has the advantage of allowing for greater HLA disparity between donor and recipient. Its disadvantage, however, is the significantly lower cell dose in UCB when compared to PBSC or BM (the cell dose in one average UCB unit is 1/10 of a typical BM allograft and 1/100 of a PBSC allograft), predictably resulting in a longer time to engraftment, and potentially greater early posttransplant complications. UCB transplants have had the best results in children where a relatively high cell dose/kg can be administered. There has been a greater risk of complications in adult recipients.

More than 500 adults have undergone UCBT worldwide [59–64], mainly for hematologic malignancies. Similar to the pediatric series, the majority of patients received HLA-mismatched grafts and myeloablative regimens. The largest series was reported by Eurocord, and contains 108 adults, with 32 cases of ALL, with a mean follow up of 20 months. The mean age was 26 years (range 15 to 53 years), mean weight 60 kg (range 35 to 110 kg), and mean number of nucleated cells infused 1.7×10^7/kg. The overall 1-year survival was 27%. Survival for early disease stage patients, including CML in chronic phase or acute leukemia in remission, was 39 vs. 17% for those transplanted with more advanced disease. The 60-day probability of neutrophil engraftment was 81% at a mean time of 32 days (range 13 to 60 days). The incidence of acute GVHD ≥II was 38%. Most deaths were due to infection or GVHD. These findings were corroborated by other series. The TRM at 100 days approached 43–54% for the myeloablative regimens, and 28–48% using nonmyeloablative regimens [59], with main reasons for TRM being regimen-related toxicity, infection, and relapse. Nucleate cell dose was a significant variable, conferring better outcome when the cell dose was $>2\times10^7$/kg and/or CD34 cells $>1.2\times10^5$/kg [60, 62]. HLA disparity had less influence on EFS [60]. In summary, despite cell dose limitations, UCBT on clinical protocols may be a viable option for selected adult patients with limited treatment options. Current research in UCB expansion may help to overcome the cell dose limitations and contribute toward reducing the TRM.

17.5.3 Source of Donor Cells: Partially Matched Related or Matched Unrelated Donors

The majority of studies indicate that the best chance for cure for refractory or high-risk ALL is allogeneic SCT with a matched related donor. Unfortunately, less than 30% of these patients have a matched sibling donor. Thus, much work continues to be done in making partially matched related donor (PMRD) and matched unrelated donor (MUD) transplantation safe and more feasible as curative therapy. Typically these transplants have been associated with a higher risk of graft rejection, GVHD, and infection. However, more precise HLA matching of donor and recipient via the use of high resolution allele-based typing for class I and II HLA molecules has allowed selection of better matched donors; this has resulted in a progressive improvement in the incidence of severe GVHD, and survival in patients undergoing MUD transplantation [65].

Two large, retrospective series compared the outcome of MUD SCT with autologous SCT. Weisdorf et al. reported the results of 517 ALL patients (median age 14 years, range 1 to 50) who received MUD-SCT and compared them to 195 patients (median age 18 years, range 1 to 50) who underwent autologous SCT between 1989 and 1998. The proportion of patients in CR1 vs. CR2 was similar for both groups. However, patients receiving MUD transplants had a greater frequency of high-risk karyotypes and elevated WBC count at presentation. TRM was higher in the MUD-SCT vs. the autologous SCT group (42 vs. 20%, $p=0.004$). Conversely, relapse was more frequent after autologous SCT (49 vs. 14% in CR1, 64 vs. 25% in CR2), resulting in net similar outcomes with either transplant approach. Three-year survival rates were 45–50% for patients transplanted in CR1 and 30–40% for patients in CR2 [66]. The Acute Leukemia Working Party of the European Cooperative Group for Blood and Marrow Transplantation (EBMT) reported very similar outcomes for ALL patients receiving MUD SCT ($n=118$) compared to those receiving an autologous transplant ($n=236$). A significantly higher TRM, from GVHD and graft failure, in the MUD-SCT group was offset by a significantly higher risk of relapse in the autologous SCT group, resulting in similar 2-year LFS for both groups (39% MUD, 32% auto) [67].

Due to the small numbers of patients and differing approaches to partially matched related donor (PMRD) transplantation, little data exists for this investigational approach. Most studies suggest a higher rate of rejection and acute GVHD, but similar overall survival for patients with donors matched for five of the six HLA A, B and DR antigens as with fully matched sibling donors [68]. Greater degrees of mismatch are associated for higher risks of rejection, GVHD and treatment related mortality. Singhal et al. reported the results of 164 patients (84 with ALL) who received a PMRD transplant between 1993 and 1999 at the South Carolina Cancer Center, and compared them to 164 patients (81 with ALL) who received an autologous transplant at the Royal Marsden Hospital, UK between 1984 and 1999 [69]. At 5 years, the cumulative TRM was 52%, incidence of relapse 32%, and DFS 16% for patients receiving PMRD transplants compared to 16%, 54%, and 30%, respectively, for those receiving autologous SCT. The retrospective nature of this study and differences in patient care that can result from two different treatment sites limit the conclusions regarding this comparative study;

it does, however, suggest that an autologous SCT may be preferable to PMRD transplantation in the absence of an HLA-matched donor. In summary, the decision to proceed with MUD or autologous transplantation, or to proceed with other "Phase I" approaches for these high-risk patients currently remains very complex, and should be based on the specific situation of each individual patient.

17.5.4 The Role of T-Cell Depletion

Studies have shown consistently that a major therapeutic effect of allogeneic SCT is derived from the GVM. There is a reduced risk of relapse in patients with GVHD, and a major difficulty lies in separating the beneficial GVM effect from the adverse consequences of GVHD. This objective is a major focus of ongoing research.

GVHD is primarily mediated by donor-derived T-lymphocytes. One approach to prevent acute GVHD, is to deplete T-cells from the donor marrow or PBSC. After initial immune reconstitution, donor T-lymphocytes (DLI) can be administered with a lower risk of GVHD to enhance the GVM anti-leukemic effect. As described previously, Campath-1H, directed against the CD52 antigen, provides a novel approach for both ex vivo and in vivo T-cell purging.

The role of T-cell depleted SCT remains controversial. While T-cell depleted SCT are associated with a lower incidence of acute and chronic GVHD, GVM effects may be reduced and leukemia-free survival has not been improved in controlled trials for either matched sibling or unrelated donor transplants. Several groups have reported a decreased risk of relapse with T-cell-depleted SCT by manipulating the preparative regimen to compensate for potential lack of a GVM effect.

Aversa et al. evaluated 54 consecutive acute leukemia patients with median age 30 (30 AML, 24 ALL) undergoing ex-vivo, T-cell-depleted BMT using bone marrow from HLA-identical or D-DR-mismatched (two patients) sibling donors [70]. Antithymocyte globulin and thiotepa were added to standard TBI/cyclophosphamide conditioning. The risk of relapse was 12% for AML patients and 28% for ALL patients. At median follow-up of 6.9 years, the EFS for AML was 74%, and 59% for ALL. Schattenberg et al. compared the outcome of HLA-identical, T-cell depleted BMT in patients less than 50 years old versus greater than 50 years old [71]. The standard conditioning regimen of TBI/cyclophosphamide was intensified with the addition of idarubicin at 42 mg/m^2. The study evaluated 131 patients, which included 34 patients with ALL. The 2-year LFS for the ALL patients in this small study was 64%, which compares very favorably with HLA-identical transplants that are not T-cell depleted.

Unmodified transplants from HLA haploidentical donors is associated with a prohibitively high risk of acute GVHD. Transplantation of high doses of CD34+ cells which are extensively depleted of T-lymphocytes has been effective to achieve engraftment without GVHD in these very high risk patients.

17.5.5 Immunomodulation with DLI

The presence of a GVM effect is based primarily on observations of lower relapse rates in patients who develop GVHD. Table 17.5 summarizes results obtained from both single institution and registry data, and demonstrates a consistent decrease in relapse rates for patients who develop GVHD vs. those who do not [20, 72, 73]. A GVM effect that is associated with the presence of GVHD has been described in ALL, AML, and CML; interestingly this effect appears most potent in ALL and is reflected by the data in Table 17.5 [74]. In distinct contrast to these consistent observations of the benefit of GVHD in reducing the relapse rate following allogeneic SCT is the marked absence of a significant GVM effect in ALL following DLI. In contrast to CML and AML where DLI often results in complete remissions in patients with relapsed disease following allogeneic transplant, DLI does not appear to be effective for ALL with relapse following an allogeneic transplant. The EBMT Working Party for Acute and Chronic Leukemia studied the effect of DLI on acute and chronic leukemia in relapse after SCT. One hundred thirty-five patients were treated, including 22 with ALL (nine in CR1, five in CR2, eight beyond CR2). The median age of the ALL patients was 21.5.

In contrast to 73% of CML patients achieving CR with DLI, no patients with ALL responded [75]. Collins et al. reviewed data on 140 patients receiving DLI at a number of transplant centers. Fifteen patients with ALL were included; three in CR and 12 with progressive disease. There was an 18% response rate to DLI seen in the ALL group in contrast to 60% seen in the CML group [76].

Table 17.5. Risk of relapse following non-T-cell depleted allogeneic transplantation in ALL

Study	No. patients		Risk of relapse (%)
Doney, 1991 [20]	192 (SCT in CR2)	No GVHD	80
		Grade II-IV GVHD	40
Sullivan, 1989 [72]	200		
	(SCT in CR)	No GVHD	56
		Acute GVHD	27
		Acute & chronic GVHD	22
	(SCT in relapse)	No GVHD	81
		Acute GVHD	39
		Acute & chronic GVHD	43
Horowitz, 1990 [73]	349 (SCT in CR1)	No GVHD	44
(IBMTR)		Acute GVHD	17
		Chronic GVHD	20
		Acute & chronic GVHD	15

Direct and indirect evidence suggests that donor T cells and NK cells are primary mediators of GVM. The target antigens for the GVM response are unknown. It is difficult to generate a T-cell response to lymphoblasts. ALL cells do not express costimulatory molecules and are poor stimulators of T-cell reactivity.

G-CSF mobilized PBSC have also been investigated as a source of donor lymphocytes for adoptive therapy. The numbers of T cells and NK cells found in PBSC are comparable to those present in a DLI. Eleven patients (four CML, five AML, one ALL) received PBSC postrelapse; all patients with acute leukemia received cytoreductive therapy prior to PBSC. All six patients with acute leukemia achieved a CR, with median remission duration of 24 weeks [77]. Perhaps the success noted in this study resulted, in part, from the cytoreduction prior to DLI, which may play an important role in the DLI efficacy. DLI has been combined with IL-2 in an attempt to augment efficacy in ALL patients. Four patients with relapsed ALL were treated with this approach and all responded [77]. No conclusions can be drawn from such small series of patients. However, these results are intriguing, and suggest that adoptive cell therapy and associated immunomodulatory therapy may be further developed as a treatment modality, and may eventually become a viable salvage option for ALL relapses following allogeneic transplants.

17.6 Long-Term Complications of Allogeneic SCT

Socie et al. analyzed the characteristics of 6691 patients listed in the IBMTR who underwent allogeneic SCT for AML, ALL, CML, or aplastic anemia between January 1980 and December 1993 [78]. The median duration of follow-up was 80 months. Mortality rates in this cohort were compared with those of an age-, sex-, and nationality-matched general population. All patients were free of disease 2 years posttransplant, with 89% survival at 5 years. Mortality rates remained significantly higher than the general population throughout the study among patients who underwent transplantation for ALL or CML, and through the ninth year for patients who had AML. Specifically, for patients with ALL, the relative mortality rate was 20.1 2 years after transplantation, 25.9 5 years after transplantation, and 15.4 10 years after transplantation. Not surprisingly, recurrent leukemia was the chief cause of death for patients who underwent SCT for leukemia and GVHD among those in either disease category, followed by infection, new cancer, and organ failure. Older age was associated with an increased risk of relapse in the ALL group, with 48% relapse observed in ALL compared with 11% relapses in the overall group. Chronic GVHD was the second leading cause of death overall, with 23% observed in the ALL cohort. A low incidence of secondary cancer was reported overall (6%), with a slightly higher rate observed in the ALL group (10%). Increased rates of secondary cancer may be noted with longer follow-up.

Quality of life and psychosocial functioning are major issues following allogeneic SCT. Broers et al. evaluated quality of life in a prospective study of 125 consecutive patients who underwent BMT between 1987 and 1992 [79]. Patients were evaluated with questionnaires measuring quality of life, functional limitations, psychological distress, anxiety, depression, and self-esteem. Questionnaires were answered prior to the BMT, 1 month after following discharge, at 6 months, 1 year, and 3 years after BMT. Nearly 90% of patients reported a good to excellent quality of life at 3 years. Changes in quality of life and psychological distress could be explained entirely by changes in functional limitations and somatic symptoms. The minority of patients who reported a worse quality of life reported experiencing continued serious functional limitations. One such limitation is the late neurotoxic effects of BMT on cognitive functioning. Harder et al. investigated this phenomenon in a consecutively treated cohort of long-term adult survivors [80]. Forty patients were included, 87.5% had undergone allogeneic transplantation. All received total body irradiation up to 12 Gy. Assessment took place 22–82 months after BMT. Mild to moderate cognitive impairment was found in 24 patients (60%). Compared with healthy population norms, selective attention and executive function, information processing speed, verbal learning, and verbal and visual memory were most likely to be affected. Therefore, cognitive functioning should be used as an outcome parameter in BMT studies, and emphasis should be placed on interventions that help patients cope with their physical limitations.

17.7 Conclusion

In conclusion, allogeneic SCT has been demonstrated to have a major therapeutic benefit for selected patients with high-risk ALL. However, much work remains to be done to improve survival for patients with this challenging disease. Results of trials of novel strategies are eagerly awaited including the incorporation of molecularly targeted chemotherapy, targeted immunotherapy using monoclonal antibodies or adoptive cellular therapy, and novel nonmyeloablative preparative regimens with promise to decrease treatment-related morbidity and improve survival.

References

1. Kantarjian HM, et al. (2000) Results of treatment with hyper-CVAD, a dose-intensive regimen, in adult acute lymphocytic leukemia. J Clin Oncol 18(3):547–561
2. Linker C, et al. (2002) Intensified and shortened cyclical chemotherapy for adult acute lymphoblastic leukemia. J Clin Oncol 20(10):2464–2471
3. Larson RA (2000) Recent clinical trials in acute lymphocytic leukemia by the Cancer and Leukemia Group B. Hematol Oncol Clin North Am 14(6):1367–1379
4. Hoelzer D, et al. (1988) Prognostic factors in a multicenter study for treatment of acute lymphoblastic leukemia in adults. Blood 71(1):123–131
5. Charrin C, Mugneret F (1996) Cytogenetics of recurrent acute leukemia. Rev Prat 46(1):37–41
6. Faderl S, et al. (1998) Clinical significance of cytogenetic abnormalities in adult acute lymphoblastic leukemia. Blood 91(11): 3995–4019
7. Wetzler M, et al. (1999) Prospective karyotype analysis in adult acute lymphoblastic leukemia: The cancer and leukemia Group B experience. Blood 93(11):3983–3993
8. Wetzler M (2000) Cytogenetics in adult acute lymphocytic leukemia. Hematol Oncol Clin North Am 14(6):1237–1249
9. Stock W, Estrov Z (2000) Studies of minimal residual disease in acute lymphocytic leukemia. Hematol Oncol Clin North Am 14(6):1289–1305, viii–ix
10. Hoelzer D (2002) Acute lymphoblastic leukemia. American Society of Hematology, Pennsylvania
11. Brisco J, et al. (1996) Relationship between minimal residual disease and outcome in adult acute lymphoblastic leukemia. Blood 87(12):5251–5256
12. Radich JP, et al. (1995) Polymerase chain reaction detection of the BCR-ABL fusion transcript after allogeneic marrow transplantation for chronic myeloid leukemia: Results and implications in 346 patients. Blood 85(9):2632–2638
13. Gehly GB, et al. (1991) Chimeric BCR-abl messenger RNA as a marker for minimal residual disease in patients transplanted for Philadelphia chromosome-positive acute lymphoblastic leukemia. Blood 78(2):458–465
14. Mitterbauer G, et al. (1999) Quantification of minimal residual disease in patients with BCR-ABL-positive acute lymphoblastic leukaemia using quantitative competitive polymerase chain reaction. Br J Haematol 106(3):634–643
15. Miyamura K, et al. (1992) Detection of Philadelphia chromosome-positive acute lymphoblastic leukemia by polymerase chain reaction: Possible eradication of minimal residual disease by marrow transplantation. Blood 79(5):1366–1370
16. Preudhomme C, et al. (1997) Good correlation between RT-PCR analysis and relapse in Philadelphia (Ph1)-positive acute lymphoblastic leukemia (ALL). Leukemia 11(2):294–298
17. Blaise D, et al. (1990) Allogeneic or autologous bone marrow transplantation for acute lymphoblastic leukemia in first complete remission. Bone Marrow Transplant 5(1):7–12
18. Chao NJ, et al. (1991) Allogeneic bone marrow transplantation for high-risk acute lymphoblastic leukemia during first complete remission. Blood 78(8):1923–1927

19. De Witte T, et al. (1994) Role of allogenic bone marrow transplantation in adolescent or adult patients with acute lymphoblastic leukaemia or lymphoblastic lymphoma in first remission. Bone Marrow Transplant 14(5):767–774
20. Doney K, et al. (1991) Treatment of adult acute lymphoblastic leukemia with allogeneic bone marrow transplantation. Multivariate analysis of factors affecting acute graft-versus-host disease, relapse, and relapse-free survival. Bone Marrow Transplant 7(6): 453–459
21. Sutton L, et al. (1993) Allogeneic bone marrow transplantation for adult acute lymphoblastic leukemia in first complete remission: Factors predictive of transplant-related mortality and influence of total body irradiation modalities. Bone Marrow Transplant 12(6):583–589
22. Vey N, et al. (1994) Bone marrow transplantation in 63 adult patients with acute lymphoblastic leukemia in first complete remission. Bone Marrow Transplant 14(3):383–388
23. Wingard JR, et al. (1990) Allogeneic bone marrow transplantation for patients with high-risk acute lymphoblastic leukemia. J Clin Oncol 8(5):820–830
24. Sebban C, et al. (1994) Allogeneic bone marrow transplantation in adult acute lymphoblastic leukemia in first complete remission: A comparative study. French Group of Therapy of Adult Acute Lymphoblastic Leukemia. J Clin Oncol 12(12):2580–2587
25. Thiebaut A, et al. (2000) Adult acute lymphocytic leukemia study testing chemotherapy and autologous and allogeneic transplantation. A follow-up report of the French protocol LALA 87. Hematol Oncol Clin North Am 14(6):1353–1366
26. Rowe J (2001) Favorable results of allogeneic bone marrow transplantation (BMT) for adults with Philadelphia (Ph)-chromosome-negative acute lymphoblastic leukemia (ALL) in first complete remission (CR): Results from the International ALL Trial (MRC UKALL XII/ECOG E2993). Blood 98:2009a
27. Report from the International Bone Marrow Transplant Registry (1989) Advisory Committee of the International Bone Marrow Transplant Registry. Bone Marrow Transplant 4(3):221–228
28. Barrett AJ, et al. (1989) Marrow transplantation for acute lymphoblastic leukemia: Factors affecting relapse and survival. Blood 74(2):862–871
29. Greinix HT, et al. (1998) Leukemia-free survival and mortality in patients with refractory or relapsed acute leukemia given marrow transplants from sibling and unrelated donors. Bone Marrow Transplant 21(7):673–678
30. Michallet M, et al. (2000) Second allogeneic haematopoietic stem cell transplantation in relapsed acute and chronic leukaemias for patients who underwent a first allogeneic bone marrow transplantation: A survey of the Societe Francaise de Greffe de moelle (SFGM). Br J Haematol 108(2):400–407
31. Forman SJ, et al. (1991) Allogeneic bone marrow transplantation as therapy for primary induction failure for patients with acute leukemia. J Clin Oncol 9(9):1570–1574
32. Biggs JC, et al. (1992) Bone marrow transplants may cure patients with acute leukemia never achieving remission with chemotherapy. Blood 80(4):1090–1093
33. Martino R, et al. (1999) Intensive salvage chemotherapy for primary refractory or first relapsed adult acute lymphoblastic leukemia: Results of a prospective trial. Haematologica 84(6):505–510
34. Druker BJ, et al. (2001) Activity of a specific inhibitor of the BCR-ABL tyrosine kinase in the blast crisis of chronic myeloid leukemia and acute lymphoblastic leukemia with the Philadelphia chromosome. N Engl J Med 344(14):1038–1042
35. Thomas DA, et al. (1999) Primary refractory and relapsed adult acute lymphoblastic leukemia: Characteristics, treatment results, and prognosis with salvage therapy. Cancer 86(7):1216–1230
36. Thomas DA, et al. (2004) Treatment of Philadelphia chromosome-positive acute lymphocytic leukemia with hyper-CVAD and imatinib mesylate. Blood 103(12):4396–4407
37. Goldstone AH, Prentice H, Durrant J, et al. (2001) Allogeneic transplant (related or unrelated donor) is the preferred treatment for adult Philadelphia chromosome positive (Ph+) acute lymphoblastic leukemia (ALL). Results from the International ALL Trial (MRC UKALLXII/ECOG E2993). American Society of Hematology, Orlando, Florida
38. Snyder DS, et al. (1999) Long-term follow-up of 23 patients with Philadelphia chromosome-positive acute lymphoblastic leukemia treated with allogeneic bone marrow transplant in first complete remission. Leukemia 13(12):2053–2058
39. Stockschlader M, et al. (1995) Bone marrow transplantation for Philadelphia-chromosome-positive acute lymphoblastic leukemia. Bone Marrow Transplant 16(5):663–667
40. Dunlop LC, et al. (1996) Bone marrow transplantation for Philadelphia chromosome-positive acute lymphoblastic leukemia. Bone Marrow Transplant 17(3):365–369
41. Sierra J, et al. (1997) Marrow transplants from unrelated donors for treatment of Philadelphia chromosome-positive acute lymphoblastic leukemia. Blood 90(4):1410–1414
42. Keil F, et al. (1997) Relapse of Philadelphia chromosome positive acute lymphoblastic leukaemia after marrow transplantation: Sustained molecular remission after early and dose-escalating infusion of donor leucocytes. Br J Haematol 97(1):161–164
43. Yazaki M, et al. (1997) Successful prevention of hematological relapse for a patient with Philadelphia chromosome-positive acute lymphoblastic leukemia after allogeneic bone marrow transplantation by donor leukocyte infusion. Bone Marrow Transplant 19(4):393–394
44. Glass B, et al. (1997) Allogeneic peripheral blood progenitor cells for treatment of relapse after bone marrow transplantation. Bone Marrow Transplant 20(7):533–541
45. Woods WG, et al. (1990) Bone marrow transplantation for acute lymphocytic leukemia utilizing total body irradiation followed by high doses of cytosine arabinoside: Lack of superiority over cyclophosphamide-containing conditioning regimens. Bone Marrow Transplant 6(1):9–16
46. Blume KG, et al. (1987) Total body irradiation and high-dose etoposide: A new preparatory regimen for bone marrow transplantation in patients with advanced hematologic malignancies. Blood 69(4):1015–1020
47. Matthews DC, et al. (1999) Phase I study of (131)I-anti-CD45 antibody plus cyclophosphamide and total body irradiation for advanced acute leukemia and myelodysplastic syndrome. Blood 94(4):1237–1247
48. Buchmann I, et al. (2002) Myeloablative radioimmunotherapy with Re-188-anti-CD66-antibody for conditioning of high-risk leukemia patients prior to stem cell transplantation: Biodistribution,

biokinetics and immediate toxicities. Cancer Biother Radiopharm 17(2):151–163

49. Copelan EA, Deeg HJ (1992) Conditioning for allogeneic marrow transplantation in patients with lymphohematopoietic malignancies without the use of total body irradiation. Blood 80(7):1648–1658
50. Gökbuget N, Hoelzer D (2004) Treatment with monoclonal antibodies in acute lymphoblastic leukemia: Current knowledge and future prospects. Ann Hematol 83(4):201–205
51. Dinndorf P, et al. (2001) Phase I trial of anti-B4-blocked ricin in pediatric patients with leukemia and lymphoma. J Immunother 24(6):511–516
52. Szatrowski TP, et al. (2003) Lineage specific treatment of adult patients with acute lymphoblastic leukemia in first remission with anti-B4-blocked ricin or high-dose cytarabine: Cancer and Leukemia Group B Study 9311. Cancer 97(6):1471–1480
53. Faderl S (2000) A broad exploratory trial of Campath-1H in the treatment of acute leukemias. American Society of Hematology, Orlando, Florida
54. Kolitz JE (1994) Treatment of acute lymphoblastic leukemia (ALL) with Campath-1H: Initial observations. American Society of Hematology, Orlando, Florida
55. Novitzky N, et al. (1999) Ex vivo depletion of T cells from bone marrow grafts with CAMPATH-1 in acute leukemia: Graft-versus-host disease and graft-versus-leukemia effect. Transplantation 67(4):620–626
56. Martino R, et al. (2003) Allogeneic hematopoietic stem cell transplantation with reduced-intensity conditioning in acute lymphoblastic leukemia: A feasibility study. Haematologica 88(5):555–560
57. Giralt S, et al. (2001) Melphalan and purine analog-containing preparative regimens: Reduced-intensity conditioning for patients with hematologic malignancies undergoing allogeneic progenitor cell transplantation. Blood 97(3):631–637
58. Champlin RE, et al. (2000) Blood stem cells compared with bone marrow as a source of hematopoietic cells for allogeneic transplantation. IBMTR Histocompatibility and Stem Cell Sources Working Committee and the European Group for Blood and Marrow Transplantation (EBMT). Blood 95(12):3702–3709
59. Barker JN, et al. (2003) Rapid and complete donor chimerism in adult recipients of unrelated donor umbilical cord blood transplantation after reduced-intensity conditioning. Blood 102(5):1915–1919
60. Laughlin MJ, et al. (2001) Hematopoietic engraftment and survival in adult recipients of umbilical-cord blood from unrelated donors. N Engl J Med 344(24):1815–1822
61. Sanz GF, et al. (2001) Standardized, unrelated donor cord blood transplantation in adults with hematologic malignancies. Blood 98(8):2332–2338
62. Gluckman E, Rocha V, Chevret S (2001) Results of unrelated umbilical cord blood hematopoietic stem cell transplantation. Rev Clin Exp Hematol 5(2):87–99
63. Cornetta K (2002) Umbilial cord blood transplantation in adults: Results of a prospective, multi-institutional, NHBLI sponsored trial. Blood 100(11):146a
64. Iseki T (2001) Unrelated cord blood transplantation in adults with hematologic malignancies: A single institution study. Blood 98(11):2729a
65. Petersdorf EW, et al. (1998) Optimizing outcome after unrelated marrow transplantation by comprehensive matching of HLA class I and II alleles in the donor and recipient. Blood 92(10):3515–3520
66. Weisdorf D, et al. (2002) Autologous versus allogeneic unrelated donor transplantation for acute lymphoblastic leukemia: Comparative toxicity and outcomes. Biol Blood Marrow Transplant 8(4):213–220
67. Ringden O, et al. (1997) Donor search or autografting in patients with acute leukaemia who lack an HLA-identical sibling? A matched-pair analysis. Acute Leukaemia Working Party of the European Cooperative Group for Blood and Marrow Transplantation (EBMT) and the International Marrow Unrelated Search and Transplant (IMUST) Study. Bone Marrow Transplant 19(10):963–968
68. Beatty PG, et al. (1985) Marrow transplantation from related donors other than HLA-identical siblings. N Engl J Med 313(13):765–771
69. Singhal S, et al. (2003) Haploidentical vs. autologous hematopoietic stem cell transplantation in patients with acute leukemia beyond first remission. Bone Marrow Transplant 31(10):889–895
70. Aversa F, et al. (1999) Improved outcome with T-cell-depleted bone marrow transplantation for acute leukemia. J Clin Oncol 17(5):1545–1550
71. Schattenberg A, et al. (2000) Outcome of T cell-depleted transplantation after conditioning with an intensified regimen in patients aged 50 years or more is comparable with that in younger patients. Bone Marrow Transplant 26(1):17–22
72. Sullivan KM, et al. (1989) Influence of acute and chronic graft-versus-host disease on relapse and survival after bone marrow transplantation from HLA-identical siblings as treatment of acute and chronic leukemia. Blood 73(6):1720–1728
73. Horowitz MM, et al. (1990) Graft-versus-leukemia reactions after bone marrow transplantation. Blood 75(3):555–562
74. Appelbaum FR (1997) Graft versus leukemia (GVL) in the therapy of acute lymphoblastic leukemia (ALL). Leukemia 11(Suppl)4:S15–17
75. Kolb HJ, et al. (1995) Graft-versus-leukemia effect of donor lymphocyte transfusions in marrow grafted patients. European Group for Blood and Marrow Transplantation Working Party Chronic Leukemia. Blood 86(5):2041–2050
76. Collins RH Jr, et al. (1997) Donor leukocyte infusions in 140 patients with relapsed malignancy after allogeneic bone marrow transplantation. J Clin Oncol 15(2):433–444
77. Slavin S, et al. (1996) Allogeneic cell therapy with donor peripheral blood cells and recombinant human interleukin-2 to treat leukemia relapse after allogeneic bone marrow transplantation. Blood 87(6):2195–2204
78. Socie G, et al. (1999) Long-term survival and late deaths after allogeneic bone marrow transplantation. Late Effects Working Committee of the International Bone Marrow Transplant Registry. N Engl J Med 341(1):14–21
79. Broers S, et al. (2000) Psychological functioning and quality of life following bone marrow transplantation: A 3-year follow-up study. J Psychosom Res 48(1):11–21
80. Harder H, et al. (2002) Cognitive functioning and quality of life in long-term adult survivors of bone marrow transplantation. Cancer 95(1):183–192

The Role of Autologous Stem Cell Transplantation in the Management of Acute Lymphoblastic Leukemia in Adults

Partow Kebriaei, Sergio Giralt

Contents

18.1 Introduction

Recent treatment strategies for adult acute lymphoblastic leukemia (ALL) have resulted in improved complete remission (CR) rates of 80–90% [1–3]. However, long-term disease-free survival (DFS) rates have remained disappointingly low at 30–40%. Current research efforts are focused on an improved understanding of the biology of the disease, and innovative postremission strategies that will prolong disease-free duration. Stem cell transplantation (SCT) is one strategy that may improve disease outcome. Allogeneic SCT has been demonstrated to improve DFS in high-risk ALL patients in multiple large series. High risk is defined by specific biologic and clinical features that have been noted to consistently influence the outcome of adult ALL (Table 18.1). Age greater than 60 years, an elevated white blood cell count at presentation, failure to achieve clinical remission within the first 4 weeks of treatment, and specific recurring cytogenetic abnormalities are all considered adverse clinical features. In a multivariate analysis of risk factors in adult ALL, karyotype was identified as the most important factor for DFS [4]. In general, patients with a normal karyotype have improved survival compared to those harboring a cytogenetic abnormality. In one series, six abnormalities were noted to result in unfavorable outcome, defined as having a 0.25 or less probability of continuous CR at 5 years. These include, in decreasing frequency, patients with t(9;22)(q34;q11), trisomy 8, t(4;11)(q21;q23), monosomy 7, a hypodiploid karyotype, and t(1;19)(q23;p13) [4–6].

However, in contrast to allogeneic SCT, most prospective, randomized studies of chemotherapy compared with autologous and allogeneic SCT have not

Table 18.1. Adverse prognostic features in Adult ALL
Age >60 yrs
WBC count >30 000/μL
Cytogenetics: t(9;22)(q34;q11), trisomy 8, t(4;11)(q21;q23), monosomy 7, a hypodiploid karyotype, t(1;19)(q23;p13)
Delayed time to CR >4 week

Table 18.2. Results of autologous transplant trials in adult ALL

Study	No. patients	Median age (yrs)	Disease status	Preparative regimen	Purging	DFS (follow-up time)
Doney, 1993	89	18.4	CR1 – 10; >CR2 – 52; relapse – 27	CY +/– TBI	None	Cr1 – 50%; CR2 – 27%; relapse – 8% (1 yr)
Uckun, 1992	14	13	CR	HiDAC/TBI	MoAb + rabbit complement + 4-HC	21% (3 yrs)
Abdallah, 2001	32	24	CR	CY +/– TBI	Mafosfamide or immuno-magnetic beads + MoAb	37.5% (4.5 yrs)
Singhal, 2003	81	18	>CR1	TBI-based; bu-sulfan-based	MoAb (13 patients)	30% (5 yrs)

No, number; CR, complete remission; DFS, disease-free survival; CY, cyclophosphamide; TBI, total body irradiation; HiDAC, dose-intensive cytarabine; MoAb, monoclonal antibody; 4-HC, 4-hydroperoxycyclophosphamide; ALL, acute lymphoblastic leukemia; AML, acute myelogenous leukemia.

shown an advantage for autologous SCT over conventional chemotherapy in any particular risk group of patients [7–9]. The two main drawbacks of autologous SCT are the absence of a graft-vs.-leukemia (GVL) effect and the potential for residual leukemic contamination of the autologous graft. Unfortunately, allogeneic SCT is limited to the approximately 30% of patients who have an appropriate human leukocyte antigen (HLA) donor, and further restricted to patients who can withstand the morbidity of the procedure. Thus, autologous SCT, in combination with novel, targeted agents and innovative posttransplant maintenance regimens, must be considered in efforts to improve disease outcome.

In this chapter, we will first review the outcomes of major clinical trials that have evaluated the efficacy of autologous SCT to identify groups of patients that may benefit most from this approach. Second, we will review the factors that affect treatment outcome, including the stem cell source, preparative regimen, and purging techniques. Finally, we will discuss novel approaches incorporating autologous SCT that are under development.

18.2 Outcome of Autologous SCT in Adult ALL

Limited conclusions can be made regarding the efficacy of autologous SCT based on small, single-center series that use a variety of purging methods. Doney, et al. reported on 89 patients with ALL, median age 18.4 years, who received autologous SCT after dose-intensive chemotherapy +/– total body irradiation (TBI). Autografts were not purged. Ten patients were in first remission, 52 were in second or greater remission, and 27 were in relapse. Disease-free survival at 1 year was 50, 27, and 8%, respectively, demonstrating the significance of disease burden on DFS [10]. The effect of purging on outcome was evaluated in three other series. Autografts were purged with mafosfamide or immunomagnetic beads [11], or monoclonal antibodies [12, 13]. Overall DFS times ranged from 27–50% for patients in remission, and the incorporation of various ex vivo purging methods did not appear to significantly alter disease outcome (Table 18.2). As described in a later section, the advent of imatinib mesylate (Gleevec, STI-571) may improve current disease outcome, as it may provide an effective in vivo purging method.

18.3 Comparison of Autologous SCT with Allogeneic SCT and Chemotherapy

Two large, multicenter, prospective, randomized studies have investigated the role of conventional chemotherapy and transplant in adult ALL patients. The French (Leucemie Aigue Lymphoblastique de l'Adulte [LALA]) study was initiated in November 1986 and completed in July 1991, and enrolled 634 patients in the LALA 87 protocol to assess the role of allogeneic SCT and autologous SCT in adult ALL. After exclusions, 572 patients were analyzed. The median age of patients entered onto this trial was 33 years, with 10-year follow-up. Patients received induction chemotherapy with cyclophosphamide, vincristine, prednisone, and one of two anthracyclines. Central nervous system (CNS) prophylaxis was administered. Four hundred thirty-six patients (76%) achieved complete remission. After CR was achieved, patients older than 50 years received postremission chemotherapy. Patients between 15 and 40 years of age were assigned to the allogeneic SCT arm if they had an HLA-matched sibling donor. Patients between ages 40 and 50, and those under the age of 40 without a matched sibling donor, were further randomized to consolidation chemotherapy or autologous SCT using bone marrow purged with antibodies or mafosfamide. Consolidation chemotherapy consisted of three monthly courses of daunorubicin or zorubicin, Ara-C, and asparaginase followed by long-term maintenance therapy. The transplant preparative regimen consisted of TBI and cyclophosphamide. There was no statistically significant difference in outcome between patients who received autologous SCT vs. consolidation chemotherapy (34% SCT, 29% chemotherapy, $p=0.6$). After stratification into high and standard risk, there was still no statistical difference between these two groups. At 10 years, only allogeneic SCT resulted in significantly greater survival among all risk groups (46% allogeneic SCT, 31% chemotherapy, $p=0.04$), and even more marked among the high-risk subset (high-risk: 44% allogeneic SCT, 11% chemotherapy, $p=0.009$; standard-risk: 49% SCT, 43% chemotherapy, $p=0.6$) [8, 14].

The United Kingdom Medical Research Council's (MRC) UKALL XII/Eastern Cooperative Oncology Group (ECOG) E2993 is an on-going international effort to prospectively define the role of allogeneic SCT, autologous SCT, and chemotherapy in adult patients with ALL in CR1. Initiated in 1993, over 1200 patients have been enrolled to date. All patients received two phases of induction therapy, and continued to allogeneic SCT if they achieved CR and had a histocompatible donor. The remaining patients were randomized to standard consolidation/maintenance therapy for 2.5 years vs. a single autologous SCT. The conditioning regimen for both allogeneic and autologous transplants was fractionated TBI (1320 cGy) and VP-16 (60 mg/kg). Based on the data presented in an abstract in 2001 [9], 239 patients received an allogeneic SCT and 291 patients received chemotherapy or autologous SCT. The overall event-free survival (EFS) for the allogeneic SCT group was 54 vs. 34% ($p=0.04$) for the chemotherapy or autologous BMT group. Excluding the t(9;22)(q34;q11) karyotype, when patients were stratified into high or standard risk, the difference in EFS becomes more dramatic in the high-risk subset (allogeneic BMT 44% vs. chemo/autologous BMT 26%, $p=0.06$). In conclusion, both of these large series defined in a prospective manner the efficacy of allogeneic SCT over chemotherapy or autologous SCT for adults with high-risk ALL in CR1.

However, as stated previously, not all patients have an available HLA-appropriate donor. Weisdorf et al. reported the results of 337 ALL patients (121 adults; 216 children) who received matched unrelated donor (MUD) SCT and compared them to 214 patients (54 adults; 160 children) who underwent autologous SCT between 1987 and 1993. For those transplanted in CR1, autologous SCT yielded a significantly higher DFS (42% autologous SCT vs. 32% MUD, $p=0.03$). In contrast, for those transplanted in CR2, MUD SCT yielded a better DFS (20% autologous SCT vs. 42% MUD, $p=0.02$). The worse outcome with autologous SCT in CR2 likely reflects the increased relapse hazard in the advanced leukemia group. When the data were analyzed separately for children and adults in CR2, MUD SCT still yielded a higher DFS when compared to autologous SCT (adults, MUD 42%+/− 22% vs. autologous SCT 0%, $p=0.006$) [15]. These results were corroborated by a study performed by the Acute Leukemia Working Party of the European Cooperative Group for Blood and Marrow Transplantation (EBMT). Data from ALL patients undergoing SCT between January 1987 and December 1994 was analyzed [16]. One hundred eighteen patients with a median age of 14 years received MUD SCT; 236 patients with a median age of 16 received autologous SCT. Disease status ranged from CR1 to CR3. There were no significant differences in the 2-year leukemia free survival (LFS) for MUD SCT vs. autologous SCT in this retrospective analysis of ALL patients matched for diagnosis, age, stage of disease, and year of transplantation (39% MUD, 32% auto). However, relapse was significantly lower in the MUD SCT group (MUD 32% vs. auto 61%, $p<0.0001$), while transplant-related mortality (TRM) was significantly higher in this group (MUD 42% vs. auto 17%, $p<0.0001$).

Finally, in an attempt to compare the outcomes of autologous SCT vs. haploidentical SCT in adults with acute leukemia beyond first remission, Singhal, et al. reported on 164 patients (ALL, n = 84) who received a partially matched related donor transplant (PMRDT) at the Division of Transplantation Medicine, South Carolina Cancer Center between February 1993 and December 1999, and compared outcomes to 131 patients (ALL, n = 81) who had received an autologous SCT at the Royal Marsden Hospital, Surrey, UK between April 1984 and November 1999 [13]. For PMRDT, patients were prepared with cyclophosphamide/TBI/methylprednisolone ± anti-thymocyte globulin (ATG), followed by cyclosporine/methylprednisolone/ATG for GVHD prophylaxis. In the autologous SCT group, patients received a variety of TBI- or busulfan-based preparative regimens. All PMRDT patients received T-cell-depleted bone marrow (BM). In the autologous SCT group, 114 patients received BM and 17 patients received peripheral blood stem cells (PBSC). Marrow was purged with anti-CD52 monoclonal antibody (MoAb) in 13 autologous SCT patients. The 5-year cumulative incidence of TRM was 52% after PMRDT vs. 16% after autologous SCT ($p < 0.0001$). The 5-year cumulative incidence of relapse was 32% after PMRDT vs. 54% after autologous SCT ($p = 0.006$). The actuarial unadjusted 5-year DFS was 16% after PMRDT vs. 30% after autologous SCT ($p = 0.006$). In conclusion, these findings suggest that the increased risk of relapse after autologous SCT is offset by the increased TRM of PMRDT, and therefore, autologous SCT is a superior option for patients with advanced leukemia who do not have an HLA-identical related donor. These conclusions are limited by the retrospective nature of this study, and the heterogeneity in the therapeutic approach of the two different institutions.

18.4 Factors Influencing Transplant Outcome

18.4.1 Source of Stem Cells

Powles et al. established the superiority of PBSC in shortening the time to hematopoietic cell recovery [17]. This is especially important since purging methods can delay hematopoietic recovery. In addition, a study by Atta, et al. demonstrated differences in leukemic contamination between PBSC and BM grafts [18]. In 40 consecutive BCR/ABL positive patients, 32% of unpurged PBSC were already BCR/ABL negative as compared to unpurged BM. Furthermore, the positive PBSC were contaminated at a lower level as compared to the BM grafts. However, other studies have not detected a difference in graft contamination, perhaps due to differences in methodology [19].

18.4.2 Preparative Regimens

Several different preparative regimens for autologous SCT have been described in attempts to decrease TRM and improve DFS. The most widely used regimen is the combination of TBI and cyclophosphamide developed by Donnall Thomas and colleagues in the 1970s. The TBI, ranging between 1200 and 1350 cGy, can be administered as a single dose, or fractionated over 3–5 days. A comparative analysis of fractionated-dose vs. single-dose TBI in adult ALL patients showed a significantly higher transplant-related mortality (TRM) in the single-dose group ($p = 0.017$), but an increase in the relapse rate of the fractionated-dose group; consequently, there were no differences in the overall LFS between the two groups [20]. A number of different chemotherapy agents, including high-dose cytarabine, vincristine, melphalan, etoposide, and/or anthracyclines have been combined with TBI with no clear advantage for any specific combination [21–24].

In attempts to intensify the antileukemic effect of the preparative regimen, the addition of a third agent to the classic cyclophosphamide/TBI combination has also been investigated. However, in contrast to results obtained with children [25, 26], the intensification of the preparative regimen improved DFS at the expense of increased TRM in adults, thereby, ultimately not improving OS [27]. Thus, novel methods to allow selective delivery of therapy to sites of leukemia without increasing systemic toxicity are currently under investigation.

Radio-immunoconjugated MoAbs with iodine-131 or yttrium-90 have already been used in advanced lymphoma patients with promising results [28]. A Phase I transplant trial using ^{131}I-labeled anti-CD45 antibody combined with cyclophosphamide/TBI was conducted in patients with advanced hematologic malignancies. The dose-limiting toxicity was grade III/IV mucositis. Nine patients with ALL (relapsed/refractory, n = 5; CR2 or CR3, n = 4) received allogeneic (n = 6) or autologous (n = 3) transplants using this preparative regimen; three patients were disease-free 19, 54, and 66 months post-transplant. A more recent study evaluated the feasibility of using ^{188}rhenium (^{188}Re)-labeled anti-CD66 in combination with standard high dose chemotherapy/TBI

(12 Gy) in 50 advanced leukemia patients, including 11 with ALL, undergoing allogeneic or autologous SCT. All patients achieved primary engraftment. After a median follow-up of 11 months, 28/50 (56%) patients were in CR, nine (5%) patients relapsed, and 13 (7%) died from treatment-related causes [29]. The ultimate benefits of this approach with respect to safety and improvements in survival will be defined by Phase II studies for patients with ALL.

Nonradiation containing regimens, most commonly busulfan and cyclophosphamide, have been investigated in hopes of decreasing radiation-related complications. Fractionated TBI/etoposide was tested against busulfan/cyclophosphamide in a prospective, randomized study conducted by the Southwest Oncology Group (SWOG 8612). One hundred twenty-two patients with leukemia beyond CR1 received either fractionated TBI/etoposide or busulfan/cyclophosphamide in preparation for SCT. One hundred fourteen (93%) proceeded to SCT. All patients received cyclosporine and prednisone for posttransplant immunosuppression. There was no significant difference with respect to toxicity, incidence of acute GVHD, overall survival, or DFS between the two groups. The leading cause for treatment failure was leukemic relapse (39%) [30]. Furthermore, retrospective analysis of registry data from the International Bone Marrow Transplant Registry (IBMTR) shows similar rates for LFS and relapse when busulfan/cyclophosphamide is compared to cyclophosphamide/TBI [31]. Careful comparisons of the incidence of second malignancies with each of these regimens have not been made but may have important consequences. Thus, a variety of preparative regimens can be used, but leukemic relapse remains the most significant factor affecting DFS.

18.4.3 Ex Vivo Purging

One major disadvantage of autologous SCT is autograft contamination leading to an increased rate of relapse. Ex vivo purging methods were developed to decrease the residual leukemic burden of the graft. Pharmacological agents include 4-hydroperoxycyclophosphamide (4-HC), mafosfamide, and edelfosine. One major concern regarding chemical purging is the potential toxic effect on normal progenitor cells [32]. In efforts to overcome this toxicity, some investigators have tested the simultaneous administration of chemoprotectant agents such as amifostine or adenosine triphosphate [33, 34].

Immunological methods of purging rely on MoAbs combined with immunotoxins [35], exposed to complement [27, 36–38], or combined with an iron-bound antibody followed by a magnetic depletion [39]. It is difficult to make any conclusions regarding the efficacy of a particular purging method based on results from multiple, single-center experiences using a variety of purging methods. Generally, immunological purging methods are able to eliminate 2–4.5 logs of leukemia cells. Between 0 and 84% of mononuclear cells are lost during the purging process; between 34 and 96% of CD34 cells are recovered after purging [27]. Although purging with monoclonal antibodies does not typically impair hematologic recovery after transplant, some studies have noted a delay in engraftment [40].

Ex vivo purging of the autograft with anti-sense oligodeoxynucleotide (ODN) or ribonucleotide interference (RNA-I) methods are still largely in preclinical phases but have great potential for certain subtypes of ALL. These methods target a specific mRNA or RNA sequence, and can effectively block the production of a protein; thus, they may be very effective therapy for leukemogenesis that is driven by a specific protein, such as in t(9;22)(q34;q11) ALL. Gewirtz et al. used ODN directed against the c-myb proto-oncogene to purge autografts of Philadelphia chromosome positive (Ph+) chronic myelogenous leukemia (CML) patients who were not eligible to receive allogeneic SCT (chronic phase, n=20; accelerated phase, n=5) [41]. Autografts were purged ex vivo with ODN for either 24 or 72 h. After purging, Myb mRNA levels declined substantially in approximately 50% of patients. However, cytogenetic response post transplant was mixed in this small pilot study, raising the issue of overall clinical efficacy. Still, the study established the feasibility of ex vivo purging with antisense ODN, and may lead to the development of more effective antisense ODN targeted against a variety of proteins.

18.5 Novel Transplant Approaches

18.5.1 Maintenance Therapy Post-SCT

Although the concept of maintenance therapy is established for the chemotherapy treatment of ALL, its use post transplant is not defined. Powles et al. reported on the use of chemotherapy after autologous SCT to prolong DFS. From July 1984 to December 1998, 77 adult

ALL patients received an autologous transplant in CR1 at the Royal Marsden Hospital. The preparative regimen consisted of melphalan and total body irradiation until December 1992; subsequently, patients received high-dose melphalan alone. Patients were scheduled to receive 6-mercaptopurine (71%), methotrexate (57%), and/or vincristine and prednisone (38%) for 2 years after the transplant. The median time to relapse post-transplant was 13 months. The cumulative incidence of relapse at 10 years was 42% (95% CI, 31–55%). The 10-year probability of DFS was 50% (95% CI, 38–62%). Age >30 years, longer than 4 weeks to attain CR, and high risk karyotype [t(9;22)(q34;q11) and t(4;11)(q21;q23)] were adverse features. Risk stratification using these features identified three prognostic risk groups with 0 (47%), 1 (36%), or 2 (17%) adverse features. The respective 10-year cumulative incidences of relapse were 20, 48, and 85% ($p<0.001$), and the probabilities of DFS were 72, 41, and 10% ($p=0.003$). Patients who received two or three maintenance drugs had a lower relapse rate than those who received only 0 or 1. Posttransplant maintenance therapy offered a benefit for low and standard risk patients, but not those with high-risk disease [42].

18.5.2 Targeted Therapies: Imatinib Mesylate

The most exciting recent development in the treatment of the t(9;22)(q34;q11), Ph+ subtype of ALL has been the promising early results observed with imatinib, a molecule specifically targeted to the BCR/ABL tyrosine kinase that is overexpressed as a result of the t(9;22)(q34;q11) in CML and Ph+ ALL. Imatinib is a specific inhibitor of the abl protein tyrosine kinase that has demonstrated remarkable targeted therapeutic efficacy in patients with the CML and ALL with increased bcr/abl activity [43]. The Cancer and Leukemia Group B (CALGB), in combination with the Southwest Oncology Group (SWOG) have recently initiated a Phase II trial of sequential chemotherapy, imatinib, and allogeneic or auto-SCT for adults with newly diagnosed Ph+ ALL. The primary objectives of this study will be to determine the ability of imatinib to produce a complete molecular response following sequential chemotherapy, imatinib, and transplantation, and to determine the ability of imatinib to prolong DFS and OS in this high-risk group of patients. The ongoing ECOG2993/UKALL 12 protocol for Ph+ ALL patients follows a similar strategy [44]. The results of these trials are eagerly anticipated.

18.5.3 Immunotherapy

In an attempt to induce an immunological response similar to GVL in allogeneic SCT, immunomodulators, such as interleukin-2 (IL-2), have been tried without success in the autologous SCT setting. Blaise, et al. conducted a prospective, randomized study to investigate the efficacy of IL-2 after autologous BMT for acute leukemia in CR1. One hundred thirty patients were enrolled (ALL, $n=52$). Analysis was based on an intent to treat, and 59% of patients randomized to IL-2 started the drug after a median of 68 days post transplant, and received 77% of the scheduled dose. With a median follow-up of 7 years, OS and LFS were not statistically different between the two study groups [45].

In vivo and ex vivo purging with MoAbs directed against surface antigens expressed by leukemic blasts, such as CD20 and CD52, are underway in many clinical trials, and results are eagerly anticipated.

Finally, active immunotherapy using dendritic cells (DCs) loaded with tumor-associated antigens to induce specific T-cell immunity is a potentially effective approach that is still in early development. Rijke, et al. investigated the use of HB-1 antigen as an autologous T-cell vaccine target, based on their previous studies that indicated HB-1 is a B-cell lineage-specific antigen that is recognized by donor-derived cytotoxic T lymphocytes (CTLs) on allogeneic B-ALL tumor cells. They demonstrated that HB-1 induces both helper and cytotoxic T-cell responses by in vitro studies [46]. This approach now needs to be evaluated in the in vivo setting.

18.6 Conclusion

In conclusion, transplantation is an effective modality in the treatment of ALL. In patients with high-risk ALL, multiple randomized trials have demonstrated the tremendous therapeutic benefit for early allogeneic SCT. However, in patients without an appropriate HLA donor, autologous SCT may be a reasonable approach to extend DFS for those in remission. The leukemic burden pretransplant will affect disease outcome, and randomized, prospective studies are necessary to determine the best pretransplant conditioning regimen and purging methods to decrease disease burden. In addition, further studies are required to determine the benefit of maintenance therapy posttransplant to decrease the rate of disease relapse. Finally, immunologic therapies currently under preclinical investigation may provide an effective alternative to the GVL phenomenon, and improve the outcome with autologous SCT in future trials.

References

1. Kantarjian HM, et al. (2000) Results of treatment with hyper-CVAD, a dose-intensive regimen, in adult acute lymphocytic leukemia. J Clin Oncol 18(3):547–561
2. Larson RA (2000) Recent clinical trials in acute lymphocytic leukemia by the Cancer and Leukemia Group B. Hematol Oncol Clin North Am 14(6):1367–1379
3. Linker C, et al. (2002) Intensified and shortened cyclical chemotherapy for adult acute lymphoblastic leukemia. J Clin Oncol 20(10):2464–2471
4. Hoelzer D, et al. (1988) Prognostic factors in a multicenter study for treatment of acute lymphoblastic leukemia in adults. Blood 71(1):123–131
5. Wetzler M, et al. (1999) Prospective karyotype analysis in adult acute lymphoblastic leukemia: The cancer and leukemia Group B experience. Blood 93(11):3983–3993
6. Wetzler M (2000) Cytogenetics in adult acute lymphocytic leukemia. Hematol Oncol Clin North Am 14(6):1237–1249
7. Horowitz MM, et al. (1991) Chemotherapy compared with bone marrow transplantation for adults with acute lymphoblastic leukemia in first remission. Ann Intern Med 115(1):13–18
8. Thiebaut A, et al. (2000) Adult acute lymphocytic leukemia study testing chemotherapy and autologous and allogeneic transplantation. A follow-up report of the French protocol LALA 87. Hematol Oncol Clin North Am 14(6):1353–1366
9. Rowe J (2001) Favorable results of allogeneic bone marrow transplantation (BMT) for adults with Philadelphia (Ph)-chromosome-negative acute lymphoblastic leukemia (ALL) in first complete remission (CR): Results from the International ALL Trial (MRC UKALL XII/ECOG E2993). Blood 98:2009a
10. Doney K, et al. (1993) Autologous bone marrow transplantation for acute lymphoblastic leukemia. Bone Marrow Transplant 12(4):315–321
11. Abdallah A, et al. (2001) Continuous complete remission in adult patients with acute lymphocytic leukaemia at a median observation of 12 years after autologous bone marrow transplantation. Br J Haematol 112(4):1012–1015
12. Uckun FM, et al. (1992) Autologous bone marrow transplantation in high-risk remission B-lineage acute lymphoblastic leukemia using a cocktail of three monoclonal antibodies (BA-1/CD24, BA-2/CD9, and BA-3/CD10) plus complement and 4-hydroperoxycyclophosphamide for ex vivo bone marrow purging. Blood 79(4):1094–1104
13. Singhal S, et al. (2003) Haploidentical vs. autologous hematopoietic stem cell transplantation in patients with acute leukemia beyond first remission. Bone Marrow Transplant 31(10):889–895
14. Sebban C, et al. (1994) Allogeneic bone marrow transplantation in adult acute lymphoblastic leukemia in first complete remission: A comparative study. French Group of Therapy of Adult Acute Lymphoblastic Leukemia. J Clin Oncol 12(12):2580–2587
15. Weisdorf DJ, et al. (1997) Autologous versus unrelated donor allogeneic marrow transplantation for acute lymphoblastic leukemia. Blood 90(8):2962–2968
16. Ringden O, et al. (1997) Donor search or autografting in patients with acute leukaemia who lack an HLA-identical sibling? A matched-pair analysis. Acute Leukaemia Working Party of the European Cooperative Group for Blood and Marrow Transplantation (EBMT) and the International Marrow Unrelated Search and Transplant (IMUST) Study. Bone Marrow Transplant 19(10):963–968
17. Powles R, et al. (2000) Allogeneic blood and bone-marrow stem-cell transplantation in haematological malignant diseases: A randomised trial. Lancet 355(9211):1231–1237
18. Atta J, et al. (2000) Purging in BCR-ABL-positive acute lymphoblastic leukemia using immunomagnetic beads: Comparison of residual leukemia and purging efficiency in bone marrow vs. peripheral blood stem cells by semiquantitative polymerase chain reaction. Bone Marrow Transplant 25(1):97–104
19. van Rhee F, et al. (1995) Quantification of residual disease in Philadelphia-positive acute lymphoblastic leukemia: Comparison of blood and bone marrow. Leukemia 9(2):329–335
20. Sutton L, et al. (1993) Allogeneic bone marrow transplantation for adult acute lymphoblastic leukemia in first complete remission: Factors predictive of transplant-related mortality and influence of total body irradiation modalities. Bone Marrow Transplant 12(6):583–589
21. Blume KG, et al. (1987) Total body irradiation and high-dose etoposide: A new preparatory regimen for bone marrow transplantation in patients with advanced hematologic malignancies. Blood 69(4):1015–1020
22. Carey PJ, et al. (1991) Autologous bone marrow transplantation for high-grade lymphoid malignancy using melphalan/irradiation conditioning without marrow purging or cryopreservation. The Northern Regional Bone Marrow Transplant Group. Blood 77(7):1593–1598
23. Kersey JH, et al. (1987) Comparison of autologous and allogeneic bone marrow transplantation for treatment of high-risk refractory acute lymphoblastic leukemia. N Engl J Med 317(8):461–467
24. Woods WG, et al. (1990) Bone marrow transplantation for acute lymphocytic leukemia utilizing total body irradiation followed by high doses of cytosine arabinoside: Lack of superiority over cyclophosphamide-containing conditioning regimens. Bone Marrow Transplant 6(1):9–16
25. Billett AL, et al. (1993) Autologous bone marrow transplantation after a long first remission for children with recurrent acute lymphoblastic leukemia. Blood 81(6):1651–1657
26. Maldonado MS, et al. (1998) Autologous bone marrow transplantation with monoclonal antibody purged marrow for children with acute lymphoblastic leukemia in second remission. Spanish Working Party for BMT in Children. Bone Marrow Transplant 22(11):1043–1047

27. Soiffer RJ, et al. (1993) Monoclonal antibody-purged autologous bone marrow transplantation in adults with acute lymphoblastic leukemia at high risk of relapse. Bone Marrow Transplant 12(3): 243–251
28. Flinn IW, Lazarus HM (2001) Monoclonal antibodies and autologous stem cell transplantation for lymphoma. Bone Marrow Transplant 27(6):565–569
29. Buchmann I, et al. (2002) Myeloablative radioimmunotherapy with Re-188-anti-CD66-antibody for conditioning of high-risk leukemia patients prior to stem cell transplantation: Biodistribution, biokinetics and immediate toxicities. Cancer Biother Radiopharm 17(2):151–163
30. Blume KG, et al. (1993) A prospective randomized comparison of total body irradiation-etoposide versus busulfan-cyclophosphamide as preparatory regimens for bone marrow transplantation in patients with leukemia who were not in first remission: A Southwest Oncology Group study. Blood 81(8):2187–2193
31. Copelan EA, Deeg HJ (1992) Conditioning for allogeneic marrow transplantation in patients with lymphohematopoietic malignancies without the use of total body irradiation. Blood 80(7):1648–1658
32. Rowley SD, et al. (1987) CFU-GM content of bone marrow graft correlates with time to hematologic reconstitution following autologous bone marrow transplantation with 4-hydroperoxycyclophosphamide-purged bone marrow. Blood 70(1):271–275
33. Douay L, et al. (1995) Amifostine improves the antileukemic therapeutic index of mafosfamide: Implications for bone marrow purging. Blood 86(7):2849–2855
34. Hatta Y, et al. (2002) Purging in autologous hematopoietic stem cell transplantation using adenosine triphosphate (ATP) and 4-hydroperoxycyclophosphamide (4-HC). Leuk Res 26(5):477–482
35. Preijers FW, et al. (1989) Autologous transplantation of bone marrow purged in vitro with anti-CD7-(WT1-) ricin A immunotoxin in T-cell lymphoblastic leukemia and lymphoma. Blood 74(3):1152–1158
36. Gilmore MJ, et al. (1991) Failure of purged autologous bone marrow transplantation in high risk acute lymphoblastic leukaemia in first complete remission. Bone Marrow Transplant 8(1): 19–26
37. Granena A, et al. (1999) Autologous bone marrow transplantation for high risk acute lymphoblastic leukemia: Clinical relevance of ex vivo bone marrow purging with monoclonal antibodies and complement. Bone Marrow Transplant 24(6):621–627
38. Morishima Y, et al. (1993) Autologous BMT in high risk patients with CALLA-positive ALL: Possible efficacy of ex vivo marrow leukemia cell purging with monoclonal antibodies and complement. Bone Marrow Transplant 11(4):255–259
39. Canals C, et al. (1997) Immunomagnetic bone marrow purging in children with acute lymphoblastic leukemia. J Hematother 6(3): 261–268
40. Mehta J, et al. (1997) Autologous transplantation with CD52 monoclonal antibody-purged marrow for acute lymphoblastic leukemia: Long-term follow-up. Leuk Lymphoma 25(5–6):479–486
41. Luger SM, et al. (2002) Oligodeoxynucleotide-mediated inhibition of c-myb gene expression in autografted bone marrow: A pilot study. Blood 99(4):1150–1158
42. Powles R, et al. (2002) The role of posttransplantation maintenance chemotherapy in improving the outcome of autotransplantation in adult acute lymphoblastic leukemia. Blood 100(5):1641–1647
43. Druker BJ, et al. (2001) Activity of a specific inhibitor of the BCR-ABL tyrosine kinase in the blast crisis of chronic myeloid leukemia and acute lymphoblastic leukemia with the Philadelphia chromosome. N Engl J Med 344(14):1038–1042
44. Avivi I, Goldstone AH (2003) Bone marrow transplant in Ph+ ALL patients. Bone Marrow Transplant 31(8):623–632
45. Blaise D, et al. (2000) Randomized study of recombinant interleukin-2 after autologous bone marrow transplantation for acute leukemia in first complete remission. Eur Cytokine Netw 11(1):91–98
46. de Rijke B, et al. (2003) Generation of autologous cytotoxic and helper T-cell responses against the B-cell leukemia-associated antigen HB-1: Relevance for precursor B-ALL-specific immunotherapy. Blood 102(8):2885–2891

Novel Therapies in Acute Lymphoblastic Leukemia

Stefan H. Faderl, Hagop Kantarjian

Contents

19.1 Introduction

Although prognosis of adult ALL has improved over the last few decades, still only 30–40% of patients achieve long-term, disease-free survival and can be considered cured [1, 2]. The remainder will eventually relapse and die from disease progression or other ALL-related consequences. New strategies, refinements of old ones, and novel agents are therefore needed. How modifications of induction regimens can positively impact the outcome in subsets of the disease is exemplified in mature B-cell ALL where short, dose-intensive chemotherapy leads to survival of 50–70% of the patients and T-cell ALL in which addition of cyclophosphamide, high-dose methotrexate and cytarabine in the induction and consolidation sequence is associated with similar survival rates [3]. Other subgroups such as Philadelphia chromosome-(Ph) positive ALL are still largely incurable with chemotherapy alone although the combination of BCR-ABL tyrosine kinase inhibitors with intensive chemotherapy is showing promising leads in this group of patients as well.

Several paths to better treatment strategies can be pursued and must not be seen isolated from each other: (1) continuous modification of current therapy programs in light of a better understanding of disease subtypes and regimen-specific components; (2) development of new drugs targeted against identifiable cytogenetic-molecular abnormalities; and (3) appreciation of the role of pharmacogenetics in ALL and developing mechanisms to overcome drug resistance. Successful implementation of any of those strategies ultimately requires a more profound understanding of the biological characteristics of ALL taking into account the heterogeneity of ALL. Given the complexity of ALL treatment programs, it can hardly be expected that there is a single new agent that will stand out on its own so that progress in ALL will require not only integration of new agents into treatment algorithms, but also to learn how to better use the armamentarium of currently available agents and combinations (Table 19.1) [4].

Table 19.1. Novel strategies in ALL

Class of agents/parameters	Examples
1. New agents	
Liposomal and pegylated formulations	Liposomal vincristine
	Pegylated asparaginase (pegaspargase)
Nucleoside analogs	Clofarabine
	Nelarabine
Purine nucleoside phosphorylase (PNP) inhibitors	Forodesine (BCX-1777)
Oligonucleotides	BCL-2 antisense
Proteasome inhibitors	Bortezomib (Velcade)
Tyrosine kinase inhibitors	Imatinib
	Nilotinib
	Dasatinib
	Semaxinib (SU5416)
Farnesyltransferase inhibitors	Tipifarnib (R115777)
	Lornafarnib (SCH66336)
Monoclonal antibodies	Rituximab (anti-CD20)
	Alemtuzumab (anti-CD52)
	Anti-CD19 + ricin/genistein/PAP
	Anti-CD7 + ricin
2. Modifications of induction regimens	
Supportive care	Laminar air flow room for older patients (>60 years)
Risk-adapted CNS prophylaxis	Adjust number of intrathecal therapy
	Examine role of craniospinal XRT
Maintenance	Duration
	Intensification
	Role of asparaginase
3. Pharmacogenetics and mechanisms of drug resistance	

19.2 New Chemotherapy Agents

19.2.1 Liposomal Preparations

Liposomal preparations of chemotherapeutic agents change the pharmacological properties of the original and active compound resulting in most cases in better efficacy with reduced toxicity. Several liposomal agents are being investigated in ALL salvage therapy among which liposomal (sphingosomal) vincristine and pegylated asparaginase (see below) have received the most attention.

Vincristine has been an active anticancer agent for many years and is widely used in the treatment of numerous malignancies, but neurotoxicity is a frequent DLT. The therapeutic activity and drug toxicity of vincristine can be improved by encapsulating vincristine into a liposomal delivery system [5]. Changes in the pharmacological properties are reflected by a comparison of plasma half-lives between the active compound and its liposomal cousin. Whereas the half-life of free vincristine is only 10 minutes, it is up to 8 h with the liposomal preparation [6]. Liposomal vincristine has been studied successfully in lymphoma salvage, as part of the CHOP (cyclophosphamide, adriamycin, vincristine, prednisone) plus rituximab regimen in Non-Hodgkin's lymphoma (NHL) patients, and in early clinical studies in ALL salvage.

Liposomal vincristine was well tolerated and achieved a response rate of 35% in patients with relapsed and refractory NHL [7]. In a more recent update important predictors of response included number of prior regimens and sensitivity to the most recent treatment regimen. Response rates of up to 64% were reported in those patients with sensitive disease and not more than two prior regimens [8]. Rodriguez et al. substituted liposomal vincristine for free vincristine and investigated the liposomal preparation as part of the CHOP plus rituximab combination in patients with previously untreated NHL [9]. Patients received standard doses of CHOP, which included liposomal vincristine at 2 mg/m^2 (no dose capping). Of 68 patients who were evaluable for response 63 (93%) responded, which included 62 patients with complete remission (CR), one with unconfirmed CR and one patient with partial response. At a median follow up of 29.5 months, median progression-free survival (PFS) and overall survival (OS) have not been reached. The treatment was well tolerated with only mild neurotoxicity. In a small study in ALL of single-agent liposomal vincristine at 2 mg/m^2 given every 2 weeks, responses occurred in two of 14 (14%) evaluable relapsed/refractory patients [10]. In a more recent phase I trial for patients with relapsed and refractory ALL, liposomal vincristine (dose range 1.5 mg/m^2 to 2.25 mg/m^2) weekly for four doses per course was given in combination with pulse dexamethasone (40 mg daily on days 1–4 and 11–14) [11]. Of 14 evaluable patients, 4 (29%) achieved CR extending through all dose levels, and another two (14%) achieved hematologic improvement. Almost all patients experienced peripheral neuropathy, which did not exceed grade 2 on the NCI Common Toxicity scale. The study is ongoing. Once the MTD has been defined, substitution of vincristine for the liposomal preparation in ALL induction protocols such as the hyper-CVAD regimen is planned.

19.2.2 Nucleoside Analogs

Since their establishment as antitumor drugs in the 1960s, nucleoside analogs have been among the most active agents for patients with cancer. In addition to the established and more traditional nucleoside analogs such as cytarabine, fludarabine, cladribine, or pentostatin, new nucleoside analogs are emerging that demonstrate additional metabolic properties and mechanisms of actions, and their activity is currently evaluated in clinical trials including in patients with ALL [12].

Nelarabine (compound 506U78, ara-G) is the water-soluble prodrug of the deoxyguanosine analog guanosine arabinoside (ara-G) [13]. Nelarabine is not active by itself and requires conversion to ara-G by the enzyme adenosine deaminase, which is an efficient enough process to result in cytotoxic levels of ara-GTP in circulating leukemia cells. It has been demonstrated that ara-GTP is accumulated at higher levels in T lymphoblasts than in myeloblasts or B lymphoblasts. In addition, it has been shown in human leukemia cell lines that cytotoxicity to T lymphoblasts was increased with greater accumulation and more prolonged retention of ara-G in these cells [14–17]. Several early clinical trials of nelarabine have been conducted in refractory acute and chronic leukemias. Using a schedule of 1200 mg/m^2 or more daily for up to 5 days, response rates of 40–50% have been reported in refractory T-cell ALL. At most of these schedules, neurotoxicity (including seizures, obtundation, ascending paralysis) was the DLT and the maximum-tolerated dose (MTD) in adults has been established at 40 mg/kg/day for 5 days [18].

Alternative schedules and doses are therefore being explored. To reduce the risk of neurotoxicity, the CALGB and SWOG investigated a nelarabine schedule of 1.5 g/m^2/day given on days 1, 3, and 5 every 21 days [19]. Forty patients (22 ALL and 18 lymphoblastic lymphoma [LL]) were enrolled. All patients were refractory to at least one induction regimen or were in first or subsequent relapse without demonstrable CNS disease. Of 21 evaluable ALL patients, the OR was 38% (including six CR patients). For the group of LL patients, 24% responded (including four CR) for an overall response rate of 38% in 38 evaluable patients. Myelosuppression was the main toxicity with minimal neurotoxicity reported. The median DFS for the CR patients was 9.8 months. The POG/CCG Intergroup investigated nelarabine in patients with relapsed and refractory T-cell malignancies <21 years of age [20]. Depending on salvage status, doses of 400 mg/m^2 up to 650 mg/m^2 daily for 5 days every 21 days were used. The initial dose of 1.2 g/m^2 daily proved too neurotoxic. Among patients with T-cell leukemia in first relapse (650 mg/m^2), response rates exceeded 50% and were lowest in those with extramedullary relapse (400 mg/m^2). Although nelarabine was well tolerated at these dose levels, peripheral neuropathy remained the most significant adverse event. The efficacy of nelarabine in T-cell leukemias notwithstanding, doses and schedules need to be further investigated in particular subsets of adults and children. Combinations of nelarabine with other nucleoside analogs such as fludarabine based on biochemical modulation of intracellular ara-GTP levels have been reported [21].

Clofarabine is a second-generation nucleoside analog that has been synthesized as a rational extension of the experience with other deoxyadenosine analogs such as fludarabine and cladribine. After cellular uptake, clofarabine is converted to the monophosphate compound by the enzyme deoxycytidine kinase whereby phosphorylation of clofarabine by deoxycytidine kinase is substantially more efficient than that of fludarabine or cladribine. Furthermore, retention of the triphosphate form of clofarabine in cells is also longer than that of fludarabine and cladribine. Clofarabine is active by inhibition of DNA synthesis, ribonucleotide reductase (resulting in depletion of normal deoxynucleotides and increased DNA incorporation of the analog referred to as self-potentiation), and various DNA polymerases [22].

In a phase I study of clofarabine in children with relapsed and refractory acute leukemias, the MTD has been established at 52 mg/m^2 daily for 5 days every month with the DLT defined by reversible hepatotoxicity and skin rash at doses of up to 70 mg/m^2 daily [23]. Out of 17 patients with heavily pretreated ALL, four (24%) achieved CR and one (6%) PR, which made for an overall response of 30%. In a subsequent larger phase II study, which included 49 children with ALL, 31% responded (six CR, four CRp, five PR) with a median survival of 42 weeks (range 7 to 63.1 +) for these patients [24]. Among the patients who were refractory to the last prior chemotherapy, 23% (7/30) patients with ALL responded. Based on the positive experience and the response rates in pediatric ALL, clofarabine received Food and Drug Administration (FDA) approval in December 2004 for children with relapsed/refractory ALL who have at least received two prior regimens. Phase I studies in adults with acute leukemias defined the MTD for clofarabine at 40 mg/m^2/day [25]. Less experience exists with clofarabine in adult ALL. A large phase II study of 62 patients with relapsed acute leukemias included 12 ALL patients, two-thirds of whom received clofarabine in their second or subsequent salvage [26]. Two patients responded (one CR, one CRp) for an overall response of 16%. The complete responder had Ph-positive disease and was primary refractory to induction with the VAD regimen. The potential of clofarabine for adult ALL remains to be explored. Clinical studies of clofarabine combinations (e.g., with cyclophosphamide) are underway.

19.2.3 Epigenetic Therapy

Aberrant methylation of promoter-associated CpG islands and silencing of tumor-related genes due to hypermethylation is an epigenetic modification that is frequently observed in human cancers and leukemias [27]. A particularly high frequency of this process has been observed in ALL both at presentation and at relapse where methylation of genes can be demonstrated in up to 80% of patients [28, 29]. Several groups have been able to identify a number of genes involved in hypermethylation, which identified subsets of patients with a "hypermethylator" phenotype that has prognostic significance. Roman-Gomez et al. evaluated the methylation status 15 genes in 251 ALL patients [30]. In more than 75% of the patients, at least one gene was hypermethylated with ≥ 4 genes hypermethylated in about 36%. Although there was no difference in CR rates among the groups with variable numbers of genes affected, DFS and overall survival were significantly different: 75.5% and 66.1%, respectively, for the nonmethylated group compared to only 9.4 and 7.8% for patients with ≥ 4 involved genes ($p < 0.0001$ and $p < 0.0004$, respectively). In a multivariate analysis, methylation status emerged as an independent prognostic factor for survival. Genes frequently involved include p73, the cyclin dependent kinase inhibitors p15, and $p57^{KIP2}$, which play an important role in cell cycle regulatory pathways. Shen et al. demonstrated that methylation of one single gene such as $p57^{KIP2}$ does not affect outcome of ALL patients, whereas methylation of at least two genes involved in cell cycle regulatory pathways resulted in unfavorable disease-free survival and overall survival [31]. Use of hypomethylating agents such as 5-aza-2′-deoxycytidine (decitabine) or 5-azacytidine may thus provide therapeutic benefit for patients with a defined methylator phenotype. Although experience with these agents in ALL remains sparse, understanding defined genetic and epigenetic changes in adult ALL may offer another dominant molecular mechanism whose targeting may lead to risk-adapted therapies.

19.2.4 Signal Transduction Inhibitors

Ph-positive ALL is the most common subtype in adult ALL and has historically been associated with one of the worst outcomes to even intense-dose multiagent chemotherapy regimens [32]. Ph-positive leukemic blasts are characterized by expression of BCR-ABL tyrosine kinases of either 210 kD (p210) or 190 kD (190) as a consequence of the reciprocal translocation between the long arms of chromosomes 9 (harboring the *ABL* gene) and 22 (*BCR*). Whereas p210 occurs most commonly in chronic myeloid leukemia (CML), p190 is more frequently expressed in Ph-positive acute leukemias and is also a more active tyrosine kinase activity than p210. Imatinib mesylate (Gleevec) is a small molecule with potent antiproliferative activity against BCR-ABL cell lines in vitro at submicromolar concentrations that are easily achievable clinically. Although imatinib has made its biggest impact in the treatment of patients with CML, p190- and p210-expressing cells are equally sensitive, making Ph-positive ALL a suitable target as well.

Although single-agent imatinib is active in Ph-positive ALL, almost all patients will eventually relapse and progress so that major efforts are being invested in combination programs of imatinib with dose-intensive chemotherapy to increase response rates and improve durability of responses. Thomas et al. were the first to combine imatinib with the ALL induction regimen hyper-CVAD (cyclophosphamide, vincristine, doxorubicin, dexamethasone alternating with high-dose methotrexate and cytarabine) [33]. In a recent update, 25 of 26 patients (96%) with active disease at study entry achieved CR at a median time to response of 21 days [34]. Thirteen of the patients were able to proceed with allogeneic stem cell transplant within a median of 3 months from start of therapy. Molecular responses as assessed by RT-PCR for BCR-ABL occurred in nine of 19 patients. Two-year DFS was 87% with the hyper-CVAD imatinib combination compared with 28% with hyper-CVAD alone in this group of patients. Similar results have been reported by the Japan Adult Leukemia Study Group (JALSG) by Towatari et al. [35]. Of 24 patients with Ph-positive ALL, all but one (96%) achieved CR after a single course of induction therapy. PCR testing was negative in almost 80% of patients during follow up. Fifteen patients (63%) were able to proceed to an allogeneic stem cell transplant. Ottmann et al. compared the efficacy of imatinib in Ph-positive ALL when given either intermittently between chemotherapy courses or concurrently [36]. Concurrent administration achieved higher CR rates (96 vs. 58%) and more profound decreases of BCR-ABL levels by PCR testing.

More potent second-generation tyrosine kinase inhibitors such as nilotinib and dasatinib have recently entered clinical trials [37]. Both agents proved more potent in proliferation assays than imatinib and also showed activity against imatinib-resistant cell lines. The role of new kinase inhibitors in Ph-positive ALL is currently investigated in clinical trials.

19.2.5 Monoclonal Antibody Therapy

Monoclonal antibody therapy has emerged as one of the most effective additions to the therapy of hematologic malignancies including the acute leukemias. The attraction of monoclonal antibodies is based on two characteristics: (1) selectivity of the tumor target by virtue of expression of more or less tumor-specific cell surface antigens; and (2) different mechanisms of actions compared to more traditional cytotoxic chemotherapy involving elements of the complement system, human effector functions, and most likely intracellular signaling pathways leading to apoptotic cell death. ALL blasts express several antigens that can serve as therapeutic targets including CD19, CD20, CD33, or CD52 [38].

Rituximab is an anti-CD20 directed chimeric monoclonal antibody that has been developed for the therapy of relapsed and refractory indolent NHL. Expression of CD20 is detected in 35% of adult ALL, particularly in elderly patients and has been associated with a worse prognosis [39]. Expression is higher in ALL subsets; up to 55% in Ph-positive ALL and almost ubiquitous in mature B ALL (Burkitt). Combination of rituximab with induction and consolidation regimens in CD20-positive ALL has been explored. Thomas et al. reported their experience with Hyper-CVAD plus rituximab in patients with Burkitt and Burkitt-like leukemia and lymphoma [40]. The CR rate among 22 evaluable non-HIV patients was 95% with no induction deaths occurring in this group. With a median follow up of 18 months, only two patients relapsed. Historical experience of hyper-CVAD alone in mature B ALL showed a CR rate of 81% with 3-year survival rates of between 17% (patients older than 60 years) and 77% (patients younger than 60 years). Rituximab has also been reported to induce molecular remissions in the setting of minimal residual disease in ALL [41].

Alemtuzumab is a humanized monoclonal antibody recognizing CD52. CD52 expression is highest on T and B lymphocytes and most frequently found in chronic lymphoproliferative disorders. Alemtuzumab has established activity in chronic lymphocytic leukemia, prolymphocytic, and other T-cell NHL. CD52 is also detected in 30–50% of ALL blasts. Experience in ALL is limited. Anecdotal reports do not support its use as single agent in relapsed and refractory disease [42]. Alemtuzumab is currently investigated as part of intense induction/consolidation programs and in combination with hyper-CVAD in aggressive T-cell malignancies including T-cell ALL.

CD19 is expressed on a large proportion of ALL blasts in most patients with B-lineage disease, and several antibodies targeting CD19 have been developed and are investigated in clinical trials. The antitumor activity of CD19 by itself is weak, but can be enhanced by conjugation with other components. Ricin is a plant toxin with potent antiribosomal activity in vitro. When conjugated as blocked ricin to CD19 (anti-B4 blocked ricin), enhanced cytotoxic activity in lymphoid malignancies has been demonstrated [43]. In a small study of relapsed childhood ALL, biologic activity (reduction in blast percentage) was observed in five of 19 patients, although no objective responses occurred. The CALGB used anti-B4 blocked ricin in B-lineage ALL after induction of residual disease [44]. Although antibody administration was feasible as part of a complex induction and consolidation regimen, no benefit could be proven with respect to remission duration or minimal residual disease levels as assessed by PCR. Experience with other conjugates (e.g., the tyrosine kinase inhibitor genistein, pokeweed antiviral protein immunotoxin) suggest antitumor activity in small studies, but experience remains limited.

19.2.6 Other Agents

19.2.6.1 Pegylated Asparaginase

L-asparaginase has been an important component of ALL therapy for many decades. Asparaginase depletes external sources of asparagine, which ALL blasts require for survival, as they are unable to synthesize asparagine. However, native asparaginase has been problematic for two reasons: (1) need for frequent injections; and (2) immunogenicity that can result in anaphylactic reactions or development of neutralizing antibodies with rapid clearance and short plasma half-lives of asparaginase [45]. To overcome these shortcomings, *E. coli* asparaginase has been covalently linked to mono-methoxy-polyethylene glycol, rendering native asparaginase less immunogenic and extending its plasma half-life to up to 6 days (5–9 times longer), enabling up to biweekly administrations and thus making therapy more convenient for patients.

When 144 children with ALL relapse were randomized to receive PEG-asparaginase either weekly or biweekly, there was, however, a significant difference in CR rate favoring weekly administration (97 vs. 82%, $p=0.003$) [46]. The CR rate was significantly associated with higher levels of asparaginase, which in turn correlated to low antibody titers. Except for infectious complications, other toxicities including hypersensitivity (4%) were infrequent. A Children's Cancer Group study conducted a randomized comparison of native *E. coli* asparaginase and PEG asparaginase in children with newly diagnosed ALL as part of induction and delayed intensification [47]. The PEG asparaginase group more rapidly cleared lymphoblasts from early marrow samples and developed less frequently antibodies, which were associated with low asparaginase activity in the native arm. No difference was noted in event-free survival. A recent study in 28 children with relapsed ALL confirmed the pharmacokinetic advantages of PEG asparaginase, which are characterized by high levels of asparaginase activity in serum and CSF and consequently effective asparagine depletion [48]. Limited experience with PEG asparaginase is available in adult ALL patients.

19.2.6.2 Forodesine (BCX-1777)

Purine nucleoside phosphorylase (PNP) catalyzes the reversible phosphorolytic cleavage of purine ribonucleosides and 2′-deoxyribose-α-1-phosphate. PNP deficiency or inhibition suppresses the proliferation of human T-cells due to subsequent accumulation of deoxyguanosine triphosphate (dGTP), which leads to allosteric inhibition of ribonucleoside diphosphate reductase (RNR), an enzyme necessary for DNA synthesis. As patients with inherited PNP deficiency are characterized by profound suppression of T-cell immunity, inhibition of this purine salvage enzyme is predominantly targeted at T-cell hematologic malignancies although in vitro studies indicated that B-lineage ALL cells are susceptible to PNP inhibition as well.

Several phase I and II trials are underway to investigate the safety profile and clinical activity of forodesine in patients with advanced T-cell malignancies. In a phase I/II multicenter dose escalation study, 15 patients with various hematologic malignancies (including six patients with B-lineage ALL) received forodesine at doses from 40 mg/m^2 up to 135 mg/m^2 intravenously (typically given every 12 h for 4 days following one single infusion in the first day) [49]. There was one complete response at 135 mg/m^2 and hematologic benefits for six other patients (including five with ALL). Maximum PNP inhibition was achieved at 40 mg/m^2. Duvic et al. treated 13 patients with cutaneous T-cell lymphoma (CTCL) or Sezary syndrome with forodesine at dose between 40 mg/m^2 and 135 mg/m^2 per infusion [50]. They report one complete and two partial responses. Overall, nine patients showed at least an improvement in skin lesions and/or a pharmacodynamic response. A phase II study of forodesine in relapsed T-cell ALL is being conducted at MD Anderson Cancer Center. An oral formulation of forodesine will become available for clinical studies in the near future.

19.3 Getting to Know Chemotherapy: The Role of Pharmacogenetics and Mechanisms of Drug Resistance

Although development of new drugs remains crucial, further understanding of the pharmacodynamics and pharmacokinetics of existing agents can help to increase their efficacy. Considerations of drug metabolism and pharmacogenetics are therefore becoming increasingly important to assess sensitivity to chemotherapy and prognosis. Many antineoplastic agents display a wide range of interpatient variability of their steady state plasma and intracellular levels, which may influence response and outcome to therapy [51]. Polymorphisms in expression of various genes account for differences in drug absorption, distribution, and metabolism. Thymidylate synthase (TS) is an important target of methotrexate. Homozygosity for a triple-tandem repeat polymorphism of the TS gene has been associated with increased levels of the enzyme, and with worse prognosis in children with ALL [52]. Polymorphisms of the methylenetetrahydrofolate reductase (MTHFR) gene have been correlated with a higher incidence of adverse events, but also greater sensitivity of leukemic blasts to methotrexate [53, 54]. In a study by Evans et al., patients with low methotrexate concentrations had significantly shorter CR durations and methotrexate clearance was an independent prognostic factor for remission duration [55]. Polymorphisms affecting the thiopurine methyltransferase (TPMT) gene may likewise lead to increased sensitivity to 6-mecaptopurine, to a higher risk of acute hematopoietic adverse events, but also to a more favorable leukemia-free survival [56]. Most of these studies have been conducted in children with ALL and it is unknown how these pharmacokinetic variables contribute to the outcome in adult ALL. There is growing interest in adult ALL as well, to designing programs that allow monitoring of pharmacogenetic properties and individualize dose and schedule of therapy accordingly.

Differences in sensitivity of ALL cells to chemotherapy are also based on cytogenetic-molecular characteristics determining, among other things, drug disposition and clearance [51]. Several karyotype abnormalities have been described that have been associated with altered responsiveness to therapy. Patients with hyperdiploid cytogenetics are highly sensitive to antimetabolite-type chemotherapy. In many cases, the leukemic cells of these patients harbor additional copies of a gene coding for cellular methotrexate transporters, and higher-than-average concentrations of intracellular methotrexate polyglutamates have been demonstrated in vitro after treatment with methotrexate in leukemic blasts of these patients [57]. Patients whose cells harbor a *TEL-AML1* fusion [as seen in translocation t(12;21)] are more sensitive to asparaginase [58]. ALL with translocation t(4;11) and *MLL* rearrangements have increased sensitivity to cytarabine possibly by overexpression of cellular cytarabine receptors [59]. Phenotypes resistant to standard doses of methotrexate include T-lineage ALL where high doses of methotrexate have been associated with better outcome and ALL associated with translocation t(1;19), which has been associated with resistance to standard antimetabolite-based therapy, but has a better prognosis using intensified chemotherapy.

19.4 Conclusion

Although remission rates in adult ALL now equal those seen in children, long-term, disease-free survival remains vastly inferior. Therapy in adult ALL thus remains a challenging task. The development of new agents that are specific for ALL is crucial, but can only be applied efficiently and to optimum benefit if paired with a thorough understanding of disease biology. Further dissection of ALL subtypes and characterization of their biological behavior therefore continues to be of crucial importance. In addition to new and targeted drugs, developments in two other aspects may provide further benefit: (1) elucidation of pharmacokinetic properties of currently used drugs; and (2) other modifications of existing combination regimens. Among the latter included are improvements in supportive care (e.g., use of laminar air flow rooms in patients over 60 years of age), risk-adaptation of CNS prophylaxis, extension and possibly intensification of maintenance therapy, or use of rituximab in CD20-positive ALL. Taken together, these approaches will allow are more sophisticated and individualized approaches to ALL therapy in adults, and hopefully an improved long-term outcome.

References

1. Larson RA, Dodge RK, Burns CP, et al. (1995) A five-drug remission induction regimen with intensive consolidation for adults with acute lymphoblastic leukemia: Cancer and Leukemia Group B study 8811. Blood 85:2025–2037
2. Kantarjian HM, O'Brien S, Smith TL, et al. (2000) Results of treatment with hyper-CVAD, a dose-intensive regimen, in adult acute lymphocytic leukemia. J Clin Oncol 18:547–561
3. Thomas DA, Cortes J, O'Brien S, et al. (1999) Hyper-CVAD program in Burkitt's-type adult acute lymphoblastic leukemia. J Clin Oncol 17:2461–2470
4. Kantarjian HM (2000) Adult acute lymphocytic leukemia: Introduction and questions related to current programs. Heme Oncol Clin North Am 14:1205–1208
5. Waterhouse DN, Madden TD, Cullis PR, et al. (2005) Preparation, characterization, and biological analysis of liposomal formulations of vincristine. Methods Enzymol 391:40–57
6. Krishna R, Webb MS, St Onge G, Mayer LD (2001) Liposomal and nonliposomal drug pharmacokinetics after administration of liposome-encapsulated vincristine and their contribution to drug tissue distribution properties. J Pharmacol Exp Ther 298:1206–1212
7. Sarris AH, Hagemeister F, Romaguera J, et al. (2000) Liposomal vincristine in relapsed non-Hodgkin's lymphomas: Early results of an ongoing phase II trial. Ann Oncol 11:69–72
8. Rodriguez MA, Winter JN (2004) Treatment response to single agent sphingosomal vincristine in patients with relapsed and/or refractory diffuse aggressive non-Hodgkin's lymphoma (NHL): Subgroup analyses. Blood 104:682a
9. Rodriguez MA, Sarris A, Dang NH, et al. (2004) Sphingosomal vincristine in CHOP +/- rituximab is a promising new treatment for patients with high risk untreated aggressive Non-Hodgkin's lymphoma (NHL): Follow-up results of a phase II study. Blood 104:234b
10. Thomas DA, Sarris A, O'Brien S, et al. (1999) Phase II study of liposomal vincristine (LipoV) in relapsed or refractory adult acute lymphoblastic leukemia (ALL). Blood 94:238b
11. Thomas DA, Garcia-Manero G, Fader S, et al. (2004) Preliminary results of phase I trial of sphingosomal vincristine (SV) and dexamethasone in relapsed or refractory acute lymphocytic leukemia (ALL). Blood 104:748a
12. Faderl S, Gandhi V, Kantarjian H, Plunkett W (2002) New nucleoside analogs in clinical development. Cancer Chemother Biol Response Modif 20:37–58
13. Lambe CU, Averett DR, Paff MT, et al. (1995) 2-amino-6-methoxypurine arabinoside: An agent for T-cell malignancies. Cancer Res 55:3352–3356
14. Gandhi V, Plunkett W, Rodriguez CO Jr, et al. (1998) Compound GW506U78 in refractory hematologic malignancies: Relationship between cellular pharmacokinetics and clinical response. J Clin Oncol 16:3607–3615
15. Cohen A, Lee JWW, Gelfand EW (1983) Selective toxicity of deoxyguanosine and arabinosyl guanine for T-leukemic cells. Blood 61:660–666
16. Ullman B, Martin DW (1984) Specific cytotoxicity of arabinosylguanine toward cultured T-lymphoblasts. J Clin Invest 74:951–955
17. Shewach DS, Daddona PE, Ashcraft E, et al. (1985) Metabolism and selective cytotoxicity of 9-β-D-arabinofuranosylguanine in human lymphoblasts. Cancer Res 45:1008–1014
18. O'Brien S, Thomas D, Kantarjian H, et al. (1998) Compound 506 has activity in mature lymphoid leukemia. Blood 92:490a
19. De Angelo DJ, Yu D, Dodge RK, et al. (2002) A phase II study of 2-amino-9-b-D-arabinosyl-6-methoxy-9H-purine (506U78) in patients with relapsed or refractory T-lineage acute lymphoblastic leukemia (ALL) or lymphoblastic lymphoma (LBL): CALGB Study 19801. Blood 198a
20. Berg SL, Blaney SM, Bernstein M, et al. (2002) Activity of compound 506U78 in patients with refractory T-cell malignancies: A POG/CCG Intergroup phase 2 study. Blood 102:211a
21. Gandhi V, Plunkett W, Weller S, et al. (2001) Evaluation of the combination of nelarabine and fludarabine in leukemias: Clinical response, pharmacokinetics, and pharmacodynamics in leukemia cells. J Clin Oncol 19:2142–2152
22. Faderl S, Gandhi V, Keating MJ, et al. (2005) The role of clofarabine in hematologic and solid malignancies – Development of a next-generation nucleoside analog. Cancer (epub ahead of print)

23. Jeha S, Gandhi V, Chan KW, et al. (2004) Clofarabine, a novel nucleoside analog, is active in pediatric patients with advanced leukemia. Blood 103(3):784–789
24. Jeha S, Razzouk BI, Rytting ME, et al. (2004) Phase II trials of clofarabine in relapsed or refractory pediatric leukemia. Blood 104:196 a
25. Kantarjian HM, Gandhi V, Kozuch P, et al. (2003) Phase I clinical and pharmacology study of clofarabine in patients with solid and hematologic cancers. J Clin Oncol 21:1167–1173
26. Kantarjian H, Gandhi V, Cortes J, et al. (2003) Phase 2 clinical and pharmacologic study of clofarabine in patients with refractory or relapsed acute leukemia. Blood 102:2379–2386
27. Santini V, Kantarjian HM, Issa J-P (2001) Changes in DNA methylation in neoplasia: Pathophysiology and therapeutic implications. Ann Intern Med 134:573–586
28. Garcia-Manero G, Bueso-Ramos C, Daniel J, et al. (2002) DNA methylation patterns at relapse in adult acute lymphocytic leukemia. Clin Cancer Res 8:1897–1903
29. Garcia-Manero G, Daniel J, Smith TL, et al. (2002) DNA methylation of multiple promoter-associated CpG islands in adult acute lymphocytic leukemia. Clin Cancer Res 8:2217–2224
30. Roman-Gomez J, Jimenez-Velasco A, Castillejo JA, et al. (2004) Promoter hypermethylation of cancer-related genes: A strong independent prognostic factor in acute lymphoblastic leukemia. Blood 104:2492–2498
31. Shen L, Toyota M, Kondo Y, et al. (2003) Aberrant DNA methylation of p57KIP2 identifies a cell-cycle regulatory pathway with prognostic impact in adult acute lymphocytic leukemia. Blood 101: 4131–4136
32. Faderl S, Kantarjian HM, Thomas DA, et al. (2000) Outcome of Philadelphia chromosome-positive adult acute lymphoblastic leukemia. Leuk Lymphoma 36:263–273
33. Thomas DA, Faderl S, Cortes J, et al. (2004) Treatment of Philadelphia chromosome-positive acute lymphocytic leukemia with hyper-CVAD and imatinib mesylate. Blood 103:4396–4407
34. Thomas DA, Faderl S, Cortes J, et al. (2004) Update of the Hyper-CVAD and imatinib mesylate regimen in Philadelphia (Ph) positive acute lymphocytic leukemia (ALL). Blood 104:748a
35. Towatari M, Yanada M, Usui N, et al. (2004) Combination of intensive chemotherapy and imatinib can rapidly induce high-quality complete remission for a majority of patients with newly diagnosed BCR-ABL-positive acute lymphoblastic leukemia. Blood 104:3507–3512
36. Ottmann OG, Wassmann B, Pfeifer H, et al. (2004) Imatinib given concurrently with induction chemotherapy is superior to imatinib subsequent to induction and consolidation in newly diagnosed Philadelphia-positive acute lymphoblastic leukemia (Ph+ ALL). Blood 104:197 a
37. Giles F, Kantarjian H, Wassmann B, et al. (2004) A phase I/II study of AMN107, a novel aminopyrimidine inhibitor of Bcr-Abl, on a continuous daily dosing schedule in adult patients (pts) with imatinib-resistant advanced phase chronic myeloid leukemia (CML) or relapsed/refractory Philadelphia chromosome (Ph+) acute lymphoblastic leukemia (ALL). Blood 104:10 a
38. Gögbuget N, Hoelzer D (2004) Treatment with monoclonal antibodies in acute lymphoblastic leukemia: Current knowledge and future prospects. Ann Hematol 83:201–205
39. Thomas DA, Cortes J, O'Brien SM, et al. (2000) Significance of CD20 positivity in de novo acute lymphocytic leukemia (ALL). Blood 96:109 a
40. Thomas DA, Cortes J, Faderl S, et al. (2004) Outcome with the Hyper-CVAD and rituximab regimen in Burkitt (BL) and Burkitt-like (BLL) leukemia/lymphoma. Blood 104:901 a
41. Ozsahin H, Fluss J, McLin V, et al. (2003) Rituximab with interleukin-2 after autologous bone marrow transplantation for acute lymphocytic leukemia in second remission. Med Pediatr Oncol 38:300–301
42. Tibes R, Keating MJ, Ferrajoli A, et al. (2006) Activity of alemtuzumab in patients with CD52-positive acute leukemia. Cancer 106: 2645–2651
43. Grossbard ML, Freedman AS, Ritz J, et al. (1992) Serotherapy of B-cell neoplasms with anti-B4-blocked ricin: A phase I trial of daily bolus infusion. Blood 79:576–585
44. Szatrowski TP, Dodge RK, Reynolds C, et al. (2003) Lineage specific treatment of adult patients with acute lymphoblastic leukemia in first remission with anti-B4-blocked ricin or high-dose cytarabine: Cancer and Leukemia Group B study 9311. Cancer 97:1471–1480
45. Graham ML (2003) Pegaspargase: A review of clinical studies. Adv Drug Delivery Rev 55:1293–1302
46. Abshire TC, Pollock BH, Billett AL, et al. (2000) Weekly polyethylene glycol conjugated L-asparaginase compared with biweekly dosing produces superior induction remission rates in childhood relapsed acute lymphoblastic leukemia: A pediatric oncology group study. Blood 96:1709–1715
47. Avramis VI, Sencer S, Periclou AP, et al. (2002) A randomized comparison of native Escherichia coli asparaginase and polyethylene glycol conjugated asparaginase for treatment of children with newly diagnosed standard-risk acute lymphoblastic leukemia: A Children's Cancer Group study. Blood 99:1986–1994
48. Hawkins D, Park JR, Thomson BG, et al. (2004) Asparaginase pharmacokinetics after intensive polyethylene glycol-conjugated L-asparaginase therapy for children with relapsed acute lymphoblastic leukemia. Clin Cancer Res 10:5335–5341
49. Furman RR, Gandhi V, Bennett JC, et al. (2004) Intravenous forodesine (BCX-1777), a novel purine nucleoside phosphorylase (PNP) inhibitor, demonstrates clinical activity in phase I/II studies in patients with B-cell acute lymphoblastic leukemia. Blood 104:750 a
50. Duvic M, Foss FM, Olsen EA, et al. (2004) Intravenous forodesine (BCX-1777), a novel purine nucleoside phosphorylase (PNP) inhibitor, demonstrates clinical activity in patients with refractory cutaneous T-cell lymphoma. Blood 104:683a
51. Pui CH, Relling MV, Evans WE (2003) Role of pharmacogenomics and pharmacodynamics in the treatment of acute lymphoblastic leukemia. Best Pract Res Clin Haematol 15:741–756
52. Krajinovic M, Costea I, Chiasson S (2002) Polymorphism of the thymidylate synthas gene and outcome of acute lymphoblastic leukemia. Lancet 359:1033–1034
53. Ulrich CM, Yasui Y, Storb R, et al. (2001) Pharmacogenetics of methotrexate: Toxicity among marrow transplantation patients varies with the methylenetetrahydrofolate reductase C677T polymorphism. Blood 98:231–234
54. Taub JW, Matherly LH, Ravindranath Y, et al. (2002) Polymorphisms in methylenetetrahydrofolate reductase and methotrexate sensi-

tivity in childhood acute lymphoblastic leukemia. Leukemia 16: 764–765
55. Evans WE, Crom WR, Abromowitch M, et al. (1986) Clinical pharmacodynamics of high-dose methotrexate in acute lymphocytic leukemia. Identification of a relation between concentration and effect. N Engl J Med 14:471–477
56. Relling MV, Hancock ML, Rivera GK, et al. (1999) Mercaptopurine therapy intolerance and heterozygosity at the thiopurine S-methyl-transferase gene locus. J Natl Cancer Inst 91:2001–2008
57. Belkow VM, Krynetski EY, Schuetz JD, et al. (1999) Reduced folate carrier expression in acute lymphoblastic leukemia: A mechanism for ploidy but not lineage differences in methotrexate accumulation. Blood 93:1643–1650
58. Ramakers-van Woerden NL, Pieters R, Loonen AH, et al. (2000) TEL-AML1 gene fusion is related to in vitro drug sensitivity for L-asparaginase in childhood acute lymphoblastic leukemia. Blood 96:1094–1099
59. Stam RW, den Boer ML, Meijerink JP, et al. (2003) Differential mRNA expression of ara-C-metabolizing enzymes explains ara-C sensitivity in MLL gene-rearranged infant acute lymphoblastic leukemia. Blood 101:1270–1276

Minimal Residual Disease Studies in Acute Lymphoblastic Leukemia

Syed Abutalib, Wendy Stock

Contents

20.1 Introduction

Considerable progress has been made in the treatment of both childhood and adult acute lymphoblastic leukemia (ALL) during the past two decades. The majority of both children and adults achieve a complete remission (CR) while the majority of children are now cured with current therapies, most adults will ultimately experience a relapse and die of their leukemia. The ability to distinguish good-risk patients who are likely to be cured with conventional chemotherapy from those who are likely to relapse has important clinical implications.

In both adult and pediatric ALL, relapse is thought to result from residual leukemia cells (as many as 10^{10}) that remain following achievement of morphologic remission and are below the limits of detection using conventional microscopic and cytogenetic assessment of the bone marrow [1–3]. A variety of sensitive techniques have been used to monitor the persistence of the leukemic clone during treatment in an attempt to identify patients who are in morphologic and cytogenetic remission, but in whom there is persistence of subclinical, or minimal residual disease (MRD), and who may be at increased risk for relapse.

Moreover, MRD studies in ALL have the potential to provide novel insights into the clinical efficacy of both standard and novel treatment strategies aimed at improving the cure rate. Recent prospective studies designed to validate the clinical significance of MRD detection in ALL are beginning to answer several important questions:

1. Does detection of MRD following achievement of clinical remission predict treatment outcome?
2. If early MRD measurements are predictive of relapse, can MRD detection be used to guide therapy (i.e., can therapy be intensified or reduced based on MRD results)?
3. What is the optimal clinical time-point(s) for MRD assessment?
4. Does clinical intervention based on MRD result improve survival?
5. Is it essential to eradicate MRD (as detected by these highly sensitive assays) in order to achieve a cure?
6. Can peripheral blood monitoring be substitute for bone marrow MRD evaluation?

Table 20.1. Characteristics of major techniques currently employed for detection of MRD in ALL

	Flow cytometric immunophenotyping	PCR analysis of chromosome aberration*	PCR analysis of IgH/TCR genes
Sensitivity	10^{-3}–10^{-4}	10^{-4}–10^{-6}	10^{-4}–10^{-5}
Applicability			
Precursor-B-ALL			
Children	80–90%	40–50%	95%
Adults	70–80%	35–45%	90%
T-ALL			
Children	>95%	10–25%	>95%
Adults	>95%	5–10%	90%
Advantages	Adequate sensitivity	Relatively easy and cheap	Minimal tissue requirements
	Applicable for most patients	Sensitive and leukemia specific	Applicable for virtually all patients if IGH, IGK-Kde, TCRG, and TCRD gene rearrangement are used as targets
	Quick: (2–3 days) and relatively cheap	Stable target during disease course	Sensitive and patient specific
	Distinguish living from dead leukemia cells	Rapid: 2–3 days	Rapid during follow up: 2–3 days (if junctional region is identified and RQ-PCR is used)
		Suitable for monitoring uniform patient groups (Ph+ ALL)	Applicable for virtually all patients if IGH, IGK-Kde, TCRG, and TCRD gene rearrangement are used as targets
		Minimal tissue requirements	Sensitive and patient specific
Disadvantages	Analysis is quite complex and depends on the expertise of the operator Difficult to distinguish between normal regenerating bone marrow progenitors and residual blasts of B-cell precursor leukemias Expert operators have to continuously be available locally since analysis can be reliably done only on fresh cells	Useful in minority of patients Cross contamination of PCR products leading to false-positive results (even at diagnosis) Risk of RNA degradation and inefficiency during conversion of mRNA to cDNA (which may reduce the sensitivity of RT-PCR monitoring leading to false-negative results)	Time-consuming at diagnosis: identification of the junctional regions and sensitivity testing Relatively expensive Need for preferably two PCR targets per patient because of chance of clonal evolution

Table 20.1 (continued)

	Flow cytometric immunophenotyping	PCR analysis of chromosome aberration	PCR analysis of IgH/TCR genes
Disadvantages	Instability of antigenic expression on leukemic cells (lineage switch, loss of antigens) during or after the treatment course (Immunophenotypic shifts)	Lack of reproducibility of results when small numbers of transcripts are present Presence of oligoclonal populations that can cause both false-negative and false-positive results Difficult quantification of MRD	Risk of RNA degradation and inefficiency during conversion of mRNA to cDNA (which may reduce the sensitivity of RT-PCR monitoring) Lack of reproducibility of results when small numbers of transcripts are present Presence of oligoclonal populations that can cause both false-negative and false-positive results

This chapter will focus on current strategies for monitoring MRD in ALL and will attempt to address these questions by summarizing some of the recent studies of MRD monitoring in ALL.

20.2 Methods for Detection of MRD

MRD detection techniques rely on the ability to identify a unique marker on the leukemia cells. The two methods that typically have been employed for MRD detection and monitoring include polymerase chain reaction (PCR) methods and flow cytometry (FC). For PCR techniques, monitoring of a leukemia-specific fusion gene (e.g., *BCR-ABL*) or a clone-specific rearrangement of the immunoglobulin heavy chain (IgH) or T-cell receptor (TCR) genes have been used. For flow cytometric MRD monitoring, an aberrant immunophenotype present on the cell surface of the leukemic blasts can be identified at diagnosis and used for MRD monitoring. These techniques have far greater sensitivity than standard cytogenetic analysis and may detect anywhere from one in ten thousand to one leukemia cell in a background of one million normal cells. General characteristics of each of these techniques are described below and summarized in Table 20.1.

20.2.1 Flow Cytometric Detection of MRD

Multiparameter flow cytometry is a widely applicable and reliable approach for monitoring MRD in ALL due to the presence of aberrant or unusual immunophenotypes expressed on the cell surface of the lymphoblast. These aberrant immunophenotypes can be the result of cross-lineage expression (e.g., presence of myeloid antigens on a lymphoid progenitor cell), asynchronous expression of lymphoid maturation antigen (e.g., when two or more antigens not normally present at the same stage of normal hematopoietic differentiation are coexpressed on the lymphoblast), antigen overexpression, absence of normal maturation antigens, and/or ectopic antigen expression [4–6].

FC detection of MRD can be utilized in the majority of cases of both B- and T-lineage ALL and is rapid, relatively sensitive, and quantitative, with the ability to detect one leukemia cell in a background of 10^3–10^4 normal cells. Disadvantages to this technique include a lack of standardization across laboratories, with significant variation depending on the expertise of the operator, difficulty in distinguishing between normal regenerating bone marrow progenitors and residual leukemic blasts, and the instability of the antigenic expression of the leukemic clone with resultant immunophenotypic shifts during treatment that can result in false-negative MRD results [7, 8]. Conversely, the selection of inappropriate antigens to distinguish leukemic cells from normal cells may result in false-positive MRD results.

20.2.2 PCR-based MRD Detection

PCR amplification of a specific DNA sequence or complementary DNA (cDNA) unique to the leukemia clone can permit identification of one malignant cell among 10^4–10^6 normal cells, making it, in general, a slightly more sensitive method of MRD detection than FC. Two types of PCR targets can be used to detect MRD in ALL patients: junctional regions of leukemia clone-specific rearranged IgH and TCR genes; or leukemia-specific breakpoint fusion regions of chromosome rearrangements. In addition to the commonly used targets which are described in detail below, several studies have suggested that the Wilms tumor suppressor gene, *WT1*, aberrantly expressed in the majority of cases of AML and ALL, may also serve as a useful target for MRD analysis [9–21].

The deletion and random insertion of nucleotides during IgH and *TCR* gene rearrangement generates unique junctional sequences that can serve as clone-specific markers of the leukemia that can be identified at the time of diagnosis and used for serially MRD assessment. The precise nucleotide sequence of the junctional region can be used in the design of oligonucleotide patient-specific primers for PCR amplification and detection of MRD during and following treatment of the leukemia [22]. The clone-specific IgH or *TCR* gene rearrangements can be identified at diagnosis in 80–95% of cases by using various PCR primer sets [22, 23]. Subsequently, patient-specific primer and probe sets based on the rearranged DNA sequence of the leukemic clone can be generated and used for MRD detection.

Leukemia-specific (chromosomal) rearrangements are also useful PCR targets for detecting MRD. Oligonucleotide primers are designed at opposite ends of the breakpoint fusion region so that the PCR product contains the tumor-specific fusion sequences. In most of the chromosome translocations common to adult ALL, the breakpoints are spread over regions larger than 2 kb of DNA, which is the maximal distance that can be reliably amplified [24]. Therefore, MRD detection of the more common fusion genes, such as *BCR-ABL* resulting from the t(9;22) and *MLL-AF4* resulting from the t(4;11), depends on identifying the resultant leukemia-specific fusion mRNA. This fusion mRNA can be used as a target for MRD analysis using PCR after the fusion mRNA (consisting of transcribed coding exons) is converted to cDNA using the enzyme reverse transcriptase (RT). This technique is known as reverse transcriptase PCR (RT-PCR). Two other fusion gene products in ALL are amenable to MRD detection using RT-PCR techniques. The *E2A/PBX1* fusion gene resulting from the t(1;19) translocation is found in approximately 5% of ALL cases, irrespective of age [25–33]. The *TEL-AML1* fusion gene product results from the cryptic translocation, t(12;21) and occurs in as many as 25% of children with precursor-B ALL [34–37]. Several studies suggest that the results of MRD detection using RT-PCR of *TEL-AML1* are concordant with MRD detection using PCR of IgH or *TCR* rearrangements [38, 39]. RT-PCR of fusion genes is highly sensitive and specific. It is also less labor intensive than PCR of clonal IgH or *TCR* gene rearrangements since a single set of primers can be utilized for each fusion gene product. Despite these advantages, the general applicability of using leukemia-specific fusion genes for MRD detection remains relatively low, since only about one-third of both pediatric and adult ALL cases harbor a recurring fusion gene for PCR amplification.

Early PCR-based MRD studies used qualitative or, at best, semiquantitative methods for detection of the leukemia-specific target. These PCR methods relied on endpoint measurements; that is, analysis of the reaction product after PCR amplification is completed. MRD measurements depended on multiple dilutions with coamplification of standards and were cumbersome, error prone, and technically demanding [40–42]. During the last several years, real-time quantitative PCR (RQ-PCR) has been introduced and has become the new standard for PCR-based MRD analysis [38, 43–45] In contrast to PCR endpoint quantification, RQ-PCR permits accurate quantification during the exponential phase of PCR amplification. This method has a very large dynamic detection range over five orders of magnitude, thereby eliminating the need for serial dilutions of follow-up samples. In addition, the quantitative data are quickly available since post-PCR processing is not necessary. Therefore RQ-PCR is suitable for quantitative detection of MRD using either junctional regions of IgH or *TCR* gene rearrangements, or using breakpoint fusion regions of chromosome aberrations.

PCR-based methods are very specific, highly sensitive, and widely applicable to the majority of patients with ALL. Recently, standardized methods for RQ-PCR analysis have been published to provide more accurate comparisons of MRD results from different laboratories [24, 46]. However, the design of primers and probes for detection of patient-specific IgH gene or *TCR* gene rearrangements can be relatively costly and time-consuming. In the latter case, to reduce the costs associated with designing fluorescent probes that match patient-specific sequences, "consensus" probes matching recurring germ line segments, such as V [47], J [48], and Kde regions [49] that are applicable to multiple patients can be used. Another concern is clonal evolution, secondary rearrangements that can occur during the disease course which may result in the loss of the specific junctional region identified at diagnosis, thereby producing false-negative MRD results. Therefore, it has been recommended that two or more independent PCR targets for each patient are used to monitor MRD [22, 23, 50].

20.3 MRD Monitoring in Clinical Trials of ALL

20.3.1 MRD Studies in Pediatric ALL

Measurements of MRD during therapy of pediatric ALL have demonstrated the ability to provide crucial information about the response to treatment and the risk of relapse. A number of large-scale prospective trials have been performed that illustrate the prognostic value of MRD measurements during the first weeks of therapy. The group at St. Jude Children's Hospital evaluated MRD on day 19 of remission induction therapy in a large cohort of 110 children treated at their center using flow cytometric techniques [51]. They found unique phenotypic markers for MRD monitoring in 90% of the children using their panel of antibodies. Interestingly, 51 of 110 patients studied achieved a profound remission by day 19 of induction therapy, defined as a MRD level of $<0.01\%$. The treatment outcome for this group of patients was outstanding, with a 3-year cumulative incidence of relapse of $1.9 \pm 1.9\%$ for this group as compared to $28.4 \pm 6.4\%$ for patients with MRD levels $\geq 0.01\%$ ($p<0.001$). The independent prognostic value of MRD quantification has also been observed when FC MRD monitoring is performed during the first weeks of remission induction therapy (Table 20.2) [52–58]. These studies emphasize the point that this technology is feasible and useful as a prognostic marker and can provide quantitative MRD information, even when samples are sent from participating clinical centers to a central referral laboratory for analysis. However, since a standardized quantitative FC protocol has not yet been developed and accepted, a careful comparison of results from different centers is difficult to accomplish.

In contrast, during the last several years, the European pediatric centers have begun to adopt a standardized protocol for PCR-based MRD quantification of *IgH* and *TCR* gene rearrangements [24, 46]. In a landmark paper, Cave and colleagues [59] demonstrated that measurement of MRD level in early remission was the most important predictor of clinical outcome in 178 children treated in a large French cooperative group study. These investigators, using a semiquantitative technique, showed that detection of high MRD levels (defined as $>10^{-2}$) after achievement of morphologic remission were strongly predictive of relapse; whereas, patients with very low levels of MRD had similarly good outcomes as those patients in whom no MRD was detected. Indeed, other investigators have also suggested that it may not be essential to eradicate all MRD in order to achieve prolonged DFS [60]. The precise nature of these residual clonal cells that do not appear to give rise to relapse remains to be defined, but may highlight the multistep pathogenesis that is presumed to be responsible for the development of acute leukemia. These studies also suggest that MRD measurement at a single treatment time-point may not provide sufficient clinical prognostic information and that serial MRD measurements augment the predictive capacity of the test. In another large study of MRD involving 240 children with ALL, van Dongen et al. [61] found that combining semiquantitative MRD information from several time-points during treatment identified three risk groups. Forty-three percent of patients were in a low-risk group with a 3-year relapse rate of only 2%; 43% were in an intermediate-risk group with a relapse rate of 23%; and 15% were in a high-risk group with a 75% relapse rate. Other studies confirm the significance of serial, quantitative measurements of MRD [41, 62–67]. These and other PCR-based MRD studies are summarized in Table 20.3.

Investigators have also compared MRD results in blood and marrow to determine whether monitoring using blood samples, which is far more accessible and tolerable for patients, yields similar results to bone marrow MRD monitoring [51, 68–75]. To date, the data suggest that blood monitoring may yield comparable results to marrow MRD levels for patients with T-lineage ALL using both flow cytometric and PCR-based methods [51, 71]. The results of blood MRD detection with precursor-B ALL, however, do not seem to be as

Table 20.2. Selected flow cytometry MRD studies

Study	N	Timing	Relapse/MRD		Major conclusion
			MRD (+)	MRD (–)	
Ciudad 1998 [56]	53C/A*	After induction therapy	27/30 (90%)	5/23 (21%)	Gradual increase in MRD levels showed a higher relapse rate and shorter median RFS
Ciudad 1999 [109]	45C*	After induction During maintenance After Rx	9/19 (47%) 13/13 (100%) 21/21 (100%)	10/41 (24%) 19/55 (34%) 9/38 (23%)	Significant increase in immature B-cell subsets or an altered B-cell differentiation predicts a high relapse rate (P <0.01) and a shorter DFS (P <0.01). MRD at specific time points during follow-up (end of induction, maintenance, or after treatment) was associated with a significantly shorter DFS (P<0.01)
Dworzak 2000 [58]	63C*	Median 4 months after CR	10/14 (71%)	10/49 (20%)	Comparative phenotype mapping proved to be a reliable method for MRD detection in pre-B ALL
Coustan 2000 [55]	195C*	End of induction Week 14 Week 32	19/42 (45%) 10/18 (55%) 4/4 (100%)	2/123 (1%) 1/14 (7%) 2/8 (25%)	Detectable MRD at each time-point was associated with a higher relapse rate (P<0.001). The incidence of relapse among patients with MRD at the end of the induction phase was 68% +/– 16% (SE) if they remained with MRD through week 14 of continuation therapy, compared with 7%+/–7% if MRD became undetectable (P=0.035)
Coustan 2002 [110]	110C*	Day 19	14/59 (23%)	3/51 (5%)	MRD <0.01% on day 19 in 46% of patients; identifies a group of patients with excellent prognosis; 3-year cumulative incidence of relapse was 1.9% ± 1.9%, as compared with 28.4% ± 6.4% for MRD+ patients
Dworzak 2002 [53]	108C*	Day 33 Week 22–24	9/38 (24%) 5/6 (83%)	4/59 (7%) 6/48 (13%)	Patients with persistent disease (1 blast/µl) at day 33 and week 12 of treatment had a 100% probability of relapse, compared with 6% in all others. It was found, however, that the sensitivity of the markers used was limited in bone marrow samples from patients who were recovering post chemotherapy
Krampera 2003 [77]	47A*	Preconsolidation Pre-third reinduction Pre-sixth reinduction	15/18 (83%) 8/11 (72%) 3/4 (75%)	15/29 (51%) 7/21 (33%) 6/20 (30%)	Adult T-ALL patients with detectable MRD at the end of induction and following induction cycles should be considered at increased risk of relapse

*C, children; *A, adults

Table 20.3. Major PCR-based MRD studies

Study	N	Method	Timing	Relapse/MRD MRD (+)	MRD (–)	Major conclusion
Brisco 1996 [76]	27A *	IgH/TCR	Day 34–43	11/18 (61%)	3/9 (33%)	ALL in adults is more drug-resistant than in children
Roberts 1997 [60]	24C *	IgH/TCR (Quantitative)	Up to 35 months after end of therapy	5/20 (25%)	0/2 (0%)	The cure of ALL may not require the elimination of all leukemia cells
Foroni 1997 [64]	30A *	IgH/TCR (Qualitative)	After induction	2/5 (40%)	2/5 (40%)	Resolution of MRD in ALL occurs more rapidly in children compared to adults
			3 months	5/8 (62%)	1/5 (20%)	Early MRD+ assessment in adult ALL may not correlate
			6 months	4/5 (80%)	1/10 (1%)	
			12 months	1/2 (50%)	3/9 (33%)	
Cave 1998 [59]	178C *	IgH/TCR (Quantitative)	After induction	25/63 (39%)	7/88 (7%)	MRD > 1% at the end of induction or MRD > 0.1% at later TP high risk of relapse
			After consolidation	15/32 (46%)	8/95 (8%)	
			6 months after consolidation	21/38 (55%)	25/215 (11%)	
Van Dongen 1998 [61]	240C *	IgH/TCR moTAL-1 (Qualöitative)	After induction	40/98 (40%)	2/71 (2%)	MRD at day 33 and day 78 defines risk of relapse:
			4–6 months	32/47 (68%)	18/166 (10%)	High risk: MRD > 1% at day 33 or MRD > 0.1% at day 78
			12 months	18/21 (85%)	14/166 (8%)	Low risk: MRD < 0.01% at day 78
			End of treatment	5/6 (83%)	9/148 (6%)	EFS: High risk = 16%; Low risk = 98%
Goulden 1998 [62]	66C *	IgH/TCR (Qualitative)	After 6 months	23/33 (69%)	5/29 (17%)	Strong correlation between clearance of MRD early in therapy and improved DFS outcome in childhood ALL
			After end of therapy	18/28 (64%)	6/30 (20%)	
Grumayer 2000 [108]	68C *	IgH/TCR (Qualitative)	Day 15	16/54 (29%)	0/14 (0%)	MRD < 0.01% on day 15 of induction therapy (in 20% of patients) identifies group of patients with excellent prognosis

Table 20.3 (continued)

Study	N	Method	Timing	Relapse/MRD MRD (+)	MRD (–)	Major conclusion
Nyvold 2002 [65]	104C*	IgH/TCR (Qualitative)	Day 15	2/34 (5%)	9/36 (25%)	MRD < 0.01% at day 29 identifies patients with extremely good prognosis
			Day 29	15/60 (25%)	0/40 (0%)	
Gameiro 2002 [66]	50C*	IgH/TCR (Qualitative)	1 month	12/25 (48%)	6/17 (35%)	MRD detection in first 24 months correlated with outcome
			2 months	3/4 (75%)	3/13 (23%)	
			3 months	7/11 (63%)	11/31 (35%)	
			5 months	3/3 (100%)	6/21 (28%)	
Mortuza 2002 [78]	50A*	IgH/TCR (Semi-quantitative)	1 months	9/13 (69%)	3/10 (30%)	% of MRD+ patients who relapsed specifical time-points 0–2 months 64%; 3–5 months 75%; 6–9 months 80%; 10–24 months 55.5%
			5 months	2/2 (100%)	3/8 (37%)	
			9 months	0/0	0/4 (0%)	
Marshall 2003 [67]	83C*	IgH/TCR (Quantitative)	1 month	22/28 (78%)	11/57 (19%)	MRD at 1 and 24 months from diagnosis can identify almost all patients who will relapse either during or after the completion of therapy
			12 months	7/20 (35%)	12/59 (20%)	
			24 months	8/22 (36%)	14/54 (25%)	

*C, children; *A, adults

straightforward; whereas one study shows equivalence of blood and marrow MRD levels [68], two studies demonstrated that MRD levels in marrow were higher than blood MRD detection [51, 71]. Based on the current data, marrow MRD monitoring remains the "gold standard" for children with precursor-B ALL.

20.3.2 MRD Studies in Adult ALL

Results of MRD evaluation in trials of adult ALL, albeit less numerous than the pediatric MRD studies, have also demonstrated the prognostic significance of MRD measurements during treatment, but with higher frequencies of persistent MRD positivity in adults [64, 76]. The results of several of these trials are also summarized in Tables 20.2 and 20.3 [54, 56, 64, 66, 76–79]. Following remission induction, high MRD levels (defined as a ratio of target gene to control gene of $>10^{-3}$) using clone-specific PCR of IgH gene rearrangements have been associated with a high risk of relapse of 89% [76]. Similar results have been found using RQ-PCR of *IgH* or *TCR* gene rearrangements for adults treated on a recent CALGB study [80]. However, even a low MRD level ($<10^{-3}$) following induction was still associated with a significant relapse risk of up to 46%. In another prospective trial using qualitative PCR monitoring of *IgH* gene rearrangements, MRD kinetics were compared in precursor-B ALL patients who achieved prolonged DFS and in those who relapsed [78].

In long-term survivors, the incidence of a MRD-positive result decreased continuously from a high of 36% following induction therapy to a low of 7% at months 10–24 of treatment. In contrast, 64% and 56% of patients who relapsed were MRD-positive following induction and at 10–24 months, respectively. MRD was a significant predictor of relapse risk at all time points; however, the predictive value of a positive result appeared the strongest between 4 and 9 months following achievement of remission. These investigators found MRD to be a significant prognostic marker in a multivariate analysis. Similarly, using flow cytometric MRD detection, high MRD level (defined as $>10^{-3}$) at any of several postremission treatment time-points was associated with a high relapse rate of 94% [56].

From these studies, it appears that MRD assessment at several time-points during treatment might enhance predictive value in adult ALL. The German Multicenter ALL study group (GMALL) found that combining the results of several MRD measurements during the first year of treatment enhances the predictive value of any single time-point. In a recent study, they evaluated the predictive value of quantitative MRD detection in 196 standard-risk ALL patients in first CR treated on a single German cooperative group study who were monitored sequentially during the first year of treatment. They found that combining MRD values from three time-points during the first 16 weeks of treatment identified three novel risk groups. Patients with a rapid MRD decline ($<10^{-4}$ at day 11 and day 24 of remission induction) had a 3-year relapse rate of 0%. In contrast, those patients with slow MRD decline (MRD of $\geq 10^{-4}$ through week 16 of therapy) had a relapse rate of 94% at three years. The remaining patients fell into an intermediate risk group where the relapse rate was 47%. Thus, MRD quantification during treatment identified new prognostic subgroups within an otherwise homogeneous standard risk subset of ALL who might benefit from risk-adapted therapeutic approaches [81].

20.3.3 MRD Monitoring in Selected Disease Subsets: t(4;11) and t(9;22)

Several smaller studies focusing on the impact of MRD detection in high-risk ALL have been performed using RT-PCR of the leukemia-specific fusion transcripts, *MLL-AF4* and *BCR-ABL*. The *MLL-AF4* fusion gene results from the t(4;11) and is found in approximately 3–6% of adults and children with ALL and is the most common cytogenetic abnormality in infants with ALL [82, 83]. The t(4;11) has been associated with a very poor prognosis when standard chemotherapy is administered, but improved survival has been reported for patients receiving an allogeneic transplant in first remission. A prospective analysis of MRD monitoring in 25 patients with the *MLL-AF4* fusion gene is the largest study of this ALL subset and demonstrated, using a qualitative RT-PCR assay, that patients who remained PCR negative 3–6 months following diagnosis enjoyed prolonged survival [84]. In contrast, this and other smaller studies showed that patients who remained PCR-positive or converted from a negative to a positive test following transplant were destined to relapse [83, 85, 86].

Beginning in the late 1990s, studies to assess MRD status following allogeneic stem cell transplantation (allo-SCT) have provided intriguing information about the risk of relapse in Philadelphia chromosome positive (Ph+) ALL patients using RT-PCR monitoring of the *BCR-ABL* fusion gene transcript [74, 87–93] (Table 20.4). Using qualitative RT-PCR testing with sensitivities reported in the 1 in 10^{5-6} range, all of these studies found that patients who were consistently PCR negative following Allo-SCT were unlikely to relapse. Conversely, patients in whom MRD was detected after allo-SCT were at very high risk of relapse. In the largest published series, Radich et al. found that the relative risk of relapse (RR) was significantly higher for patients with detectable *BCR-ABL* fusion gene transcript following transplantation than for those without detectable transcript ($RR=5.7$, $p=0.025$) [90]. The prognostic significance of the PCR assay remained after controlling for other clinical variables (e.g., stem cell source, presence of graft-vs.-host disease) that could influence relapse risk. Interestingly, the genetic context of MRD may also be of relevance. In their study, Radich noted that the risk of relapse was greatest for PCR+ patients with a p190 *BCR-ABL* transcript in comparison to patients who had detectable p210 *BCR-ABL* transcripts after transplantation. The median time from detection of a positive PCR result to relapse was 94 days.

MRD detection prior to transplant for Ph+ ALL is also a good predictor of relapse-free survival after Allo-SCT [90, 94]. Based on these data, there has been a concerted effort to eradicate MRD prior to moving forward with transplant for these high-risk patients.

Table 20.4. MRD and outcome: Pre- and Posttransplant

Study	N	Relapse/MRD MRD positive	MRD negative	Major outcome
Vervoordeldonk 1997 [103]	13C	8/8 (100%)	0/5 (0%)	MRD in harvested BM predicts relapse after transplantation with autologous purged BM in children in 2nd remission of pre-B-ALL
Knechtli 1998 [99]	64C	12/12 (100%)	8/38 (21%)	2-year EFS for these groups was 0%, and 73%, respectively (P <0.001)
Uzunel 2001 [100]	30C	8/15 (53%)	0/5 (0%)	Match to Allo-SCT had higher relapse rate than MRD– patients
Van der Velden 2001 [102]	17C	4/6 (66%)	4/11 (36%)	MRD before Allo-SCT predicts outcome in children with ALL
Bader 2002 [98]	38C	11/17 (64%)	2/14 (14%)	5-year EFS for these groups was 23% and 78% (P=0.022)
Mortuza 2002 [78]	15A	6/6 (100%)	1/9 (11%)	Detection of MRD prior to auto-SCT predicted relapse but not predictive of outcome with Allo-SCT
Goulden 2002 [104]	64C	12/12 (100%)	8/41 (19%)	The prognostic value of any MRD result is dependent upon the treatment received both prior to and following Allo-SCT
Radich 1995 [93]	20	11/13 (84%)	1/7 (14%)	Detection of MRD in ALL predicts relapse after Allo-BMT
Vervoordeldonk 1997 [103]	23C	9/9 (100%)	6/14 (42%)	PCR-positivity in harvested bone marrow predicts relapse after transplantation with autologous purged bone marrow in children in second remission of precursor B-cell acute leukemia
Knechtli 1998 [106]	68C	28/32 (87%)	8/36 (22%)	MRD after Allo-BMT is a poor prognostic sign
Mortuza 2002 [78]	13A	2/2 (100%)	1/11 (9%)	Detection of MRD following Allo-SCT predicted relapse
Uzunel 2003 [107]	32C	8/9 (88%)	6/23 (26%)	MRD detection after Allo-SCT is correlated to relapse in patients with ALL

To achieve this goal, several studies have now incorporated imatinib mesylate, a potent inhibitor of the *abl* tyrosine kinase into front-line therapy for Ph+ ALL. RQ-PCR analysis demonstrates a rapid reduction in MRD when imatinib is added to front-line therapy with the majority of patients (82%) becoming PCR negative prime to Allo-SCT [95, 96]. Moreover, with a median follow-up of 25 months after Allo-SCT, outcome in these patients appears to be improved with a DFS of 78% [97].

20.3.4 Prognostic Significance of MRD in Patients Undergoing Stem Cell Transplantation

The prognostic significance of MRD measurements before and following Allo-SCT have extended beyond the studies described above for Ph+ ALL. In both children and adults, MRD measurements using clone-specific PCR of *IgH* and/or *TCR* gene rearrangements for all disease subsets have demonstrated prognostic significance of pre- and posttransplant MRD measurements (Table 20.5) [66, 78, 93, 98–105]. Using semiquantitative PCR methods, two large studies in pediatric ALL were able to identify three risk groups based on pretransplant MRD status [98, 99]. For patients who were MRD negative prior to transplant, DFS was 78% in both series; for those with intermediate-level MRD, DFS was 48% and 36%, respectively; and for those with high levels of MRD (but in clinical remission) prior to Allo-SCT, DFS was only 23% and 0%, respectively. The majority of studies reported and summarized in Table 20.5 also suggest that the presence of MRD prior to transplant is associated with significantly higher relapse rates following transplant. In contrast, only one study in adult ALL patients found that MRD detection prior to transplant had no predictive value; whereas, MRD detection following Allo-SCT in this series was highly predictive of relapse [78]. Of the several studies where serial MRD measurements were taken, the presence of MRD following Allo-SCT was an ominous sign, with the majority of these patients relapsing within months following transplant [78, 93, 103, 106, 107]. Taken together with the results described above for the subset of patients with Ph+ ALL, the data suggest that MRD analysis prior to transplant can contribute significant prognostic information and that the goal of pretransplant therapy should be to achieve MRD negative status. Whether RQ-PCR methods will help to refine the prognostic capabilities and guide therapeutic interventions pre- and posttransplant (e.g., novel molecular targeted therapy, early withdrawal of immunosuppressive therapy, posttransplant immunotherapy) remains an open question.

20.3.5 The Future: Risk-Adapted Therapy Based on MRD

The demonstration that MRD measurement provides valuable and validated independent prognostic information has led to the implementation of MRD-based risk-adapted therapy based on MRD in several pediatric and adult ALL trials. Two general strategies are being evaluated: intensification of postremission treatment (e.g., allogeneic stem cell transplant in first remission) for patients with high levels of MRD, or decreased duration or intensity of treatment for patients with low or undetectable levels of MRD. The Children's Oncology Group in North America plans to combine two prognostic markers to assign postremission therapy: results of a remission induction day 14 bone marrow examination and a day 29 MRD evaluation. MRD measurements will be performed using a 4-color flow cytometric assay in two central reference laboratories. Patients defined as "high risk" based on these two tests will be assigned to an intensified postremission course of treatment. The Dana Farber ALL consortium also plans to use MRD detection to further stratify postremission therapy. Using RQ-PCR following induction therapy, patients will be assigned to receive additional postremission therapy with daunorubicin and/or cytarabine. In these North American studies, there will be no de-escalation of therapy based on MRD. In contrast, the ongoing European BFM-AEIOP uses the results of RQ-PCR performed in reference laboratories to assign "MRD-high level" patients to Allo-SCT in first remission, while "MRD-low level" patients will receive a reduced course of postremission therapy. In adult ALL, the GMALL group is performing a prospective study with MRD-based treatment decisions after 1 year of chemotherapy in patients considered standard risk according to conventional risk factors described above [81]. For MRD low-risk patients, defined as MRD levels of $<10^{-4}$ at all postremission time-points, treatment will be stopped after 1 year and maintenance therapy will be omitted; whereas, MRD high risk patients, defined as patients with MRD $>10^{-4}$ at any postremission time-point, will have treatment intensification, focusing on Allo-SCT.

20.4 Summary

In conclusion, MRD evaluation provides independent prognostic information in both children and adults with ALL. To date, there is quite convincing evidence in both pediatric and adult ALL studies of MRD that a high level of MRD at the end of induction therapy is associated with a higher relapse rate. Furthermore, the continuous detection of high levels of MRD during consolidation and maintenance therapy, the re-emergence, or increase in MRD levels all appear to herald relapse. In contrast, declining or negative MRD results are associated with a favorable prognosis. From the studies that have been completed over the last decade, there appear to be sufficient data to justify the incorporation of MRD status into decisions about postremission treatment assignment and several studies outlined in the section above are now underway using this strategy. MRD evaluation

Table 20.5. MRD studies in Ph+ALL

Study	N	Rx	Relapsed MRD-status		Major conclusion
			MRD+	MRD–	
Gehly 1991 [92]	4	Allo	1/1 (100%)	0/3 (0%)	Interval between MRD detection and relapse in Ph+ALL may be relatively short and quite different from Ph+ CML post transplant
	2	Auto	1/1 (100%)	1/1 (100%)	
Miyamura 1992 [91]	9	Allo	5/5 (100%)	1/4 (25%)	Median interval between PCR positivity and clinical relapse was only 4 weeks
	6	Auto	2/2 (100%)	0/4 (0%)	
Radich 1995 [93]	8	Auto	1/8 (12%)	–	PCR+ following Allo-SCT predictive of relapse
Mitterbauer 1995 [88]	7	–	6/6 (100%)	1/1 (100%)	One-step combined with two-step RQ-PCR analysis gives valuable information about the efficacy of treatment and the dynamics of the leukemia
Radich 1997 [90]	30	Allo	8/21 (38%)	0/9 (0%)	Median time from first PCR-positive test to relapse was 94 days
	6	Auto	2/2 (100%)	2/4 (50%)	p190 confers higher risk of relapse than p210
Sierra 1997 [89]	18	Allo	5/18 (62%)	–	PCR+ following match Allo-SCT correlates with relapse
Preudhomme 1997 [87]	8	CT	6/7 (85%)	0/1 (0%)	Relapse is always preceded by switch to PCR positivity of Ph+ by 4 to 6 months
	5	Allo	3/3 (100%)	0/2 (0%)	Lower sensitivity of RT-PCR in PB compared with BM
	4	Auto	2/3 (66%)	0/1 (0%)	
Mitterbauer 1999 [74]	4	CT	4/4 (100%)	–	Relapse is preceded by 5 to 15 weeks by one step PCR
	3	Allo	2/3(66%)	–	
	2	Auto	0/2 (0%)	–	

CT=Chemotherapy
Auto=Autologous stem cells transplant
Allo=Allogeneic stem cell transplant

also has begun to provide important insights into the efficacy of treatment for specific molecular cytogenetic subsets of ALL.

Several important issues remain to be answered in carefully controlled trials. If MRD measurements are to be incorporated into clinical trials and used for treatment stratification and evaluation of treatment efficacy, the unresolved issues of technique standardization and quality control must be addressed. The Europe Against Cancer (EAC) and BIOMED initiatives have resulted in the development of standardized and validated methodology for quantitative PCR analysis in order to permit accurate comparison of MRD data [46]. Adoption of this approach in future trials and standardization of methodologies for flow cytometric MRD studies will be essential to accurately evaluate data from different clinical trials, and to help to answer important questions that remain including: (1) what level of MRD is clinically important; (2) when are the critical treatment time-points for MRD evaluation; (3) will MRD-based treatment intervention improve outcome. Finally, any MRD result must be interpreted in the context of the treatment administered and the clinical context in which it is being evaluated. Prospective MRD monitoring may enhance our ability to interpret the efficacy of these new treatment strategies. Only by addressing these issues using standardized methods for MRD evaluation will the clinical promise of this important bio-marker be realized.

References

1. Miller CB, et al. (1991) Correlation of occult clonogenic leukemia drug sensitivity with relapse after autologous bone marrow transplantation. Blood 78(4):1125–1131
2. Potter MN, et al. (1993) Molecular evidence of minimal residual disease after treatment for leukaemia and lymphoma: An updated meeting report and review. Leukemia 7(8):1302–1314
3. Pui CH, Campana D (2000) New definition of remission in childhood acute lymphoblastic leukemia. Leukemia 14(5):783–785
4. Campana D, Pui CH (1995) Detection of minimal residual disease in acute leukemia: Methodologic advances and clinical significance. Blood 85(6):1416–1434
5. Szczepanski T, et al. (2001) Minimal residual disease in leukaemia patients. Lancet Oncol 2(7):409–417
6. Vidriales MB, et al. (2003) Minimal residual disease monitoring by flow cytometry. Best Pract Res Clin Haematol 16(4):599–612
7. Campana D, Coustan-Smith E (2002) Advances in the immunological monitoring of childhood acute lymphoblastic leukaemia. Best Pract Res Clin Haematol 15(1):1–19
8. Coustan-Smith E, et al. (1998) Immunological detection of minimal residual disease in children with acute lymphoblastic leukaemia. Lancet 351(9102):550–554
9. Inoue K, et al. (1994) WT1 as a new prognostic factor and a new marker for the detection of minimal residual disease in acute leukemia. Blood 84(9):3071–3079
10. Inoue K, et al. (1997) Aberrant overexpression of the Wilms tumor gene (WT1) in human leukemia. Blood 89(4):1405–1412
11. Miyagi T, et al. (1993) Expression of the candidate Wilm's tumor gene, WT1, in human leukemia cells. Leukemia 7(7):970–977
12. Bergmann L, et al. (1997) High levels of Wilms' tumor gene (wt1) mRNA in acute myeloid leukemias are associated with a worse long-term outcome. Blood 90(3):1217–1225
13. Sugiyama H (1998) Wilms tumor gene (WT1) as a new marker for the detection of minimal residual disease in leukemia. Leuk Lymphoma 30(1–2):55–61
14. Miwa H, Beran M, Saunders GF (1992) Expression of the Wilms' tumor gene (WT1) in human leukemias. Leukemia 6(5):405–409
15. Menssen HD, et al. (1995) Presence of Wilms' tumor gene (wt1) transcripts and the WT1 nuclear protein in the majority of human acute leukemias. Leukemia 9(6):1060–1067
16. Inoue K, et al. (1996) Long-term follow-up of minimal residual disease in leukemia patients by monitoring WT1 (Wilms tumor gene) expression levels. Blood 88(6):2267–2278
17. Tamaki H, et al. (1996) Increased expression of the Wilms tumor gene (WT1) at relapse in acute leukemia. Blood 88(11):4396–4398
18. Ogawa H, et al. (2003) The usefulness of monitoring WT1 gene transcripts for the prediction and management of relapse following allogeneic stem cell transplantation in acute type leukemia. Blood 101(5):1698–1704
19. Garg M, et al. (2003) Prognostic significance of quantitative analysis of WT1 gene transcripts by competitive reverse transcription polymerase chain reaction in acute leukaemia. Br J Haematol 123(1):49–59
20. Cilloni D, et al. (2002) Quantitative assessment of WT1 expression by real time quantitative PCR may be a useful tool for monitoring minimal residual disease in acute leukemia patients. Leukemia 16(10):2115–2121
21. Kreuzer KA, et al. (2001) Fluorescent 5'-exonuclease assay for the absolute quantification of Wilms' tumour gene (WT1) mRNA: Implications for monitoring human leukaemias. Br J Haematol 114(2):313–318
22. Pongers-Willemse MJ, et al. (1999) Primers and protocols for standardized detection of minimal residual disease in acute lymphoblastic leukemia using immunoglobulin and T cell receptor gene rearrangements and TAL1 deletions as PCR targets: Report of the BIOMED-1 CONCERTED ACTION: Investigation of minimal residual disease in acute leukemia. Leukemia 13(1):110–118
23. van Dongen JJ, Wolvers-Tettero IL (1991) Analysis of immunoglobulin and T cell receptor genes. Part II: Possibilities and limitations in the diagnosis and management of lymphoproliferative diseases and related disorders. Clin Chim Acta 198(1–2):93–174
24. van Dongen JJ, et al. (1999) Standardized RT-PCR analysis of fusion gene transcripts from chromosome aberrations in acute leukemia for detection of minimal residual disease. Report of the BIOMED-1 Concerted Action: Investigation of minimal residual disease in acute leukemia. Leukemia 13(12):1901–1928
25. Hunger SP (1996) Chromosomal translocations involving the E2A gene in acute lymphoblastic leukemia: Clinical features and molecular pathogenesis. Blood 87(4):1211–1224
26. Hunger SP, et al. (1998) E2A-PBX1 chimeric transcript status at end of consolidation is not predictive of treatment outcome in childhood acute lymphoblastic leukemias with a t(1;19)(q23;p13): A Pediatric Oncology Group study. Blood 91(3):1021–1028
27. Privitera E, et al. (1992) Different molecular consequences of the 1;19 chromosomal translocation in childhood B-cell precursor acute lymphoblastic leukemia. Blood 79(7):1781–1788
28. Devaraj PE, et al. (1995) Expression of the E2A-PBX1 fusion transcripts in t(1;19)(q23;p13) and der(19)t(1;19) at diagnosis and in remission of acute lymphoblastic leukemia with different B lineage immunophenotypes. Leukemia 9(5):821–825
29. Lanza C, et al. (1996) Persistence of E2A/PBX1 transcripts in t(1;19) childhood acute lymphoblastic leukemia: Correlation with chemotherapy intensity and clinical outcome. Leuk Res 20(5):441–443
30. Group Francais de Cytogenetique Hematologique (1996) Cytogenetic abnormalities in adult acute lymphoblastic leukemia: Correlations with hematologic findings outcome. A Collaborative Study of the Group Francais de Cytogenetique Hematologique. Blood 87(8):3135–3142
31. Gabert J, et al. (2001) Improved outcome of Adult patients with E2A PBX1/t(1;19) positive ALL after intensive therapy: Results of the LAL-94 multicentric protocol. Blood 98:840a
32. Secker-Walker LM, et al. (1997) Cytogenetics adds independent prognostic information in adults with acute lymphoblastic leukaemia on MRC trial UKALL XA. MRC Adult Leukaemia Working Party. Br J Haematol 96(3):601–610

33. Foa R, et al. (2003) E2A-PBX1 fusion in adult acute lymphoblastic leukaemia: Biological and clinical features. Br J Haematol 120(3): 484–487
34. Romana SP, et al. (1995) High frequency of t(12;21) in childhood B-lineage acute lymphoblastic leukemia. Blood 86(11):4263–4269
35. Shurtleff SA, et al. (1995) TEL/AML1 fusion resulting from a cryptic t(12;21) is the most common genetic lesion in pediatric ALL and defines a subgroup of patients with an excellent prognosis. Leukemia 9(12):1985–1989
36. Raynaud S, et al. (1996) The 12;21 translocation involving TEL and deletion of the other TEL allele: Two frequently associated alterations found in childhood acute lymphoblastic leukemia. Blood 87(7):2891–2899
37. Borkhardt A, et al. (1997) Incidence and clinical relevance of TEL/AML1 fusion genes in children with acute lymphoblastic leukemia enrolled in the German and Italian multicenter therapy trials. Associazione Italiana Ematologia Oncologia Pediatrica and the Berlin-Frankfurt-Munster Study Group. Blood 90(2):571–577
38. de Haas V, et al. (2002) The TEL-AML1 real-time quantitative polymerase chain reaction (PCR) might replace the antigen receptor-based genomic PCR in clinical minimal residual disease studies in children with acute lymphoblastic leukaemia. Br J Haematol 116(1):87–93
39. Pine SR, et al. (2003) Real-time quantitative PCR: Standardized detection of minimal residual disease in pediatric acute lymphoblastic leukemia. Polymerase chain reaction. J Pediatr Hematol Oncol 25(2):103–108
40. Sykes PJ, et al. (1992) Quantitation of targets for PCR by use of limiting dilution. Biotechniques 13(3):444–449
41. Cave H, et al. (1994) Prospective monitoring and quantitation of residual blasts in childhood acute lymphoblastic leukemia by polymerase chain reaction study of delta and gamma T-cell receptor genes. Blood 83(7):1892–1902
42. Ouspenskaia MV, et al. (1995) Accurate quantitation of residual B-precursor acute lymphoblastic leukemia by limiting dilution and a PCR-based detection system: A description of the method and the principles involved. Leukemia 9(2):321–328
43. Pallisgaard N, et al. (1999) Rapid and sensitive minimal residual disease detection in acute leukemia by quantitative real-time RT-PCR exemplified by t(12;21) TEL-AML1 fusion transcript. Genes Chromosomes Cancer 26(4):355–365
44. Chen X, et al. (2001) Quantification of minimal residual disease in T-lineage acute lymphoblastic leukemia with the TAL-1 deletion using a standardized real-time PCR assay. Leukemia 15(1):166–170
45. Pongers-Willemse MJ, et al. (1998) Real-time quantitative PCR for the detection of minimal residual disease in acute lymphoblastic leukemia using junctional region specific TaqMan probes. Leukemia 12(12):2006–2014
46. Gabert J, et al. (2003) Standardization and quality control studies of "real-time" quantitative reverse transcriptase polymerase chain reaction of fusion gene transcripts for residual disease detection in leukemia – A Europe Against Cancer program. Leukemia 17(12): 2318–2357
47. Donovan JW, et al. (2000) Immunoglobulin heavy-chain consensus probes for real-time PCR quantification of residual disease in acute lymphoblastic leukemia. Blood 95(8):2651–2658
48. Bruggemann M, et al. (2000) Improved assessment of minimal residual disease in B cell malignancies using fluorogenic consensus probes for real-time quantitative PCR. Leukemia 14(8):1419–1425
49. van der Velden VH, et al. (2002) Immunoglobulin kappa deleting element rearrangements in precursor-B acute lymphoblastic leukemia are stable targets for detection of minimal residual disease by real-time quantitative PCR. Leukemia 16(5):928–936
50. Beishuizen A, et al. (1994) Analysis of Ig and T-cell receptor genes in 40 childhood acute lymphoblastic leukemias at diagnosis and subsequent relapse: Implications for the detection of minimal residual disease by polymerase chain reaction analysis. Blood 83(8):2238–2247
51. Coustan-Smith E, et al. (2002) Use of peripheral blood instead of bone marrow to monitor residual disease in children with acute lymphoblastic leukemia. Blood 100(7):2399–2402
52. Griesinger F, et al. (1999) Leukaemia-associated immunophenotypes (LAIP) are observed in 90% of adult and childhood acute lymphoblastic leukaemia: Detection in remission marrow predicts outcome. Br J Haematol 105(1):241–255
53. Dworzak MN, et al. (2002) Prognostic significance and modalities of flow cytometric minimal residual disease detection in childhood acute lymphoblastic leukemia. Blood 99(6):1952–1958
54. Farahat N, et al. (1998) Detection of minimal residual disease in B-lineage acute lymphoblastic leukaemia by quantitative flow cytometry. Br J Haematol 101(1):158–164
55. Coustan-Smith E, et al. (2000) Clinical importance of minimal residual disease in childhood acute lymphoblastic leukemia. Blood 96(8):2691–2696
56. Ciudad J, et al. (1998) Prognostic value of immunophenotypic detection of minimal residual disease in acute lymphoblastic leukemia. J Clin Oncol 16(12):3774–3781
57. Borowitz MJ, et al. (2003) Minimal residual disease detection in childhood precursor-B-cell acute lymphoblastic leukemia: Relation to other risk factors. A Children's Oncology Group study. Leukemia 17(8):1566–1572
58. Dworzak MN, et al. (2000) Detection of residual disease in pediatric B-cell precursor acute lymphoblastic leukemia by comparative phenotype mapping: Method and significance. Leuk Lymphoma 38(3–4):295–308
59. Cave H, et al. (1998) Clinical significance of minimal residual disease in childhood acute lymphoblastic leukemia. European Organization for Research and Treatment of Cancer—Childhood Leukemia Cooperative Group. N Engl J Med 339(9):591–598
60. Roberts WM, et al. (1997) Measurement of residual leukemia during remission in childhood acute lymphoblastic leukemia. N Engl J Med 336(5):317–323
61. van Dongen JJ, et al. (1998) Prognostic value of minimal residual disease in acute lymphoblastic leukaemia in childhood. Lancet 352(9142):1731–1738
62. Goulden NJ, et al. (1998) Minimal residual disease analysis for the prediction of relapse in children with standard-risk acute lymphoblastic leukaemia. Br J Haematol 100(1):235–244
63. Brisco MJ, et al. (1994) Outcome prediction in childhood acute lymphoblastic leukaemia by molecular quantification of residual disease at the end of induction. Lancet 343(8891):196–200
64. Foroni L, et al. (1997) Molecular detection of minimal residual disease in adult and childhood acute lymphoblastic leukaemia

reveals differences in treatment response. Leukemia 11(10): 1732–1741

65. Nyvold C, et al. (2002) Precise quantification of minimal residual disease at day 29 allows identification of children with acute lymphoblastic leukemia and an excellent outcome. Blood 99(4):1253–1258
66. Gameiro P, et al. (2002) Polymerase chain reaction (PCR)- and reverse transcription PCR-based minimal residual disease detection in long-term follow-up of childhood acute lymphoblastic leukaemia. Br J Haematol 119(3):685–696
67. Marshall GM, et al. (2003) Importance of minimal residual disease testing during the second year of therapy for children with acute lymphoblastic leukemia. J Clin Oncol 21(4):704–709
68. Brisco MJ, et al. (1997) Monitoring minimal residual disease in peripheral blood in B-lineage acute lymphoblastic leukaemia. Br J Haematol 99(2):314–319
69. Yokota S, et al. (1991) Use of polymerase chain reactions to monitor minimal residual disease in acute lymphoblastic leukemia patients. Blood 77(2):331–339
70. Martin H, et al. (1994) In patients with BCR-ABL-positive ALL in CR peripheral blood contains less residual disease than bone marrow: Implications for autologous BMT. Ann Hematol 68(2):85–87
71. van der Velden VH, et al. (2002) Minimal residual disease levels in bone marrow and peripheral blood are comparable in children with T cell acute lymphoblastic leukemia (ALL), but not in precursor-B-ALL. Leukemia 16(8):1432–1436
72. Lal A, et al. (2001) Detection of minimal residual disease in peripheral blood prior to clinical relapse of childhood acute lymphoblastic leukaemia using PCR. Mol Cell Probes 15(2):99–103
73. van Rhee F, et al. (1995) Quantification of residual disease in Philadelphia-positive acute lymphoblastic leukemia: Comparison of blood and bone marrow. Leukemia 9(2):329–335
74. Mitterbauer G, et al. (1999) Quantification of minimal residual disease in patients with BCR-ABL-positive acute lymphoblastic leukaemia using quantitative competitive polymerase chain reaction. Br J Haematol 106(3):634–643
75. Brisco MJ, et al. (2001) Molecular relapse can be detected in blood in a sensitive and timely fashion in B-lineage acute lymphoblastic leukemia. Leukemia 15(11):1801–1802
76. Brisco J, et al. (1996) Relationship between minimal residual disease and outcome in adult acute lymphoblastic leukemia. Blood 87(12):5251–5256
77. Krampera M, et al. (2003) Outcome prediction by immunophenotypic minimal residual disease detection in adult T-cell acute lymphoblastic leukaemia. Br J Haematol 120(1):74–79
78. Mortuza FY, et al. (2002) Minimal residual disease tests provide an independent predictor of clinical outcome in adult acute lymphoblastic leukemia. J Clin Oncol 20(4):1094–1104
79. Nizet Y, et al. (1991) Follow-up of residual disease (MRD) in B lineage acute leukaemias using a simplified PCR strategy: Evolution of MRD rather than its detection is correlated with clinical outcome. Br J Haematol 79(2):205–210
80. Sher D, et al. (2002) Clone-specific quantitative real-time PCR of IgH or TCR gene rearrangements in adult ALL following induction chemotherapy identifies patients with poor prognosis: Pilot study from the Cancer and Leukemia Group B (CALGB 20101). Blood 100:153 a
81. Bruggemann M, et al. (2006) Clinical significance of minimal residual disease quantification in adult patients with standard-risk acute lymphoblastic leukemia. Blood 107:1116–1123
82. Biondi A, et al. (1993) Detection of ALL-1/AF4 fusion transcript by reverse transcription-polymerase chain reaction for diagnosis and monitoring of acute leukemias with the t(4;11) translocation. Blood 82(10):2943–2947
83. Ludwig WD, et al. (1998) Immunophenotypic and genotypic features, clinical characteristics, and treatment outcome of adult pro-B acute lymphoblastic leukemia: Results of the German multicenter trials GMALL 03/87 and 04/89. Blood 92(6):1898–1909
84. Cimino G, et al. (2000) A prospective study of residual-disease monitoring of the ALL1/AF4 transcript in patients with t(4;11) acute lymphoblastic leukemia. Blood 95(1):96–101
85. Janssen JW, et al. (1994) Pre-pre-B acute lymphoblastic leukemia: High frequency of alternatively spliced ALL1-AF4 transcripts and absence of minimal residual disease during complete remission. Blood 84(11):3835–3842
86. Cimino G, et al. (1996) Clinical relevance of residual disease monitoring by polymerase chain reaction in patients with ALL-1/AF-4 positive-acute lymphoblastic leukaemia. Br J Haematol 92(3):659–664
87. Preudhomme C, et al. (1997) Good correlation between RT-PCR analysis and relapse in Philadelphia (Ph1)-positive acute lymphoblastic leukemia (ALL). Leukemia 11(2):294–298
88. Mitterbauer G, et al. (1995) PCR-monitoring of minimal residual leukaemia after conventional chemotherapy and bone marrow transplantation in BCR-ABL-positive acute lymphoblastic leukaemia. Br J Haematol 89(4):937–941
89. Sierra J, et al. (1997) Marrow transplants from unrelated donors for treatment of Philadelphia chromosome-positive acute lymphoblastic leukemia. Blood 90(4):1410–1414
90. Radich J, et al. (1997) Detection of bcr-abl transcripts in Philadelphia chromosome-positive acute lymphoblastic leukemia after marrow transplantation. Blood 89(7):2602–2609
91. Miyamura K, et al. (1992) Detection of Philadelphia chromosome-positive acute lymphoblastic leukemia by polymerase chain reaction: Possible eradication of minimal residual disease by marrow transplantation. Blood 79(5):1366–1370
92. Gehly GB, et al. (1991) Chimeric BCR-abl messenger RNA as a marker for minimal residual disease in patients transplanted for Philadelphia chromosome-positive acute lymphoblastic leukemia. Blood 78(2):458–465
93. Radich J, Ladne P, Gooley T (1995) Polymerase chain reaction-based detection of minimal residual disease in acute lymphoblastic leukemia predicts relapse after allogeneic BMT. Biol Blood Marrow Transplant 1(1):24–31
94. Dombret H, et al. (2002) Outcome of treatment in adults with Philadelphia chromosome-positive acute lymphoblastic leukemia – Results of the prospective multicenter LALA-94 trial. Blood 100(7):2357–2366
95. Towatari M, et al. (2004) Combination of intensive chemotherapy and imatinib can rapidly induce high-quality complete remission for a majority of patients with newly diagnosed BCR-ABL-positive acute lymphoblastic leukemia. Blood 104(12):3507–3512
96. Thomas DA, et al. (2004) Treatment of Philadelphia chromosome-positive acute lymphocytic leukemia with hyper-CVAD and imatinib mesylate. Blood 103(12):4396–4407

97. Lee S, et al. (2002) The impact of first-line imatinib interim therapy on the outcome of allogeneic stem cell transplantation in adults with newly diagnosed Philadelphia chromosome-positive acute lymphoblastic leukemia. Blood 105(9):3449–3457
98. Bader P, et al. (2002) Minimal residual disease (MRD) status prior to allogeneic stem cell transplantation is a powerful predictor for post-transplant outcome in children with ALL. Leukemia 16(9): 1668–1672
99. Knechtli CJ, et al. (1998) Minimal residual disease status before allogeneic bone marrow transplantation is an important determinant of successful outcome for children and adolescents with acute lymphoblastic leukemia. Blood 92(11):4072–4079
100. Uzunel M, et al. (2001) The significance of graft-versus-host disease and pretransplantation minimal residual disease status to outcome after allogeneic stem cell transplantation in patients with acute lymphoblastic leukemia. Blood 98(6):1982–1984
101. Uckun FM, et al. (1993) Pretransplantation burden of leukemic progenitor cells as a predictor of relapse after bone marrow transplantation for acute lymphoblastic leukemia. N Engl J Med 329(18):1296–1301
102. van der Velden VH, et al. (2001) Real-time quantitative PCR for detection of minimal residual disease before allogeneic stem cell transplantation predicts outcome in children with acute lymphoblastic leukemia. Leukemia 15(9):1485–1487
103. Vervoordeldonk SF, et al. (1997) PCR-positivity in harvested bone marrow predicts relapse after transplantation with autologous purged bone marrow in children in second remission of precursor B-cell acute leukaemia. Br J Haematol 96(2):395–402
104. Goulden N, Steward C (2002) Clinical relevance of MRD in children undergoing allogeneic stem cell transplantation for ALL. Best Pract Res Clin Haematol 15(1):59–70
105. Sanchez J, et al. (2002) Clinical value of immunological monitoring of minimal residual disease in acute lymphoblastic leukaemia after allogeneic transplantation. Br J Haematol 116(3): 686–694
106. Knechtli CJ, et al. (1998) Minimal residual disease status as a predictor of relapse after allogeneic bone marrow transplantation for children with acute lymphoblastic leukaemia. Br J Haematol 102(3):860–871
107 Uzunel M, et al. (2003) Minimal residual disease detection after allogeneic stem cell transplantation is correlated to relapse in patients with acute lymphoblastic leukaemia. Br J Haematol 122(5):788–794
108. Panzer-Grumayer ER, et al. (2000) Rapid molecular response during early induction chemotherapy predicts a good outcome in childhood acute lymphoblastic leukemia. Blood 95(3):790–794
109. Ciudad J, et al. (1999) Detection of abnormalities in B-cell differentiation pattern is a useful tool to predict relapse in precursor-B-ALL. Br J Haematol 104(4):695–705
110. Coustan-Smith E, et al. (2002) Prognostic importance of measuring early clearance of leukemic cells by flow cytometry in childhood acute lymphoblastic leukemia. Blood 100(1):52–58

Central Nervous System Involvement in Adult Acute Lymphocytic Leukemia

Ricardo H. Alvarez, Jorge E. Cortes

Contents

21.1 Introduction

Central nervous system (CNS) involvement is identified at the time of diagnosis in less than 5% of children with acute lymphoblastic leukemia (ALL) [1]. However, prior to the institution of adequate CNS prophylaxis, it was a major obstacle to cure in childhood ALL as 50–75% of patients would eventually relapse in the CNS [1, 2]. The routine use of CNS prophylaxis has improved the long-term prognosis of patients, and CNS relapse occurs in less than 10% of patients treated with contemporary protocols [3]. Effective means of CNS prophylaxis include cranial irradiation, intrathecal chemotherapy (IT), and high-dose systemic chemotherapy (HDCT) with agents that can cross the blood-brain barrier [4]. A risk-oriented approach has been developed for childhood CNS prophylaxis, in an attempt to reduce the occurrence of CNS relapse while minimizing the potentially serious adverse effects of radiotherapy and chemotherapy [4].

Less than 10% of adults with ALL have CNS involvement at presentation [5, 6]. However, without CNS prophylaxis, approximately one third of patients will eventually have CNS involvement [6–8], with a 5-year CNS event-free survival rate of 42% [5]. These data may be an underestimation as CNS disease has been identified at autopsy in patients who were thought to have bone marrow disease only [9]. CNS prophylaxis in adults has mostly been patterned after studies in childhood ALL, but several features are unique to adult ALL. Unfortunately, few studies dealing with CNS leukemia in adult ALL have been reported. Herein we review some of the relevant aspects of CNS disease in adult ALL including diagnostic and prognostic criteria, current prophylaxis and treatment options.

21.2 Diagnosis

Cytologic examination of the CSF is the most important tool for the diagnosis of meningeal localization of lymphoid malignancies. However, early meningeal involvement may be difficult to detect and false-negative rates up to 40% for the first lumbar puncture have been reported [10]. Patients with leukemia often develop CSF lymphocytosis. Staining for terminal deoxynucleotidyl transferase (TdT) is helpful to distinguish between leukemic lymphoblasts and normal lymphocytes [11, 12]. However, unequivocal identification of leukemic cells in nontraumatic lumbar puncture in the CSF, regardless of cell count, signifies clinical meningeal leukemia.

CNS involvement among children with ALL has historically been defined at most institutions by either the presence of at least 5 leukocytes per microliter of cerebrospinal fluid (CSF) associated with the presence of leukemic blasts (identified on a cytocentrifuged preparation) or the presence of a cranial nerve palsy on physical examination [13]. A large trial conducted at St. Jude's Hospital introduced a new classification of patients with ALL and CNS status at diagnosis: CNS1 denotes the absence of identifiable leukemic blast cells in CSF; CNS2, the presence of blast in a sample that contains <5 WBC/μl; and CNS3, a nontraumatic sample that contains ≥5 WBCs/μl with identifiable blasts, or the presence of a cerebral mass or cranial nerve palsy with leukemic cells in CSF [14]. The probability of 5-year CNS leukemia-free survival for CNS1 was significantly higher than for CNS2 and CNS3 (96% vs. 87% vs. 74% respectively) ($p<0.001$). The projected 5-year survival rates for these groups of patients were 75%, 49%, and 53% respectively [14].

Although the adverse prognosis of CNS2 status was confirmed by the Pediatric Oncology Group [15] several other investigators could not confirm this association among patients classified as having intermediate-risk ALL [16–18]. This discrepancy can be explained by differences in treatment regimens and in the clinical characteristics of the patients studied.

It has been argued that leukemic blasts may be iatrogenically introduced into the cerebrospinal fluid by a traumatic lumbar puncture (defined as more than 10 red blood cells per μl of CSF). A recent report by Gajjar et al. [19] provides evidence of the adverse impact of a traumatic lumbar puncture at the time of diagnosis on treatment outcome of children with ALL. The EFS for patients with one CSF sample contaminated with blasts was worse that that for patients with no contaminated CSF (5-year EFS estimates 76±6% and 60±6% respectively, $p=0.026$); for those patients with two consecutive contaminated CSF the 5-year EFS was 46±9%. In a Cox multiple regression analysis, the strongest prognostic indicator was two consecutive contaminated CSF samples, with a hazard ratio of 2.39 [95% confidence interval (CI) 1.36–4.20]. Investigators from Germany published a large retrospective study among 2,021 pediatric patients with ALL, enrolled in the BMF-95 trial [18]. Patients were analyzed according to type of CNS involvement and traumatic lumbar puncture (TLP) with (+) or

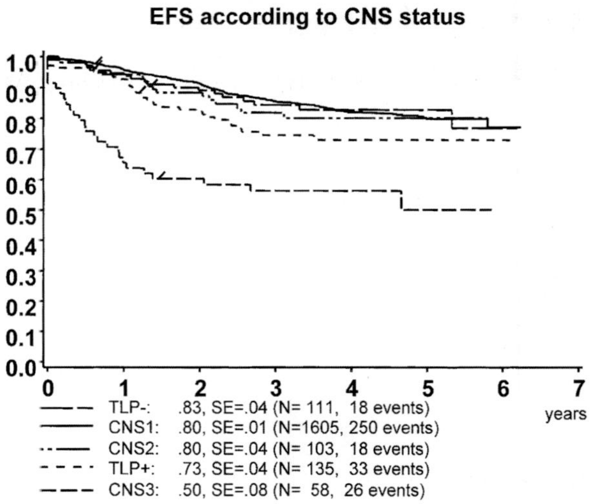

Fig. 21.1. Event-free survival (EFS) for the five CNS status groups is shown.

without (–) CNS blasts. CNS2, CNS3, and TLP+ groups contained a higher percentage of patients with unfavorable characteristics. Cox regression analysis identified TLP+ and CNS3 status as prognostically significant. The CNS3 risk ratio was 2.3 with 95% CI, 1.4 to 3.6, $p=0.0005$; the TLP+ risk ratio was 1.5 with 95% CI, 1.02 to 2.2; $p=0.04$. Five-year event-free survival (EFS) was 79% overall, 80% for CNS1, and 83% for TLP–. CNS2 patients have an EFS of 80%, but the cumulative incidence of relapses with CNS involvement is higher compared with CNS1 patients (0.10 vs. 0.04). TLP+ patients have a significantly reduced EFS (73%, $p=0.003$) because of an increased incidence of CNS relapses. CNS3 patients suffer from more systemic and CNS relapses (EFS 50%) (Fig. 21.1). These data emphasize the importance of a properly performed lumbar puncture by an experienced clinician particularly at diagnosis, when higher numbers of blast cells are circulating in the peripheral blood [20].

There has been no organized analysis of these or other criteria for adult ALL. Currently, CNS leukemia is defined by the presence of >5 WBC/μl in the CSF, with morphologically unequivocal lymphoblasts in cytocentrifuged sample [21]. However, the presence of blasts in the CSF when the WBC is <5/μl may have a similar clinical significance [14].

Several markers of CNS disease have been investigated to substitute or complement the results of cytology. DNA content may be abnormal and has a high specificity (95%) but low sensitivity [22]. High serum β2-microglobulin (B2M) levels in patients with ALL are associated with lower CR rates ($p=0.02$), shorter survival ($p<0.01$), and higher incidence of CNS leukemia ($p<0.001$) [23]. Serial determination of CSF B2M correlated well with the presence of CNS involvement. These data suggest that serial and simultaneous determinations of B2M in serum and CSF may be useful in early diagnosis of CNS involvement and in monitoring intrathecally in patients with acute leukemia [24].

CD27 is a transmembrane disulfide-linked 55-kD homodimer present on most peripheral blood T cells and on a subset of B cells and is also a member of the TNF-receptor family. CD27 is also expressed on human malignant B cells and high levels of soluble CD27 can be present in the serum of patients with B-cell malignancies [25]. Soluble CD27 (sCD27) has been reported elevated in patients with CNS involvement from lymphoid malignancies [26]. In one study, sCD27 had a higher sensitivity and specificity than CSF B2M. Other CSF tumor markers, such us fibronectin and tumor necrosis factor α (TNF) have a low specificity [27, 28].

Molecular techniques have also been investigated as a way to detect CNS disease. T-cell receptor delta rearrangements were identified in the CSF in nine of 21 patients studied and were identical to those identified in the bone marrow [29]. The long-term significance of these findings remains to be determined.

Imaging techniques, in particular magnetic resonance imaging (MRI), have also been used as aids in the diagnosis of CNS leukemia [30]. Fourteen patients with leptomeningeal compromise from several solid tumors were evaluated with both MRI and with standard computerized tomography (CT). The results suggested that MRI might be more accurate in identifying leptomeningeal metastasis compared to CT. However, all of these imaging techniques have a false-negative rate of up to 30%.

21.3 Pathology

Meningeal leukemia arises from neoplastic lymphocytes or myelocytes in the cranial arachnoid tissue [31]. These proliferating cells extend through the superficial arachnoid tissue into the arachnoid surrounding blood vessels: arteries, veins, arterioles, and venules [13] causing cerebral hypoperfusion secondary to the leukemic mass clogging these vessels. Eventually, they can burst out of the arachnoid trabeculae into the CSF, resulting in leukemic meningitis that leads to symptoms including headache, vomiting, meningismus, and papilledema [32]. With further increase of leukemic cell mass, the malignant cells are able to penetrate into the cerebral parenchyma leading to further cerebral dysfunction. The vasculature of the cranial nerves can be compressed and damaged by leukemic nerves infiltrates as the nerves traverse the leptomeninges, resulting in clinical neuropathy [33]. Endocrine abnormalities such as Cushing's syndrome and diabetes insipidus may result from malignant invasions of the hypothalamus and pituitary gland, respectively. Spinal leptomeningeal leukemia can extend to dorsal nerve roots, producing tabetic symptoms, or to the cauda equina, causing paraparesis [13].

21.4 Prognostic Factors

Several risk factors have been associated with the development of CNS leukemia. Age is an important factor. Infants and preschool children are more susceptible than adolescent or adults, possibly because a higher proportion of their vasculature is in the leptomeninges [1].

ALL with mature B-cell immunophenotype (L3 of the FAB classification) have a high risk of CNS involvement, with 12–42% of patients presenting with CNS involvement at diagnosis. They also have a higher risk of CNS relapses, isolated or with BM relapse occurring in 17–57% of patients [34, 35]. The T-cell immunophenotype is also associated with a high risk of CNS leukemia [36].

The translocation t(9,22) (q34;q11.2), which represents the Philadelphia chromosome (Ph+), occurs in 3–5% of children and 20–30% of adults with ALL [37]. The presence of the Ph+ chromosome has been considered a high-risk feature for CNS disease in some reports. However, some investigators suggest that in this type of ALL, the prognosis is determined by the use of treatment with glucocorticoids and IT with methotrexate given with induction chemotherapy, or by other factors (age and leukocyte count at diagnosis) in children treated only with intensive chemotherapy [38].

The expression of CD7 and CD56 in leukemia cells has been suggested to have prognostic implications with respect to CNS and other extramedullary disease. One study showed that CD7 and CD56 positivity at diagnosis is associated with a lower probability of achieving complete remission [39]. Ravandi et al. [40] found that CD56

Table 21.1. Risk groups for CNS leukemia in adult ALL [33, 34]

LDH (U/l)	S + G2M (%)	Estimated (%) CNS leukemia at 1 year	B2M (mg/l)	Estimated (%) CNS leukemia at 1 year
<600	<14	4	NS	NS
<600	≥14	13	NS	NS
>600	<14	29	<4	21
>600	≥14	56	≥4	67

NS, Not significant

expression, although infrequently found, was associated with a higher incidence of CNS disease at diagnosis (19% vs. 4%, p=0.016) in adult patients with ALL. The incidence of CNS disease at any time was also higher in patients with CD56+ disease (31 vs. 14%, p= 0.057). Among the 109 patients uniformly treated with the HyperCVAD regimen, CD56 expression was associated with a statistically significant higher incidence of CNS disease (33 vs. 9%, p=0.026). The authors concluded that CD56 expression may be used in combination with other high-risk features (e.g., LDH, S-phase fraction, mature B-cell phenotype) to design a risk-oriented approach to CNS prophylaxis [40].

Race has been considered an important prognostic factor for CNS disease in some reports, but it may be related to the presence of other high-risk features. In a recent retrospective analysis of 412 children and adolescents (68 African American, 338 Caucasian, and six other race) with newly diagnosed ALL, African American children were significantly more likely than Caucasian children to have higher risk features, including an initial leukocyte count greater than 100×10^9/l, a T-cell immunophenotype, a translocation t(1;19) with E2A-PBX1 fusion, and were less likely to have hyperdiploid karyotype, a favorable prognostic factor in childhood ALL. Still, the clinical outcomes for these cohorts were not significantly different: 5-year event-free and overall survival rates were 80.7% (95% CI, 70.3–91.1%) and 86.2% (95% CI, 77.2–95.2%) for African American children respectively, compared to 79.4% (95% CI, 74.7–84.1%) and 85.0% (95% CI, 80.9–89.1%) for Caucasian children. The lack of a racial effect on the long-term outcome of therapy was still apparent in a multivariate Cox regression analysis. The authors concluded that with an equal access to effective antileukemic therapy, African American and Caucasian children with ALL can expect the same high rate of cure [41].

In a review of the natural history of CNS acute leukemia in adults, elevated serum LDH, alkaline phosphatase, and uric acid are all strongly correlated with the development of CNS leukemia. In a multivariate analysis, LDH proved to be the best predictor of the risk of CNS disease [42].

By incorporating all significant clinical variables associated with increased risk of CNS disease in adults with ALL into a multivariate analysis, a prognostic model has been proposed [43]. Mature B-cell disease, serum LDH levels, and the proportion of bone marrow cells in the S+G2M phases had independent prognostic value. The risk of developing CNS leukemia within 1 year was 5% when LDH was normal (i.e., <600 U/l) and the proportion of cells in S+G2M phase was <14% in the bone marrow. In contrast, the risk was 20% when either variable was above these values, and 56% when both were elevated [43]. The major disadvantage of this model is that the S+G2M fraction is not measured routinely and is not readily accessible. Interestingly, serum B2M levels could discriminate two groups with different risks within the high-risk group (as defined above) [44]. Only seven of 60 (12%) low-risk patients had elevated B2M levels and an increased risk could not be demonstrated for this group (Table 21.1).

21.5 CNS Prophylaxis

Three therapeutic modalities can be used to prevent meningeal leukemia: intrathecal injection of antileukemia antimetabolites with or without corticosteroids, high-dose systemic administration of high doses of the antimetabolites or other agents that can cross the blood-brain barrier (BBB) sufficient to achieve therapeutic levels in the CSF (HDCT), and cranial irradiation [45, 46].

IT involves the direct injection of drugs into the CSF and is an obvious way to bypass the BBB. Relatively small doses of a drug given by intrathecal injection can achieve high local concentrations, due to the small volume of CSF. Furthermore, because of intrinsically low levels of metabolizing enzymes in the CSF, agents that are subject to rapid metabolism in blood may avoid degradations in the CSF [47]. For example, one of the principal mechanisms of inactivation of cytarabine in the bloodstream is deamination catalyzed by cytidine deaminase. Cytidine deaminase is present at much lower concentration in CSF, which results in an eightfold longer half-life of the drug in CSF than in plasma. In addition, more unbound drug is available to diffuse from CSF to brain tissue because of the very low protein content in the CSF [48].

IT has historically employed methotrexate single agent or methotrexate combined with cytarabine, with or without steroids. Liposomal cytarabine (DepoCyt) is a slow-release formulation of cytarabine that is manufactured by encapsulating the aqueous drug solution in spherical multivesicular particles known as DepoFoam, which consist of 96% water and 4% biodegradable lipid. A recent trial of intrathecal DepoCyt in children with neoplastic meningitis showed that eight of the 14 assessable patients demonstrated evidence of benefit manifested by prolonged disease stabilization or response [49].

The importance of IT for CNS prophylaxis in adults with ALL was first established in a randomized trial comparing CNS chemo-prophylaxis with cranial irradiation with 2,400 rads plus IT methotrexate versus cranial irradiation alone [8]. Three of 28 evaluable patients (11%) receiving IT had a CNS relapse, compared with 11 of 34 patients (32%) not receiving any prophylaxis.

Several chemotherapy agents used systemically may have CNS activity when used at adequate doses. Systemic administration of high-dose cytarabine reaches therapeutic levels in the CSF, which is slowly degraded to ara-U due to the absence of cytidine deaminase in this compartment [45]. Thus, systemic administration of high-dose methotrexate or high-dose cytarabine can effectively eradicate CNS leukemia [50, 51], although there is patient-to-patient variability in the drug concentrations of these agents achieved in the CSF.

Systemic administration of dexamethasone and prednisone have been utilized in combination with IT, and have significant antileukemic activity. Dexamethasone is five to six times more potent than prednisone [52]; in addition dexamethasone achieves higher CSF levels and has longer half-life in the CSF than prednisone [53].

Although cytarabine, methotrexate, and steroids (particularly dexamethasone) are the most important systemically administered agents used for CNS prophylaxis, other agents may have some role. Etoposide administered intravenously or as low-dose orally prolonged administration achieves effective concentration in the CSF and may contribute to successful CNS prophylaxis in same pediatric regimens [54].

The oral absorption of 6-mercaptopurine (6-MP) is highly variable. However, prolonged IV infusion can reach therapeutic levels in the CSF and is associated with improved antileukemic activity in vitro [55]. A recent report from Children's Cancer Group in standard-risk ALL patients compared daily oral versus weekly intravenous 6-MP. The 6-year EFS were similar in both groups. However, patients receiving IV 6-MP had unexplained shorter survival after relapse than oral 6-MP patients [56].

IV administration of L-asparaginase can deplete the CSF of L-asparagine for prolonged periods of time [57, 58]. Pegylated L-asparaginase has a prolonged half-life that may result in high plasma levels of asparaginase, and prolonged asparagine depletion in serum and CSF is achieved [59].

Cranial irradiation has been frequently utilized in patients with high-risk CNS disease [60, 61], but CNS regimens without cranial irradiation have also achieved excellent results [62, 63]. The Pediatric Oncology Group published a clinical study where two different regimens of intrathecal and systemic chemotherapy were used for CNS prophylaxis in children with acute leukemia. The standard regimen (S) consisted on six injections of triple intrathecal chemotherapy (TIC) with methotrexate, hydrocortisone, and cytarabine administered during intensification treatment and at 8-week intervals throughout the maintenance phase for 17 additional doses. The second regimen, standard and methotrexate pulses (SAM), also specified six TIC administrations during intensification, but substituted pulses of intermediate-dose parenteral methotrexate (IDM, 1 g/m^2) every 8 weeks for the 17 maintenance TIC injections, with a low-dose IT methotrexate boost administered with the first four maintenance IDM pulses. Otherwise, systemic therapy on regimen SAM was identical to regimen S. The 5-year of an isolated CNS relapse was regimen S: good risk 2.8%, and poor risk 7.7%; for the regimen

SAM: good risk 9.6%, and poor risk 12.7%. In poor-risk patients, approximately one third of the isolated CNS relapses occurred before preventive CNS therapy was begun at week 9. Hence, regimen S has provided better CNS preventive therapy for both good- and poor-risk patients ($p < 0.001$ overall) [62].

Several issues remain debatable: which drugs are the best IT combinations, the preferred schedule of administration, and the use of a risk-oriented strategy. Some of the lessons learned from childhood ALL have been analyzed in an attempt to answer these questions. A risk-oriented approach is clearly indicated.

In low-risk childhood ALL patients, IT alone can effectively prevent CNS disease, and this is the preferred method for CNS prophylaxis for this group of patients because of toxicities of cranial irradiation in a growing child [61, 64]. Although the definition of low-risk disease varies, CNS relapse rates in this group are ≤5% in most studies. For intermediate-risk patients two studies have combined IT with HDCT [65, 66] whereas others combined low-dose (1200 rads) cranial irradiation with IT [61]. Both approaches have similar response rates with long-term CNS disease-free survival (DFS) rates about 90% with or without cranial irradiation.

There are few studies regarding CNS prophylaxis in adult ALL and they vary considerably with respect to inclusion criteria, dose of radiation, dose of chemotherapy, and timing of prophylaxis. A summary of selected trials is presented in Table 21.2.

It is clear that at least two modalities are required for adequate prophylaxis. Most trials have used a combination of IT and cranial irradiation. However, an approach combining high-dose IV methotrexate, cytarabine, and dexamethasone in conjunction with 16 doses of IT methotrexate alternating with cytarabine has been reported to greatly reduce the risk of CNS leukemia [5, 67].

Analysis of multiple chemotherapy approaches without cranial irradiation from a single institution was published by Cortes et al. [5]. Patients at low risk for CNS leukemia were given high-dose cytarabine and intermediate-dose methotrexate. Their 5-year CNS event-free rate was 85%, which compares favorably to the historical 65% with no prophylaxis ($p = 0.05$). Comparatively, for patients with high-risk CNS leukemia who had no prophylaxis, the 5-year CNS event-free rate was 28%, compared to 67% with HDST, 70% with HDST plus late (at the time of CR) IT, and 98% (at 3-year EFS) with HDST and early (starting with induction chemotherapy) IT [5]. This study emphasizes the importance of early start of prophylaxis (i.e., at the start of induction chemotherapy) and the use of a risk-oriented approach for prophylaxis. In this study risk was determined by the serum LDH level and the percentage of cells in S + G2M phase in the bone marrow.

Mature B-cell ALL is by definition associated with high risk for CNS disease. Between 10 to 40% of patients

Table 21.2. CNS prophylaxis by induction treatment regimen

Treatment regimen[a]	CNS prophylaxis Low risk	High risk
VAD	High-dose systemic chemotherapy[b]	High-dose Systemic chemotherapy[b]
Modified VAD	High-dose systemic chemotherapy[c]	High-dose systemic[c] + IT (×22) chemotherapy
Hyper-CVAD	High-dose systemic[e] + IT (×4) chemotherapy[f]	High-dose systemic[e] + IT (×4) chemotherapy[f]

CNS, central nervous system; high-risk, mature B-cell immunophenotype, or the presence of either elevated serum levels of lactate dehydrogenase or high proliferative index in the bone marrow (i.e., ≥14% cells in S and G2M phase; all others were low risk); VAD, Vincristine, doxorubicin, and dexamethasone; IT, intrathecal.

a IT started in complete response for patients on the modified VAD regimen and during induction for patients on the hyper-CVAD regimen.

b High-dose cytosine arabinoside (ara-C) (3 g/m^2 every 12 h for six doses) and moderate dose methotrexate (MTX) (400–1600 mg/m^2).

c High-dose ara-C (3 g/m^{2}every 12 h for six doses).

d Ara-C 100 mg weekly ×8, then every other week ×8, then monthly ×6 (22 IT doses in 12 months).

e High-dose ara-C (3 g/m^2 every 12 h for four doses) and high-dose MTX (1 g/m^2).

f MTX 12 mg on day 2, ara-C 100 mg on day 8 with each hyper-CVAD or MTX/ara-C course. High-risk patients received 16 IT doses, low-risk patients received four IT doses.

with this form of ALL have CNS leukemia at the time of diagnosis [34, 35, 68]. Hoelzer et al. [34] used IT and cranial irradiation and the rate of isolated CNS relapse decreased from 20 to 0% with the introduction of triple IT (methotrexate, cytarabine, and dexamethasone). At MD Anderson Cancer Center (MDACC) [35] the HyperCVAD regimen includes HDCT (methotrexate, cytarabine, dexamethasone, cyclophosphamide, doxorubicin, and vincristine) together with eight alternating IT doses of methotrexate and cytarabine for a total of 16 doses. No isolated CNS relapses were observed among 26 patients treated with this regimen.

In conclusion, CNS prophylaxis in adult ALL can be achieved without cranial irradiation. For patients with low-risk for CNS disease, prophylaxis with HDST alone and an abbreviated course of IT (e.g., 4–6 doses) may provide effective prophylaxis. For those patients with high-risk for CNS disease, early HDST and IT virtually eliminates the risk of CNS relapse. The risk-oriented approach is an excellent tool to minimize risk and optimize efficacy.

21.6 CNS Treatment

The treatment of patients who develop CNS leukemia has unfortunately not been standardized, and there is little information about the optimal management of adult patients. There are two different scenarios of occurrence of CNS leukemia: at the time of diagnosis and CNS relapse. Patients, who present at the time of diagnosis with CNS involvement, are treated with a more intensive IT regimen than the one used for prophylaxis. This may also include cranial irradiation. Kantarjian et al. [67] treated patients with CNS leukemia with twice-weekly IT doses, alternating methotrexate and cytarabine, until the CSF had no more identifiable leukemia cells in two consecutive determinations. Patients then followed the standard IT prophylaxis schedule consisting of an IT methotrexate and cytarabine dose with each of the eight courses of chemotherapy. CNS irradiation was not incorporated into this treatment program, except for those patients with cranial-nerve root involvement who received 2400 to 3000 rads of radiation in 10–12 fractions directed to the base of the skull or to the whole brain. Using this approach, the presence of CNS leukemia at the time of diagnosis did not have an adverse impact on outcome, suggesting that the strategy was effective.

Another approach used 3000 rads cranial irradiation and IT for patients with CNS leukemia at the time of induction [69, 70]. Linker et al. [70] treated 109 adult patients with ALL excluding patients who were more than 50 years old, and Burkitt's leukemia. CNS prophylaxis was initiated within 1 week of the achievement of CR. Eighteen hundred rads of cranial irradiation were delivered in 10 fractions over 12–14 days. Six weekly doses of 12 mg of IT methotrexate were administered by lumbar puncture. Patients with CNS involvement at diagnosis began their weekly IT methotrexate during the induction chemotherapy and received 10 weekly doses. Thereafter, these high-risk patients received IT methotrexate monthly during the first year of therapy and their dose of cranial irradiation was increased to 2,800 rads. This study accrued 109 patients who ranged in age from 16 to 49 years, with a median age of 25 years. Seven patients presented with CNS disease at diagnosis. The results of this therapeutic approach showed that neither sex, WBC count, or the presence of CNS disease were predictive of outcome. Patients with no leukemia evidence on day 14 of induction (receiving three doses of daunorubicin) had projected CCR rate of 51% ± 8% compared with 40% ± 8% for patients achieving remission after four doses of daunorubicin [70].

CNS disease is present at the time of diagnosis more frequently among patients with mature B-cell ALL. Good results have been obtained with a regimen using intensive IT and high-dose systemic chemotherapy [34, 35]. In one recent study, 26 adults with newly diagnosed mature B-cell ALL received Hyper-CVAD and CNS prophylaxis alternated IT methotrexate and cytarabine on days 2 and 7 of each course for a total eight courses [35]. Their median age was 58 years (range 17 to 79 years), and 46% were ≥60 years. Complete hematologic remission (CR) was obtained in 21 patients (81%). There were five induction deaths (19%). Eleven (42%) patients had CNS disease at the time of diagnosis and had a similar outcome. The presence of CNS disease at diagnosis was not associated with a lower probability of remission or survival. No isolated CNS relapses were observed.

CNS relapse can occur in three clinical settings: isolated CNS relapse, concomitant bone marrow (BM) and CNS relapse, and CNS relapse after BM recurrence. Over 80% of children with isolated CNS recurrence will die or will have a subsequent recurrence if there is no change in their systemic therapy [71]. A similar outcome can be expected in adults. In one study, all 18 patients who had an isolated CNS recurrence eventually had a recurrence in the BM or died despite responding to treatment for CNS disease but with no change in systemic therapy [6]. This suggests that even when the disease is not readily identified in the blood or BM at the time of CNS relapse, there is residual disease. Indeed, Neale et al. [72] identified molecular evidence of minimal residual disease in BM from four of six patients with T-cell ALL and seemingly isolated CNS recurrence. Goulden et al. [73] found evidence of minimal residual disease by polymerase chain reaction analysis in BM from 12 of 13 children with B-lineage ALL who were otherwise considered to have isolated extramedullary disease.

Using intensive systemic reinduction regimens together with IT with or without cranial irradiation at the time of isolated CNS relapse has resulted in remarkably improved results. With intensive regimens, children who had isolated CNS recurrences had a better survival compared with patients who had BM recurrences. Ribeiro et al. [74] treated 20 children who had isolated CNS recurrences with triple IT therapy given weekly for at least 4 weeks, until two consecutive CSF examinations showed no CNS disease, and then every 6 weeks. In addition, patients received cranial irradiation (the cranium was treated with 2400 rads and spine with 1500 rads) and systemic chemotherapy. Five drugs systemic reinduction treatment included standard dose prednisone, vincristine, and asparaginase plus teniposide and cytarabine. After reinduction therapy, continuation therapy consisted of four drug pairs (etoposide plus cyclophosphamide, methotrexate plus mercaptopurine, teniposide plus cytarabine, and vincristine plus prednisone) administered sequentially every 5 weeks. All patients achieved CR and the estimated 5-year EFS rate was 70%. A similar approach was used by Ritchey et al. [75] in 83 patients (median age 4.1 years) who had isolated recurrences. All patients achieved second CR, and the 4-year event free survival rate was 71%. Thus, patients with "isolated" CNS disease should receive systemic reinduction chemotherapy together with IT. With this strategy, children with isolated CNS relapse have a significant probability of being cured and this group constitutes indeed a favorable subset among those with CNS relapse.

The experience in adults has not been as favorable. In a recent series from MDACC [76] thirty-two adult patients with CNS recurrence were analyzed. The timing of CNS recurrences were: 17 patients isolated (53%), eight patients after BM recurrence (24%), and seven patients simultaneous BM and CNS recurrence (21%). Seventeen patients (53%) had no neurologic symptoms at the time of CNS recurrence and their diagnosis was made on a routine lumbar puncture. The majority of patients (88%) were treated with VAD (vincristine, adriamycin, and dexamethasone) regimen for induction and the rest received Hyper-CVAD. All patients received IT to treat the CNS recurrence. The majority received alternating IT agents twice weekly until CSF was negative, although the specific sequence and frequency of administration varied. The IT agents used were cytarabine in all 32 patients, methotrexate in 26 patients, hydrocortisone in 19 patients, and thiotepa in one patient. The 15 patients with cranial palsies or motor and sensory deficits also received cranial irradiation. IT was effective in achieving a CNS CR in 30 patients (94%), but 10 patients (31%) had a second CNS recurrence. However, the median survival was only 6 months. Only 28% of patients were alive at 1 year, and only 6% were alive at 4 years. This single institution study demonstrated that adults patients with ALL and isolated CNS recurrence had a slightly better outcome compared to others with CNS recurrence concomitant or after BM relapse. However, the prognosis for isolated CNS recurrence clearly is worse for adults than for children. Isolated CNS recurrences occur much earlier in adults than in children. This may be due at least in part to the earlier occurrence of CNS relapse in adults. The median duration of first CR in the MDACC series was 21 weeks, compared with 2 years in children with isolated CNS recurrence, and only 15–17% had a first CR duration of <1 year [75, 77]. A short CR duration has been proposed as the single most important prognostic variable for children with isolated CNS recurrence [75]. Thus, CNS relapse confers a very poor prognosis to adult patients, even in the setting of isolated CNS relapse and despite the use of systemic chemotherapy at the time of relapse. New approaches are needed for this setting.

Bone marrow transplantation (BMT) is unfortunately also ineffective in the management of CNS leukemia. Thompson et al. [78] reported the probability of CNS relapse was 52% for patients with a history of and/or active CNS disease at the time of BMT. The probability was 17% for patients receiving IT Mtx after BMT, although IT significantly increased the risk of leukoencephalopathy. However, in a study by van Besien et al. [79] all four patients with active CNS disease at the time of BMT, and 16 of 20 with history of CNS disease relapsed despite receiving IT methotrexate for 9 months post transplant.

21.7 Toxicity of CNS Prophylaxis and Treatment

CNS-directed therapy involving single- or multiple-agent IT approaches, whether alone or particularly when combined with cranial irradiation, can induce significant toxicities [1]. The earliest understanding of the effects of ALL and its treatments on the CNS was based on autopsy studies. Price et al. [80, 81] described major neuropathologic findings including subacute leukoencephalopathy, mineralizing microangiopathy, and subacute necrotizing leukomyelopathy. Multiple retrospective outcome studies have been published concerning cognitive, motor, and behavioral functioning of surviving ALL patients. These include mostly patients that were initially diagnosed and treated during their childhood. Some of these effects may be attenuated with lower doses of irradiation (e.g., 1800 rads) more frequently used in recent trials [82, 83].

A recent study including 1612 consecutive pediatric patients with newly diagnosed ALL treated on sequential protocols at St. Jude Children's Research Hospital [84] between 1967 and 1988 analyzed the long-term effects of cranial irradiation. With a median follow-up duration of 15.9 years, the cumulative incidence of brain tumors at 20 years was 1.39%. Twenty- two brain tumors (10 high-grade gliomas, one low-grade glioma, and 11 meningiomas) were diagnosed in 21 patients after a median latency of 12.6 years (high-grade gliomas, 9.1 years; meningiomas, 19 years). The use of dose-intensive antimetabolite therapy together with cranial irradiation also increased the risk of brain tumors [77]. The psychosocial outcomes of surviving cancer as a child or adolescent are complex. Among 9535 young adults who survived ALL [85], 17% had depressive, somatic, or anxious symptoms. About 10% reported moderate to extreme pain as a result of their cancer therapy, and 13% expressed frequent fears related to their cancer experience. The role CNS therapy had in the genesis of these symptoms is difficult to estimate.

The Children's Cancer Group also investigated the impact of CNS treatment on scholastic performance of 593 adult survivors of ALL and compared them with 409 sibling controls [86]. Survivors treated with 2400 rads cranial irradiation were much more likely to enter special education or learning disabled programs. In general, survivors were as likely to finish high school and enter college as the controls, but those treated with 2400 rads or treated before the age of 6 years were less likely to enter college than those who received less amounts of radiation. There were no gender differences in educational achievements. In addition, moderate doses of radiation (2400 rads) are associated with obesity, particularly in female patients treated at a young age. In an analysis of 1765 adult survivors of childhood ALL, female survivors who had received cranial irradiation with >2000 rads were two to three times more likely to be obese in comparison with siblings of childhood cancer survivors [87].

Although less well studied, significant toxicity has also been reported with CNS prophylaxis in adults, including neurologic changes, acute and chronic neurotoxicity, decreased tolerance to systemic chemotherapy, and infections associated with therapy-related immunosuppression. The use of prophylactic cranial irradiation in patients with small lung cancer has resulted in borderline dementia in 25% of patients, moderate to marked neuropsychologic deficits in 50%, and significant emotional distress in 16% [88]. In adults with leukemia and lymphoma, minor but significant neuropsychological symptoms are also frequently detected.

Because spinal irradiation can result in growth retardation [89], long-term neurologic changes and cardiac dysfunction [90], it is now used less frequently. In addition, as mentioned earlier, strategies using IT and high-dose systemic chemotherapy have significantly reduced the incidence of CNS leukemia.

21.8 Conclusions

Without CNS prophylaxis, CNS leukemia will occur in approximately 30–50% of patients with ALL in CR. With effective CNS prophylaxis, most adults with ALL will remain free of CNS leukemia. During the last decades, multiple approaches for CNS prophylaxis have been developed with combination of IT, HDST, and cranial irradiation. Excellent results can be achieved with regimens that do not include radiation therapy. The exclusion of radiotherapy decreases acute and long-term toxicities.

A prophylactic approach tailored to the risk of CNS leukemia has proven valuable in childhood ALL, and in at least one adult study. Further studies should focus on defining risk groups for CNS leukemia, and designing effective prophylaxis for each group. In view of the poor prognosis of patients with CNS relapse, adequate prophylaxis is critical. Still, new agents and approaches are needed for patients who develop CNS disease as their outcome is uniformly poor with the strategies investigated to date.

References

1. Bleyer WA, Poplack DA (1985) Prophylaxis and treatment of leukemia in the central nervous system and other sanctuaries. Sem Oncol 12:131–148
2. Evans AE, Gilbert ES, Zandstra R (1970) The increasing incidence of central nervous system leukemia in children. Children's Cancer Study Group A. Cancer 26:404–409
3. Pui CH (2000) Acute lymphoblastic leukemia in children. Current Op Oncol 12:3–12
4. Bleyer WA (1988) Central nervous system leukemia. Pediatr Clin North Am 35:789–814
5. Cortes J, O'Brien SM, Pierce S, et al. (1995) The value of high-dose systemic chemotherapy and intrathecal therapy for central nervous system prophylaxis in different risk groups of adult acute lymphoblastic leukemia. Blood 86:2091–2097
6. Larson RA, Dodge RK, Burns CP, et al. (1995) A five-drug remission induction regimen with intensive consolidation for adults with acute lymphoblastic leukemia: Cancer and leukemia group B study 8811. Blood 85:2025–2037
7. Keating MJ, Gehan EA, Smith TL, et al. (1987) A strategy for evaluation of new treatments in untreated patients: Application to a clinical trial of AMSA for acute leukemia. J Clin Oncol 5:710–721
8. Omura GA, Moffitt S, Vogler WR, et al. (1980) Combination chemotherapy of adult acute lymphoblastic leukemia with randomized central nervous system prophylaxis. Blood 55:199–204
9. Stewart DJ, Keating MJ, McCredie KB, et al. (1981) Natural history of central nervous system acute leukemia in adults. Cancer 47: 184–196
10. Glass JJP, Melamed M, Chernik NL, et al. (1979) Malignant cells in cerebrospinal fluid: The meaning of a positive CSF cytology. Neurol 29:1369
11. Bradstock KF, Papageorgiou ES, Janossy G (1981) Diagnosis of meningeal involvement in patients with acute lymphoblastic leukemia: Immunofluorescence for terminal transferase. Cancer 47:2478
12. Lauer SJ, Kirchner PA, Camitta BM (1989) Identification of leukemia cells in the cerebrospinal fluid from children with acute lymphoblastic leukemia: Advances and dilemmas. Am J Pediatr Hematol Oncol 11:65
13. Pinkel D, Woo S (1994) Prevention and treatment of meningeal leukemia in children. Blood 84:355–366
14. Mahmoud HH, Rivera GK, Hancock ML, et al. (1993) Low leukocyte counts with blast cells in cerebrospinal fluid of children with newly diagnosed acute lymphoblastic leukemia. N Engl J Med 329:314–319
15. Lauer S, Shuster J, Kirschner P, et al. (1994) Prognostic significance of cerebrospinal fluid lymphoblast at diagnosis in children with acute lymphoblastic leukemia. Proc Am Soc Clin Oncol 13:317 (abstr 1041)
16. Gilchrist GS, Tubergen DG, Sather HN, et al. (1994) Low numbers of CSF blasts at diagnosis do not predict the development of CNS leukemia in children with intermediate-risk acute lymphoblastic leukemia: A Children's Cancer Group report. J Clin Oncol 12: 2594–2600
17. van der Berg H, Vet R, den Ouden E, et al. (1995) Significance of lymphoblast in cerebrospinal fluid in newly diagnosed pediatric acute lymphoblastic malignancies with bone marrow involvement: Possible benefit of dexamethasone. Med Pediatr Oncol 25:22–27
18. Burger B, Zimmermann M, Mann G, et al. (2003) Diagnostic cerebrospinal fluid examination in children with acute lymphoblastic leukemia: Significance of low leukocyte counts with blast or traumatic lumbar puncture. J Clin Oncol 21:184–188
19. Gajjar A, Harrison PL, Sandlund JT, et al. (2000) Traumatic lumbar puncture at diagnosis adversely affects outcome in childhood acute lymphoblastic leukemia. Blood 96:3381–3384
20. Kebelmann-Betzing C, Seeger K, Wolf R, et al. (2001) Traumatic lumbar puncture at diagnosis and outcome in childhood acute lymphoblastic leukemia. Letter. Blood 98:3496–3497
21. Mastrangelo R, Poplack D, Bleyer A, et al. (1986) Report and recommendations for the Rome workshop concerning poor-prognosis acute lymphoblastic leukemia in children: Biologic bases for staging, stratification, and treatment. Med Pediatric Oncol 14:191–194
22. Cibas ES, Malkin MG, Posner JB, et al. (1987) Detection of DNA abnormalities by flow cytometry in cells form cerebrospinal fluid. Am J Clin Path 88:570–577
23. Mavlight GM, Stuckey SE, Cabanillas FF, et al. (1980) Diagnosis of leukemia or lymphoma in the central nervous system by beta 2-microglobulin determination. N Engl J Med 303:718–722
24. Kantarjian H, Smith T, Estey E, et al. (1992) Prognostic significance of elevated serum β2-microglobulin levels in acute lymphocytic leukemia. Am J Med 93:599–604
25. Hintzen RQ, de Jong R, Hack CE, et al. (1991) A soluble form of the human T cell differentiation antigen CD27 is released after triggering of the TCR/CD3 complex. J Immunol 35:211
26. Kertern MJ, Evers LM, Dellemijn PL, et al. (1996) Elevation of cerebrospinal fluid soluble CD27 levels in patients with meningeal localization of lymphoid malignancies [published erratum appears in Blood 1996 Oct 1;88(7):2818]. Blood 87:1985–1989
27. Weller M, Stevens A, Sommer N, et al. (1992) Humoral CSF parameters in the differential diagnosis of hematologic CNS neoplasia. Acta Neurol Scan 86:129
28. Twijnstra A, Ongerboer de Visser BW, van Zantern PP (1987) Diagnosis of leptomeningeal metastasis. Clin Neurol Neurosurg 98:79
29. Januszkiewicz DA, Nowak JS (1995) Molecular evidence for central nervous system involvement in children with newly diagnosed acute lymphoblastic leukemia. Hematol Oncol 13:201–206
30. Chamberlain MC, Sandy AD, Press GA (1990) Leptomeningeal metastasis: A comparison of gadolinium-enhanced MR and contrast-enhanced CT of the brain. Neurol 40:435–438
31. Price RA, Johnson WW (1973) The central nervous system in childhood with leukemia: I. The arachnoid. Cancer 31:520
32. Prochedly C (1977) Neurologic manifestations of leukemia. In: Prochedly C (ed) Leukemia and lymphoma in the central nervous system. Charles C. Thomas, Springfield, IL, p 3

33. Ingram LC, Fairclough DL, Furman WL, et al. (1991) Cranial nerve palsy in childhood acute lymphoblastic leukemia and non-Hodgkin's lymphoma. Cancer 67:2262
34. Hölzer D, Ludwig WD, Thiel E, et al. (1996) Improved outcome in adult B-cell acute lymphoblastic leukemia. Blood 87:495–508
35. Thomas DA, Cortes J, O'Brien S, et al. (1999) Hyper-CVAD program in Burkitt's-type adult acute lymphoblastic leukemia. J Clin Oncol 17:2461–2470
36. Pavlovsky S, Eppinger-Helft M, Sackmann Muriel F (1973) Factors that influence the appearance of central nervous system leukemia. Blood 42:935–939
37. Schlieben S, Borkhardt A, Reinisch I, et al. (1996) Incidence and clinical outcome of children with BCR/ABL-positive acute lymphoblastic leukemia (ALL): A prospective RT-PCR study based on 673 patients enrolled in the German pediatric multicenter therapy trials ALL-BFM 90 and CoALL-05-92. Leukemia 10:957–963
38. Schrappe M, Arico M, Harbott J, et al. (1998) Philadelphia chromosome-positive (Ph+) childhood acute lymphoblastic leukemia: Good initial steroid response allows early prediction of a favorable treatment outcome. Blood 92:2730–2741
39. Tiftik N, Bolaman Z, Batun S (2004) The importance of CD7 and CD56 antigens in acute leukemias. Int J Clin Pract 58(2):149–152
40. Ravandi F, Cortes J, Estrov Z, et al. (2002) CD56 expression predicts occurrence of CNS disease in acute lymphoblastic leukemia. Leukemia Res 26:643–649
41. Pui CH, Sandlund JT, Pei D, et al. (2003) Results of therapy for acute lymphoblastic leukemia in black and white children. JAMA 290:2061–2063
42. Stewart DJ, Keating MJ, McCredie KB, et al. (1981) Natural history of central nervous system acute leukemia in adults. Cancer 47:187–196
43. Kantarjian HM, Walters RS, Smith TL, et al. (1988) Identification of risk groups for development of central nervous system leukemia in adults with acute lymphocytic leukemia. Blood 72:1784–1789
44. Kantarjian HM, Smith T, Estey E, et al. (1992) Prognostic significance of elevated serum beta 2-microglobulin levels in adult acute lymphocytic leukemia [see comments]. Am J Med 93: 599–604
45. Blaney SM, Balis FM, Poplack DG (1991) Current pharmacological treatment approaches to central nervous system leukemia. Drugs 41:702–716
46. Balis FM, Poplack DG (1989) Central nervous system pharmacology of antileukemic drugs. Am J Pediatr Hematol Oncol 11:74–86
47. Greig NH (1987) Optimizing drug delivery to brain tumors. Cancer Treat Rev 14:1
48. Harbaugh RE (1989) Novel CNS-directed drug delivery systems in Alzheimer's disease and other neurological disorders. Neurobiol Aging 10:623
49. Bomgaars L, Geyer JR, Franklin J, et al. (2004) Phase I of intrathecal liposomal cytarabine in children with neoplastic meningitis. J Clin Oncol 22:3916–3921
50. Balis FM, Savitch JL, Bleyer WA, et al. (1985) Remission induction of meningeal leukemia with high-dose intravenous methotrexate. J Clin Oncol 3:485–489
51. Morra E, Lazzarino M, Inverardi D, et al. (1986) Systemic high-dose ara-C for the treatment of meningeal leukemia in adult acute lymphoblastic leukemia and non-Hodgkin's lymphoma. J Clin Oncol 4:1207–1211
52. Ito C, Evans WE, McNinch L, et al. (1996) Comparative cytotoxicity of dexamethasone and prednisolone in childhood acute lymphoblastic leukemia. J Clin Oncol 14:2370–2376
53. Balis FM, Lester CM, Chrousos GP, et al. (1987) Differences in cerebrospinal fluid penetration of corticosteroids: Possible relationship to the prevention of meningeal leukemia. J Clin Oncol 5:202–207
54. Relling MV, Mahmoud HH, Pui CH, et al. (1996) Etoposide achieves potentially cytotoxic concentrations in CSF of children with acute lymphoblastic leukemia. J Clin Oncol 14:399–404
55. Zimm S, Ettinger LJ, Holcenberg JC, et al. (1985) Phase I and clinical pharmacological study of mercaptopurine administered as a prolonged intravenous infusion. Cancer Res 45:1869–1873
56. Bostrom BC, Sensel MR, Sather HN, et al. (2003) Dexamethasone versus prednisone and daily oral versus weekly intravenous mercaptopurine for patients with standard-risk acute lymphoblastic leukemia: A report from the Children's Cancer Group. Blood 101:3809–3817
57. Dibenedetto SP, Di Cataldo A, Ragusa R, et al. (1995) Levels of L-asparagine in CSF after intramuscular administration of asparaginase form Erwinia in children with acute lymphoblastic leukemia. J Clin Oncol 13:339–344
58. Riccardi R, Holcenberg JS, Glaubiger DL, et al. (1981) L-asparaginase pharmacokinetics and asparagines levels in cerebrospinal fluid of rhesus monkeys and humans. Cancer Res 41:4554–4558
59. Hawkins DS, Park JR, Thomson BJ, et al. (2004) Asparaginase pharmacokinetics after intensive polyethylene glycol-conjugated L-asparaginase therapy for children with relapsed acute lymphoblastic leukemia. Clin Cancer Res 10:5335–5341
60. Pui CH, Mahmoud HH, Rivera GK, et al. (1998) Early intensification of intrathecal chemotherapy virtually eliminates central nervous system relapse in children with acute lymphoblastic leukemia. Blood 92:411–415
61. Schrappe M, Reiter A, Ludwig WD, et al. (2000) Improved outcome in childhood acute lymphoblastic leukemia despite reduced use of anthracyclines and cranial radiotherapy: Results of trial ALL-BFM 90. Blood 95:3310–3322
62. Pullen J, Boyett J, Shuster J, et al. (1993) Extended triple intrathecal chemotherapy trial for prevention of CNS relapse in good-risk and poor-risk patients with B-progenitor acute lymphoblastic leukemia: A Pediatric Oncology Group study. J Clin Oncol 11:839–849
63. Krance RA, Newman EM, Ravindranath Y, et al. (1991) A pilot study of intermediate-dose methotrexate and cytosine arabinoside, "spread-out" or "up-front," in continuation therapy for childhood non-T, non-B acute lymphoblastic leukemia. A Pediatric Oncology Group study. Cancer 67:550–556
64. Mahoney DH Jr, Shuster JJ, Nitschke R, et al. (1998) Acute neurotoxicity in children with B-precursor acute lymphoid leukemia: An association with intermediate-dose intravenous methotrexate and intrathecal triple therapy – A Pediatric Oncology Group study. J Clin Oncol 16:1712–1722
65. Kamps WA, Bokkerink JP, Hahlen K, et al. (1999) Intensive treatment of children with acute lymphoblastic leukemia according to ALL-BFM-86 without cranial radiotherapy: Results of Dutch Childhood Leukemia Study Group Protocol ALL-7 (1988–1991). Blood 94:1226–1236
66. Tubergen DG, Gilchrist GS, O'Brien RT, et al. (1993) Prevention of CNS disease in intermediate-risk acute lymphoblastic leukemia:

Comparison of cranial radiation and intrathecal methotrexate and the importance of systemic therapy: A Childrens Cancer Group report. J Clin Oncol 11:520–526
67. Kantarjian HM, O'Brian S, Smith TL, et al. (2000) Results of treatment with hyper-CVAD, a dose-intensive regimen, in adult acute lymphocytic leukemia. J Clin Oncol 18:547–561
68. Gururangan S, Sposto R, Cairo MS, et al. (2000) Outcome of CNS disease at diagnosis in disseminated small noncleaved-cell lymphoma and B-cell leukemia: A Children's Cancer Group study. J Clin Oncol 18:2017–2025
69. Hoelzer D, Thiel E, Loffler H, et al. (1984) Intensified therapy in acute lymphoblastic and acute undifferentiated leukemia in adults. Blood 64:38–47
70. Linker CA, Levitt LJ, O'Donnell M, et al. (1991) Treatment of adult acute lymphoblastic leukemia with intensive cyclical chemotherapy: A follow-up report. Blood 78:2814–2822
71. George SL, Ochs JJ, Mauer AM, et al. (1985) The importance of an isolated central nervous system relapse in children with acute lymphoblastic leukemia. J Clin Oncol 3:776–781
72. Neale GA, Pui CH, Mahmoud HH, et al. (1994) Molecular evidence for minimal residual bone marrow disease in children with isolated extramedullary relapse of T-cell acute lymphoblastic leukemia. Leukemia 8:768–775
73. Goulden N, Langlands K, Steward C, et al. (1994) PCR assessment of bone marrow status in isolated extramedullary relapse of childhood B-precursor acute lymphoblastic leukemia. Brit J Haematol 87:282–285
74. Ribeiro RC, Rivera GK, Hudson M, et al. (1995) An intensive retreatment protocol for children with an isolated CNS relapse of acute lymphoblastic leukemia. J Clin Oncol 13:333–338
75. Ritchey AK, Pollock BH, Lauer SJ, et al. (1999) Improved-survival of children with isolated CNS relapse of acute lymphoblastic leukemia: A Pediatric Oncology Group study. [Published erratum appears in Journal of Clinical of Oncology 18:703, 2000] J Clin Oncol 17:3745–3752
76. Surapanemi UR, Cortes J, Thomas D, et al. (2002) Central nervous system relapses in adults with acute lymphoblastic leukemia. Cancer 94:773–779
77. Relling MV, Rubnitz JE, Rivera GK, et al. (1999) High incidence of secondary brain tumors after radiotherapy and antimetabolites [see comments]. Lancet 354:34–39
78. Thompson CB, Sanders JE, Flournoy N, et al. (1986) The risk of central nervous system relapse and leukoencephalopathy in patients receiving marrow transplants for acute leukemia. Blood 67:195–199
79. van Besien K, Przepiorka D, Mehra R, et al. (1996) Impact of preexisting CNS involvement on the outcome of bone marrow transplantation in adult hematologic malignancies. J Clin Oncol 14:3036–3042
80. Price RA, Johnson WW, et al. (1973) The central nervous system in childhood leukemia. I. The arachnoid. Cancer 31:520–532
81. Price RA, Birdwell DA, et al. (1978) The central nervous system in childhood leukemia. III. Mineralizing microangiopathy and dystrophic calcification. Cancer 42:717–728
82. Waber DP, Tarbell NJ (1997) Toxicity of CNS prophylaxis for childhood leukemia. Oncology (Huntington) 11:259–264; discussion 264–265
83. Mulhern RK, Fairclough D, Ochs J (1991) A prospective comparison of neuropsychologic performance of children surviving leukemia who received 1,800 rads, 2,400 rads, or no cranial irradiation. [Published erratum appears in Journal of Clinical Oncology 9: 1922, 1991] J Clin Oncol 9:1348–1356
84. Walter AW, Hancock ML, Pui CH, et al. (1998) Secondary brain tumors in children treated for acute lymphoblastic leukemia at St. Jude Children's Research Hospital. J Clin Oncol 16:3761–3767
85. Hudson MM, Mertens AC, Yasui Y, et al. (2003) Health status of adult long-term survivors of childhood cancer: A report from the Childhood Cancer Survivor Study. JAMA 290:1583–1592
86. Haupt R , Fears TR, Robison LL, et al. (1994) Educational attainment in long-term survivors of childhood acute lymphoblastic leukemia. JAMA 272:1427–1432
87. Oeffinger KC, Mertens AC, Sklar CA, et al. (2003) Obesity in adult survivors of childhood acute lymphoblastic leukemia: A report from the Childhood Cancer Survivor Study. J Clin Oncol 21: 1359–1365
88. Crossen JR, Garwood D, Glatstein E, et al. (1994) Neurobehavioral sequela of cranial irradiation in adults: A review of radiation-induced encephalopathy. J Clin Oncol 12:627–642
89. Shalet SM, Gibson B, Swindell R, et al. (1987) Effect of spinal irradiation of growth. Arch Dis Childhood 62:461–464
90. Jakacki RI, Goldwein JW, Larsen RL, et al. (1993) Cardiac dysfunction following spinal irradiation during childhood. J Clin Oncol 11:1033–1038

Relapsed Acute Lymphoblastic Leukemia

Nicole Lamanna, Melissa von Hassel, Mark Weiss

Contents

22.1 Introduction

Treatment of acute lymphoblastic leukemia in children is one of the great success stories of combination chemotherapy. Unfortunately, adults fare much worse and the majority of adult patients ultimately fail their initial treatment program. Most current induction regimens obtain complete responses (CRs) in 65–90% of newly diagnosed adult patients with acute lymphoblastic leukemia (ALL). Early deaths account for some of the induction failures, but in most studies 10–25% of patients have disease resistant to vincristine/prednisone-based regimens. In addition to these primary refractory patients, 60–70% of patients who achieve a CR relapse. Treatment of relapsed and refractory patients is therefore an important and common problem. Numerous regimens have been reported in the setting of relapsed ALL. There are two widely tested approaches to reinduction therapy for adult patients with recurrent or refractory ALL. One option is to treat the patient with a regimen that is similar to their original induction therapy (this strategy is obviously not used for primary refractory patients). Combinations of vincristine, prednisone, and an anthracycline intensified with cyclophosphamide and/or L-asparaginase represent traditional induction therapy, and variations on this approach are employed frequently in the salvage setting. Patients who have had a long first remission or who develop recurrent disease after completing maintenance chemotherapy occasionally can achieve a second CR with a repetition of their initial induction regimen [1].

Unfortunately most patients develop recurrent disease within the first 12–24 months of achieving their first remission, at a time when they are still receiving maintenance chemotherapy [2–5]. For these patients, the likelihood of achieving a second CR with reinduction therapy similar to their initial regimen is low. In addition, for the 10–25% of patients whose disease is primarily refractory to standard induction therapy, simply repeating the same induction treatments offers essentially no hope of obtaining a CR. A second option for these patients is to employ an active salvage regimen that relies on agents that are relatively distinct from traditional induction treatments. The most commonly tested regimens of this type are based on high-dose cytarabine, which, as a single agent, may induce a CR in approximately 30% of patients with recurrent or refractory ALL. In combination with other agents, particularly anthracyclines, high-dose cytarabine-based regimens appear to yield even higher response rates.

An example of the type of regimen that reiterates the initial treatment program was the report by Koller et al. using "hyper-CVAD." This regimen is patterned after the style of therapy developed to treat Burkitt's lymphoma/leukemia and utilizes fractionated cyclophosphamide, high-dose cytarabine, and high-dose methotrexate [6]. Sixty-six adults with relapsed ALL received this regimen consisting of eight courses of alternating chemotherapy with growth factor support followed by oral maintenance chemotherapy. The authors reported a frequency of CR of 44% with a median survival of approximately 8 months. Three-year survival was poor at approximately 10%.

High-dose cytarabine has been used alone and in combination with a number of different agents. In combination with L-asparaginase [2–4], doxorubicin [5], idarubicin [7, 8], or mitoxantrone [9–12], CRs as high as 72% have been reported in relapsed patients with ALL. Issues of patient mix make it difficult to assess if a specific regimen is superior to others, but in general a combination of high-dose cytarabine and an anthracycline has the greatest likelihood of achieving a second CR in relapsed patients (or a first CR in refractory patients). The toxicity of these regimens should be balanced against the benefits of achieving a CR. An example of such a regimen is the combination of high-dose cytarabine with a single high dose of idarubicin. We reported that this active regimen produced CRs in 44% of patients [13, 14].

However, second CRs are notoriously difficult to maintain and typically each succeeding response (if one can be achieved) is briefer than the preceding one. In general, patients with a suitable allogeneic transplant option should be referred for such a transplant in second CR.

22.2 Bone Marrow Transplant in Adult Acute Lymphoblastic Leukemia

Human leukocyte antigen- (HLA) matched identical sibling bone marrow transplants have been used in adults with ALL in a variety of settings. This dose-intense treatment has the ability to eradicate leukemia in a small subset of patients with disease refractory to conventional chemotherapy. In general, there are three main prerequisites for performing an allogeneic transplant. The patient must be in acceptable physical condition to withstand the rigors of the transplant. Secondly, the disease should be in a minimal disease state (preferably complete remission) to reduce the risk of relapse posttransplant. Finally, a suitable donor must be identified. HLA typing should be performed on the patient and the patients' immediate family at the time of diagnosis. Early HLA typing is preferred because this typing may take up to 2 weeks to complete and if deferred until relapse, unwanted delays in identifying a donor may occur. If a suitable related donor is not identified, we recommend no further testing until a transplant is recommended. At that time extended family members may be typed, but in addition, a preliminary search of unrelated donors should be initiated. This initial search through the National Marrow Donor Registry is performed free of charge to the patient. This is a one-time search of over ten million adult donors and more than 190 000 cord blood units to help identify potential candidates. In addition to the preliminary domestic search, an international search may also be initiated depending on the patient's racial and ethnic background. If a potential donor is identified, additional testing will be necessary, and this is known as the "formal" search. Once an unrelated donor is identified, logistical planning for the transplant can begin.

However, the lack of availability of HLA-matched donors and the toxicity and mortality seen with transplant often limits the utility of this approach. Davies et al. [15] studied the outcome of 115 consecutive patients with recurrent ALL over a 2-year period from 1991–1993. A matched, related donor was identified in 35% of which 75% made it to transplant (26% of the original cohort). Of the 75 patients without a related donor, 58 patients had an unrelated donor search initiated. An unrelated donor was identified for 22 (37%) of those whom a search was performed and 15 of these patients proceeded to a matched, unrelated donor transplant [15]. Fortunately, the likelihood of finding a suitable matched, unrelated donor has improved; however, there are still some patients for whom a suitable donor cannot be identified.

Unfortunately allogeneic transplant is not a panacea for treating relapsed ALL. In part, the limits of transplant can be seen by reviewing patterns of failure. Patterns of failure with allogeneic transplant in ALL are dissimilar to that of patients transplanted for AML. In AML, patients treated with allogeneic transplant often fail therapy because of treatment-related mortality (infectious complications, GVHD, etc.). In contrast, patients with ALL who undergo allogeneic transplant suffer from both treatment-related mortality and a significant rate of relapse. Ultimately, few patients are long-term disease-free survivors. A major cause of this high degree of relapse is related to the modest "graft-versus-leukemia" effect associated with treating ALL. Graft-versus-leukemia is the process by which the transplanted (donor) immune system eliminates residual leukemic cells and as such is a type of graft-versus-host reaction. Graft-versus-leukemia appears to be less active in ALL than in AML or CML. Supporting this concept are data from the International Bone Marrow Transplant Registry that compared identical twin (syngeneic) transplants to HLA-identical sibling transplants [16]. Graft-versus-leukemia should be more pronounced in the allogeneic transplants as compared with the syngeneic transplants, and in this study there was a significantly higher relapse rate in the syngeneic transplants for AML and CML, but not for ALL. This implies that graft-versus-leukemia is less important in ALL. A second indication that graft-versus-leukemia is less active in ALL comes from an analysis of studies of donor T-cell infusions used to treat leukemia that has relapsed after allogeneic bone marrow transplant. In this study, donor lymphocyte infusions produced complete responses in 73% of patients with CML, 29% of patients with AML, and 0% of patients with ALL [17]. There is however, a mild graft-versus-leukemia effect in ALL and a report of 1132 patients with ALL demonstrated that acute and chronic graft-versus-host disease are associated with lower overall rates of relapse compared to those patients without graft-versus host disease [18].

There is significant controversy over the use and timing of allogeneic transplant in adult ALL. The results of 192 adults with ALL transplanted at the Fred Hutchinson Cancer Center report a 5-year disease-free survival of only 15% for patients transplanted in second CR or beyond [19]. Another study suggested more favorable results, but this is difficult to interpret as the results combined both pediatric and adult patients, or patients in first CR (who may already be cured) with higher-risk patients [20]. As only a small subset of patients with relapsed disease are cured with allogeneic transplant, many investigators have chosen to evaluate this modality in patients in first CR. However, two large comparisons of allogeneic transplant versus standard chemotherapy for patients in first CR have failed to demonstrate an improved survival for the transplant arm [21, 22]. In one of these studies, subset analysis suggests a benefit for certain high-risk patients [21]. However, this benefit was not confirmed in the other study [22]. Thus, currently the only patients for whom allogeneic transplant in first CR can be routinely recommended are in patients with t(9;22) and t(4;11). For other adult patients, we recommend that allogeneic transplant be reserved for second CR.

Autologous transplant for adult ALL is even less effective than allogeneic transplant [23]. The extremely poor results in patients in second CR led to testing this modality in patients in first CR. However, both a non-randomized [24] and randomized trial [25] have shown no benefit to autologous transplant compared with maintenance chemotherapy in patients in first CR. This modality should therefore be considered investigational at this time and not routinely performed in patients in first CR.

22.3 Philadelphia Chromosome-Positive Adult Acute Lymphoblastic Leukemia

Philadelphia-chromosome positive (Ph+) disease carries a very poor prognosis, and long-term survival, even with high-dose chemotherapy, is rare. Thus, for patients with Ph+ disease, allogeneic transplant in first CR is commonly recommended and may be curative in a minority of patients [26, 27]. The development of imatinib (Gleevec®, formerly STI-571), a tyrosine kinase inhibitor with relative specificity for bcr-abl, has dramatically changed the treatment and outcome of patients with CML [28]. This agent also has activity in Ph+ ALL [29]. In this setting, however, it is less active than it is in CML with only 29% of relapsed or refractory patients achieving a CR [29]. Unfortunately, the median time to progression is only 2.2 months, demonstrating the development of resistance to imatinib in this patient group [30, 31]. Currently, many investigators are assessing combination therapy with imatinib and chemotherapy in both the initial treatment [32] or in the relapsed setting [33].

22.4 CNS Relapsed in Adult Acute Lymphoblastic Leukemia

CNS relapse occurs in approximately 10% of patients who have received appropriate prophylaxis. In the majority of these patients, simultaneous bone marrow relapse can be documented. In occasional patients, CNS relapse may occur without demonstrable systemic relapse ("isolated CNS relapse"); however, this event almost always predicts subsequent bone marrow relapse, and patients with isolated CNS relapse should receive reinduction chemotherapy following treatment of their CNS disease. Treatment of established CNS disease requires a combination of radiotherapy and intrathecal chemotherapy. Radiotherapy should consist of 1800–2400 cGy (in 150–200 cGy fractions) administered to the whole brain. Higher doses should be avoided because of the risk of late toxicity and the fact that some patients may later require total body irradiation as part of a conditioning regimen for an allogeneic transplant. Despite encouraging results in children, spinal radiotherapy should be avoided in adults because the dose of radiotherapy to marrow-bearing areas subsequently limits the ability to administer necessary systemic chemotherapy. Furthermore, though this approach can help control the CNS disease it does not prolong survival as these patients will typically succumb to refractory systemic disease [34]. Intrathecal therapy with methotrexate (12 mg) for patients with established CNS disease should be administered intraventricularly, preferably via an Ommaya reservoir. Intrathecal chemotherapy can be administered as often as two or even three times per week with at least 1 day off between doses until the CSF is cleared of leukemic blasts, then twice a week for 2–3 weeks, and then twice a month for 2 or 3 additional months. Patients who develop CNS disease despite prophylaxis with intrathecal methotrexate, or those who do not clear the blasts from the CSF promptly (within two treatments) with methotrexate, should receive intraventricular therapy with cytarabine at a dose of 60 mg.

22.5 Newer Agents

Given the poor overall long-term results for adult patients with relapsed ALL, newer agents are being evaluated. Clofarabine, a nucleoside analog that is a hybrid of fludarabine and cladribine, has been reported in a small group of patients (n=12) with ALL [35]. One patient (8%) achieved a complete response that lasted 4 months. Another investigational agent, perhaps with greater promise is nelarabine, a pro-drug of ara-G. This arabinosyl analog of deoxyguanosine has shown activity [36, 37]. Nelarabine, the prodrug of ara-G, was evaluated in a phase I multicenter trial of 26 patients [36]. Complete (n=5) or partial remission (n=5) was achieved in patients; seven out of eight patients with T cell ALL, one with T lymphoid blast crisis of CML, and one with T cell lymphoma, and one with B cell CLL. Interestingly, responses were not seen in patients with B-lineage ALL.

22.6 Conclusions

The treatment of adult patients with relapsed acute lymphoblastic leukemia remains a daunting task. As we gain a better understanding of the biology that distinguishes relapsing patients from those who are successfully treated, we hope to develop novel, targeted therapies to improve the initial treatment of the patients and thereby minimize the number of patients requiring treatment in the relapsed setting. Currently, the only realistic chance for long-term, disease-free survival is to induce a second CR (we favor high dose cytarabine with high dose anthracycline approach) followed by an allogeneic transplant.

References

1. Woodruff R, Lister T, Paxton A, Whitehouse J, Malpas J (1978) Combination chemotherapy for hematologic relapse in adult acute lymphoblastic leukemia (ALL). Am J Hematol 4:173–177
2. Capizzi RI, Poole M, Cooper MR, et al. (1984) Treatment of poor risk acute leukemia with sequential high-dose Ara-C and asparaginase. Blood 63:694–700
3. Amadori S, Papa F, Avisati G, et al. (1984) Sequential combination high-dose Ara-C and asparaginase for the treatment of advanced acute leukemia and lymphoma. Leuk Res 8:729–735
4. Wells RJ, Feusner J, Devney R, et al. (1985) Sequential high-dose cytosine arabinoside-asparaginase treatment in advance childhood leukemia. J Clin Oncol 3:998–1004
5. Ishii E, Mara T, Ohkubo K, et al. (1986) Treatment of childhood acute lymphoblastic leukemia with intermediate-dose cytosine arabinoside and adriamycin. Med Pediatr Oncol 14:73
6. Koller CA, Kantarjian HM, Thomas D, et al. (1997) The hyper-CVAD regimen improves outcome in relapsed acute lymphoblastic leukemia. Leukemia 11:2039–2044
7. Giona F, Testi A, Amadori G, et al. (1990) Idarubicin and high-dose cytarabine in the treatment of refractory and relapsed acute lymphoblastic leukemia. Ann Oncol 1:51–55
8. Tan C, Steinherz P, Meyer P (1990) Idarubicin in combination with high-dose cytosine arabinoside in patients with acute leukemia in relapse. Proc Annu Meet Am Assoc Cancer Res 31:A1133 (abstr)
9. Hiddemann W, Kreutzman H, Straif K, et al. (1987) High-dose cytosine arabinoside in combination with mitoxantrone for the treatment of refractory acute myeloid and lymphoblastic leukemia. Semin Oncol 14:73

10. Leclerc J, Rivard G, Blanch M, et al. (1988) The association of once a day high-dose Ara-C followed by mitoxantrone for 3 days induces a high rate of complete remission in children with poor prognosis acute leukemia. Blood 72(Suppl):210 (abstr)
11. Kantarjian H, Walters R, Keating M, et al. (1990) Mitoxantrone and high-dose cytosine arabinoside for the treatment of refractory acute lymphocytic leukemia. Cancer 65:5–8
12. Feldman EJ, Alberts DS, Arlin Z, et al. (1993) Phase I clinical and pharmacokinetic evaluation of high-dose mitoxantrone in combination with cytarabine in patients with acute leukemia. J Clin Oncol 11:2002–2009
13. Weiss MA, Drullinsky P, Maslak P, et al. (1998) A phase I trial of a single high dose of idarubicin combined with high-dose cytarabine as induction therapy in relapsed or refractory adult patients with acute lymphoblastic leukemia. Leukemia 12(6):865–868
14. Weiss MA, Aliff TB, Tallman MS, et al. (2002) A single, high dose of idarubicin combined with cytarabine as induction therapy for adult patients with recurrent or refractory acute lymphoblastic leukemia. Cancer 95(3):581–587
15. Davies SM, Ramsay NK, Weisdorf DJ (1996) Feasibility and timing of unrelated donor identification for patients with ALL. Bone Marrow Transplant 17:737–740
16. Gale RP, Horowitz MM, Ash RC, et al. (1994) Identical-twin bone marrow transplants for leukemia. Ann Intern Med 120:646–652
17. Kolb H-J, Schattenberg A, Goldman JM, et al. (1995) Graft-versus-leukemia effect of donor lymphocyte transfusions in marrow grafted patients. Blood 86:2041
18. Passweg JR, Tiberghien P, Cahn J-Y, et al. (1998) Graft-versus-leukemia effects in T lineage and B lineage acute lymphoblastic leukemia. Bone Marrow Transplant 21:153–158
19. Doney K, Fisher LD, Appelbaum FR, et al. (1991) Treatment of adult acute lymphoblastic leukemia with allogeneic bone marrow transplantation. Multivariate analysis of factors affecting acute graft-versus-host disease, relapse, and relapse-free survival. Bone Marrow Transplant 7:453–459
20. Weisdorf DJ, Woods WG, Nesbit ME Jr, et al. (1994) Allogeneic bone marrow transplantation for acute lymphoblastic leukemia: Risk factors and clinical outcome. Br J Haematol 86:62–69
21. Sebban C, Lepage E, Vernant J-P, et al. (1994) Allogeneic bone marrow transplantation for acute lymphoblastic leukemia in first complete remission: A comparative study. J Clin Oncol 12:2580–2587
22. Zhang M-J, Hoelzer D, Horowitz MM, et al. (1995) Long-term follow-up of adults with acute lymphoblastic leukemia in first remission treated with chemotherapy or bone marrow transplantation. Ann Intern Med 123:428–431
23. Attal M, Blaise D, Marit G, et al. (1995) Consolidation treatment of adult acute lymphoblastic leukemia: A prospective, randomized trial comparing allogeneic versus autologous bone marrow transplantation and testing the impact of recombinant interleukin-2 after autologous bone marrow transplant. Blood 86:1619–1628
24. Thiebaut A, Vernant JP, Degos L, et al. (2000) Adult acute lymphocytic leukemia study testing chemotherapy and autologous and allogeneic transplantation. A follow-up report of the French protocol LALA 87 (Review). Hematol Oncol Clin N Amer 14:1353–1366
25. Fiere D, Lepage E, Sebban C, et al. (1993) Adult acute lymphoblastic leukemia: A multicentric randomized trial testing bone marrow transplantation as postremission therapy. J Clin Oncol 11:1990–2001
26. Barrett AJ, Horowitz, MM, Ash RC, et al. (1992) Bone marrow transplantation for Philadelphia chromosome-positive acute lymphoblastic leukemia. Blood 79:3067–3070
27. Dombret H, Gabert J, Boiron JM, et al. (2002) Outcome of treatment in adults with Philadelphia chromosome-positive acute lymphoblastic leukemia: Results of the prospective multicenter LALA-94 trial. Blood 100:2357–2366
28. Druker BJ, Talpaz M, Resta DJ, et al. (2001) Efficacy and safety of a specific inhibitor of the BCR-ABL tyrosine kinase in chronic myeloid leukemia. N Engl J Med 344:1031–1037
29. Ottmann OG, Druker BJ, Sawyers CL, et al. (2002) A phase 2 study of imatinib in patients with relapsed or refractory Philadelphia chromosome-positive acute lymphoid leukemias. Blood 100: 1965–1971
30. Hoffman WK, Jones JC, Lemp NA, et al. (2002) Ph+ acute lymphoblastic leukemia resistant to the tyrosine kinase inhibitor STI571 has a unique BCR-ABL gene mutation. Blood 99:1860–1862
31. Hoffman WK, Komor M, Wassman B, et al. (2003) Presence of the BCR-ABL mutation Glu255Lys prior to STI571 (imatinib) treatment in patients with Ph+ acute lymphoblastic leukemia. Blood 102: 659–661
32. Thomas DA, Faderl S, Cortes J, et al. (2004) Treatment of Philadelphia chromosome-positive acute lymphocytic leukemia with hyper-CVAD and imatinib mesylate. Blood 103(12):4396–4407
33. Wassmann B, Scheuring U, Pfeifer H, et al. (2003) Efficacy and safety of imatinib mesylate (Glivec) in combination with interferon-alpha (IFN-alpha) in Philadelphia chromosome-positive acute lymphoblastic leukemia (Ph+ ALL). Leukemia 17:1919–1924
34. Sanders KE, Ha CS, Cortes-Franco JE, et al. (2004) The role of craniospinal irradiation in adults with a central nervous system recurrence of leukemia. Cancer 100:2160–2180
35. Kantarjian H, Gandhi V, Cortes J, et al. (2001) Phase 2 clinical and pharmacologic study of clofarabine in patients with refractory or relapsed acute leukemia. Blood 103:2379
36. Gandhi V, Plunkett W, Rodriguez CO Jr, et al. (1998) Compound GW506U78 in refractory hematologic malignancies: Relationship between cellular pharmacokinetics and clinical response. J Clin Oncol 16:3607–3615
37. Gandhi V, Plunkett W, Weller S, et al. (2001) Evaluation of the combination of nelarabine and fludarabine in leukemias: clinical response, pharmacokinetics, and pharmacodynamics in leukemia cells. J Clin Oncol 19(8):2142–2152

Emergencies in Acute Lymphoblastic Leukemia

Olga Frankfurt, Martin S. Tallman

Contents

23.1 Introduction

The clinical presentation of acute lymphoblastic leukemia (ALL) may range from nonspecific symptoms such as progressive malaise, fever, and fatigue to severe life-threatening manifestations, requiring immediate medical intervention.

23.2 Metabolic Complications

Severe metabolic disturbances may accompany the initial diagnosis of ALL as well as the first phase of the induction chemotherapy [1].

Patients with high leukemic burden are at risk of developing acute tumor lysis syndrome (ATLS), manifesting by hyperuricemia, hyperkalemia, hyperphosphatemia, and secondary hypocalcemia. Such electrolyte abnormalities may lead to the development of oliguric renal failure due to the tubular precipitation of urate and calcium phosphate crystals, fatal cardiac arrhythmias, hypocalcemic tetany, and seizures.

Administration of vigorous intravenous hydration of 2–4 times daily fluid maintenance (approximately 3 l/m^2/d), sodium bicarbonate to alkalinize the urine (must be given with caution since it may potentiate hypocalcemia), oral or intravenous allopurinol to control hyperuricemia, and phosphate binders to treat hyperphosphatemia remain the standard therapy for management of ATLS in the USA.

Although urine alkalinization (urine pH >7) historically has been recommended for the prophylaxis and treatment of ATLS [2], it remains controversial. Since maximum uric acid solubility occurs at the pH of 7.5, alkalinization of urine promotes the urinary excretion of the urate. However, solubility of urate precursors – xanthine and hypoxanthine – is dramatically reduced at such pH, leading to the development of urinary xanthine crystals and xanthine obstructive uropathy [2, 3].

A xanthine analog allopurinol, which competitively inhibits xanthine oxidase and the conversion of xanthine and hypoxanthine to uric acid, has been demonstrated to effectively decrease the formation of uric acid and reduce the incidence of uric acid obstructive uropathy [4, 5]. However, allopurinol has several significant limitations. First, allopurinol only prevents further uric acid formation and has no effect of already existing uric acid. Second, administration of allopurinol increases the serum levels of the purine precursors, xanthine and hypoxanthine, which may lead to xanthine nephropathy and obstructive uropathy [4, 6]. Third, allopurinol reduces the degradation of other purines, including 6-mercaptopurine (6-MP) and azathioprine, requiring 50–70% of their dose reduction [6].

An alternative to preventing uric acid formation by inhibiting xanthine oxidase with allopurinol is to promote the catabolism of uric acid to much more soluble allantoin by urate oxidase [7]. Urate oxidase (UO) is an endogenous enzyme commonly found in many mammalian species, but not in humans, due to a nonsense mutation in the coding region of the urate oxidase-encoding gene [8]. A nonrecombinant UO, extracted from *Aspergillus flavus* species, has been demonstrated to reduce uric acid levels in patients at risk for ATLS and has been available in France since 1975 and in Italy since 1984 [9–11]. Subsequently, the gene coding for the UO was isolated from the *A. flavus* species and expressed in the yeast *Saccharomyces cerevisiae* strain to yield large quantities of the pure recombinant form of UO [12].

Recombinant UO (rasburicase) [12], which recently became available in the USA, was demonstrated to be a safe and effective alternative to allopurinol in several multicenter clinical trials [5, 13, 14]. In a randomized clinical trial rasburicase was shown to significantly reduce the exposure to uric acid in patients with hyperuricemia compared to allopurinol [5]. Although the recommended dose of rasburicase is 0.15–0.2 mg/kg/day for 5 days, at our institution, an excellent control of hyperuricemia was achieved with a lower dose of 3 mg/day. Administration of 3 mg of rasburicase to 18 patients with hyperuricemia secondary to leukemia/lymphoma resulted in the normalization of the uric acid in 11 patients with just a single dose of rasburicase, in six patients with two doses, and in one patient with three doses [15].

Patients with ALL, who either present with or are at high risk of developing ATLS (high tumor burden with WBC $>50\times10^9$/L, high LDH, or mediastinal mass; elevated uric acid level; renal infiltration with leukemic cells, or renal insufficiency) are good candidates for rasburicase therapy [6].

Hypocalcemia, one of the most dangerous sequelae of ATLS, may result in potentially lethal cardiac (ventricular arrhythmias, heart block) and neurological (hallucination, seizures, coma) manifestations [16]. In an asymptomatic patient with laboratory evidence of hypocalcemia and hyperphosphatemia, calcium replacement is not recommended, since it may precipitate metastatic calcifications [16]. However, in a patient with symptomatic hypocalcemia, calcium gluconate may be carefully administered to correct the clinical symptoms.

Hyperkalemia, defined by a potassium level of >6 mmol/l, caused by massive cellular degradation, may precipitate significant neuromuscular (muscle weakness, cramps, paresthesias) and potentially life-threatening cardiac (asystole, ventricular tachycardia, and ventricular fibrillation) abnormalities [16]. Patients should be treated with oral sodium-potassium exchange resin, such as kayexalate 15–30 g every 6 h and/or combined glucose/insulin therapy [17].

Serum electrolytes, uric acid, phosphorus, calcium, and creatinine should be monitored several times a day, depending on the severity of the clinical condition and degree of metabolic abnormality. Early hemodialysis may be required in patients who develop oliguric renal failure or recalcitrant electrolyte disturbances. The electrocardiogram should be obtained and cardiac rhythm monitored while these abnormalities are corrected.

23.3 Lactic Acidosis

Primary leukemia-induced lactic acidosis (LA) is a rare yet potentially fatal event, characterized by low arterial pH due to the accumulation of blood lactate. It has been suggested that LA occurring in the setting of hematological malignancy is associated with an extremely poor prognosis [18]. Lactate, the end product of anaerobic glycolysis, is metabolized to glucose by the liver and kidneys. Because leukemic cells have a high rate of glycolysis even in the presence of oxygen and produce a large quantity of lactate, LA may result from an imbalance between lactate production and hepatic lactate utilization [18]. Several factors may contribute to the high rate of glycolysis. Overexpression or aberrant expression of glycolytic enzymes, such as hexokinase, the first rate-limiting enzyme in the glycolytic pathway [19], allows tumor cells to proliferate rapidly and survive for prolonged periods [20]. Although insulin normally regulates the expression of this enzyme, insulin-like growth factors (IGFs), which are overexpressed by malignant leukemic cells, can mimic insulin activity [21–23]. Lactate production may also be increased by the paracrine and systemic action of TNF-α [24].

LA is frequently associated with ATLS and its extent is correlated with the severity of ATLS. There is laboratory evidence to suggest that loss of mitochondrial function induced by cytotoxic therapy, leads to compensatory glycolysis and subsequently to lactate accumulation and acidosis [25]. In a review of twenty-five cases of lactic acidosis attributed to underlying malignancy, more than two-thirds were associated with leukemia and lymphoma [26]. Twenty-five cases of LA associated with acute leukemia has been reported by Sillos et al. with eight cases of ALL [18]. Typically, the patient with lactic acidosis presents with weakness, tachycardia, nausea, mental status changes, hyperventilation, and hypotension, which may progress to frank shock as acidosis worsens. Laboratory studies show decreased blood pH (<7.37), a widened anion gap (>18), and low serum bicarbonate.

The most important therapy for lactic acidosis is the treatment of the underlying leukemia. The role of sodium bicarbonate in the treatment of lactic acidosis remains controversial. The deleterious effect of severe acidemia on cardiovascular function can potentially be ameliorated by sodium bicarbonate administration; however, no study has shown a convincing survival advantage for alkali therapy in this condition [27]. In addition, there are several reports suggesting that administration of sodium bicarbonate may increase lactate and CO_2 production, impair oxygen delivery, and worsen lactic acidosis [28]. Hemodialysis and hemofiltration with bicarbonate-based replacement fluid is a successful therapy for severe LA not associated with malignancy [29, 30]. Hemofiltration with bicarbonate-based replacement fluid used in a patient with LA and underlying acute leukemia resulted in rapid correction of acidosis; however, plasma lactate level decreased only after the initiation of chemotherapy [18].

23.4 Hypercalcemia

Severe hypercalcemia is a rare serious manifestation of ALL, reported in 2.5–4.8% patients at diagnosis [31]. Patients may experience severe malaise, diffuse abdominal pain, emesis, and changes in mental status. Both humoral and local mechanisms have been implicated in the pathogenesis of hypercalcemia in ALL [32]. Paraneoplastic production of parathyroid hormone-related protein (PTHrP) is thought to be responsible for hypercalcemia via a humoral effect, while osteolytic skeletal metastasis and cytokines, such as TNF-α, IL-6 and IL-2, may be responsible for local osteolytic hypercalcemia [33, 34]. Occasionally a combination of high calcium and phosphorus level leads to the calcinosis cutis – an aberrant deposition of calcium salts in the skin [35]. The combination of hydration, loop diuretics, intravenous bisphosphonates, corticosteroids, and calcitonin is usually sufficient to achieve adequate control of hypercalcemia [36]. Patients who do not respond to bisphosphonate infusions should be considered for additional therapy with gallium nitrate, which is a potent inhibitor of bone resorption [37]. Randomized double-blinded studies have demonstrated superiority of gallium nitrate compared to calcitonin, etidronate, and pamidronate for acute treatment of resistant hypercalcemia. Administered as a continuous intravenous infusion at a dose of 200 mg/m^2/day over 24 h for up to 5 days, gallium nitrate induces normocalcemia in 70–90% of patients [38].

However, cutaneous lesions are usually resistant to the initial therapy, causing significant morbidity. Patients experience severe resting and mechanical pain usually requiring a combination of morphine, tricyclic antidepressants, and anti-inflammatory medications for adequate pain control. Cases of calcinosis cutis have been described to resolve over a period of time, once control of the calcium and phosphate levels have been established, which would imply successful therapy for the underlying ALL [39, 40].

23.5 Hyperleukocytosis

Although hyperleukocytosis is a common presenting feature (10–30%) in patients with ALL, symptomatic leukostasis is exceedingly rare [41, 42]. However, when present, it constitutes a medical emergency and efforts should be made to lower white blood cell count (WBC) rapidly. Historically, leukapheresis has been used in ALL patients (especially children) with high WBC count ($>200\,000$/mm^3) and neurological and pulmonary symptoms suggestive of leukostasis [43]. Theoretically, leukapheresis should reduce the end organ damage by decreasing tumor burden and alleviating metabolic complications associated with leukostasis. Unfortunately the short- and long-term benefits of this procedure remain controversial and there are no data to suggest that the response rate or overall outcome are improved in an asymptomatic patient [44, 45]. Cautious preinduction therapy with glucocorticoids, adding vincristine and cyclophosphamide in cases of B-cell ALL, is a preferred means for the amelioration of hyperleukocytosis [46, 47]. Preinduction chemotherapy in combination with urate oxidase has dramatically decreased the frequency of tumor lysis syndrome and the need for hemodialysis in patients with B-ALL [48].

If administration of chemotherapy is not feasible in a patient with hyperleukocytosis and symptoms of leukostasis, or it must be delayed secondary to the significant metabolic abnormalities, renal insufficiency, or possibly pregnancy, emergency leukapheresis may be used to decrease or stabilize WBC count. However, based on the available data, leukapheresis cannot be recommended as a routine therapy or as a form of tumor debulking in an asymptomatic adult patient with ALL.

23.6 SVC/Mediastinal Mass

Patients with ALL (particularly T-ALL) may present with symptoms of cough, dyspnea, stridor, or dysphagia from the tracheal and esophageal compression by a mediastinal mass. More than 27% of children who presented with mediastinal mass have acute airway compromise [49]. Compression of great vessels by a bulky mediastinal mass may also lead to the life-threatening superior vena cava syndrome. In addition to the above-mentioned symptoms, patients might develop cyanosis, facial edema, increased intracranial pressure, and syncope.

The prognosis of patients with SVC syndrome is strongly correlated with the prognosis of underlying disease. Diagnosis of primary condition must be established promptly, and therapy with steroids, radiation, and/or chemotherapy must be initiated without delay. When the therapeutic goal is only palliation of SVC syndrome, or if emergent treatment of the venous obstruction is required, direct opening of the occlusion with endovascular stenting and angioplasty with possible thrombolysis should provide prompt relief of symptoms [50]. Other medical measures such as head elevation and oxygen administration, which can reduce cardiac output and venous pressure, might be helpful.

23.7 DIC

Disseminated intravascular coagulation (DIC) is a known complication of ALL in children [51–53] and adults [54]. The frequency of DIC in adults is reported to be 10–16% at presentation and 36–78% during remission induction therapy [55–57]. Hypofibrinogenemia (<100 mg/dl) was detected in 41% of patients with ALL at the time of diagnosis and after initiation of therapy [58]. Hemorrhagic symptoms are usually mild; however, serious hemorrhage occurs in 20% of patients with laboratory evidence of DIC [55].

Patients who develop DIC tend to have a higher WBC (77 900/mm^3 vs. 9400/mm^3) counts and a higher frequency of palpable splenomegaly than the patients who do not develop DIC. However, no statistically significant relationship was established between DIC and age, FAB subtype, immunophenotype, karyotype, LDH, and percentage of blasts in the bone marrow. An etiologic link between CD34 expression and DIC has been suggested [57].

ALL patients who developed DIC after the initiation of chemotherapy had a lower platelet level and higher level of the E-fragment of serum fibrinogen/fibrin degradation products (FDP) at presentation, suggesting that they already had DIC at presentation. These findings indicate that perhaps patients with high WBC counts, higher FDP level, a low platelet count, and splenomegaly at presentation require closer monitoring for DIC after the initiation of chemotherapy.

The best way to treat DIC is to treat the underlying ALL. However, exacerbation of DIC may occur during induction therapy and with ATLS.

The coagulation profile must be obtained at the time of diagnosis and repeated frequently, especially when laboratory evidence of DIC is detected, to guide the replacement therapy in DIC. Theoretical concerns for exacerbating DIC with blood products have not been substantiated clinically, and hemostatic competence to avoid severe bleeding must be maintained. It is reasonable to keep activated partial thromboplastin time (aPTT) at about 1.5 times normal level with FFP, platelets at about 50 000/µl with platelet transfusions, and fibrinogen level over 100 mg/dl with cryoprecipitate. Heparin therapy is rarely indicated in the patient with ALL and DIC. However, if required, heparin levels should be followed, since the monitoring aPTT may lead to over- or under-treatment of the patient.

23.8 L-Asparaginase and Coagulopathy

L-asparaginase (L-asp), an enzyme from bacteria that destroys the amino acid asparagine, required primarily by leukemic cells, is an important component of combination chemotherapy for ALL. L-asp can produce depletion of many of the hemostatic, anticoagulant, and fibrinolytic factors such as fibrinogen, factors IX, XI, antithrombin III, proteins C and S, and plasminogen with an associated risk of thrombosis and hemorrhage [59–61]. These effects are likely due to the decreased protein synthesis by the liver, rather than clotting factor consumption or the production of the abnormal molecules [60, 62, 63]. This reduction of the synthesis of the clotting factors appears to be proportional to the elimination of asparagine from the plasma, and normalizes as soon as L-asp is discontinued [64].

Although marked reductions in fibrinogen and factors IX and XI due to L-asp occurs frequently, excessive bleeding is rare [60]. There is no prospective data to suggest a fibrinogen level at which replacement is required. It is reasonable to temporarily discontinue the L-asp when fibrinogen level decreases to 50–70 mg/dl. However, in general, we do not recommend fibrinogen replacement therapy in an asymptomatic patient regardless of fibrinogen level. When clinically significant bleeding occurs or a patient is required to undergo a surgical procedure, therapy with cryoprecipitate or FFP is usually successful in correcting the hemostatic defect [65].

The concentration of the anticoagulant proteins AT III, protein C, and protein S can decrease to 30% of normal level in patients treated with L-asp, levels low enough to predispose to thrombosis. The low level of circulating fibrinogen does not appear to offset the risk of thrombosis, since cases of severe central nervous system (CNS) thrombosis are reported in patients with a fibrinogen level of 29 mg/dl [66]. Prophylactic use of FFP was ineffective in preventing the decrease in antithrombin III level induced by L-asp [67].

In a setting of L-asp therapy, the presence of an inherited hypercoagulable state such as Factor V Leiden, or the prothrombine gene mutation was shown to increase the risk of thrombosis in some studies [68], but not in others [69]. The presence of the antiphospholipid antibody increases the risk of thrombosis in patients treated with L-asp [69].

CNS thrombosis occurs in approximately 4% of adult patients with ALL, usually 2–3 weeks after the initiation of therapy with L-asp. Although most patients recover without significant neurological consequences, death and permanent neurological defects have been reported [70–72]. While the risk of thrombosis is greatest during the remission induction phase of chemotherapy with L-asp, it may occur at any stage of therapy [73].

Pegaspargase, a modified form of native *E. coli* asparaginase, has been reported to cause hypofibrinogenemia in more than 50% of patients, however the clinical evidence of thrombosis were rarely encountered [73a, 73b]. Pancreatitis was reported in approximately 15% of patients treated with *E. coli* L-asparaginase and in 1–4% of patients receiving pegaspargase [73c]. Hepatotoxicity and hyperbilirubinemia are common complications of asparaginase therapy, although typically are grades 1–2 and are reversible with the discontinuation of therapy [73b]. However, in one study grade 4 hyperbilirubinemia was reported in 54% of patients who received 1–4 doses of pegasparaginase [73a]. The rate of allergic reaction appears to be less frequent in patients receiving pegasparaginase compared to ones treated with *E. coli* L-asparaginase [73d].

23.9 Neurological Complications

Five to ten percent of adult patients with ALL may present with clinically significant neurological findings related to the leukemic infiltration of CNS [74]. CNS involvement may manifest as generalized headache and papilledema from raised intracranial pressure, blindness due to the bilateral optic nerve infiltration, trigeminal neuralgia secondary to 7th cranial nerve infiltration and lymphomatous meningitis, transverse myelopathy, and epidural spinal cord compression [75–78].

Significance of such symptoms must be recognized immediately and chemotherapy with systemic and intrathecal methotrexate or cytarabine, steroids, and radiation therapy should be administered promptly in hopes to prevent permanent damage.

In a study of 36 patients with leukemic involvement of the nervous system (46 episodes of CNS involvement) 21.7% of the episodes involved the cranial nerve, most commonly the bulbar motor, facial, and optic nerves [79]. Although CNS involvement is likely to require radiation therapy, the optimal protocol for radiation administration is yet to be determined. Patients with symptomatic cranial nerve palsy are recommended to receive a total radiation dose of 3000 cGy, with 1000–1,500 cGy of it applied to the nerve sheath and the cranial base [80].

23.10 Other Organ Involvement

Leukemic cells may infiltrate virtually any organ system, especially in mature B-cell ALL (32%) and T-cell ALL, and usually do not cause significant morbidity. However, patients presenting with diffuse abdominal pain require immediate evaluation by the surgeon, due to high mortality rate (100%) from bowel perforation attributable to leukemic infiltrates [81]. Cases of splenic rupture form leukemic infiltrate and priapism due to leukostasis in corpora cavernosa and dorsal vein and sacral involvement in ALL have been described [82, 83].

References

1. O'Regan S, Carson S, Chesney RW, Drummond KN (1977) Electrolyte and acid-base disturbances in the management of leukemia. Blood 49(3):345–353
2. Ten Harkel AD, Kist-Van Holthe JE, Van Weel M, Van der Vorst MM (1998) Alkalinization and the tumor lysis syndrome. Med Pediatr Oncol 31(1):27–28
3. Jones DP, Mahmoud H, Chesney RW (1995) Tumor lysis syndrome: Pathogenesis and management. Pediatr Nephrol 9(2):206–212
4. Spector T (1977) Inhibition of urate production by allopurinol. Biochem Pharmacol 26(5):355–358
5. Goldman SC, Holcenberg JS, Finklestein JZ, et al. (2001) A randomized comparison between rasburicase and allopurinol in children with lymphoma or leukemia at high risk for tumor lysis. Blood 97(10):2998–3003
6. Cairo MS, Bishop M (2004) Tumour lysis syndrome: New therapeutic strategies and classification. Br J Haematol 127(1):3–11
7. Brogard JM, Coumaros D, Franckhauser J, Stahl A, Stahl J (1972) Enzymatic uricolysis: A study of the effect of a fungal urate-oxydase. Rev Eur Etud Clin Biol 17(9):890–895
8. Yeldandi AV, Yeldandi V, Kumar S, et al. (1991) Molecular evolution of the urate oxidase-encoding gene in hominoid primates: Nonsense mutations. Gene 109(2):281–284
9. Masera G, Jankovic M, Zurlo MG, et al. (1982) Urate-oxidase prophylaxis of uric acid-induced renal damage in childhood leukemia. J Pediatr 100(1):152–155
10. Pui CH, Relling MV, Lascombes F, et al. (1997) Urate oxidase in prevention and treatment of hyperuricemia associated with lymphoid malignancies. Leukemia 11(11):1813–1816
11. Patte C, Sakiroglu C, Ansoborlo S, et al. (2002) Urate-oxidase in the prevention and treatment of metabolic complications in patients with B-cell lymphoma and leukemia, treated in the Societe Francaise d'Oncologie Pediatrique LMB89 protocol. Ann Oncol 13(5): 789–795
12. Legoux R, Delpech B, Dumont X, et al. (1992) Cloning and expression in Escherichia coli of the gene encoding Aspergillus flavus urate oxidase. J Biol Chem 267(12):8565–8570
13. Coiffier B, Mounier N, Bologna S, et al. (2003) Efficacy and safety of rasburicase (recombinant urate oxidase) for the prevention and treatment of hyperuricemia during induction chemotherapy of aggressive non-Hodgkin's lymphoma: Results of the GRAAL1 (Groupe d'Etude des Lymphomes de l'Adulte Trial on Rasburicase Activity in Adult Lymphoma) study. J Clin Oncol 21(23):4402–4406
14. Lee AC, Li CH, So KT, Chan R (2003) Treatment of impending tumor lysis with single-dose rasburicase. Ann Pharmacother 37(11): 1614–1617
15. Trifilio S, Tallman M, Singhal S, Gordon L, Evens A, Mehta J (2004) Low-dose recombinant urate oxidase (rasburicase) is effective in hyperuricemia. 46th ASH Annual Meeting
16. Jeha S (2001) Tumor lysis syndrome. Semin Hematol 38(4 Suppl 10):4–8
17. Kelly KM, Lange B (1997) Oncologic emergencies. Pediatr Clin North Am 44(4):809–830
18. Sillos EM, Shenep JL, Burghen GA, Pui CH, Behm FG, Sandlund JT (2001) Lactic acidosis: A metabolic complication of hematologic malignancies: Case report and review of the literature. Cancer 92(9):2237–2246
19. Mazurek S, Boschek CB, Eigenbrodt E (1997) The role of phosphometabolites in cell proliferation, energy metabolism, and tumor therapy. J Bioenerg Biomembr 29(4):315–330
20. Mathupala SP, Rempel A, Pedersen PL (1997) Aberrant glycolytic metabolism of cancer cells: A remarkable coordination of genetic, transcriptional, post-translational, and mutational events that lead to a critical role for type II hexokinase. J Bioenerg Biomembr 29(4):339–343
21. Elmlinger MW, Wimmer K, Biemer E, Blum WF, Ranke MB, Dannecker GE (1996) Insulin-like growth factor binding protein 2 is differentially expressed in leukaemic B- and T-cell lines. Growth Regul 6(3):152–157
22. Cohick WS, Clemmons DR (1993) The insulin-like growth factors. Annu Rev Physiol 55:131–153
23. Werner H, LeRoith D (1996) The role of the insulin-like growth factor system in human cancer. Adv Cancer Res 68:183–223
24. Durig J, Fiedler W, de Wit M, Steffen M, Hossfeld DK (1996) Lactic acidosis and hypoglycemia in a patient with high-grade non-Hodgkin's lymphoma and elevated circulating TNF-alpha. Ann Hematol 72(2):97–99
25. Tiefenthaler M, Amberger A, Bacher N, et al. (2001) Increased lactate production follows loss of mitochondrial membrane potential during apoptosis of human leukaemia cells. Br J Haematol 114(3):574–580
26. Sculier JP, Nicaise C, Klastersky J (1983) Lactic acidosis: A metabolic complication of extensive metastatic cancer. Eur J Cancer Clin Oncol 19(5):597–601
27. Stacpoole PW (1986) Lactic acidosis: The case against bicarbonate therapy. Ann Intern Med 105(2):276–279
28. Cooper DJ, Walley KR, Wiggs BR, Russell JA (1990) Bicarbonate does not improve hemodynamics in critically ill patients who have lactic acidosis. A prospective, controlled clinical study. Ann Intern Med 112(7):492–498

29. Hingorani AD, Macdougall IC, Browne M, Walker RW, Tomson CR (1993) Successful treatment of acute D-lactate encephalopathy by haemodialysis. Nephrol Dial Transplant 8(11):1283–1285
30. Barton IK, Streather CP, Hilton PJ, Bradley RD (1991) Successful treatment of severe lactic acidosis by haemofiltration using a bicarbonate-based replacement fluid. Nephrol Dial Transplant 6(5): 368–370
31. Fukasawa H, Kato A, Fujigaki Y, Yonemura K, Furuya R, Hishida A (2001) Hypercalcemia in a patient with B-cell acute lymphoblastic leukemia: A role of proinflammatory cytokine. Am J Med Sci 322(2):109–112
32. Schneider T, Seydlitz F, Zimmermann U, Sontag B, Boesken WH (2001) [Life threatening hypercalcemia in a young man with ALL]. Dtsch Med Wochenschr 126(1/2):7–11
33. Lankisch P, Kramm CM, Hermsen D, Wessalowski R (2004) Hypercalcemia with nephrocalcinosis and impaired renal function due to increased Parathyroid hormone secretion at onset of childhood acute lymphoblastic leukemia. Leuk Lymphoma 45(8): 1695–1697
34. Esbrit P (2001) Hypercalcemia of malignancy – New insights into an old syndrome. Clin Lab 47(1/2):67–71
35. Tan AW, Ng HJ, Ang P, Goh YT (2004) Extensive calcinosis cutis in relapsed acute lymphoblastic leukaemia. Ann Acad Med Singapore 33(1):107–109
36. Schmid I, Stachel D, Schon C, Bauer M, Haas RJ (2001) Pamidronate and calcitonin as therapy of acute cancer-related hypercalcemia in children. Klin Padiatr 213(1):30–34
37. Bockman R (2003) The effects of gallium nitrate on bone resorption. Semin Oncol 30(2 Suppl 5):5–12
38. Warrell RP Jr, Murphy WK, Schulman P, O'Dwyer PJ, Heller G (1991) A randomized double-blind study of gallium nitrate compared with etidronate for acute control of cancer-related hypercalcemia. J Clin Oncol 9(8):1467–1475
39. Chaves Alvarez AJ, Herrera Saval A, Marquez Enriquez J, Camacho Martinez F (2000) Metastatic calcinosis cutis in multiple myeloma. Br J Dermatol 142(4):820–822
40. Cochran RJ, Wilkin JK (1983) An unusual case of calcinosis cutis. J Am Acad Dermatol 8(1):103–106
41. Porcu P, Farag S, Marcucci G, Cataland SR, Kennedy MS, Bissell M (2002) Leukocytoreduction for acute leukemia. Ther Apher 6(1):15–23
42. Porcu P, Cripe LD, Ng EW, et al. (2000) Hyperleukocytic leukemias and leukostasis: A review of pathophysiology, clinical presentation and management. Leuk Lymphoma 39(1/2):1–18
43. Strauss RA, Gloster ES, McCallister JA, Jimenez JF, Neuberg RW, Berry DH (1985) Acute cytoreduction techniques in the early treatment of hyperleukocytosis associated with childhood hematologic malignancies. Med Pediatr Oncol 13(6):346–351
44. Bunin NJ, Kunkel K, Callihan TR (1987) Cytoreductive procedures in the early management in cases of leukemia and hyperleukocytosis in children. Med Pediatr Oncol 15(5):232–235
45. Maurer HS, Steinherz PG, Gaynon PS, et al. (1988) The effect of initial management of hyperleukocytosis on early complications and outcome of children with acute lymphoblastic leukemia. J Clin Oncol 6(9):1425–1432
46. Harousseau JL, Tobelem G, Schaison G, et al. (1980) High risk acute lymphocytic leukemia: A study of 141 cases with initial white blood cell counts over 100,000/cu mm. Cancer 46(9): 1996–2003
47. Lichtman MA, Heal J, Rowe JM (1987) Hyperleukocytic leukaemia: Rheological and clinical features and management. Baillieres Clin Haematol 1(3):725–746
48. Patte C, Philip T, Rodary C, et al. (1991) High survival rate in advanced-stage B-cell lymphomas and leukemias without CNS involvement with a short intensive polychemotherapy: Results from the French Pediatric Oncology Society of a randomized trial of 216 children. J Clin Oncol 9(1):123–132
49. Lam JC, Chui CH, Jacobsen AS, Tan AM, Joseph VT (2004) When is a mediastinal mass critical in a child? An analysis of 29 patients. Pediatr Surg Int 20(3):180–184
50. Schindler N, Vogelzang RL (1999) Superior vena cava syndrome. Experience with endovascular stents and surgical therapy. Surg Clin North Am 79(3):683–694, xi
51. Abshire TC, Gold SH, Odom LF, Carson SD, Hathaway WE (1990) The coagulopathy of childhood leukemia. Thrombin activation or primary fibrinolysis? Cancer 66(4):716–721
52. Champion LA, Luddy RE, Schwartz AD (1978) Disseminated intravascular coagulation in childhood acute lymphocytic leukemia with poor prognostic features. Cancer 41(4):1642–1646
53. Ribeiro RC, Pui CH (1986) The clinical and biological correlates of coagulopathy in children with acute leukemia. J Clin Oncol 4(8):1212–1218
54. Guarini A, Baccarani M, Corbelli G, Gugliotta L, Tura S (1980) Defibrination in adult acute lymphoblastic leukaemia. Report of four cases. Nouv Rev Fr Hematol 22(2):115–123
55. Sarris AH, Kempin S, Berman E, et al. (1992) High incidence of disseminated intravascular coagulation during remission induction of adult patients with acute lymphoblastic leukemia. Blood 79(5):1305–1310
56. Sarris A, Cortes J, Kantarjian H, et al. (1996) Disseminated intravascular coagulation in adult acute lymphoblastic leukemia: Frequent complications with fibrinogen levels less than 100 mg/dl. Leuk Lymphoma 21(1/2):85–92
57. Higuchi T, Mori H, Niikura H, Omine M, Okada S, Terada H (1998) Disseminated intravascular coagulation in acute lymphoblastic leukemia at presentation and in early phase of remission induction therapy. Ann Hematol 76(6):263–269
58. Solano C, Lopez J, Gomez N, Fernandez-Ranada JM (1992) Acute lymphoblastic leukemia: Hypofibrinogenemia with a low incidence of clinical complications is often found during induction remission therapy. Blood 80(5):1366–1368
59. Bezeaud A, Drouet L, Leverger G, Griffin JH, Guillin MC (1986) Effect of L-asparaginase therapy for acute lymphoblastic leukemia on plasma vitamin K-dependent coagulation factors and inhibitors. J Pediatr 108(5 Pt 1):698–701
60. Ramsay NK, Coccia PF, Krivit W, Nesbit ME, Edson JR (1977) The effect of L-asparaginase of plasma coagulation factors in acute lymphoblastic leukemia. Cancer 40(4):1398–1401
61. Priest JR, Ramsay NK, Bennett AJ, Krivit W, Edson JR (1982) The effect of L-asparaginase on antithrombin, plasminogen, and plasma coagulation during therapy for acute lymphoblastic leukemia. J Pediatr 100(6):990–995
62. Bushman JE, Palmieri D, Whinna HC, Church FC (2000) Insight into the mechanism of asparaginase-induced depletion of antithrom-

bin III in treatment of childhood acute lymphoblastic leukemia. Leuk Res 24(7):559–565
63. Bettigole RE, Himelstein ES, Oettgen HF, Clifford GO (1970) Hypofibrinogenemia due to L-asparaginase: Studies of fibrinogen survival using autologous 131-I-fibrinogen. Blood 35(2):195–200
64. Nowak-Gottl U, Ahlke E, Klosel K, Jurgens H, Boos J (1997) Changes in coagulation and fibrinolysis in childhood acute lymphoblastic leukaemia re-induction therapy using three different asparaginase preparations. Eur J Pediatr 156(11):848–850
65. Cairo MS, Lazarus K, Gilmore RL, Baehner RL (1980) Intracranial hemorrhage and focal seizures secondary to use of L-asparaginase during induction therapy of acute lymphocytic leukemia. J Pediatr 97(5):829–833
66. Priest JR, Ramsay NK, Latchaw RE, et al. (1980) Thrombotic and hemorrhagic strokes complicating early therapy for childhood acute lymphoblastic leukemia. Cancer 46(7):1548–1554
67. Halton JM, Mitchell LG, Vegh P, Eves M, Andrew ME (1994) Fresh frozen plasma has no beneficial effect on the hemostatic system in children receiving L-asparaginase. Am J Hematol 47(3):157–161
68. Mauz-Korholz C, Junker R, Gobel U, Nowak-Gottl U (2000) Prothrombotic risk factors in children with acute lymphoblastic leukemia treated with delayed E. coli asparaginase (COALL-92 and 97 protocols). Thromb Haemost 83(6):840–843
69. Mitchell LG, Andrew M, Hanna K, et al. (2003) A prospective cohort study determining the prevalence of thrombotic events in children with acute lymphoblastic leukemia and a central venous line who are treated with L-asparaginase: Results of the Prophylactic Antithrombin Replacement in Kids with Acute Lymphoblastic Leukemia Treated with Asparaginase (PARKAA) Study. Cancer 97(2): 508–516
70. Gugliotta L, Mazzucconi MG, Leone G, et al. (1992) Incidence of thrombotic complications in adult patients with acute lymphoblastic leukaemia receiving L-asparaginase during induction therapy: A retrospective study. The GIMEMA Group. Eur J Haematol 49(2):63–66
71. Benzon HT, Iqbal M, Tallman MS, Boehlke L, Russell EJ (2003) Superior sagittal sinus thrombosis in a patient with postdural puncture headache. Reg Anesth Pain Med 28(1):64–67
72. Duru F, Ertem U, Dagdemir A, et al. (1997) Coexistence of life threatening chemotherapy related leukoencephalopathy, sagittal sinus thrombosis and multiple organ failure in a child with acute lymphoblastic leukemia: An unusual case with clinical recovery. Leuk Lymphoma 26(3/4):377–385
73. Corso A, Castagnola C, Bernasconi C (1997) Thrombotic events are not exclusive to the remission induction period in patients with acute lymphoblastic leukemia: A report of two cases of cerebral sinus thrombosis. Ann Hematol 75(3):117–119
73a. Wetzler MS, Sanford BL, Owzar K (2005) Effective asparagine depletion with pegylated asparaginase results in improved outcomes in adult lymphoblastic leukemia (ALL)-CALGB 9511. Blood 106:519a
73b. Douer D, et al. (2007) Pharmacodynamics and safety of intravenous pegaspargase during remission induction in adults aged 55 years or younger with newly diagnosed acute lymphoblastic leukemia. Blood 109(7):2744–2750
73b. Graham ML (2003) Pegaspargase: a review of clinical studies. Adv Drug Deliv Rev 55(10):1293–1302
73d. Silverman LB, et al. (2001) Improved outcome for children with acute lymphoblastic leukemia: results of Dana-Farber Consortium Protocol 91-01. Blood 97(5):1211–1218
74. Gokbuget N, Hoelzer D (1998) Meningeosis leukaemica in adult acute lymphoblastic leukaemia. J Neurooncol 38(2/3):167–180
75. Kaikov Y (1996) Optic nerve head infiltration in acute leukemia in children: An indication for emergency optic nerve radiation therapy. Med Pediatr Oncol 26(2):101–104
76. Kataoka A, Shimizu K, Matsumoto T, et al. (1995) Epidural spinal cord compression as an initial symptom in childhood acute lymphoblastic leukemia: Rapid decompression by local irradiation and systemic chemotherapy. Pediatr Hematol Oncol 12(2):179–184
77. Schattner A, Kozack N, Sandler A, Shtalrid M (2001) Facial dysplasia as the presenting manifestation of acute lymphoblastic leukemia. Mt Sinai J Med 68(6):406–409
78. Mayo GL, Carter JE, McKinnon SJ (2002) Bilateral optic disk edema and blindness as initial presentation of acute lymphocytic leukemia. Am J Ophthalmol 134(1):141–142
79. Beslac-Bumbasirevic L, Boskovic D, Tomin D, Colovic M, Kovacevic M, Bumbasirevic V (1996) Neuroleukemia in adults. Srp Arh Celok Lek 124(3/4):82–86
80. Leibel SA, Phillips TL (1998) Textbook of radiation oncology. WB Saunders, Philadelphia
81. Storti S, Marra R, Pagano L, et al. (1988) Emergency abdominal surgery in patients with acute leukemia and lymphoma. Ital J Surg Sci 18(4):361–363
82. Ferrara F, D'Ambrosio V, Di Noto R, Mele G, Giovine S, Romano L (1998) Spontaneous splenic rupture in a patient with acute lymphoblastic leukemia of Burkitt type. Leuk Lymphoma 29(5/6):613–616
83. Choo-Kang LR, Jones DM, Fehr JJ, Eskenazi AE, Toretsky JA (1999) Cerebral edema and priapism in an adolescent with acute lymphoblastic leukemia. Pediatr Emerg Care 15(2):110–112

Subject Index

A

B

C

D

E

F

G

H

I

K

L

M

N

O

P

Q

R

S